THE AIRWAYS

LUNG BIOLOGY IN HEALTH AND DISEASE

Executive Editor: **Claude Lenfant**

Director, National Heart, Lung, and Blood Institute
National Institutes of Health
Bethesda, Maryland

Volume 1 IMMUNOLOGIC AND INFECTIOUS REACTIONS IN THE LUNG, *edited by Charles H. Kirkpatrick and Herbert Y. Reynolds*

Volume 2 THE BIOCHEMICAL BASIS OF PULMONARY FUNCTION, *edited by Ronald G. Crystal*

Volume 3 BIOENGINEERING ASPECTS OF THE LUNG, *edited by John B. West*

Volume 4 METABOLIC FUNCTIONS OF THE LUNG, *edited by Y. S. Bakhle and John R. Vane*

Volume 5 RESPIRATORY DEFENSE MECHANISMS (in two parts), *edited by Joseph D. Brain, Donald F. Proctor, and Lynne M. Reid*

Volume 6 DEVELOPMENT OF THE LUNG, *edited by W. Alan Hodson*

Volume 7 LUNG WATER AND SOLUTE EXCHANGE, *edited by Norman C. Staub*

Volume 8 EXTRAPULMONARY MANIFESTATIONS OF RESPIRATORY DISEASE, *edited by Eugene Debs Robin*

Volume 9 CHRONIC OBSTRUCTIVE PULMONARY DISEASE, *edited by Thomas L. Petty*

Volume 10 PATHOGENESIS AND THERAPY OF LUNG CANCER, *edited by Curtis C. Harris*

Volume 11 GENETIC DETERMINANTS OF PULMONARY DISEASE, *edited by Stephen D. Litwin*

Volume 12 THE LUNG IN THE TRANSITION BETWEEN HEALTH AND DISEASE, *edited by Peter T. Macklem and Solbert Permutt*

Volume 13 EVOLUTION OF RESPIRATORY PROCESSES: A COMPARATIVE APPROACH, *edited by Stephen C. Wood and Claude Lenfant*

Volume 14 PULMONARY VASCULAR DISEASES, *edited by Kenneth M. Moser*

Volume 15 PHYSIOLOGY AND PHARMACOLOGY OF THE AIRWAYS, *edited by Jay A. Nadel*

Volume 16 DIAGNOSTIC TECHNIQUES IN PULMONARY DISEASE (in two parts), *edited by Marvin A. Sackner*

Volume 17 REGULATION OF BREATHING (in two parts), *edited by Thomas F. Hornbein*

Volume 18 OCCUPATIONAL LUNG DISEASES: RESEARCH APPROACHES AND METHODS, *edited by Hans Weill and Margaret Turner-Warwick*

Volume 19 IMMUNOPHARMACOLOGY OF THE LUNG, *edited by Harold H. Newball*

Volume 20 SARCOIDOSIS AND OTHER GRANULOMATOUS DISEASES OF THE LUNG, *edited by Barry L. Fanburg*

Volume 21 SLEEP AND BREATHING, *edited by Nicholas A. Saunders and Colin E. Sullivan*

Volume 22 *PNEUMOCYSTIS CARINII* PNEUMONIA: PATHOGENESIS, DIAGNOSIS, AND TREATMENT, *edited by Lowell S. Young*

Volume 23 PULMONARY NUCLEAR MEDICINE: TECHNIQUES IN DIAGNOSIS OF LUNG DISEASE, *edited by Harold L. Atkins*

Volume 24 ACUTE RESPIRATORY FAILURE, *edited by Warren M. Zapol and Konrad J. Falke*

Volume 25 GAS MIXING AND DISTRIBUTION IN THE LUNG, *edited by Ludwig A. Engel and Manuel Paiva*

Volume 26 HIGH-FREQUENCY VENTILATION IN INTENSIVE CARE AND DURING SURGERY, *edited by Graziano Carlon and William S. Howland*

Volume 27 PULMONARY DEVELOPMENT: TRANSITION FROM INTRAUTERINE TO EXTRAUTERINE LIFE, *edited by George H. Nelson*

Volume 28 CHRONIC OBSTRUCTIVE PULMONARY DISEASE, second edition, revised and expanded
edited by Thomas L. Petty

Volume 29 THE THORAX (in two parts),
edited by Charis Roussos and Peter T. Macklem

Volume 30 THE PLEURA IN HEALTH AND DISEASE,
edited by Jacques Chrétien, Jean Bignon, and Albert Hirsch

Volume 31 DRUG THERAPY FOR ASTHMA: RESEARCH AND CLINICAL PRACTICE ,
edited by John W. Jenne and Shirley Murphy

Volume 32 PULMONARY ENDOTHELIUM IN HEALTH AND DISEASE
edited by Una S. Ryan

Volume 33 THE AIRWAYS: NEURAL CONTROL IN HEALTH AND DISEASE
edited by Michael A. Kaliner and Peter J. Barnes

Volume 34 PATHOPHYSIOLOGY AND TREATMENT OF INHALATION INJURIES
edited by Jacob Loke

Volume 35 RESPIRATORY FUNCTION OF THE UPPER AIRWAY
edited by Oomen P. Mathew and Giuseppe Sant'Ambrogio

Other volumes in preparation

CHRONIC OBSTRUCTIVE PULMONARY DISEASE: A BEHAVIORAL PERSPECTIVE
edited by John A. McSweeney and Igor Grant

IMMUNOLOGY OF LUNG CANCER: DIAGNOSIS AND TREATMENT
edited by Steven T. Rosen, James L. Mulshine, Frank Cuttitta, and Paul G. Abrams

LUNG CELL BIOLOGY
edited by Donald Massaro

PULMONARY VASCULAR PHYSIOLOGY AND PATHOPHYSIOLOGY
edited by E. Kenneth Weir and John T. Reeves

THE AIRWAYS

NEURAL CONTROL IN HEALTH AND DISEASE

Edited by

MICHAEL A. KALINER

National Institute of Allergy and Infectious Diseases
National Institutes of Health
Bethesda, Maryland

PETER J. BARNES

The Cardiothoracic Institute
Brompton Hospital
London, United Kingdom

MARCEL DEKKER, INC. New York • Basel

Library of Congress Cataloging-in-Publication Data

The Airways, neural control in health and disease.

(Lung biology in health and disease ; v. 33)
Includes bibliographies and indexes.
1. Respiratory organs–Innervation–Congresses.
2. Respiration-Regulation–Congresses. 3. Asthma–
Etiology–Congresses. I. Kaliner, Michael A.
II. Barnes, Peter J. III. Series.
[DNLM: 1. Airway Obstruction. 2. Airway Resistance.
3. Respiratory System–innervation. 4. Respiratory
System–physiology. W1 LU62 v.33 / WF 102 A2985]
QP123.A37 1988 616.2 87-24431
ISBN 0-8247-7779-4

MARCEL DEKKER, INC.
270 Madison Avenue, New York, New York 10016

Current printing (last digit):
10 9 8 7 6 5 4 3 2 1

PRINTED IN THE UNITED STATES OF AMERICA

INTRODUCTION

The lungs are the origin of the breath and the dwelling of the animal spirits or impervious soul.

Ch'i Po 2600 BC
Minister of the Yellow Emperor*

If the atmospheric air is to arrive in suitable quantity and composition at the seat of respiration . . . it is absolutely necessary that the road through the air passages should be unobstructed, that these canals should be pervious.

Julius Cohnheim, 1839-1884†

In the nineteenth century, there were many misconceptions about the permeability of the air passages and what might reduce it. Although asthma was first described by physicians in ancient Greece, it was really only at the beginning of the twentieth century that investigators began to focus on the innervation of the airways. Since the original description of tracheobronchial neuroreceptors by Widdicombe in 1954, the study of the neural regulation of the airways has been a progressive and fertile field of investigation. It has been well served by such newer approaches to neurobiology as neurochemistry and neurophysiology. Research in molecular biology will open the way to new discoveries and even greater summits. Moreover, there are few areas of investigation that are as international in their pursuit and their impact. The progress, excitement, plurality of approaches, and internationality that are characteristic of this field are reflected in this new monograph, *The Airways: Neural Control in Health and Disease,* in the series, "Lung Biology in Health and Disease." Drs. Michael Kaliner, from Bethesda, and Peter Barnes, from London, have done a truly remarkable job in

---

**The Yellow Emperor's Classic of Internal Medicine.* Translated by Ieza Veith. University of California Press, Berkeley, 1949.

†Julius Cohnheim. *Lectures on General Pathology.* Translated by A. B. McKee. The New Sydenham Society, London, 1889.

assembling a group of investigators who represent the "best of the best" in the field.

This volume has an important new feature: it is the proceedings of a conference where the authors discussed their research. These discussions are included because they present points or emphases that may not be as completely covered in the chapters.

It is my understanding that this conference was made possible through an educational grant from Abbott Laboratories, a contribution that is greatly appreciated.

As the Executive Editor of the series, "Lung Biology in Health and Disease," I want to express my deepest appreciation to Drs. Kaliner and Barnes for organizing and editing this volume. I also thank the many contributors for making it both informative for the reader and challenging for the student of this area of research. They will find inspiration and ideas to pave the way for their future pursuits.

Claude Lenfant, M.D.

PREFACE

It has long been suspected that neural mechanisms may be important in diseases of the airways, such as asthma. Although neurogenic theories of asthma were popular in the last century, they subsequently have received less attention than immunologic theories based on mediator release. Over the last few years, there has been a revival of interest in neural control of the airways, particularly with the recognition that, in addition to classical cholinergic and adrenergic pathways, there are also nonadrenergic noncholinergic (NANC) nerves and several neuropeptides in the respiratory tract. Recently, there have been considerable advances in our understanding of autonomic regulation of the airways. This has been made possible by improvement in histochemical and ultrastructural techniques for mapping innervation, by the application of radioligand binding studies which have advanced our understanding of airway autonomic receptors, and by physiologic methods which have been refined for measuring functional effects in airway smooth muscle, glands, and the bronchial circulation.

Autonomic neural control is likely to be abnormal in airways disease and it seems likely that there is a complex interplay between inflammation in the asthmatic airway and neural control, since it is known that several inflammatory mediators may affect airway neurotransmission. It is also becoming increasingly apparent that nerves in the airway may themselves contribute to the inflammatory response.

Because of all the new information on neural control of airways it was decided to hold a workshop to discuss new developments and to assess the significance of neural mechanisms in airway disease. This was held in Cancun, Mexico, in February 1986 and was attended by leading international authorities, some of whom have worked on airways and some on other autonomic systems, so that parallels could be drawn. The workshop was lively and informative, generating many new ideas. We hope some of this flavor has been transmitted in the edited discussion which follows each chapter. We are most grateful to Abbott Laboratories and Mr. Robert Schoellhorn, Chairman, for generously sponsoring the workshop.

The book that has evolved from the workshop is the first publication devoted to this important topic and brings together a large amount of previously widely dispersed information.

Michael A. Kaliner, M.D.
Peter J. Barnes, M.D.

CONTRIBUTORS

Ralph J. Altiere, Ph.D.* Assistant Professor, University of Kentucky College of Pharmacy, Lexington, Kentucky

A. Änggård, M.D., Ph.D. Department of Oto-Rhino-Laryngology, Karolinska Institute, Stockholm, Sweden

Peter J. Barnes, M.A., D.M., F.R.C.P.[†] Professor and Director, Department of Clinical Pharmacology, The Cardiothoracic Institute, Brompton Hospital, London, United Kingdom

Jeffrey L. Benovic, Ph.D. Research Associate, Department of Biochemistry, Duke University Medical Center, Durham, North Carolina

Stephen R. Bloom, M.A., M.D., D.Sc., F.R.C.P. Professor of Endocrinology, Department of Medicine, Royal Postgraduate Medical School, Hammersmith Hospital, London, United Kingdom

D. Benjamin Borson, Ph.D. Lecturer, Department of Physiology and Cardiovascular Research Institute, University of California, San Francisco, California

Jean Bousquet, M.D. Clinique des Maladies Respiratoires, Centre Hospitalier Universitaire, Montpellier, France

Geoffrey Burnstock, B.Sc., Ph.D., M.Sc. (Honorary), D.Sc. Professor of Anatomy, Head, Department of Anatomy and Embryology, and Convenor of Centre for Neuroscience, University College London, London, United Kingdom

---

Present affiliations:

*Associate Professor of Pharmacology, University of Colorado School of Pharmacy, Boulder, Colorado

†Professor and Chairman, Department of Thoracic Medicine, The Cardiothoracic Institute, Brompton Hospital, London, United Kingdom

Marc G. Caron, Ph.D. Associate Professor Department of Physiology and Medicine, Duke University Medical Center, Durham, North Carolina

Thomas B. Casale, M.D. Assistant Professor, Department of Internal Medicine, University of Iowa, Iowa City, Iowa

Anne-Marie Clauzel, M.D. Clinique des Maladies Respiratoires, Centre Hospitalier Universitaire, Montpellier, France

Ronald F. Coburn, M.D. Professor, Department of Physiology, University of Pennsylvania School of Medicine, Philadelphia, Pennsylvania

Edwin E. Daniel, Ph.D. Professor of Neurosciences and Coordinator of Smooth Muscle Research Program, Department of Neurosciences, McMaster University, Faculty of Health Sciences, Hamilton, Ontario, Canada

Pamela B. Davis, M.D., Ph.D. Associate Professor of Pediatrics and Medicine, Department of Pediatrics, Case Western Reserve University School of Medicine, Cleveland, Ohio

Richard D. Dey, Ph.D. Associate Professor, Department of Anatomy, West Virginia University Medical Center, Morgantown, West Virginia

Louis Diamond, Ph.D.* Professor and Director, Pharmacology and Toxicology Division, University of Kentucky College of Pharmacy, Lexington, Kentucky

Ingrid A-L. Erjefält, Pharm. Engr. Pharmacological Engineer, Pharmacological Department, AB Draco, Lund, Sweden

Nicholas A. Flavahan, Ph.D.† Senior Research Fellow, Department of Physiology and Biophysics, Mayo Clinic and Mayo Foundation, Rochester, Minnesota

Hans-L. Hahn, M.D. Medizinische Poliklinik, University of Würzburg, Würzburg, West Germany

---

Present affiliations:

*Professor and Dean, University of Colorado School of Pharmacy, Boulder, Colorado

†Visiting Scientist, Department of Anatomy and Embryology, University College London, London, United Kingdom

Tomas G. Hökfelt, M.D. Professor, Department of Histology, Karolinska Institute, Stockholm, Sweden

Michael A. Kaliner, M.D. Head, Allergic Diseases Section, National Institute of Allergy and Infectious Disease, National Institutes of Health, Bethesda, Maryland

Lauri A. Laitinen, M.D., Ph.D.* Visiting Professor, Department of Physiology, St. George's Hospital Medical School, University of London, London, United Kingdom

Robert J. Lefkowitz, M.D. James B. Duke Professor of Medicine, Department of Medicine, Howard Hughes Medical Institute at Duke University Medical Center, Durham, North Carolina

Jan M. Lundberg, M.D. Associate Professor, Department of Pharmacology, Karolinska Institute, Stockholm, Sweden

Lars Lundblad, M.D., Ph.D. Department of Oto-Rhino-Laryngology, Karolinska Institute, Stockholm, Sweden

Gabriel M. Makhlouf, M.D., Ph.D. Professor of Medicine, Director of Gastroenterology Research, Department of Medicine, Medical College of Virginia, Richmond, Virginia

Zvi Marom, M.D. Associate Professor of Medicine, Pulmonary Division, Mt. Sinai Medical Center, New York, New York

C-R. Martling, M.D. Department of Anesthesiology, Karolinska Institute, Stockholm, Sweden

François-Bernard Michel, M.D. Clinique des Maladies Respiratoires, Centre Hospitalier Universitaire, Montpellier, France

Jay A. Nadel, M.D. Professor of Medicine, Physiology and Radiation, Cardiovascular Research Institute, University of California, San Francisco, California

---

Present affiliation:
*Chairman, Research Institute of Military Medicine, Central Military Hospital, Helsinki, Finland

Albert K. Oehling, Prof. Dr. Director, Department of Allergology, Clinica Universitaria de Navarra, Pamplona, Spain

Carl A. Patow, M.D. Instructor, Department of Surgery (Otolaryngology), Uniformed Services University of the Health Sciences, Bethesda, Maryland

Carl G. A. Persson, Ph.D. Professor, Department of Clinical Pharmacology, University Hospital of Lund and Research Advisor, Pharmacological Laboratory, A. B. Draco, Lund, Sweden

Julia M. Polak, Ph.D. Professor, Histochemistry Unit, Department of Histopathology, Royal Postgraduate Medical School, Hammersmith Hospital, London, United Kingdom

John B. Richardson, M.D., Ph.D. Professor, Departments of Pathology and Pharmacology, McGill University, Montreal, Quebec, Canada

Sami I. Said, M.D.* Professor of Medicine and Chief, Pulmonary Disease & Critical Care Section, Department of Medicine, University of Oklahoma Health Sciences Center and VA Medical Center, Oklahoma City, Oklahoma

Alois Saria, M.D. Univ. Doz., Institute for Experimental and Clinical Pharmacology, University of Graz, Graz, Austria

Kaspar Sertl, M.D.† Guest Worker, National Institute of Allergy and Infectious Disease, National Institutes of Health, Bethesda, Maryland

James H. Shelhamer, M.D. Senior Investigator, Department of Critical Care Medicine, National Institutes of Health, Bethesda, Maryland

Bengt-Eric Skoogh, M.D. Assistant Professor, Department of Pulmonary Medicine, University of Göteborg, Göteborg, Sweden

David R. Springall, M.D. Lecturer, Histochemistry Unit, Department of Histopathology, Royal Postgraduate Medical School, Hammersmith Hospital, London, United Kingdom

Present affiliations:

*Professor, Department of Medicine, University of Illinois School of Medicine, Chicago, Illinois

†Fellow, Max Kade Foundation, Vienna, Austria

Pär Stjärne, M.D. Department of Oto-Rhino-Laryngology, Karolinska Institute, Stockholm, Sweden

Ruth H. Strasser, M.D., Ph.D.* Research Associate, Department of Medicine, Duke University Medical Center, Durham, North Carolina

Elvar Theodorsson-Norheim, M.D., Ph.D. Department of Clinical Chemistry, Karolinska Institute, Stockholm, Sweden

Paul M. Vanhoutte, M.D., Ph.D. Professor of Physiology and Pharmacology, and Consultant, Department of Physiology and Biophysics and Cardiovascular Medicine, Mayo Clinic, Mayo Medical School and Mayo Graduate School of Medicine, Rochester, Minnesota

Adam Wanner, M.D. Chief, Pulmonary Division, Department of Medicine, University of Miami School of Medicine, Miami, Florida

John G. Widdicombe, D.M., M.A., D.Phil., F.R.C.P. Professor, Chairman and Head, Department of Physiology, St. George's Hospital Medical School, London, United Kingdom

---

Present affiliation:
*Assistant Professor, Department of Cardiology, University of Heidelberg, Heidelberg, West Germany

CONTENTS

THE AIRWAYS

1

Autonomic Neural Control Mechanisms
With Special Reference to the Airways

GEOFFREY BURNSTOCK

University College London
London, United Kingdon

I. The Autonomic Neuroeffector Junction

The autonomic neuroeffector junction is not a "synapse" where there are *both* pre- and postsynaptic specializations typified by the skeletal neuromuscular junction or presynaptic terminals in ganglion cells, but a "junction" where transmitter is released en passage from varicosities in extensive branching terminal nerve fibers (Fig. 1). The varicosities are probably labile and have variable separations from effector cells (20 nm to 2 μm), which have no distinctive postjunctional specializations (see Burnstock, 1986a,b). Thus absence of boutons on an effector cell does not mean that it is not innervated, since transmitter released from a distance to reach any cell that has the appropriate receptors is, in effect, innervated. For example, although mast cells do not have neuronal boutons, they are often in close apposition to varicosities of passing autonomic nerve fibers (Heine and Förster, 1975; Wiesner-Menzel et al., 1981; Newson et al., 1983). Consequently, adenosine 5′-triphosphate (ATP), released as a cotransmitter with norepinephrine from many sympathetic nerves (see Burnstock and Sneddon, 1985), would be a potent degranulator of mast cells, while substance P (and/or ATP) released from some sensory nerve collaterals during an axon reflex would also degranulate mast cells (Diamant and Kruger,

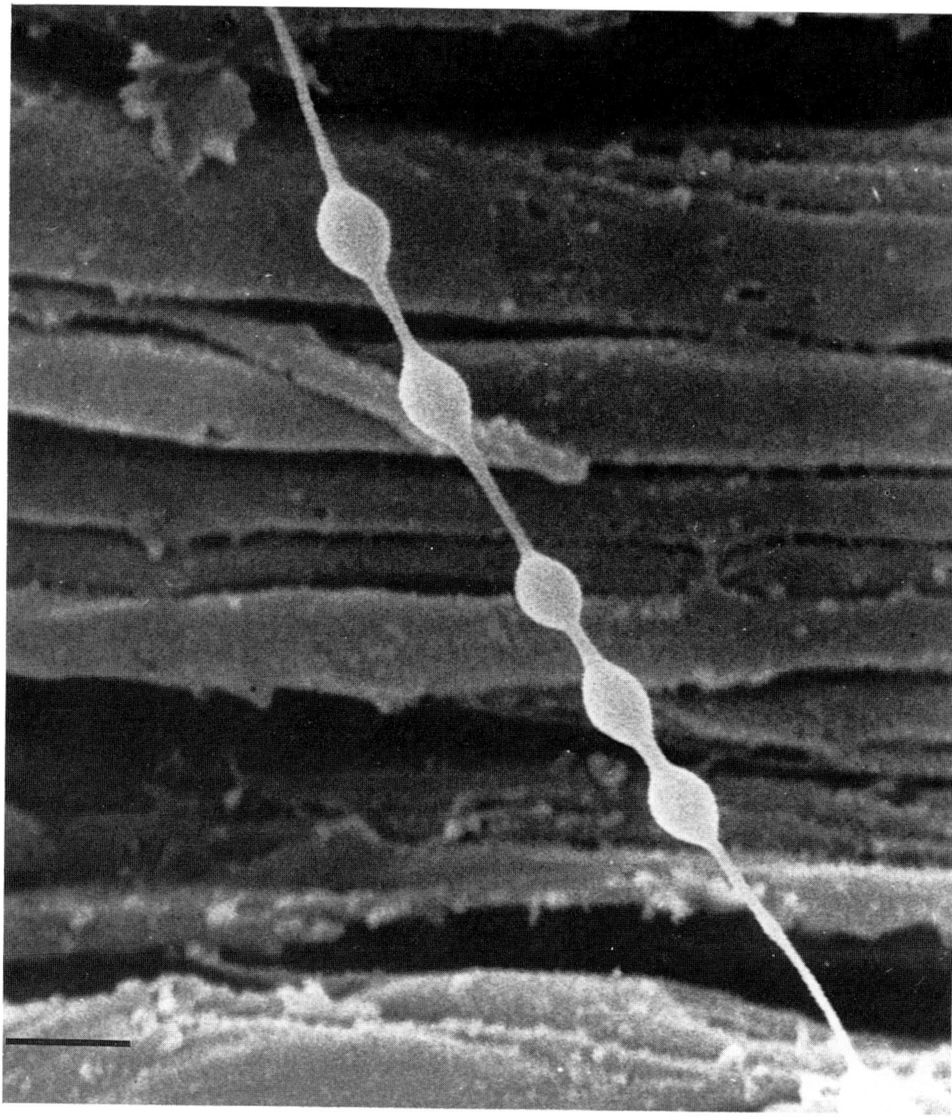

Figure 1 A scanning electron micrograph of a single terminal varicose nerve fiber lying over smooth muscle of the small intestine of the rat. The intestine was pretreated to remove connective tissue components by digestion with trypsin and hydrolysis with HCl. Scale bar = 3 μm. (Courtesy of T. Komuro, unpublished.)

1967; Kiernan, 1972; Burnstock, 1977; Hagermark et al., 1978; Pernow, 1983; Foreman and Jordan, 1983). Since it has been calculated that there are 10^7-10^8 mast cells in the lung (monkey) (Guerzon et al., 1979), this could be an important consideration. Transmitters released from passing autonomic nerves might influence capillary endothelial cells and venous and capillary pericytes.

Autonomic neuroeffector junctions appear to be particularly open to neuromodulatory influences, including prejunctional modulation of transmitter release and postjunctional modulation of transmitter action (Fig. 2).

Another feature of autonomic neuromuscular transmission is that some smooth muscle cells are not directly activated by transmitter released from autonomic varicosities, but are activated indirectly via gap junctions between neighboring muscle cells within muscle effector bundles (Uehara and Burnstock, 1970; Fry et al., 1977). Gap junctions form low-resistance pathways that allow

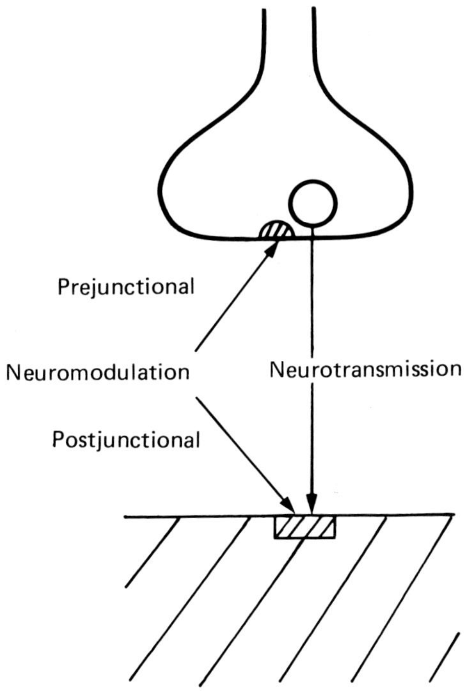

Figure 2 Diagrammatic representation of neuromodulation. Prejunctional neuromodulators increase or decrease release of transmitter; postjunctional neuromodulators alter the extent and/or time course of transmitter action. (From Burnstock, 1982c, by permission of Pitman Publishing Ltd., London.)

electrotonic coupling of activity between cells; therefore in smooth muscles such as those in the airways, which are relatively sparsely innervated (compared, for example to vas deferens or iris), spread of excitation from directly innervated cells to smooth muscle cells remote from nerves is an important mechanism (Burnstock, 1970).

II. Classic Cholinergic and Adrenergic Autonomic Nerves

At cholinergic neuroeffector junctions, synthesis of acetylcholine (ACh) by choline acetyltransferase occurs both in the neuron body and in the terminal axon varicosities. The ACh is stored in electron-transparent agranular vesicles, 30-60 nm in diameter, and released into the junctional cleft probably by a process of exocytosis. Inactivation of ACh following its interaction with the postjunctional receptors is mainly due to local hydrolysis by postjunctionally situated acetylcholinesterase, although a small fraction of ACh may diffuse away from the junctional cleft to be hydrolyzed by cholinesterases elsewhere in the effector tissue or in the circulation. Reuptake of ACh itself into the nerve terminals does not occur. However, choline produced by ACh hydrolysis is actively taken up into varicosities and is important in maintaining continued transmitter synthesis.

At adrenergic neuroeffector junctions, all the enzymes involved in the synthesis and breakdown of norepinephrine (NE), namely tyrosine hydroxylase, DOPA decarboxylase, dopamine β-hydroxylase, monoamine oxidase (MAO), and probably some catechol-O-methyltransferase (COMT), are present throughout the adrenergic neuron. Tyrosine hydroxylase forms the rate-limiting step in NE synthesis, and control is mediated by feedback inhibition of its activity by an extravesicular pool of NE that rapidly equilibrates with vesicular stores. During transmission, NE is released into the junctional cleft, probably by a process of exocytosis. Following its action on the postsynaptic muscle membrane, NE is removed largely by reuptake into the nerves, where it is either reincorporated into vesicular stores or degraded by MAO. Some NE is taken up by smooth muscle cells and inactivated by intracellular MAO or COMT, while any NE that leaks away into the circulation is inactivated by the same enzymes, largely in the liver or kidney (see Burnstock and Costa, 1975).

There is an anatomical basis for interactions or "cross talk" between adrenergic and cholinergic nerves in visceral and vascular systems, since examples of close apposition of adrenergic and cholinergic nerve varicosities, often enclosed within the same Schwann's cell sheath, have been described. ACh has an inhibitory effect on responses to sympathetic nerve stimulation via prejunctional muscarinic receptors, and NE released from sympathetic nerve terminals reduces the release of ACh from cholinergic nerves in the gut, thereby inhibiting gastrointestinal motility. As far as I am aware, examples of adrenergic and cholinergic "cross-talk" have not yet been described in the airways, but may prove to be an important mechanism (see Burnstock, 1986a).

III. Nonadrenergic, Noncholinergic (NANC) Autonomic Nerves

Although there was recognition by Langley and his colleagues at the turn of the century of atropine-resistant responses in both gastrointestinal tract and bladder to parasympathetic nerve stimulation, it was generally assumed that these could be explained within the classic framework of adrenergic and cholinergic transmitters. However, new observations in the early 1960s changed this view. My colleagues and I in Melbourne were able to show that when the responses to both adrenergic and cholinergic nerve stimulation had been blocked in guinea pig intestinal preparations, large transient hyperpolarizations and relaxations were produced, even with single pulses. Since these responses were abolished by tetrodotoxin, they were established as inhibitory junction potentials resulting from stimulation of NANC neurons (Burnstock et al., 1963). At about the same time, Martinson and Muren (1963) in Göteborg presented evidence for NANC responses of the cat stomach following stimulation of the vagus nerves. By the end of the 1960s, NANC nerves were recognized in a wide variety of organs including urinary bladder, lung, esophagus, seminal vesicles, trachea, and parts of the vascular system (see Burnstock, 1969).

The next step was to try to determine the principal transmitter in these nerves. The following criteria are generally regarded as necessary for establishing a substance as a neurotransmitter: synthesis and storage of transmitter in nerve terminals; release of transmitter during nerve stimulation; postjunctional responses to exogenous transmitter that mimic responses to nerve stimulation; enzymes that inactivate the transmitter and/or an uptake system for the transmitter or its breakdown products; and drugs that produce parallel blocking or potentiating effects on the responses of both exogenous transmitter and nerve stimulation. NANC nerves were considered the "third nervous system" at that time, which turned out to be too simplistic a view, since it became clear that a number of different neurotransmitter substances are utilized by NANC nerves supplying different organs and effector cells.

A. Purinergic Nerves

Evidence was presented in the early 1970s that the principal transmitter utilized by intramural neurons supplying the smooth muscle of the intestine and urinary bladder was a purine nucleotide, probably ATP (Burnstock et al., 1970, 1972).

NANC nerves using ATP were termed "purinergic" (Burnstock, 1972). It was proposed that ATP is synthesized in the terminal nerve varicosities and stored in vesicles. After its release and activation of purinergic receptors in the postjunctional membrane, ATP is rapidly broken down by magnesium-activated ATPase and 5′-nucleotidase to adenosine. Adenosine is taken up into the nerve terminals by a high-affinity uptake system, converted to ATP, and reincorporated into physiological stores. Since this hypothesis was put forward, there has been much debate with further evidence presented for and against (see Burnstock, 1979, 1981, 1985; Stone, 1981; Gillespie, 1982). Much of the negative evidence is not so much against the hypothesis per se, but rather supports the view that some NANC nerves do not utilize ATP as the principal transmitter. On the other hand, evidence has been presented that confirms and extends knowledge of purinergic transmission from intrinsic neurons to the smooth muscle of the gut, bladder, and rabbit portal vein. In addition to these examples where ATP is claimed to be the principal transmitter, there is now evidence for ATP as a purinergic cotransmitter with NE in sympathetic nerves (see below).

Lars Olson and his colleagues (1976) have shown that quinacrine, which binds strongly to ATP, can be used as a fluorescent histochemical marker for some NANC nerves that appear to be purinergic (Burnstock et al., 1978, 1979). As far as I am aware, quinacrine histochemical analysis has not yet been applied to the intramural ganglia of the airways.

The suggestion that purinergic receptors could be classified into subclasses (Burnstock, 1978) has contributed to a proliferation of interest in the roles of purines in a wide range of tissues (Baer and Drummond, 1979; Burnstock, 1981; Daly, 1983; Berne et al., 1983). The P_1-purinoceptors are most sensitive to adenosine and adenosine 5′-monophosphate (AMP), which usually act via an adenylate cyclase system and are antagonized by methylxanthines such as caffeine and theophylline in lower concentrations than are needed to produce phosphodiesterase inhibition. The P_2-purinoceptors are most sensitive to ATP and adenosine 5′-phosphate (ADP), do not act via adenylate cyclase, and one subgroup is antagonized by arylazidoaminoproprionyl-ATP ($ANAPP_3$) and selectively desensitized by α,β-methylene ATP. The P_2-purinoceptors mediate transmission while P_1-purinoceptors are present on both adrenergic and cholinergic nerve terminals, where they mediate neuromodulation of transmitter release, as well as on cell membranes of many different cell types. Both P_1- and P_2-purinoceptors have been shown to be stereoselective and further subclassification of both receptor types has been proposed (Burnstock and Brown, 1981; Burnstock and Buckley, 1985; Burnstock and Kennedy, 1985). Table 1 summarizes the basis of current subclassifications of purinoceptors, and includes selective agonists and antagonists for each subtype.

There are hints that purinoceptors may be of particular importance in the airways. For example, theophylline, a selective P_1-purinoceptor antagonist, in lower concentrations than produces phosphodiesterase inhibition, has been the drug of choice for treatment of asthma in the United States over the past few years. Furthermore, it has been shown recently that adenosine is a potential broncho-constrictor in asthmatic, but not normal, patients (Cushley et al., 1983; Holgate et al., 1984; Marmo et al., 1985). However, it should be noted that enprofylline, which is claimed to be a weak P_1-purinoceptor antagonist, also appears to be effective in asthma (Lunell et al., 1982; but see also Lagercrantz et al., 1984). Our own autoradiographic studies of the localization of adenosine receptors have shown them to be present largely on epithelial cells, with few in the bronchial musculature (Buckley and Burnstock, unpublished data). It has been shown recently that adenosine produces a dose-related increase in respiration in healthy human subjects; it was speculated that adenosine is a mediator in the carotid body of the ventilatory response to hypoxia (Watt and Routledge, 1985). Pulmonary arteries are particularly sensitive to ATP, which may be involved in the vasoconstrictor response to hypoxia in this vascular bed (see Burnstock, 1980a, 1982a; Burnstock and Kennedy, 1986). P_1-purinoceptors are present in both sympathetic and parasympathetic nerve terminals that act as potent prejunctional modulators of release of NE (De Mey et al., 1979) and ACh (Burnstock, 1980b), respectively. The large number of mast cells present in the lung may be degranulated by ATP released as a cotransmitter with NE from sympathetic nerves or with substance P from sensory nerves via purinoceptors known to be present in the mast cell membrane (Diamant and Kruger, 1967; Burnstock, 1977; Cockcroft and Gomperts, 1980). ATP receptors have also been shown recently to be present on fibroblasts (Okada et al., 1984); since sympathetic innervation of fibroblasts has been claimed (Soares da Silva and Azevedo, 1985), release of ATP as a cotransmitter may be involved in the fibroproliferative activity that occurs after adrenoceptor blockade (Marigold et al., 1982) or sympathectomy (Branco et al., 1984). Finally, the possibility that there are receptors for purines on epithelial cells in the airways, by analogy with those claimed for ACh, serotonin (5-hydroxytryptamine; 5-HT), and histamine (Flavahan et al., 1985; Barnes et al., 1985), should be explored.

B. Peptidergic and Aminergic Nerves

Between 1975 and 1977, important new findings suggested that it was likely that some NANC nerves utilized transmitter substances other than ATP. Systematic electron microscope studies of the enteric plexuses (Cook and Burnstock, 1976) revealed up to nine morphologically distinguishable types of neurons. Some nerve profiles contained a complex mixture of vesicles, suggesting that they may contain more than one transmitter. These findings were followed by numerous investigations based on immunohistochemical methods for localizing various biologically active polypeptides. Autonomic nerves contain-

Table 1 Characteristics of Proposed Subtypes of P_1- and P_2-Purinoceptors

	Subclass	Actions	Rank order of agonist potency	Antagonists	Adenylate cyclase activity	Prostaglandin synthesis
P_1 (AD/AMP)	A_1 (R_i)	*Prejunctional inhibition of neurotransmitter release* Rat vas deferens, anococcy-geus, guinea pig ileum	L-PIA > NECA > 2-chloro-adenosine > adenosine	Caffeine Theophylline 8-Phenyltheophylline PACPX	↓	–
		–Ve inotropy and chronotropy Guinea pig and rat atria	L-PIA >> D-PIA			
	A_2 (R_a)	*Relaxation* Guinea pig *taenia coli,* aorta, trachea	NECA > 2-chloroadeno-sine > L-PIA > adenosine		↑	–
		Prejunctional inhibition of neurogenic twitch Rat portal vein	L-PIA > D-PIA			

Receptor	Subtype	Response / tissue	Agonist potency	Antagonist		
P_2 (ATP/ADP)	Subtype 1 (P_2X)	*Contraction* Guinea pig vas deferens, urinary bladder, rabbit portal vein *+Ve inotropy and chronotropy* Frog atria, ventricles, rat ventricles	α,β-meATP, β,γ-meATP > ATP = 2-methylthioATP	$ANAPP_3$ Desensitization by α,β-meATP	–	↑
	Subtype 2 (P_2Y)	*Relaxation* Guinea pig *taenia coli,* rabbit portal vein *Endothelium-dependent vasodilation* Guinea pig aorta, rat femoral artery *–Ve inotropy* Rat ventricle	2-MethylthioATP >> ATP > α,β-meATP, β,γ-meATP	Reactive blue II (an anthraquinone-sulphonic acid derivative)	–	↑

AD, adenosine; $ANAPP_3$, arylazidoaminoproprionyl-ATP; meATP, methylene ATP; NECA, 5′-N-ethylcarboxamidoadenosine; PACPX, 1,3-dipropyl-8-(2-amino-4-chlorophenyl)xanthine; L-PIA, N^6-[R(–)-L-methyl-2-phenethyl] adenosine (L-N^6-phenylisopropyladenosine); D-PIA, D-N^6-phenylisopropyladenosine.

Table 2 Transmitters Proposed in the Autonomic Nervous System

Acetylcholine
Norepinephrine
Adenosine 5′-triphosphate
Serotonin (5-hydroxytryptamine)
γ-Aminobutyric acid
Dopamine
Peptides
Enkephalin/endorphin
Vasoactive intestinal polypeptide/peptide HI
Substance P
Gastrin-releasing peptide/bombesin
Somatostatin
Neurotensin
Luteinizing hormone-releasing hormone
Cholecystokinin/gastrin
NeuropeptideY/pancreatic polypeptide
Galanin
Angiotensin
Adrenocorticotrophic hormone
Calcitonin gene-related peptide

ing enkephalin, substance P, vasoactive intestinal polypeptide (VIP), neurotensin, somatostatin, gastrin-releasing peptide/bombesin, cholecystokinin, neuropeptide Y/pancreatic polypeptide, calcitonin gene-related peptide, and, most recently, galanin have been described (Hökfelt et al., 1980; Furness and Costa, 1982; Melander et al., 1985). In addition to polypeptides, there is evidence that 5-HT or a related indoleamine (see Gershon, 1979; Furness and Costa, 1979; Wood and Mayer, 1979) and γ-aminobutyric acid (Jessen et al., 1979) may be transmitters in some neurons of the gastrointestinal tract. Other experiments have led to the suggestion that dopamine is an autonomic transmitter in some blood vessels (Bell, 1982). Finally, Gillespie and his colleagues have extracted a potent vasodilator and smooth muscle inhibitory substance (as yet unidentified) from bovine retractor penis that they consider to be a putative neurotransmitter for some NANC nerves (Gillespie and martin, 1980; Bowman and Gillespie, 1982). A list of the substances currently considered to be transmitters or putative transmitters in autonomic nerve fibers is given in Table 2.

It should be noted that the criteria for establishing a neurotransmitter listed earlier have not been rigorously satisfied for a number of these substances and it seems likely that many more putative transmitters will be put forward in the future on the basis of the sensitive techniques of immunohistochemistry. In a recent study of the development of peptide- and catecholamine-containing nerves supplying blood vessels of the guinea pig, we showed that while the density of adrenergic nerves in mesenteric and carotid arteries reached a peak at about 4-6 weeks and was maintained at this level until old age, nerves containing vasoactive intestinal polypeptide and calcitonin gene-related peptide reached a density peak at birth and declined thereafter (Dhall et al., 1986). This poses the possibility that some neuropeptides may play a "trophic" role in development (see also Burnstock, 1982b).

Although vasoactive intestinal polypeptide, neuropeptide Y, and substance P have been shown to be strongly represented in nerve fibers in the lung (see chapters by Said, Laitinen, and Springall in this volume), immunohistochemical localization of some peptides and monoamines has not been thoroughly described yet in the human lung; this is partly because of the difficulty of seeing specific fluorescence in nerves against the high background autofluorescence characteristic of human tissues. We have recently developed a method of counterstaining autofluorescence with pontamine sky blue, which allows the labeled nerves to be seen clearly (Cowen et al., 1985); this method may prove useful in studies of the innervation of the human airways.

IV. Cotransmission

The suggestion that some nerve cells store and release more than one transmitter (Burnstock, 1976) was based largely on the early studies of Burn and Rand (1965), comparative studies of the evolution of the autonomic nervous system (Burnstock, 1969), and evidence for the coexistence of biologically active substances on some invertebrate nerves (e.g., Brownstein et al., 1974; Cottrell, 1976). There is now considerable experimental support for coexistence of peptides or purine nucleotides together with classic neurotransmitters (see Cuello, 1982; Osborne, 1983; Chan-Palay and Palay, 1984). Some examples of cotransmission that may be particularly pertinent to the airways are described in the following sections.

A. Serotonin and Peptides

Double immunolabeling techniques have been used to demonstrate coexistence of 5-HT and substance P in single intramural enteric neurons (Legay et al., 1984) and 5-HT and neuropeptide Y in single intramural neurons in the heart (Hassall and Burnstock, unpublished data). No double immunostaining has been described yet on intramural neurons of the airways.

B. Norepinephrine and ATP

There is strong evidence for NE and ATP coexisting and acting as cotransmitters in sympathetic nerves supplying the vas deferens (Fedan et al., 1981; Sneddon et al., 1982; Meldrum and Burnstock, 1983; Sneddon and Burnstock, 1984a; Sneddon and Westfall, 1984), nictitating membrane (Duval et al., 1985), heart (Hoyle and Burnstock, 1986), seminal vesicles (Meldrum and Burnstock, 1985), and a number of blood vessels (Su, 1978; Muramatsu et al., 1981; Sneddon and Burnstock, 1984b; Suzuki, 1985; Hicks et al., 1985; Kügelgen and Starke, 1985; Muramatsu, 1986). The prazosin-resistant component of the responses to sympathetic nerve stimulation is blocked by the P_2-purinoceptor antagonist $ANAPP_3$ or by selective desensitization with α,β-methylene ATP and is mimicked by local application of ATP, but not by NE. Both prazosin-sensitive and prazosin-resistant responses are abolished by sympathectomy or guanethidine, but only the prazosin-sensitive component is abolished following reserpine depletion of NE.

C. Acetylcholine and VIP

Cotransmission from parasympathetic nerves releasing both ACh and VIP during control of the salivary secretion has also been examined (Lundberg et al., 1979; Bloom and Edwards, 1980). The essential feature appears to be that different quantities of ACh and VIP can be released at different nerve discharge frequencies, perhaps because they are stored in different synaptic vesicles. This contrasts with sympathetic nerves, where different postjunctional responses to NE and ATP, perhaps released from the same synaptic vesicles, take place when sympathetic nerves fire for different frequencies and periods.

V. Sensory Nerves

Many sensory nerve endings have been recognized in the airways, particularly in the epithelial cell layer (e.g., Das et al., 1978; Lauweryns and Van Lommel, 1983; Laitinen, 1985). "Axon reflexes", in which antidromic impulses pass down collateral branches of primary afferent sensory fibers, have been recognized for many years to be involved in local vasodilation of the skin (Lewis, 1927). This concept has been extended recently to "axon reflex" activity in stomach (Delbro et al., 1982) and it seems likely to be an important mechanism in other organs, including the lung (Lundberg et al., 1983). Both substance P (Hagermark et al., 1978, Lembeck et al., 1982) and ATP (Holton and Holton, 1954; Jahr and Jessel, 1983; Fyffe and Perl, 1984), and/or possibly a combination of these two substances (Burnstock, 1977), have been claimed as transmitters in different populations of primary afferent sensory fibers and these may turn out to represent important "sensory-motor" neurotransmitters in the nervous control of the airways. Another feature of axon reflexes in the skin that may be relevant to the lung is that antidromic release of sensory transmitters leads to the release or synthesis of local agents such as histamine, bradykinin, and prostaglandins (Burnstock, 1977; Hellewell and Pearson, 1984).

VI. Endothelial- and Epithelial-Mediated Responses

Receptors to a number of neurotransmitters including ACh, ATP, substance P, and 5-HT are present in vascular endothelial cells, occupation of which leads to release of endothelium-derived relaxing factor and subsequent vasodilatation (Furchgott and Zawadzki, 1980; Vanhoutte and Rimele, 1982-1983; Furchgott, 1984). This important discovery has opened up the possibility that endothelial cells, perhaps containing some of these substances (see Parnavelas et al., 1985) are involved in the pathophysiology of blood flow in vascular beds during ischemia and hypoxia (Burnstock and Kennedy, 1986).

This concept has been followed recently with observations on the epithelial layer of the airways and evidence has been presented from several laboratories that removal of the epithelium from tracheal or bronchial preparations results in increased contractile responses evoked by ACh, histamine, and 5-HT (Flavahan et al., 1985; Barnes et al., 1985; Holroyde, 1986). It is suggested that respiratory epithelial cells may generate an inhibitory signal to decrease the responsiveness of bronchial smooth muscle to contractile agents and/or augment the effectiveness of inhibitory stimulii.

VII. Intramural Ganglia

Intramural ganglia in visceral organs have been much neglected and one often reads in physiology texts that "following denervation of the heart, bladder or lung" such and such occurs. This is clearly a misnomer, since all these organs contain many thousands (and in the case of the gut, millions) of intramural neurons that survive following section of the extrinsic sympathetic and parasympathetic nerves. One of the reasons for this neglect is that intramural ganglia are not easily accessible for functional studies in situ, although Coburn and his colleagues have made some progress in the airways by selecting the ferret tracheal ganglia for their electrophysiology studies (see Coburn's chapter, this volume). The development of culture preparations of intramural ganglia in the heart (Hassall and Burnstock, 1984, 1986) and bladder (Crowe et al., 1986) has allowed analysis of the interactions of extrinsic and intrinsic neuron activity within these ganglia and we are now extending this work to cultured tracheal ganglia. The projections of neurons and these ganglia and the possibility that they mediate intramural reflexes, independent of central control, are important questions to answer.

VIII. Future Directions

I have pointed out the substantial changes in our understanding of autonomic neuroeffector mechanisms, many aspects of which have not been systematically applied to the airways. The involvement of many of the putative autonomic transmitter substances, and in particular in cotransmitter combinations, remains to be clarified in the neural control of the airways. Few studies of the distribution of the receptors to these transmitters in different cell types in the airways have yet been carried out with modern autoradiographic methods. Investigation of the possible roles of epithelial cells, their receptors, and the many biologically active substances contained within them is in its infancy, as are studies of the possibility that sympathetic and sensory nerves control release of histamine and other substances from mast cells. Our understanding of the local control of pulmonary blood pressure by perivascular nerves and endothelium-mediated stimuli is only just beginning. A particularly prominent gap is our lack of knowledge of the types, projections, roles, and interactions of the intramural neurons present in the airways.

Until more is known of these normal mechanisms, it will be difficult to recognize the changes that have occurred in pathologic conditions and to develop therapeutic strategies to overcome them. Neither must we neglect the "trophic" influences that lead to long-term changes in autonomic nerves, receptors, and effector cells during development, regeneration, and during compensatory changes that occur after surgery and disease.

Discussion

Nadel. What is known about the mechanisms of release of neuropeptides from sensory nerves?

Burnstock. In view of the description of vesicular storage organelles in many sensory terminals it is assumed that release mechanisms are likely to be comparable to those in motor nerve terminals.

Barnes. Is there evidence for plasticity in the autonomic nervous system, and can chronic nerve stimulation lead to structural changes?

Burnstock. There is evidence for considerable plasticity in the autonomic nervous system. Thus, chronic stimulation of hypogastric nerves for several days in vivo leads to significant changes in neurotransmuscular transmission in the vas deferens (Jones et al., *Cell Tissue Res.*, 1983; *232*:265-279), and there is an increase in substance P immunoreactivity in nerve fibers of rabbit iris 1 month after sympathetic denervation (Cole et al., *Exp. Eye Res.*, 1983; *37*:191-197).

Coburn. Is there any evidence that the same postganglionic neuron may have both excitatory and inhibitory transmitters?

Burnstock. In most examples of sympathetic cotransmission the transmitters act synergistically (e.g., norepinephrine and ATP in blood vessels and vas deferens). There are instances where cotransmitters may have opposite effects. Thus, in perivascular nerves one cotransmitter may constrict smooth muscle in a low-tone preparation, while another dilates it in a high-tone preparation (Morris et al., *Neurosci. Lett.*, 1985; *62*:31-37).

References

Baer, H. P., and Drummond, G. I. (Eds.) (1979). *Physiological and Regulatory Functions of Adenosine and Adenine Nucleotides.* New York, Raven Press.

Barnes, P. J., Cuss, F. M., and Palmer, J. B. (1985). The effect of airway epithelium on smooth muscle contractility in bovine trachea. *Br. J. Pharmacol.* **86**:685-691.

Bell, C. (1982). Dopamine as a postganglionic autonomic neurotransmitter. *Neuroscience* **7**:1-8.

Berne, R. M., Rall, T. W., and Rubio, R. (Eds.) (1983). *Regulatory Function of Adenosine.* The Hague, Martinus Nijhoff.

Bloom, S. R., and Edwards, A. V. (1980). Vasoactive intestinal peptide in relation to atropine resistant vasodilatation in the submaxillary gland of the cat. *J. Physiol. (Lond.)* **300**:41-53.

Bowman, A., and Gillespie, J. S. (1982). Block of some non-adrenergic inhibitory responses of smooth muscle by a substance from haemolysed erythocytes. *J. Physiol. (Lond.)* **328**:11-25.

Branco, D., Albino Teixeira, A., Azevedo, I., and Osswald, W. (1984). Structural and functional alterations caused at the extraneuronal level by sympathetic denervation of blood vessels. *Arch. Pharmacol.* **326**:302-312.

Brownstein, M. J., Saavedra, J. M., Axelrod, J., Zeman, G. H., and Carpenter, D. O. (1974). Coexistence of several putative neurotransmitters in single identified neurons of *Aplysia. Proc. Natl. Acad. Sci. U.S.A.* **71**: 4662-4665.

Burn, J. H., and Rand, M. J. (1965). Acetylcholine in adrenergic transmission. *Annu. Rev. Pharmacol.* **5**:163-182.

Burnstock, G. (1969). Evolution of the autonomic innervation of visceral and cardiovascular systems in vertebrates. *Pharmacol. Rev.* **21**:247-324.

Burnstock, G. (1970). Structure of smooth muscle and its innervation. In *Smooth Muscle.* Edited by E. Bülbring, A. Brading, A. Jones and T. Tomita. London, Edward Arnold, pp. 1-69.

Burnstock, G. (1972). Purinergic nerves. *Pharmacol. Rev.* **24**:509-581.

Burnstock, G. (1976). Do some nerve cells release more than one transmitter? *Neuroscience* **1**:239-248.

Burnstock, G. (1977). Autonomic neuroeffector junctions—reflex vasodilatation of the skin. *J. Invest. Dermatol.* **69**:47-57.

Burnstock, G. (1978). A basis for distinguishing two types of purinergic receptor. In *Cell Membrane Receptors for Drugs and Hormones: A Multidisciplinary Approach.* Edited by L. Bolis and R. W. Straub. New York, Raven Press, pp. 107-118.

Burnstock, G. (1979). Past and current evidence for the purinergic nerve hypothesis. In *Physiological and Regulatory Functions of Adenosine and Adenine Nucleotides.* Edited by H. P. Baer and G. I. Drummond. New York, Raven Press, pp. 3-32.

Burnstock, G. (1980a). Cholinergic and purinergic regulation of blood vessels. In *Handbook of Physiology,* Section 2. The Cardiovascular System. Vol. II. Vascular Smooth Muscle. Edited by D. F. Bohr, A. D. Somlyo, H. W. Sparks and S. R. Geiger. Baltimore, American Physiological Society/ Waverly Press, pp. 567-612.

Burnstock, G. (1980b). Purinergic modulation of cholinergic transmission. *Gen. Pharmacol.* **11**:15-18.

Burnstock, G. (1981). Neurotransmitters and trophic factors in the autonomic nervous system. *J. Physiol. (Lond.)* **313**:1-35.

Burnstock, G. (1982a). Adenine nucleotides and nucleosides in cerebral hypoxia. In *Cerebral Hypoxia in the Pathogenesis of Migraine.* Progress in Neurobiology Series. Edited by F. C. Rose and W. K. Amery. Bath, Pitman Press, pp. 77-81.

Burnstock, G. (1982b). Neuropeptides as trophic factors. In *Systemic Role of Regulatory Peptides.* Symposia Medica Hoechst, No. 18. Stuttgart, Schattauer, pp. 423-446.

Burnstock, G. (1982c). Neuromuscular transmitters and trophic factors. In *Advanced Medicine,* Vol. 18. Edited by M. Sarner. London, Pitman Medical, pp. 143-148.

Burnstock, G. (1985). Purinergic mechanisms broaden their sphere of influence. *Trends Neurosci.* **8**:5-6.

Burnstock, G. (1986a). The changing face of autonomic neurotransmission. (The First von Euler Lecture in Physiology.) *Acta Physiol. Scand.* **126**:67-91.

Burnstock, G. (1986b). Autonomic neuromuscular junctions: current developments and future directions. (The Anatomical Society Review Lecture.) *J. Anat.* **146**:1-30.

Burnstock, G., and Brown, C. (1981). An introduction to purinergic receptors: history, classification and future developments. In *Purinergic Receptors.* Edited by G. Burnstock. London, Chapman and Hall, pp. 1-45.

Burnstock, G., and Buckley, N. (1985). The classification of receptors for adenosine and adenine nucleotides. In *Methods used in Adenosine Research.* Methods in Pharmacology, Vol. 6. Edited by D. M. Paton. New York, Plenum Press, pp. 193-212.

Burnstock, G., Campbell, G., Bennett, M., and Holman, M. E. (1963). Inhibition of the smooth muscle of the *taenia coli. Nature* **200**:581-582.

Burnstock, G., Campbell, G., Satchell, D. G., and Smythe, A. (1970). Evidence that adenosine triphosphate or a related nucleotide is the transmitter substance released by non-adrenergic inhibitory nerves in the gut. *Br. J. Pharmacol.* **40**:668-688.

Burnstock, G., Cocks, T., Crowe, R., and Kasakov, L. (1978). Purinergic innervation of the guinea-pig urinary bladder. *Br. J. Pharmacol.* **63**:125-138.

Burnstock, G., and Costa, M. (1975). *Adrenergic Neurons: Their Organisation, Function and Development in the Peripheral Nervous System.* London, Chapman and Hall.

Burnstock, G., Crowe, R., and Wong, H. K. (1979). Comparative pharmacological and histochemical evidence for purinergic inhibitory innervation of the portal vein of the rabbit, but not guinea-pig. *Br. J. Pharmacol.* **65**:377-388.

Burnstock, G., Dumsday, B. H., and Smythe, A. (1972). Atropine-resistant excitation of the urinary bladder: the possibility of transmission via nerves releasing a purine nucleotide. *Br. J. Pharmacol.* **44**:451-461.

Burnstock, G., and Kennedy, C. (1985). Is there a basis for distinguishing two types of P_2-purinoceptor? *Gen. Pharmacol.* **16**:433-440.

Burnstock, G., and Kennedy, C. (1986). A dual function for adenosine 5′-triphosphate in the regulation of vascular tone: excitatory cotransmitter with noradrenaline from perivascular nerves and locally released inhibitory intravascular agent. *Circ. Res.* **58**:319-330.

Burnstock, G., and Sneddon, P. (1985). Evidence for ATP and noradrenaline as cotransmitters in sympathetic nerves. *Clin. Sci.* **68**:89S-92S.

Chan-Palay, V., and Palay, S. L. (Eds.) (1984). *Co-existence of Neuroactive Substances in Neurones.* New York, John Wiley.

Cockcroft, S., and Gomperts, B. D. (1980). The ATP^{4-} receptor of rat mast cells. *Biochem. J.* **188**:789-798.

Cook, R. D., and Burnstock, G. (1976). The ultrastructure of Auerbach's plexus in the guinea-pig. I. Neuronal elements. *J. Neurocytol.* **5**:171-194.

Cottrell, G. A. (1976). Does the giant cerebral neurone of *Helix* release two transmitters: ACh and serotonin? *J. Physiol. (Lond.)* **259**:44P-45P.

Cowen, T., Haven, A. J., and Burnstock, G. (1985). Pontamine sky blue: a counter stain for background autofluorescence in fluorescence and immunofluorescence histochemistry. *Histochemistry* **82**:205-208.

Crowe, R., Haven, A. J., and Burnstock, G. (1986). Intramural neurones of the guinea-pig urinary bladder: histochemical localization of putative neurotransmitters in cultures and newborn animals. *J. Autonom. Nerv. Syst.* **15**:319-339.

Cuello, A. C. (Ed.) (1982). *Co-transmission.* London, Macmillan Press.

Cushley, M. J., Tattersfield, A. E., and Holgate, S. T. (1983). Inhaled adenosine and guanosine on airway resistance in normal and asthmatic subjects. *Br. J. Clin. Pharmacol.* **15**:161-165.

Daly, J. W. (1983). Role of ATP and adenosine receptors in physiologic processes: summary and prospectus. In *Physiology and Pharmacology of Adenosine Derivatives.* Edited by J. W. Daly, Y. Kuroda, J. W. Phillis and M. Ui. New York, Raven Press, pp. 275-290.

Das, R. M., Jeffery, P. K., and Widdicombe, J. G. (1978). The epithelial innervation of the lower respiratory tract of the cat. *J. Anat.* **126**:123-131.

Delbro, D., Fändriks, L., Lisander, B., and Andersson, S. A. (1982). Gastric atropine-sensitive excitation by peripheral vagal stimulation after hexamethonium. Antidromic activation of afferents? *Acta Physiol. Scand.* **114**:433-440.

De Mey, J., Burnstock, G., and Vanhoutte, P. M. (1979). Modulation of the evoked release of noradrenaline in canine saphenous vein via presynaptic receptors for adenosine but not ATP. *Eur. J. Pharmacol.* **55**:401-405.

Dhall, U., Cowen, T., Haven, A. J., and Burnstock, G. (1986). Perivascular noradrenergic and peptide-containing nerves show different patterns of changes during development and ageing in the guinea-pig. *J. Autonom. Nerv. Syst.* **16**:109-126.

Diamant, B., and Kruger, P. G. (1967). Histamine release from isolated rat peritoneal mast cells induced by ATP. *Acta Physiol. Scand.* 77:291-302.

Duval, N., Hicks, P. E., and Langer, S. Z. (1985). Inhibitory effects of α,β-methylene ATP on nerve-mediated contractions of the nictitating membrane in reserpinised cats. *Eur. J. Pharmacol.* **110**:373-377.

Fedan, J. S., Hogaboom, G. K., O'Donnell, J. P., Colby, J., and Westfall, D. P. (1981). Contributions by purines to the neurogenic response of the vas deferens of the guinea-pig. *Eur. J. Pharmacol.* **69**:41-53.

Flavahan, N. A., Aarhus, L. L., Rimele, T. J., and Vanhoutte, P. M. (1985). Respiratory epithelium inhibits bronchial smooth muscle tone. *J. Appl. Physiol.* **58**:834-838.

Foreman, J. C., and Jordan, C. C. (1983). Histamine release and vascular changes induced by neuropeptides. *Agents Actions* **13**:105-116.

Fry, G. N., Devine, C. E., and Burnstock, G. (1977). Freeze fracture studies of nexuses between smooth muscle cells; close relationship to sarcoplasmic reticulum. *J. Cell Biol.* **72**:26-34.

Furchgott, R. F. (1984). Role of endothelium in responses of vascular smooth muscle to drugs. *Annu. Rev. Pharmacol. Toxicol.* **24**:175-197.

Furchgott, R. F., and Zawadzki, J. V. (1980). The obligatory role of endothelial cells in the relaxation of arterial smooth muscle by acetylcholine. *Nature* **288**:373-376.

Furness, J. B., and Costa, M. (1979). Actions of somatostatin on excitatory and inhibitory nerves in the intestine. *Eur. J. Pharmacol.* **56**:69-74.

Furness, J. B., and Costa, M. (1982). Identification of gastrointestinal neurotransmitters. In *Handbook of Experimental Pharmacology,* Vol. 59. Edited by G. Bertaccini. Berlin, Springer, pp. 383-460.

Fyffe, R. E. W., and Perl, E. R. (1984). Is ATP a central synaptic mediator for certain primary afferent fibres from mammalian skin? *Proc. Natl. Acad. Sci. U.S.A.* **81**:6890-6893.

Gershon, M. D. (1979). Non-adrenergic, non-cholinergic autonomic neurotransmission mechanisms. In *Neurosciences Research Program Bulletin,* Vol. 17. Edited by G. Burnstock, T. Hökfelt, M. D. Gershon, L. L. Iversen, H. W. Kosterlitz and J. H. Szurszewski. Cambridge, MIT Press, pp. 414-424.

Gillespie, J. S. (1982). Non-adrenergic, non-cholinergic inhibitory control of gastrointestinal motility. In *Motility of the Digestive Tract.* Edited by M. Wienbeck. New York, Raven Press, pp. 51-66.

Gillespie, J. S., and Martin, W. (1980). A smooth muscle inhibitory material from the bovine retractor penis and rat anococcygeus muscles. *J. Physiol. (Lond.)* **309**:55-64.

Guerzon, G. M., Paré, P. D., Michoud, M.-C., and Hogg, J. C. (1979). The number and distribution of mast cells in monkey lungs. *Am. Rev. Respir. Dis.* **119**:59-66.

Hagermark, O., Hökfelt, T., and Pernow, B. (1978). Flare and itch induced by substance P in human skin. *J. Invest. Dermatol.* **71**:233-235.

Hassall, C. J. S., and Burnstock, G. (1984). Neuropeptide Y-like immunoreactivity in cultured intrinsic neurones of the heart. *Neurosci. Lett.* **52**:111-115.

Hassall, C. J. S., and Burnstock, G. (1986). Intrinsic neurones and associated cells of the guinea-pig heart in culture. *Brain Res.* **364**:102-113.

Heine, H., and Förster, F. J. (1975). Relationships between mast cells and preterminal nerve fibres. *Z. Mikrosk. Anat. Forsch.* **89**:934-937.

Hellewell, P. G., and Pearson, J. D. (1984). Purinoceptor mediated stimulation of prostacyclin release in the porcine pulmonary vasculature. *Br. J. Pharmacol.* **83**:457-462.

Hicks, P. E., Langer, S. Z., and Vidal, M. J. (1985). α,β-Methylene ATP inhibits the vasoconstriction to periarterial field stimulation in SHR but not WKY tail arteries *in vitro*. *Br. J. Pharmacol.* **85**:225P.

Hökfelt, T., Johansson, O., Ljungdahl, A., Lundberg, J. M., and Schultzberg, M. (1980). Peptidergic neurones. *Nature* **284**:515-521.

Holgate, S. T., Mann, J. S., and Cushley, M. J. (1984). Adenosine as a bronchoconstrictor mediator in asthma and its antagonism by methylxanthines. *J. Allergy Clin. Immunol.* **74**:302-306.

Holroyde, M. C. (1986). The influence of epithelium on the responsiveness of guinea-pig isolated trachea. *Br. J. Pharmacol.* **87**:501-507.

Holton, F. A., and Holton, P. (1954). The capillary dilator substances in dry powders of spinal roots: a possible role of adenosine triphosphate in chemical transmission from nerve endings. *J. Physiol. (Lond.)* **126**:124-140.

Hoyle, C. H. V., and Burnstock, G. (1986). Evidence that ATP is a neurotransmitter in the frog heart. *Eur. J. Pharmacol.* **124**:285-289.

Jahr, C. E., and Jessel, T. M. (1983). ATP excites a subpopulation of rat dorsal horn neurones. *Nature* **304**:730-733.

Jessen, K. R., Mirsky, R., Dennison, M., and Burnstock, G. (1979). GABA may be a neurotransmitter in the vertebrate peripheral nervous system. *Nature* **281**:71-74.

Kiernan, J. A. (1972). The involvement of mast cells in vasodilatation due to axon reflexes in injured skin. *Q. J. Exp. Physiol.* **57**:311-317.

Kügelgen, I. v., and Starke, K. (1985). Noradrenaline and adenosine triphosphate as co-transmitters of neurogenic vasoconstriction in rabbit mesenteric artery. *J. Physiol. (Lond.)* **367**:435-455.

Lagercrantz, H., Yamamoto, Y., Fredholm, B. B., Prabhakar, N. R., and von Euler, C. (1984). Adenosine analogues depress ventilation in rabbit neonates. Theophylline stimulation of respiration via adenosine receptors? *Pediatr. Res.* **18**:387-390.

Laitinen, A. (1985). Ultrastructural organisation of intraepithelial nerves in the human airway tract. *Thorax* **40**:488-492.

Lauweryns, J. M., and Van Lommel, A. (1983). The intrapulmonary neuroepithelial bodies after vagotomy: demonstration of their sensory neuroreceptor-like innervation. *Experientia* **39**:1123-1124.

Legay, C., Saffrey, M. J., and Burnstock, G. (1984). Coexistence of immunoreactive substance P and serotonin in neurones of the gut. *Brain Res.* **302**: 379-382.

Lembeck, F., Donnerer, J., and Barthó, L. (1982). Inhibition of neurogenic vasodilatation and plasma extravasation by substance P antagonists, somatostatin and (D-Met^2, Pro^5)-enkephalinamide. *Eur. J. Pharmacol.* **85**:171-176.

Lewis, J. (1927). *The Blood Vessels of the Human Skin and their Responses.* London, Shaw.

Lundberg, J. M., Brodin, E., and Saria, A. (1983). Effects and distribution of vagal capsaicin-sensitive substance P neurons with special reference to the trachea and lungs. *Acta Physiol. Scand.* **119**:243-252.

Lundberg, J. M., Hökfelt, T., Schultzberg, M., Uvnaswald, K., Kohler, C., and Said, S. I. (1979). Occurrence of vasoactive intestinal polypeptide (VIP)-like immunoreactivity in certain cholinergic neurons of the cat: evidence from combined immunohistochemistry and acetylcholinesterase staining. *Neuroscience* **4**:1539-1559.

Lunell, E., Svedmyr, N., Andersson, K.-E., and Persson, C. G. A. (1982). Effects of enprofylline, a xanthine lacking adenosine receptor antagonism, in patients with chronic obstructive lung disease. *Eur. J. Clin. Pharmacol.* **22**: 395-402.

Muramatsu, I. (1986). Evidence for sympathetic, purinergic transmission in the mesenteric artery of the dog. *Br. J. Pharmacol.* **87**:478-480.

Muramatsu, I., Fujiwara, M., Miura, A., and Sakakibara, Y. (1981). Possible involvement of adenine nucleotides in sympathetic neuroeffector mechanisms of dog basilar artery. *J. Pharmacol. Exp. Ther.* **216**:401-409.

Marigold, J. H., Pounder, R. E., Pemberton, J., and Thompson, R. P. H. (1982). Propranolol, oxprenolol and sclerosing peritonitis. *Br. Med. J.* **284**:870.

Marmo, E., Cazzola, M., Chieppa, S., Lampa, E., Lobefalo, G., and Filippelli, A. (1985). Documentation of presence of a purinergic reactivity at tracheobronchial level in man. *Curr. Ther. Res.* **38**:118-134.

Martinson, J., and Muren, A. (1963). Excitatory and inhibitory effects of vagus stimulation on gastric motility in the cat. *Acta Physiol. Scand.* **57**:309-316.

Melander, T., Hökfelt, T., Rökaeus, A., Fahrenkrug, J., Tatemoto, K., and Mutt, V. (1985). Distribution of galanin-like immunoreactivity in the gastrointestinal tract of several mammalian species. *Cell Tissue Res.* **239**:253-270.

Meldrum, L. A., and Burnstock, G. (1983). Evidence that ATP acts as a cotransmitter with noradrenaline in sympathetic nerves supplying the guinea-pig vas deferens. *Eur. J. Pharmacol.* **92**:161-163.

Meldrum, L. A., and Burnstock, G. (1985). Evidence that ATP is involved as a cotransmitter in the hypogastric nerve supplying the seminal vesicle of the guinea-pig. *Eur. J. Pharmacol.* **110**:363-366.

Newson, B., Dahlström, A., Enerbäck, L., and Ahlman, H. (1983). Suggestive evidence for a direct innervation of mucosal mast cells. An electron microscopic study. *Neuroscience* **10**:565-570.

Okada, Y., Yada, T., Ohno-Shosaku, T., Oiki, S., Ueda, S., and Machida, K.

(1984). Exogenous ATP induces electrical membrane responses in fibroblasts. *Exp. Cell Res.* **152**:552-557.

Olson, L., Ålund, M., and Norberg, K-A. (1976). Fluorescence microscopical demonstration of a population of gastrointestinal nerve fibres with a selective affinity for quinacrine. *Cell Tissue Res.* **171**:407-423.

Osborne, N. N. (Ed.) (1983). *Dale's Principle and Communication between Neurones.* Oxford, Pergamon Press.

Parnavelas, J., Kelly, W., and Burnstock, G. (1985). Ultrastructural localisation of choline acetyltransferase in vascular endothelial cells in rat brain. *Nature* **316**:724-725.

Pernow, B. (1983). Substance P—a putative mediator of antidromic vasodilatation. *Gen. Pharmacol.* **14**:13-16.

Sneddon, P., and Burnstock, G. (1984a). Inhibition of excitatory junction potentials in guinea-pig vas deferens by α,β-methylene-ATP: further evidence for ATP and noradrenaline as cotransmitters. *Eur. J. Pharmacol.* **100**:85-90.

Sneddon, P., and Burnstock, G. (1984b). ATP as a neurotransmitter in rat tail artery. *Eur. J. Pharmacol.* **106**:149-152.

Sneddon, P., and Westfall, D. P. (1984). Pharmacological evidence that adenosine triphosphate and noradrenaline are co-transmitters in the guinea-pig vas deferens. *J. Physiol. (Lond.)* **347**:561-580.

Sneddon, P., Westfall, D. P., and Fedan, J. S. (1982). Co-transmitters in the motor nerves of the guinea-pig vas deferens: electrophysiological evidence. *Science* **218**:693-695.

Soares da Silva, P., and Azevedo, I. (1985). Fibroblasts and sympathetic innervation of blood vessels. *Blood Vessels* **22**:278-285.

Stone, T. W. (1981). Physiological roles for adenosine and adenosine 5′-triphosphate in the nervous system. *Neuroscience* **6**:523-555.

Su, C. (1978). Purinergic inhibition of adrenergic transmission in rabbit blood vessels. *J. Pharmacol. Exp. Ther.* **204**:351-361.

Suzuki, H. (1985). Electrical responses of smooth muscle cells of the rabbit ear artery to adenosine triphosphate. *J. Physiol. (Lond.).* **359**:401-415.

Uehara, Y., and Burnstock, G. (1970). Demonstration of 'gap junctions' between smooth muscle cells. *J. Cell Biol.* **44**:215-217.

Vanhoutte, P. M., and Rimele, T. J. (1982-1983). Role of endothelium in the control of vascular smooth muscle function. *J. Physiol. (Paris)* **78**:681-686.

Watt, A. H., and Routledge, P. A. (1985). Adenosine stimulates respiration in man. *Br. J. Clin. Pharmacol.* **20**:503-506.

Wiesner-Menzel, L., Schulz, B., Vakilzadeh, F., and Czarnetzki, B. M. (1981). Electron microscopical evidence for a direct contact between nerve fibres and mast cells. *Acta Derm. Venereol. (Stockh.)* **61**:465-469.

Wood, J. D., and Mayer, C. J. (1979). Serotonergic activation of tonic-type enteric neurons in guinea-pig small bowel. *J. Neurophysiol.* **42**:582-593.

2

Innervation of the Lung

JOHN B. RICHARDSON

McGill University
Montreal, Quebec, Canada

The mammalian lung has at least three efferent neural pathways to the smooth muscle and the secretory cells and three basic afferent neural pathways have been delineated by physiological studies (Widdicombe, 1981). Two of the efferent pathways, the cholinergic and the adrenergic, have been extensively studied and characterized while the third, the nonadrenergic, noncholinergic pathways remain largely undefined due to the lack of both a suitable inhibitor for this pathway and knowledge of its neurotransmitter (Richardson, 1979, 1983). The efferent neural pathways pathways are classified into excitatory and inhibitory and this basic pattern has been found in all animals studied to date, with obvious species variation. In the human lung, the principal neural pathway is the cholinergic, which is excitatory and the inhibitory pathway is the nonadrenergic, noncholinergic (NAIS) pathway with no detectable adrenergic component (Richardson and Béland, 1976; Davis et al., 1982), whereas in the well-studied canine airways the only inhibitory neural pathway is the adrenergic (Russell, 1980). This basic pattern is not consistent throughout the airways in either the density of innervation or receptor population (O'Donnel et al., 1978; Doidge and Satchell, 1982; Leff et al., 1983; Nadel and Barnes, 1984). The reasons for these differences between the central and the peripheral airways are not known and this is an area of current investigation. While the NAIS and the adrenergic neural pathways are predominantly inhibitory in their actions on the airways smooth muscle, both have been shown to have an excitatory action under certain circumstances. Nonadrenergic, noncholinergic excitation has been demonstrated in the guinea pig tracheobronchial tree and this excitatory action can be inhibited by $alpha_2$ adrenergic receptor activation (Grundström et al., 1984). It is not clear, however, if this is the same neural pathway also capable of inhibiting the smooth muscle in the guinea pig. The likely mediator of the excitatory pathway is substance P (Sub P), which may be released from the afferent neurons present in the airways of the guinea pig (Grundström et al., 1984; Lundberg et al., 1984). If the neurotransmitter is not substance P, the neurotransmitter that normally results in inhibition may also be capable of excitation in a manner similar to that seen in the muscle of the urogenital system (Burnstock et al., 1978). The adrenergic neural pathway, or circulating catecholamines, are capable of excitation in the smooth muscle by activating alpha receptors. These receptors have an unequal distribution throughout the tracheobronchial tree, with the bronchi being much more responsive to alpha stimulation than the tracheal smooth muscle (Leff et al., 1983).

In some species, such as *Aves*, the only inhibitory pathway demonstrated is the NAIS. In these animals this pathway is dominant as reflected in field stimulation, which causes relaxation of the smooth muscle (Bhatla et al., 1980), while stimulation of irritant receptors in geese causes bronchodilatation (Callanan et al., 1974). This latter response, if the goose resembles the chicken and the duck, indicates that stimulation of irritant receptors causes reflex activation of the inhibitory system over the excitary cholinergic system. This is the reverse of the situation found in mammals. What advantage there is to bronchodilatation instead of bronchoconstriction remains obscure but birds, with their predominant inhibitory system, are interesting models for the study of this neural pathway and also as a source for the neurotransmitter. Several animals, such as the guinea pig (Coburn and Tomita, 1973) and the cat (Diamond and O'Donnell, 1980; Irvin et al., 1980), have two inhibitory neural pathways, the adrenergic and the nonadrenergic. In cats, the NAIS preferentially dilates the middle-sized airways, which are the same ones maximally constricted by vagal stimulation, while the trachea and the smallest bronchi are only slightly affected by either the adrenergic or the NAIS pathways (Matsumoto et al., 1985). Such a response pattern might be expected if the inhibitory neurons migrate with the cholinergic neurons, as has been demonstrated for the gastrointestinal tract (Gershon and Thompson, 1973). In humans and other primates (Richardson, 1979; Doidge and Satchell, 1982; Middendorf and Russell, 1980) there appears to be only one inhibitory pathway, the NAIS. To date, no definite abnormalities in the NAIS have been demonstrated in a large series of patients with pulmonary disease.

The central control of the airways has been further delineated through studies on reflex pathways (Roberts et al., 1981; Rao et al., 1981; Davis et al., 1982b; Kaufman et al., 1982; Shultz et al., 1985) and direct pathways in the vagus (Mitchell et al., 1985). In the latter study, in cats, cholinergic nerves were found which fired during inspiration and were considered to be a major excitatory input to the tracheal smooth muscle (Mitchell et al., 1985). The central neurons were localized to the dorsal motor vagal nuclei, the nucleus ambiguus, and the reticular formation by studies that involved exposing the cut vagal nerves from anesthetized cats and dogs to horseradish peroxidase and then examining the brain stems for the presence of the histochemical reaction product (Bennett et al., 1981). The same authors also suggest that there may be a separation of the somata with myelinated fibers from the nucleus ambiguus and nonmyelinated fibers from the dorsal vagal motor nuclei and that the bronchomotor activity may arise from the nucleus ambiguus (Bennett et al., 1981). This finding confirms the earlier suggestion that a group of such fibers may innervate the smooth muscle of the airways (Widdicombe, 1966). The control of the airways motor activity by inspiratory neurons in the brain stem is similar to the phenomenon of swallowing that usually occurs during expiration. The area responsible for the esophageal control is located in the same area in the brain stem as that for the inspiratory control; the area of the nucleus ambiguus (Doty, 1968). Inspiration, expiration, sucking, and swallowing are even more coordinated in the human infant, where a 1:1:1 relationship exists between sucking, breathing, and swallowing (Doty, 1968). What role, if any, this central control of airway motor activity may have in disease remains to be clarified but it is an important observation for the understanding of airway smooth muscle tone.

Several recent studies on pulmonary reflexes have shown that stimulation of bronchial C fibers with bradykinin results in a reflex contraction of the airways smooth muscle (Roberts et al., 1981) and can also increase the tracheal gland secretions (Davis et al., 1982b; Schultz et al., 1985). Other studies have demonstrated bradykinin-induced changes in expiratory duration and inhibition of inspiration with distention of the trachea (Rao et al., 1981). These studies all show the varied functions of reflex pathways but also point out our lack of understanding of the role of the afferent nerves in the lung and their influence on breathing and airway calibre. The earlier suggestion that neuroepithelial bodies might have a sensory role as chemoreceptors (Lauweryns and Peuskens, 1972) has been given support by a recent morphologic study on the innervation of the neuroepithelial bodies in the rabbit lung (Lauweryns et al., 1985). This was a quantitative and qualitative study on denervated lungs in which the vagus was sectioned both above and below the nodose ganglion and the effects of these operations observed on the neuroepithelial bodies in the airways as well as on the nerve endings adjacent to the neuroepithelial bodies. The infranodosal vagotomy markedly decreased the neuroepithelial body innervation. The authors concluded that the neuroepithelial bodies were innervated by sensory fibers (Lauweryns et al., 1985). While the neural connection for these bodies suggests that they are sensory in nature, the role of these interesting bodies remains elusive. A recent study on the mouse lung, with particular attention to the trachea and the primary bronchi, with and without unilateral cervical vagotomy, demonstrated that vagotomy resulted in degeneration of 70% of the nerves in the smooth muscle of the primary bronchi (Pack et al., 1984). This study demonstrated a very complex neural network within the smooth muscle fibers, which the authors presumed represented stretch receptors. The very large sensory component in the smooth muscle, some portions of which apparently contained vesicles, further complicates our understanding of the innervation of the smooth muscle by efferent neuronal pathways and makes the afferent pathway appear all the more important in the control of the smooth muscle tone.

There is recent interest in pulmonary nerves that contain neuropeptides and many peptides have been localized to both the nerves and the ganglia by use of immunohistochemical techniques (Ghatei et al., 1982; Hakanson et al., 1983). Several of these peptides have been proposed as modulators of pulmonary physiology, and their potential effects on smooth muscle (Said, 1982) and inflammatory changes in the mucosa have been stressed (Lundberg et al., 1984). The two peptides that have received the most attention are vasoactive intestinal peptide (VIP) and substance P (Sub P), due to their actions on relaxing and contracting smooth muscle, vascular permeability, and gland secretion (Said, 1982; Lundberg et al., 1984). Substance P immunoreactive nerves have been demonstrated in the respiratory tract of many species, particularly sensory nerve endings (Polak and Bloom, 1982; Hakanson et al., 1983). Vagal stimulation results in vasodilatation and edema of the tracheal mucosa, which can be prevented either by prior treatment with capsaicin or through the use of Sub P antagonists (Lundberg et al., 1984). Capsaicin treatment results in the loss of Sub P from the nerves (Jessel et al., 1978). The treatment of neonatal animals with this extract results in degeneration of the chemoreceptive neurons (Jancso et al., 1977). In untreated animals, Sub P is thought to be released following stimulation of the irritant receptors in the airways. This reflex may have a central connection mediated by Sub P (Jessel, 1982) and is thought to be similar to cutaneous vasodilatory responses (Lundberg et al., 1984). The released Sub P produces vasodilatation, increased permeability, and mucosal edema. Bronchoconstriction may also be produced by Sub P either by a direct effect (Lundberg et al., 1983, 1984) or through an indirect action causing the release of acetylcholine from nerves in the airways (Tanaka and Grunstein, 1984). The role of these peptide-containing nerves in the pathogenesis of asthma and other inflammatory diseases of the airways remains to be clarified, but the presence of this potent peptide in the submucosal nerves and its release through irritation of the mucosa argues for an important role.

Vasoactive intestinal peptide has been demonstrated in nerve trunks and neurons of pulmonary ganglia (Dey et al., 1981; Polak and Bloom, 1982; Hakanson et al., 1983). Its presence in these nerves plus its relaxant effect on airway smooth muscle has led to the proposition that this peptide is the neurotransmitter of the nonadrenergic inhibitory neural pathway (Said et al., 1980; Fahrenkrug and Emson, 1982; Nadel and Barnes, 1984). There is evidence to support this proposal both in animal and human subjects (Matsuzaki et al., 1980; Barnes and Dixon, 1984; Cameron et al., 1983). However, there is evidence against VIP as the NAIS neurotransmitter (Karlsson and Persson, 1983; Altiere and Diamond, 1985; Satchell, 1984; Davis et al., 1982a) and even suggestions that its actions on smooth muscle are indirect (Regal and Johnson, 1983). It is possible that VIP may be a regulatory or modulating substance in the neural control of smooth muscle, as has been demonstrated for the leucine and methionine enkephalins that inhibit the release of acetylcholine from postganglionic neurons (Russell and Simons, 1985).

The intrapulmonary ganglia have been studied from several aspects and we now have some understanding of their structure and possible function. A technique for the vital staining of ganglion cells, similar to that used in the gastrointestinal tract, has allowed for the direct study of pulmonary ganglia (Grillo and Nadel, 1980). One study has shown that norepinephrine can inhibit cholinergic neurotransmission in pulmonary ganglia (Baker et al., 1982) and another has demonstrated depression of neurotransmission in ganglia by barbiturates (Skoogh, 1983).

The structure of ganglia in the human trachea resembles intestinal ganglia, with a dense neurophil and many axon profiles filled with agranular and granular vesicles and supporting glial cells (Richardson, 1983). This morphologic pattern resembles central more than peripheral nervous tissue and has been well described in the intestine (Gabella, 1972, 1981). These ganglia receive central imput from the nucleus ambiguus and the doral vagal nuclei (Mitchell et al., 1985).

Modulation of pulmonary neural responses has been an area of great interest in the past few years. Many agents including the enkephalins (Russell and Simons, 1985), substances derived from the epithelium (Flavahan et al., 1985; Barnes et al., 1985), or inflammatory products (Holtzman, et al., 1983) have been shown to influence these neural pathways, either by an augmentation or a depression of the output of transmitters.

The innervation of the glands in the lung has been studied in the human, ferret, and cat lung. In the human bronchus, field stimulation of the tissue resulted in mucus secretion. This secretion was blocked by tetrodotoxin and atropine, which indicated a selective cholinergic innervation of the glands (Baker et al.,

1985). The finding of selective cholinergic innervation was puzzling due to the presence of adrenergic nerves located in the human bronchi and the response of the glands to adrenergic agonists (Pack and Richardson, 1983). It was suggested that the adrenergic innervation may modulate cholinergic innervation (Baker et al., 1985). In the ferret and the cat there is evidence for participation by cholinergic, adrenergic, and nonadrenergic, noncholinergic neural pathways in control of mucus secretion (Peatfield and Richardson, 1983; Borson et al., 1984; Baker et al., 1985). The nonadrenergic, noncholinergic component involves VIP, which inhibits mucus secretion (Baker et al., 1985). However, this peptide has been shown to stimulate the secretion of mucus in the ferret (Peatfield et al., 1983).

There has been a steady increase in our knowledge of the innervation of the lung in the past few years, but fundamental problems are still not resolved. The central control of the airways is of great interest, as is the possible modulatory role of the peptides present in the pulmonary neural tissue. The exact role of both of these components in health and disease remains to be shown but they certainly offer some interesting possibilities. The problem of hyperreactive airways and the role of neural innervation in their pathogenesis remains unsolved. The neural control of mucus production in both normal and disease states is not understood. Finally the morphology of the airways needs further study to allow us to establish if there are definite differences between the central and the distal airways, as suggested by physiological studies, and by the innervation patterns, and to delineate further the role of the neuropeptides.

Discussion

Burnstock. There is an increase in gap junctions in denervated vas deferens (Westfall, D. P., 1977), which supports the view that there is a reciprocal relationship between density of innervation and frequency of gap junctions. Small gap junction sites may not be detected by transmission electron microscopy but may be observed by freeze-fracture techniques.

Barnes. Are there any differences in frequency of gap junctions or in the density of innervation in airway smooth muscle of horses with heaves compared with normal animals?

Richardson. Preliminary observations suggest differences in smooth muscle cell size, but it is not yet certain whether the innervation or gap junction frequency is different.

Widdicombe. The majority of nerves in large airway smooth muscle are afferent (pulmonary stretch receptors), so the decrease in innervation in small airways may represent the "dropping out" of sensory nerves. Have you performed any degeneration studies?

Richardson. No degeneration studies have yet been performed.

Laitinen. In human airway smooth muscle 300 nerve profiles were examined; 299 contained many vesicles and few mitochondria, suggesting that they were motor nerves, and only 1 had many mitochondria characteristic of a sensory nerve.

Widdicombe. Perhaps the presence of sensory neuropeptides might be useful to identify nonmyelinated afferent nerves in airways.

Lundberg. Afferent nerves containing substance P and CGRP represent only a subpopulation of sensory nerves (unmyelinated C fibers).

References

Altiere, R. J., and Diamond, L. (1985). Effect of alpha-chymotrypsin on the nonadrenergic noncholinergic inhibitory system in cat airways. *Eur. J. Pharmacol.* **114**:75-80.

Baker, D. G., Herbert, D. A., and Mitchell, R. A. (1982). Cholinergic neurotransmission in airway ganglia: inhibition by norepinephrine. *Physiologist* **25**: 225.

Baker, B., Peatfield, A. C., and Richardson, P. S. (1985). Nervous control of mucin secretion into human bronchi. *J. Physiol.* **365**:297-305.

Barnes, P. J., and Dixon, C. M. (1984). The effect of inhaled vasoactive intestinal peptide on bronchial reactivity to histamine in humans. *Am. Rev. Respir. Dis.* **130**:162-166.

Barnes, P. J., Cuss, F. M., and Palmer, J. B. (1985). The effect of airway epithelium on smooth muscle contractility in bovine trachea. *Br. J. Pharmacol.* **86**:685-691.

Bhatla, R., Ferguson, C., and Richardson, J. (1980). The innervation of smooth muscle in the primary bronchus of the chicken. *Can. J. Physiol. Pharmacol.* **58**:310-315.

Bennett, J. A., Kidd, C., Latif, A. B., and McWilliam, P. N. (1981). A horseradish peroxidase study of vagal motoneurones with axons in cardiac and pulmonary branches of the cat and dog. *Q. J. Exp. Physiol.* **66**:145-154.

Borson, D. B., Charlin, M., Gold, B. D., and Nadel, J. A. (1984). Neural regulation of $^{35}SO_4$ macromolecule secretion from tracheal glands of ferrets. *J. Appl. Physiol.* **57**:457-466.

Burnstock, G., Cocks, T., Crowe, R., and Kasakov, L. (1978). Purinergic innervation of the guinea pig urinary bladder. *Br. J. Pharmacol.* **63**:125-138.

Callanan, D., Dixon, M., Widdicombe, J. G., and Wise, J. C. M. (1974). Responses of geese to inhalation of irritant gases and injections of phenyl diguanide. *Respir. Physiol.* **22**:157-166.

Cameron, A. R., Johnston, C. F., Kirkpatrick, C. T., and Kirkpatrick, M. C. (1983). The quest for the inhibitory neurotransmitter in bovine tracheal smooth muscle. *Q. J. Exp. Physiol.* **68**:413-326.

Coburn, R. F., and Tomita, T. (1973). Evidence for nonadrenergic inhibitory nerves in the guinea pig trachealis muscle. *Am. J. Physiol.* **224**:1072-1080.

Davis, C., Kannan, M. S., Jones, T. R., and Daniel, E. E. (1982). Control of human airway smooth muscle: in vitro studies. *J. Appl. Physiol.* **53**:1080-1087.

Davis, B., Roberts, A. M., Coleridge, H. M., and Coleridge, J. C. G. (1982). Reflex tracheal gland secretion evoked by stimulation of bronchial C-fibers in dogs. *J. Appl. Physiol.* **53**:985-991.

Dey, D. A., Shannon, W. A., and Said, S. I. (1981). Localization of VIP-immunoreactive nerves in airways and pulmonary vessels of dogs, cats and human subjects. *Cell Tissue Res.* **220**:231-238.

Diamond, L., and M. O'Donnell (1980). A nonadrenergic vagal inhibitory pathway to feline airways. *Science* **208**:185-188.

Doidge, J. M., and Satchell, D. G. (1982). Adrenergic and nonadrenergic inhibitory nerves in mammalian airways. *J. Auton. Nerv. Syst.* **5**:83-99.

Doty, R. W. (1968). Neural organization of deglutition. In *Handbook of Physiology,* Section 6, Alimentary Canal, Vol. IV. Motility. Washington, D.C., American Physiological Society, pp. 1861-1902.

Fahrenkrug, J., and Emson, P. C. (1982). Vasoactive intestinal polypeptide: functional aspects. *Br. Med. Bull.* **38**:265-270.

Flavahan, N. A., Aarhus, L. L., Rimele, T. J., and Vanhoutte, P. M. (1985). Respiratory epithelium inhibits bronchial smooth muscle tone. *J. Appl. Physiol.* **58**:853-858.

Gabella, G. (1972). Fine structure of the myenteric plexus in the guinea pig ileum. *J. Anat.* **111**:69-97.

Gabella, G. (1981). Structure of muscles and nerves in the gastrointestinal tract. In *Physiology of the Gastrointestinal Tract.* Edited by L. R. Johnson. New York, Raven Press, pp. 197-241.

Gershon, M. D., and Thompson, E. B. (1973). The maturation of neuromuscular function in a multiple innervated structure: development of the longitudinal smooth muscle of the foetal mammalian gut and its cholinergic excitatory, adrenergic inhibitory and non-adrenergic inhibitory innervation. *J. Physiol.* **234**:257-278.

Ghatei, M. A., Sheppard, N., O'Shaughnessy, D. J., Adrian, T. E., McGregor, G. P., Polak, J. M., and Bloom, S. R. (1982). Regulatory peptides in the mammalian respiratory tract. *Endocrinology* **111**:1248-1254.

Grillo, M. A., and Nadel, J. A. (1980). Vital staining of tracheal ganglia. *Physiologist* **23**:77.

Grundström, N., Andersson, R. G., and Wikberg, J. E. (1984). Inhibition of the excitatory non-adrenergic, non-cholinergic neurotransmission in the guinea pig tracheobronchial tree mediated by alpha 2 adrenoceptors. *Acta Pharmacol. Toxicol.* **54**:8-14.

Hakanson, R., Sundler, F., Moghimzadeh, E., and Leander, S. (1983). Peptide-containing nerve fibers in the airways: distribution and functional implications. *Eur. J. Respir. Dis.* **63**:115-140.

Holtzman, M. J., Fabbri, L. M., O'Byrne, P. M., Gold, B. D., Aizawa, H., Walters, E. H., Alpert, S. E., and Nadel, J. A. (1983). Importance of airway inflammation for hyperresponsiveness induced by ozone. *Am. Rev. Respir. Dis.* **127**:686-690.

Irvin, C. G., Boileau, R., Tremblay, J., Martin, R. R., and Macklem, P. T. (1980). Bronchodilation: noncholinergic, nonadrenergic mediation demonstrated in vivo in the cat. *Science* **207**:791-792.

Jancso, N., Kiraly, E., and Jancso-Gabor, A. (1977). Pharmacologically induced selective degeneration of chemosensitive primary sensory neurons. *Nature* **270**:741-743.

Jessell, T. M. (1982). Fifty years of substance P. *Nature* **295**:551-553.

Jessell, T. M., Iverson, L. L., and Cuello, A. C. (1978). Capsaicin induced depletion of substance P from primary sensory neurons. *Brain Res.* **152**:183-188.

Karlsson, J. A., and Persson, C. G. A. (1983). Evidence against vasoactive intestinal peptide (VIP) as a dilator and in favour of substance P as a constrictor in airway neurogenic responses. *Br. J. Pharmacol.* **79**:634-636.

Kaufman, M. P., Ordway, G. A., Longhurst, J. C., and Mitchell, J. H. (1982). Reflex relaxation of tracheal smooth muscle by thin-fiber muscle afferents in dogs. *Am. J. Physiol.* **243**:R383-R388.

Lauweryns, J. M., and Peuskens, J. C. (1972). Neuro-epithelial bodies (neuro-receptor or secretory organs?) in human infant bronchial and bronchiolar epithelium. *Anat. Res.* **172**:471-482.

Lauweryns, J. M., Van Lommel, A. T., and Dom, R. J. (1985). Innervation of rabbit intrapulmonary neuroepithelial bodies. *J. Neurol. Sci.* **67**:81-92.

Leff, A. R., Munoz, N. M., and Hendrix, S. G. (1983). Parasympathetic and adrenergic contractile response in canine trachea and bronchus. *J. Appl. Physiol.* **55**:113-120.

Lundberg, J. M., Brodin, E., Hua, X., and Saria, A. (1984). Vascular permeability changes and smooth muscle contraction in relation to capsaicin-sensitive substance P afferents in the guinea pig. *Acta Physiol. Scand.* **120**:217-227.

Lundberg, J. M., Martling, C. R., and Saria, A. (1983). Substance P and capsaicin-induced contraction of human bronchi. *Acta Physiol Scand.* **119**:49-53.

Matsumoto, N., Inoue, H., Ichinose, M., Ishii, M., Inoue, C., Saraki, H., and Takishima, T. (1985). Effective sites by sympathetic beta-adrenergic and vagal nonadrenergic inhibitory stimulation in constricted airways. *Am. Rev. Respir. Dis.* **132**:1113-1117.

Matsuzaki, Y., Hamasaki, Y., and Said, S. I. (1980). Vasoactive intestinal peptide: a possible transmitter of non-adrenergic relaxation of guinea pig airways. *Science* **210**:1252-1253.

Middendorf, W. F., and Russell, J. A. (1980). Innervation of airway smooth muscle in the baboon: evidence for a nonadrenergic inhibitory system. *J. Appl. Physiol.* **48**:947-956.

Mitchell, R. A., Herbert, D. A., and Baker, D. G. (1985). Inspiratory rhythm in airway smooth muscle tone. *J. Appl. Physiol.* **58**:911-920.

Nadel, J. A., and Barnes, P. J. (1984). Autonomic regulation of the airways. *Annu. Rev. Med.* **35**:451-467.

O'Donnell, S. R., Saar, N., and Wood, L. J. (1978). The density of adrenergic nerves at various levels in the guinea pig lung. *Clin. Exp. Pharmacol. Physiol.* **5**:325-332.

Pack, R. J., Al-Ugaily, L. H., and Widdicombe, J. G. (1984). The innervation of the trachea and extrapulmonary bronchi of the mouse. *Cell Tissue Res.* **238**:61-68.

Pack, R. J., and Richardson, P. S. (1984). The aminergic innervation of the human bronchus: a light and electron microscopic study. *J. Anat.* **138**:493-502.

Peatfield, A. C., and Richardson, P. S. (1983). Evidence of non-cholinergic, non-adrenergic nervous control of mucous secretion into the cat trachea. *J. Physiol.* **342**:315-345.

Polak, J. M., and Bloom, S. R. (1982). Regulatory peptides and neuron-specific enolase in the respiratory tract of man and other mammals. *Exp. Lung. Res.* **3**:313-328.

Rao, S. V., Sant'Ambrogio, F. B., and Sant'Ambrogio, G. (1981). Respiratory reflexes evoked by tracheal distention. *J. Appl. Physiol.* **50**:421-427.

Regal, J. F., and Johnson, D. E. (1983). Indomethacin alters the effects of substance P and VIP on isolated airway smooth muscle. *Peptides* **4**:581-584.

Richardson, J. B. (1979). Nerve supply to the lungs. *Am. Rev. Respir. Dis.* **119**:785-802.

Richardson, J. B. (1983). Recent progress in pulmonary innervation. *Am. Rev. Respir. Dis.* **128**:S65-S68.

Richardson, J. B., and Béland, J. (1976). Nonadrenergic inhibitory nervous system in human airways. *J. Appl. Physiol.* **41**:764-771.

Roberts, A. M., Kaufman, M. P., Baker, D. G., Brown, J. K., Coleridge, H. M., and Coleridge, J. C. G. (1981). Reflex tracheal contraction induced by stimulation of bronchial C-fibers in dogs. *J. Appl. Physiol.* **51**:485-493.

Russell, J. A. (1980). Noradrenergic inhibitory innervation of canine airways. *J. Appl. Physiol.* **48**:16-22.

Russell, J. A., and Simons, E. J. (1985). Modulation of cholinergic neurotransmission in airways by enkephalin. *J. Appl. Physiol.* **58**:859-868.

Said, S. I. (1982). Vasoactive peptides in the lung with special reference to vasoactive intestinal peptide. *Exp. Lung. Res.* **3**:343-348.

Said, S. I., Giachetti, A., and Nicosia, S. (1980). VIP: possible functions as a neural peptide. In *Neural Peptides and Neuronal Communication.* Edited by E. Costa and M. Trabucchi. New York, Raven Press, pp. 75-82.

Satchell, D. G. (1984). Adenosine deaminase antagonizes inhibitory responses to adenosine and non-adrenergic, non-cholinergic inhibitory nerve stimulation in isolated preparations of guinea-pig trachea. *Br. J. Pharmacol.* **83**: 329-336.

Schultz, H. D., Roberts, A. M., Bratcher, C., Coleridge, H. M., Coleridge, J. C., and Davis, B. (1985). Pulmonary C-fibers reflex increase secretion by tracheal submucosal glands in dogs. *J. Appl. Physiol.* **58**:907-910.

Skoogh, B. E. (1983). Transmission through airway ganglia. *Eur. J. Respir. Dis.* **131**:159-170.

Tanaka, D. T., and Grunstein, M. M. (1984). Mechanisms of substance P induced contraction of rabbit airway smooth muscle. *J. Appl. Physiol.* **57**: 1551-1557.

Widdicombe, J. G. (1966). Action potentials in parasympathetic and sympathetic efferent fibers to the trachea and lungs of dogs and cats. *J. Physiol.* **186**:56-88.

Widdicombe, J. G. (1981). Nervous receptors in the respiratory tract and lungs. In *Lung Biology in Health and Disease.* Part 1, *Regulation of Breathing.* Edited by T. Hornbein. New York, Marcel Dekker, pp. 429-472.

3

Detailed Analysis of Neural Elements in Human Airways

LAURI A. LAITINEN*

St. George's Hospital Medical School
University of London
London, United Kingdom

I. Introduction

The earlier concepts of innervation of human airways have recently been undergoing change due to expanded research. Histochemical and electron microscopic studies have revealed the presence of acetylcholinesterase-positive nerve fibers and "cholinergic" nerve profiles in the human bronchial tree (Richardson, 1979). Recently the concept of nerves in human airway tract has been widened to include adrenergic nerves as well (Partanen et al., 1982b). The bronchial smooth muscle tone is known to be regulated by acetylcholine via muscarinic receptors (Richardson and Beland, 1976) and by catecholamines via α- and β-receptors (Simonsson et al., 1972; Richardson and Beland, 1976), while in vitro studies with human bronchial smooth muscle strips have also revealed a third neural system, a nonadrenergic inhibitory regulatory mechanism (Richardson and Beland, 1976). Vasoactive intestinal peptide (VIP) has been suggested as a possible relaxant of bronchial smooth muscle tone (Said et al., 1974), and, in this respect, may serve as a neurotransmitter for the nonadrenergic inhibitory system in human respiratory tract as well (Barnes, 1984).

Sensory receptors of the airways can be described as those primarily in-

---

**Present affiliation*: Central Military Hospital, Helsinki, Finland

volved in the physiological control of breathing pattern (slowly adapting pulmonary stretch receptors) and those primarily concerned with changes in pathologic conditions (rapidly adapting irritant and C-fiber receptors) (Sant'Ambrogio, 1982). Neuroepithelial bodies may also be receptors with afferent nerves (Lauweryns and Peuskens, 1972; Hung et al., 1973) responding to changes in the partial pressure of oxygen (Lauweryns and Cocelaere, 1973). Complete understanding of airway receptors is handicapped, however, by the fact that their histologic appearance has not been completely analyzed (Widdicombe, 1982). Therefore, studies on structure-function relationships of the airway receptors have been difficult to conduct.

It is evident that both the quality and quantity of innervation vary so much between humans and animal species that results from animal experiments should be interpreted with caution. Therefore, in this chapter I have concentrated on what is known of the neural elements in the human airways from the larynx to the periphery. Of the progressively increasing number of neuropeptides, I have selected only vasoactive intestinal peptide for this review.

II. Smooth Muscle

A. Cholinergic Innervation: AchE-Containing and Cholinergic-Like Nerve Fibers

In all mammals studies, AChE-containing fibers are found in the airway smooth muscle (Richardson, 1979), but differences exist in the density of the nerve fibers (Mann, 1971). In humans, AChE-containing nerve fibers have been described in the smooth muscle of the newborn (Pessacq, 1971), and recently it has been shown (Partanen et al., 1982b) that the bronchial smooth muscle of adults also receives a rich AChE-positive network of nerve fibers that extends from lobar bronchi to terminal bronchioli. These fibers originate mainly from the peribronchial plexuses, but the possibility of an additional supply from the periarterial plexus cannot be excluded.

After glutaraldehyde fixation and staining with lead citrate and uranyl acetate, the nerve profiles containing only predominantly small agranular vesicles (SAGV) and some large granular vesicles (LGV) are considered cholinergic (Richardson, 1966; Hökfelt and Jonsson, 1968). On the basis of these morphologic criteria, cholinergic nerve profiles are present in the smooth muscle layer of the human respiratory tract (Laitinen et al., 1985b). The importance of cholinergic nerves in human bronchial smooth muscle and their bronchoconstrictive effect have been widely accepted (Richardson, 1979; Daniel et al., 1980; Orehek, 1981). Laitinen et al. (1985b) found that some nerve profiles in humans contained mainly LGV and differed from classic cholinergic nerves. They resemble the p-type nerves defined by Burnstock (1972) or the small p-type nerves defined by Baumgarten et al. (1970) and Gibbins and Haller (1979). These have been considered to represent nonadrenergic noncholinergic (NANC) nerves. Laitinen et al. (1985b) did not classify the nerves into two groups based on the difference between the number of LGV. Because of the great variability in the proportion of SAGV and LGV as well as in the size of LGV in the nerves, it may be an oversimplification to classify them into different groups (cholinergic and NANC) and thus exclude the possible coexistence of neural transmitters.

B. Sympathetic Innervation: Catecholamine-Containing and Adrenergic-Like Nerve Fibers

Catecholamine-containing nerve fibers have been found in airway smooth muscle in several animal species (Doidge and Satchell, 1982) but not in humans (Richardson and Beland, 1976; Doidge and Satchell, 1982). One reason for the difficulty in demonstrating the adrenergic nerves, especially in human tissue, is the extensive autofluorescence due to collagen fibers. Therefore, in a recent study, a method was selected based on glyoxylic acid (de la Torre, 1980), although the method is not specific only to norepinephrine of the monoamines. This method enabled demonstration of catecholamine-containing nerves in smooth muscle, from lobar bronchi to terminal bronchioli (Partanen et al., 1982b). Although adrenergic nerves evidently are present in the smooth muscle layer of adult human airways, their number is much lower than that of AChE-containing nerve fibers. Catecholamine-containing fibers represented only a few percent of those innervating smooth muscle in humans (Partanen et al., 1982b).

In an electron microscopic study, nerves considered adrenergic by ultrastructural criteria have also been found in the proximity of the smooth muscle (Laitinen et al., 1982; 1985b; Pack and Richardson, 1984). In these studies, the nerve endings of autonomic axons have been distinguished by their distinct population of vesicles (see Richardson, 1966; Hökfelt, 1967). According to these criteria, nerve fibers that after conventional fixation predominantly exhibit small granular vesicles (30-50 nm in diameter) are considered adrenergic. Thus, electron microscopic findings confirm the histochemical findings (Partanen et al., 1982b) and demonstrate the close association of adrenergic nerves with smooth muscle cells. The number of adrenergic profiles is small, however, which may explain the difficulty in finding these nerves in earlier studies.

Human bronchial smooth muscle cells have numerous cell-to-cell connections of the gap-junction type (Richardson and Ferguson, 1979; Daniel et al., 1980), which implies that smooth muscle cells are electrically coupled and may act in a single unit rather than in a multiunit fashion (Richardson and Ferguson, 1979). Thus every cell need not be innervated. In this respect, a sparse innervation may have physiological significance in the regulation of bronchial smooth muscle tone in humans, either directly or by reducing cholinergic transmission (Nadel and Barnes, 1984).

C. Nonadrenergic Noncholinergic Innervation

Richardson and Beland (1976) have described a nonadrenergic inhibitory nervous system in human lung. Recent immunohistochemical studies on neuropeptides have revealed that VIP-containing nerve fibers are present in the airway smooth muscle layer (Dey et al., 1981; Partanen et al., 1982a) and that their density exceeds that of adrenergic nerves (Partanen et al., 1982a). Since VIP also exhibits general features of a neurotransmitter (Said et al., 1980) and is a potent relaxant of tracheal smooth muscle (Said et al., 1974), the neuronally mediated smooth muscle relaxation could mainly be derived from a VIP-containing nervous system.

Based on the light microscopic observations on the VIP-like immunoreactivity in the human airways, immunohistochemical and electron microscopic investigations have been combined to get more information about the localization of VIP. These studies have led to the demonstration of VIP-like immunoreactivity in the vesicles of nerve profiles close to airway smooth muscle. Under electron microscopy, VIP-like immunoreactivity has been found in large granular vesicles ranging from 90 to 210 nm. The number of LGV varies between nerve profiles. The majority of nerve profiles contain several LGV (120-210 nm), but profiles containing only a few smaller VIP-positive large granules (90-150 nm) are also present (Laitinen et al., 1985c). Larsson (1977), in his ultrastructural study of the cat colon, has suggested that VIP is localized in nerve terminals of p-type neurons. Conversely, Johansson and Lundberg (1981) have reported that ultrastructurally VIP-like immunoreactivity in cat salivary glands is in LGV (mean 90 nm) of "cholinergic-type" nerve profiles, and they have suggested a possible coexistence of acetylcholine and VIP in the same neurons. In the study by Laitinen et al. (1985c), VIP-like immunoreactivity was located in LGV of variable size. When only a few LGV were present in the nerve profile, the size of the LGV was smaller. Based upon the size and number of LGV, these nerve profiles corresponded to classic "cholinergic-type" nerve profiles, when several LGV were present, the sizes were larger and the profiles corresponded to "p-type" nerve profiles.

On the basis of these results, it cannot be concluded whether a separate type of VIP nerve exists and/or if several transmitters coexist in some nerves. This concept is supported by the findings of Wharton et al. (1981) who found nerve profiles in cat ureter that contained a mixed population of vesicles, characteristic of both cholinergic and p-type nerves. To get more finite information, a simultaneous immunohistochemical demonstration of two different transmitters in the same nerve or cell body is needed. However, the present results show that VIP-like immunoreactivity found by light microscopy is ultrastructurally localized in nerves in humans (Laitinen et al., 1985c). Also these ultrastructural results show a great anatomical variation between different VIP-containing nerve profiles, which may indicate more than one type of VIP-containing nerve.

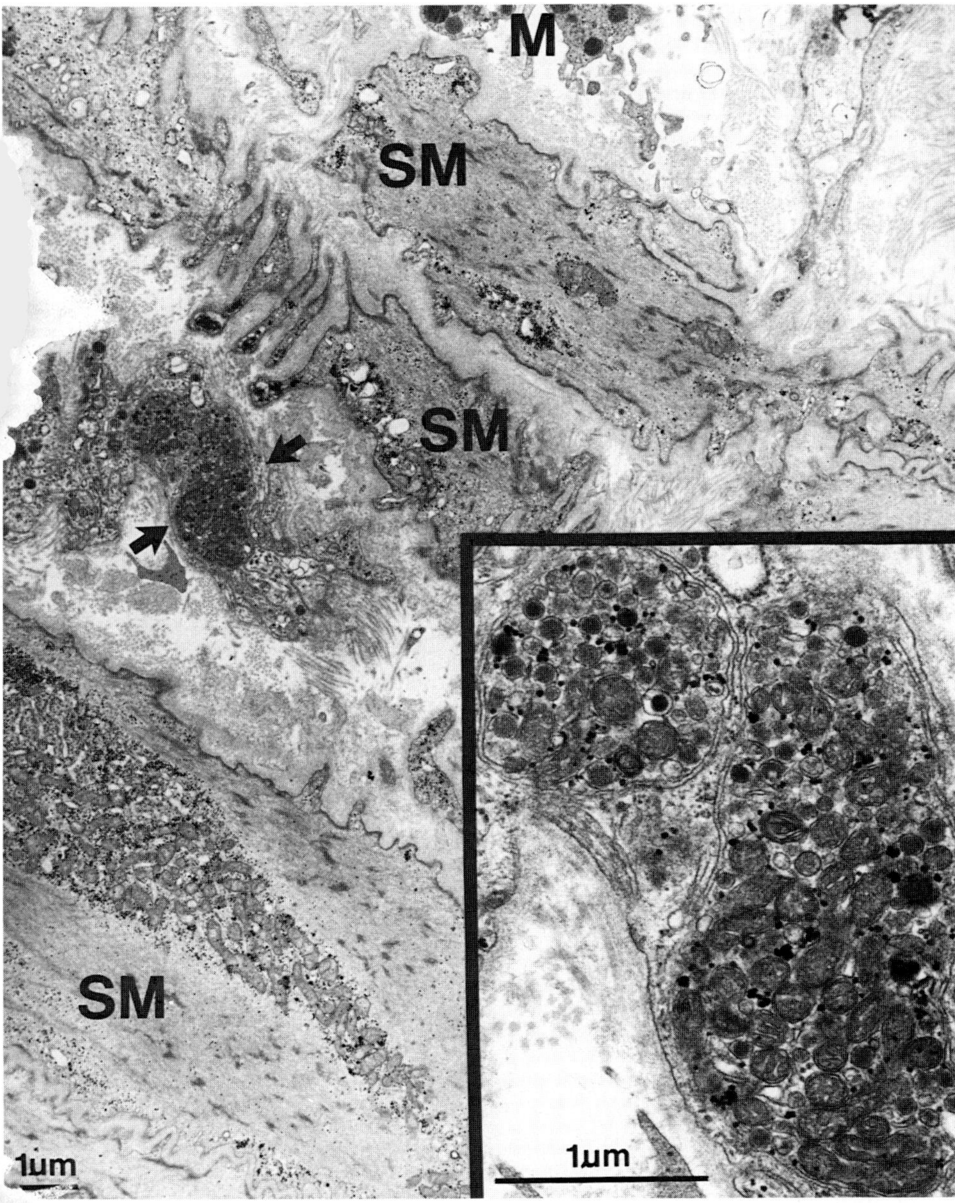

Figure 1 An electron micrograph of normal human airway smooth muscle layer. A presumed afferent nerve fiber packed with mitochondria is seen between smooth muscle cells of human lobar bronchus. Smooth muscle cells (SM) are seen at both sides of the nerve (arrows). Parts of a mast cell (M) are seen at the top of the picture. Magnification ×9,700. Inset: the nerve with a greater magnification ×39,000; bar = 1 μm.

D. Afferent Innervation

Physiological evidence indicates that the slowly adapting stretch receptors lie within or are associated with the smooth muscle of the airways (Widdicombe, 1954; Bartlett et al., 1976; Bradley and Scheuermier, 1977; Sant'Ambrogio et al., 1977). Afferent nerves have been identified at this location in several species by light and electron microscopy (Von Düring et al., 1974; Krauhs, 1984; Pack et al., 1984). In human bronchial smooth muscle only a few studies of afferent terminals are available (Larsell and Dow, 1933; Jabonero and Sabadell, 1972).

In a morphologic study of nerve fibers found close to smooth muscle cells (Laitinen et al., 1985b) nearly all fibers (of 300 analyzed) mainly contained vesicles with few mitochondria and therefore resembled motor nerves. One exceptional axon profile (Fig. 1) was packed with 37 mitochondria. Because it clearly differed from all of the efferent axonal fibers, having features characteristic of afferent nerves, it may represent an afferent nerve responding to slowly adapting pulmonary stretch receptors.

III. Bronchial Glands

A. Cholinergic and Sympathetic Innervation: AChE- and Catecholamine-Containing and Cholinergic- and Adrenergic-Like Nerve Fibers

The innervation of bronchial glands differs between mammals. In sheep the glands receive both AChE- and catecholamine-containing nerve fibers; in goat only AChE-positive fibers; and in calf, pig, and rabbit no AChE- or catecholamine-containing nerves exist (Mann, 1971). In humans the presence and distribution of AChE- and catecholamine-containing nerve fibers in bronchial glands have been recently reported (Partanen et al., 1982b; Pack and Richardson, 1984). On the basis of these studies the human bronchial glands receive both an AChE-containing and an adrenergic nerve supply. According to Spencer and Leof (1964) the nerve supply to the bronchial glands in humans is derived mainly from the nerve plexus around the bronchial arteries, while Larsell and Dow (1933) support the concept that they arise mainly from adjacent intrabronchial ganglia. I suggest that nerves in bronchial glands are derived from several sources. The supply of adrenergic fibers is mainly from the plexus around bronchial arteries, while the AChE-containing fibers are mainly from both extrachondrial and/or subchondrial microganglia and from the corresponding nerve plexuses, and represent the cholinergic innervation of the gland.

On the basis of morphologic criteria (Richardson, 1966; Hökfelt and Jonsson, 1968), cholinergic nerve profiles are also present in the glands of the human respiratory tract. The importance of cholinergic nerves in human bronchial glands has been widely accepted (Orehek, 1981). Nerve profiles containing SGV are considered adrenergic (Richardson, 1966; Hökfelt and Jonsson, 1968), and these also have been found in the bronchial glands in human airways (Laitinen et al., 1985b). In the bronchial glands nerve profiles were found between acini as well as in the acini between gland cells.

B. Nonadrenergic Noncholinergic Innervation

VIP-like immunoreactive nerves have also been found in bronchial glands in human airways (Dey et al., 1981). Ultrastructurally, VIP-like immunoreactivity was localized in LGV ranging from 90 to 210 nm (Laitinen et al., 1985c).

IV. Airway Blood Vessels: Sympathetic Innervation via Catecholamine-Containing and Adrenergic-Like Nerve Fibers

Human bronchial blood vessels are innervated by adrenergic nerves (Doidge and Satchell, 1982; Partanen et al., 1982b), whereas AChE-positive nerves have not been found in the bronchial vessels (Partanen et al., 1982b). Catecholamine-containing nerve fibers innervate bronchial blood vessels of different sizes which are located in the connective tissue as well as subepithelially. Electron microscopy has revealed nerves close to the walls of small arteries (Fig. 2).

V. Microganglia

A. Cholinergic and Sympathetic Innervation: AChE- and Catecholamine-Containing Nerve Fibers

The nerve plexuses present in human lung are periarterial and peribronchial and the latter can be subdivided into extrachondrial and subchondrial plexuses. The intrapulmonary microganglia are mostly located inside the extrachondrial plexuses, but a few are also present subchondrially as well as close to periarterial plexuses. These plexuses contain AChE-positive fibers, and the nerve cell bodies inside the microganglia also give a positive reaction. Extrachondrially the microganglia are located inside the plexuses, while subchondrially the AChE-positive nerve cell bodies are either inside or beside the nerve bundles emerging in the tissue (Partanen et al., 1982b).

Catecholamine-positive nerve fibers have been located around the nerve cell bodies in some microganglia in human airways (Partanen et al., 1982b).

B. Nonadrenergic Noncholinergic Innervation

In the human upper respiratory tract, VIP-immunoreactive nerve cell bodies have been observed in local microganglia (Uddman and Sundler, 1979; Dey et al.,

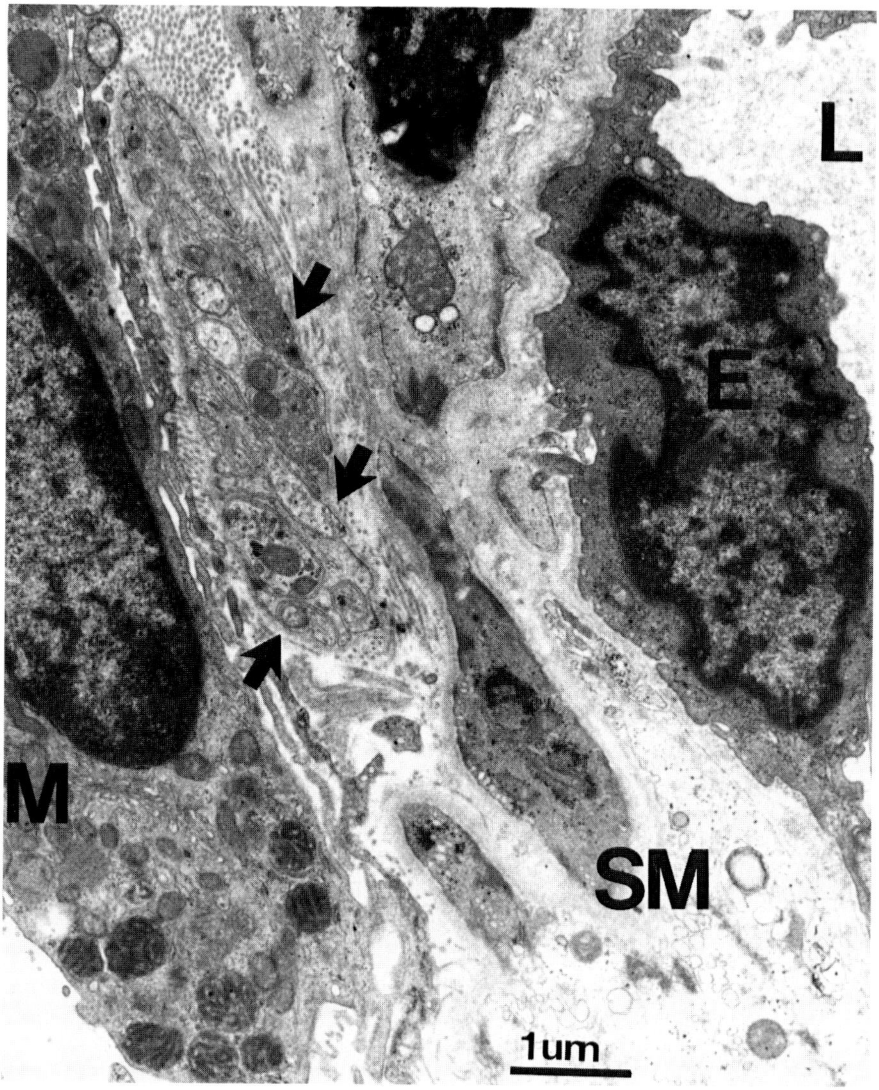

Figure 2 An electron micrograph of normal human tracheal mucosa. Nonmyelinated nerve axons (arrows) containing synaptic vesicles and mitochondria are seen close to smooth muscle cells (SM) in the wall of a small arteriole (luminal diameter approximately 15 μm). A partly degranulated mast cell (M) is adjacent to the vessel and nerves. L, lumen of the arteriole; E, endothelium. Magnification ×16,000; bar = 1 μm.

1981). VIP-immunoreactive nerve fibers have also been reported in the human vagus nerve (Lundberg et al., 1979). Laitinen and co-workers (1985c) did not observe any VIP-immunoreactive nerve cell bodies in the microganglia of the lower respiratory tract, but a dense network of VIP-immunoreactive nerve fibers was found scattered around the nerve cell bodies of these microganglia. However, in the study by Laitinen et al. (1985c), negative nerve cell bodies do not exclude the possible VIP-ergic nature of these cells; these nerve cell bodies may contain VIP in concentrations undetectable by this method.

VIP-immunoreactive nerve fibers in the human lower respiratory tract may originate from upper local microganglia, where VIP-positive cell bodies exist (Uddman and Sundler, 1979; Dey et al., 1981), or via the vagus nerve from nerve cell bodies located more centrally, or from local microganglia. In the human trachea, VIP-positive nerve cell bodies are also present locally, which suggests a local origin of VIP-immunoreactive nerves (Uddman and Sundler, 1979). Since the VIP-immunoreactive nerve fibers are also scattered around nerve cell bodies in the microganglia of the human lower respiratory tract, these nerves may also control the function of microganglia as well.

VI. Airway Epithelium

A. Afferent Innervation

Nerves in human airway epithelium have been studied by light microscopy by Larsell and Dow (1933), Gaylor (1934), Spencer and Leof (1964), and Pessacq (1971), and by electron microscopy by Rhodin (1966) and Laitinen and coworkers (Heino et al., 1982; Laitinen, 1985; Laitinen et al., 1985a, 1985d). The human bronchial epithelium receives terminal fibers from the peribronchial plexus (Larsell and Dow, 1933; Gaylor, 1934; Pessacq, 1971). In human tracheal epithelium, Rhodin (1966), using electron microscopy, described nonmyelinated axons that contained only neurotubuli and no vesicles.

The concentration of intraepithelial nerves at various airway levels in humans has recently been established (Laitinen, 1985). In the epithelium, axon profiles seem to have two predominant locations: either close to the airway lumen or at the base of the epithelium close to the basement membrane. Nerve fibers penetrating the basement membrane and traversing the epithelium from the base to the luminal side are also present. Since only a few nerves are seen to penetrate the basement membrane and enter the epithelium, probably the nerve fibers entering the airway epithelium divide further and form several axon profiles.

There is a difference between different airway levels in the location of intraepithelial nerves. Nerves near the lumen are mostly found in the larger airways and relatively few are observed in the smaller airways (Laitinen, 1985). This is in accordance with the findings of previous animal studies (Fillenz and Woods, 1970; Jeffery and Reid, 1973; King et al., 1974; Das et al., 1978). Ultrastructural studies in animals have rarely shown nerves in the intrapulmonary airways (Richardson, 1979).

When the ultrastructure of nerves in the airway epithelium of humans is analyzed further, the variation in the number of mitochondria suggests two populations of axon profiles (Laitinen, A., Partanen, M., Mattila, S., and Laitinen, L. A., unpublished observations). The "mitochondrial type," containing mainly mitochondria, is found only at the base of the epithelium. The "vesicle type," containing many vesicles and only some mitochondria, is found near the airway lumen in central airways (Fig. 3) and at the base of the epithelium at all airway levels studied (trachea, upper lobe, and segmental bronchus).

The only definitive morphologic methods of locating and identifying afferent nerves in the airways are the use of intracellular labels (Bower et al., 1978; Lacey, 1978) and degeneration studies (Das et al., 1979; Pack et al., 1984). Since such studies are very difficult to perform in humans, the ultrastructure of axon profiles in human airway epithelium has to be compared with more definitive findings in other species, and with nerves in some sensory organs in humans. The axons close to the basement membrane containing many mitochondria, and especially those associated with granular cells, conform well to the classic morphologic criteria for afferent axonal fibers King et al., 1974; Das et al., 1978; Hoyes and Barber, 1981). The "mitochondrial type" axon profile has been described by several authors in the airway epithelium of several animal species (Hung et al., 1973, Jeffery and Reid, 1973; King et al., 1974; Das et al., 1978). These nerves may represent a part of a sensory unit arising from the lung and representing the so-called rapidly adapting "irritant receptors."

In humans the "vesicle type" of axon profile has rarely been illustrated intraepithelially, and only in larger airways (Jeffery, 1982), whereas in several laboratory animals it has frequently been found (Jeffery and Reid, 1973; King et al., 1974; Das et al., 1978). In a recent study (Laitinen, A., Partanen, M., Mattila, S., and Laitinen, L. A., unpublished observations) these axonal profiles resembled the intraepithelial endings noted by Cauna et al. (1969) and the horizontal dermal and intradermal endings of Cauna (1966). Although it should be safe to assume that intraepidermal endings are afferent, one cannot exclude the possibility that these axons in the respiratory epithelium might be efferent to either ciliated or mucous cells. Nevertheless, histochemical studies have not revealed AChE- (Partanen et al., (1982b) or catecholamine-positive (Partanen et al., 1982b; Pack and Richardson, 1984) nerve fibers in human airway epithelium. Moreover, the human epithelium of secondary bronchi or of the more distal parts of the bronchial tree do not receive VIP-like immunoreactive nerve fibers (Dey et al., 1981; Laitinen et al., 1985c).

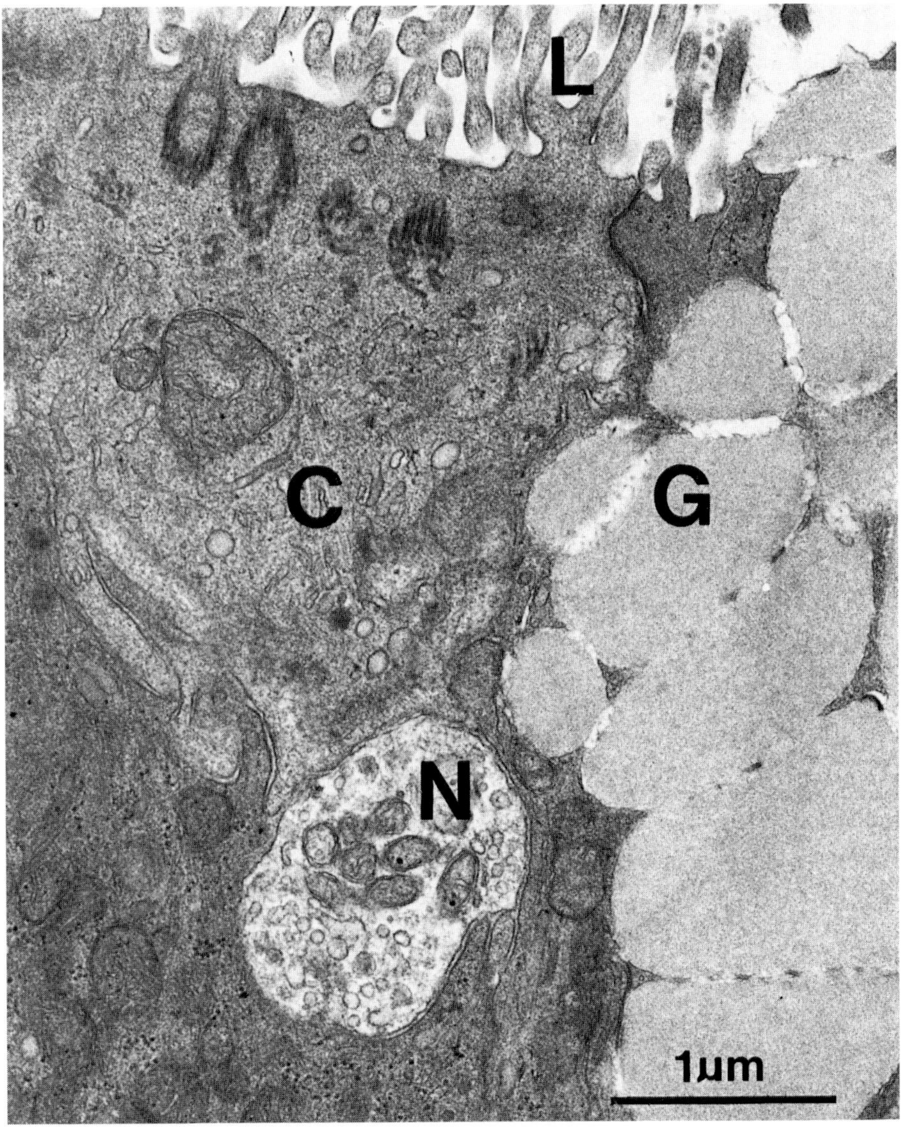

Figure 3 An electron micrograph of normal tracheal epithelium. An axon profile (N) is located between ciliated (C) and goblet (G) cells close to the airway lumen (L). The profile contains many small agranular vesicles and some mitochondria. Magnification ×30,000; bar = 1 μm.

B. Granule-Containing (APUD) Cells

Granule-containing (GC) cells have been described in adult (Bensch et al., 1965; Lauweryns and Goddeeris; Partanen et al., 1986) and fetal (Lauweryns et al., 1970) human lung. They are found from trachea to segmental bronchi (Partanen et al., 1986). Their frequency in the human airway epithelium has been estimated using quantitative electron microscopic methods: 6 cells in the trachea, 4 cells in the upper lobe bronchus, and 2.4 cells in the segmental bronchus per mm basement membrane (Partanen, M., Laitinen, A., Pelto-Huikko, M., Laitinen, L. A., and Hervonen, A., unpublished observations). One function of CG cells may be sensory: a GC cell body sends a long narrow "fingertip" (Fig. 4) through thick epithelium to reach the lumen, and this fingertip may act as a receptor unit for stimuli coming through the airways.

In humans, GC cells contain biogenic monoamine (Lauweryns et al., 1970), and peptide hormones (DiAugustine and Sonstegard, 1984). By cytochemical characteristics the GC cell was earlier also classified as a member of the widespread amine precursor uptake and decarboxylation (APUD) cell system (Pearse, 1969). These APUD cells may have a neurosecretory function and secrete monoamines and/or bioactive peptides (Pearse, 1976; Reichlin, 1980). Partanen and co-workers (unpublished observations) found that the cell body of a GC cell located close to the basement membrane contained several neurosecretory granular vesicles. In these anatomical regions fenestrated capillaries came close to the epithelial basement membrane and GC cells (Fig. 5). The GC cells may secrete their contents through fenestrated capillaries into the microcirculation and affect tissue lying nearly (epithelium, smooth muscle, vascular beds).

The GC cells of human airways are also in close association with basal intraepithelial nerves (Fig. 5). These nerve profiles coming to GC cells contain clear vesicles of variable size, a few larger vesicles, and mitochondria. Although the nerve profiles containing small clear vesicles have earlier been considered motor in function (Richardson, 1966; Tranzer and Richards, 1976), recently they have been found to be associated with sensory function (King et al., 1974; McDonald, 1977). When synaptic organizations were found between GC cells and neuronal profiles, the dense projections were observed on each side of the synapses (Partanen et al., unpublished observations).

VII. Conclusions

1. Acetylcholinesterase-positive nerve fibers and nerve profiles of cholinergic type are found in the smooth muscle and glands from the lobar bronchi to the terminal bronchioli (Partanen et al., 1982b; Laitinen et al., 1985b).

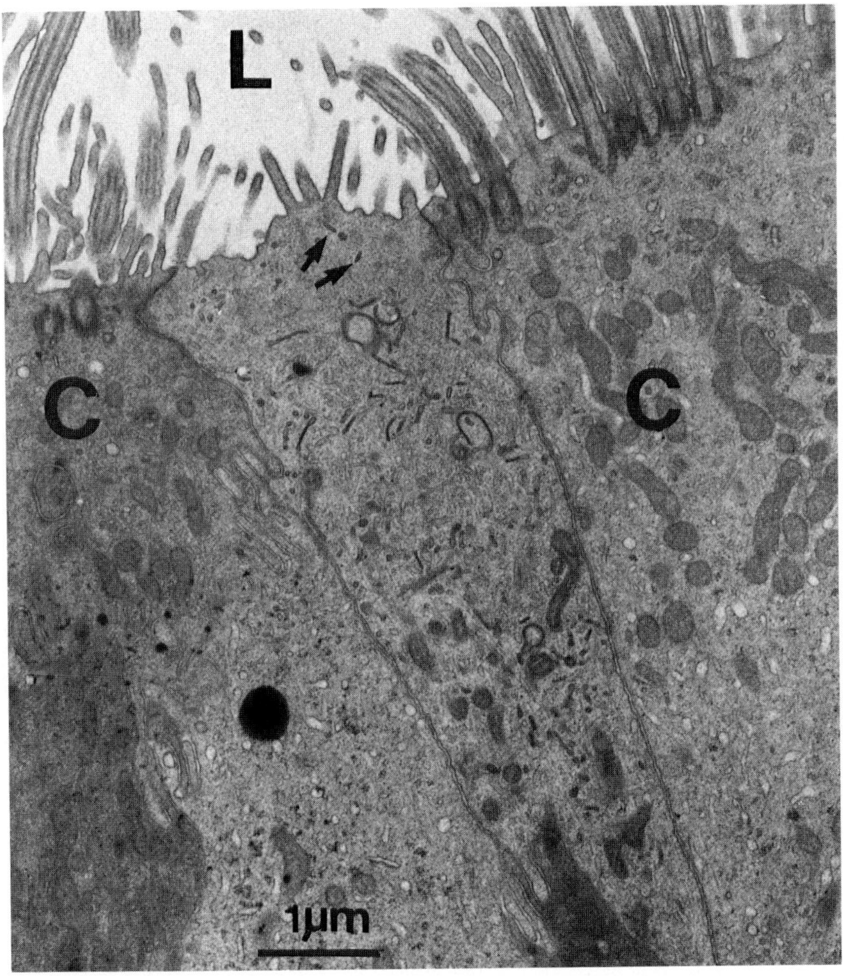

Figure 4 An electron micrograph of a luminal part of an APUD cell between two ciliated cells (C). It contains cytoplasmic tubules (arrows) and small microvilli. The luminal part is connected by a narrow neck to a larger basal portion of the APUD cell. Only the basal cellular area contains neurosecretory vesicles. L, lumen: Magnification ×15,600; bar = 1 μm.

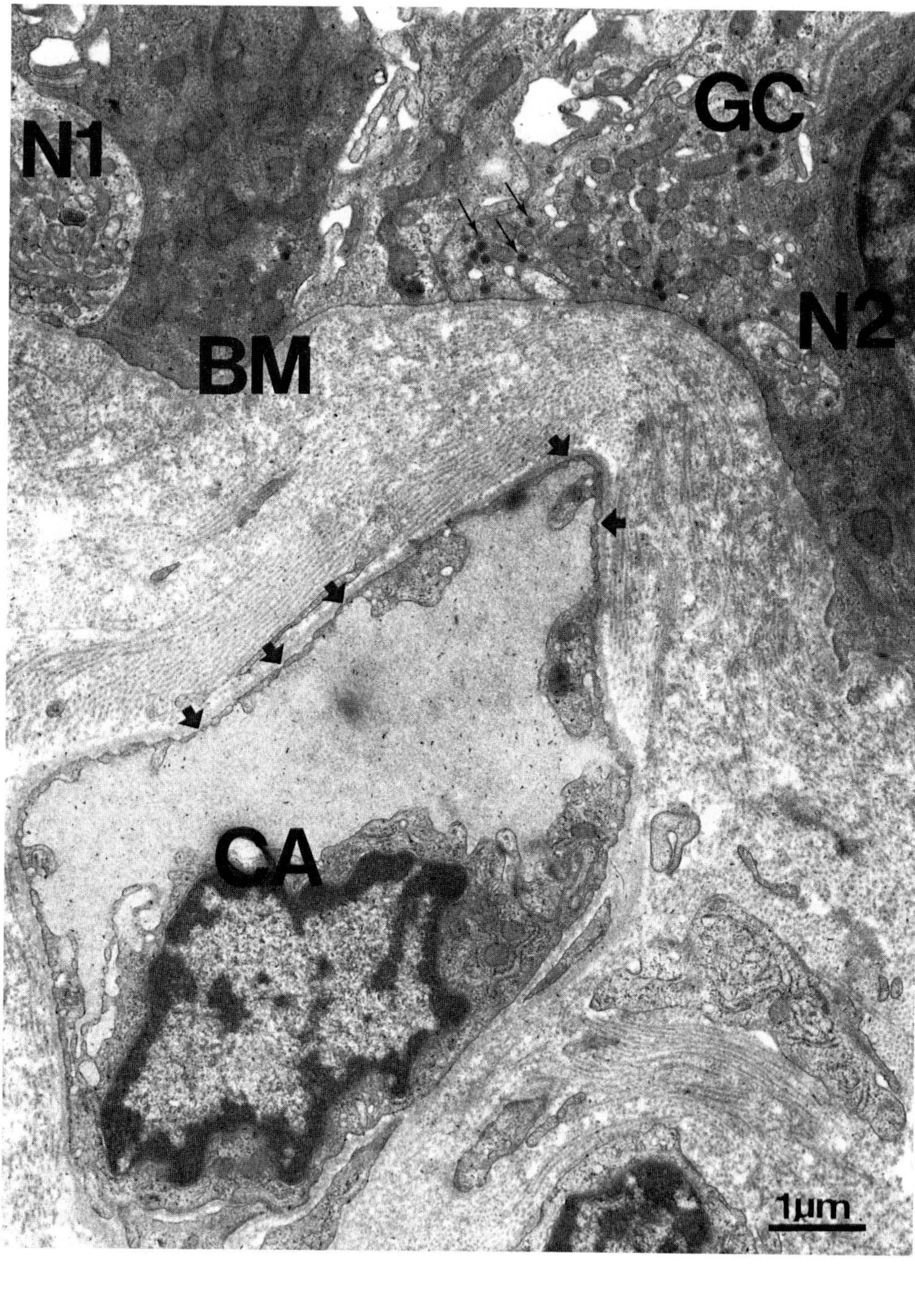
N1
GC
N2
BM
CA
1μm

2. Catecholamine-positive nerve fibers and nerve profiles of adrenergic type are found in smooth muscle (sparse), glands, and vessels from the lobar bronchi to the terminal bronchioli (Partanen et al., 1982b; Pack and Richardson, 1984; Laitinen et al., 1985b).
3. Nerve fibers containing VIP immunoreactivity are found in the smooth muscle, glands, vessels, and microganglia (Dey et al., 1981). VIP-like immunoreactivity is localized in large granules or vesicles of nerve profiles (Laitinen et al., 1985c).
4. The concentration and structure of the intraepithelial nerves and APUD cells are established (Laitinen, 1985; Partanen, M., Laitinen, A., Pelto-Huikko, M., Laitinen, L. A., and Hervonen, A., unpublished observations). The intraepithelial nerves seem to have two predominant locations: either close to the airway lumen or near the basement membrane.

Of the variety of neuropeptides, only VIP has been included in this review.

Acknowledgments

This work was written during a Visiting Professorship at the Department of Physiology, St. George's Hospital Medical School, London, U.K., which was supported by grants from the Sigrid Juselius Foundation (Finland) and the Wellcome Trust (U.K.). I would like to thank Dr. Annika Laitinen for her help in the preparation of this chapter.

Figure 5 An electron micrograph of normal human airway mucosa in the right upper lobe bronchus. A capillary (CA) containing numerous fenestrae (thick arrows) is seen in the lamina propria "extending" towards the epithelial basement membrane (BM). In the epithelium at this point a granule-containing (GC) APUD-like cell is seen containing many dense-cored neurosecretory vesicles (thin arrows). Two nerves (N1 and N2) containing mitochondria and vesicles are located intraepithelially close to the basement membrane. The nerve N2 comes in close contact with the granule-containing cell. Magnification ×13,000; bar = 1 μm.

Discussion

Wanner. Mast cells may be closely related to nerves; is there any evidence that they communicate with each other?

Laitinen. Mast cells are found adjacent to nerves in normal and asthmatic airways but the functional association is uncertain.

Burnstock. Both ATP from adrenergic nerves and substance P could theoretically degranulate mast cells.

Widdicombe. Furthermore, mast cell mediators may have effects on the nerve.

Burnstock. Time-lapse recordings of cocultures of explants of rat sympathetic ganglia and mast cells from rat peritoneum show that mast cells may become aligned to growing sympathetic nerve fibers and move slowly down their length.

Vanhoutte. In blood vessels, histamine could have profound prejunctional inhibition or the release of norepinephrine. This could explain "histaminergic neurogenic vasodilatation."

Lundberg. In skin, capsaicin pretreatment, which causes local sensory denervation, reduces the wheal and flare response to injected allergen in atopic individuals. This clearly indicates that sensory nerves are involved in the response to mast cell degranulation.

Nadel. High densities of mast cells are found near airway cholinergic ganglia and so might have effects on ganglionic neurotransmission.

Richardson. Few adrenergic nerve profiles have been demonstrated in human airway smooth muscle, but there does not appear to be any function.

Makhlouf. In the gut, adrenergic innervation projects to intrinsic plexuses and acts presynaptically.

Burnstock. A major problem is that the nerve varicosity profile cannot necessarily be equated with a neurotransmitter type. For example, many nerve profiles in the gut that are immunoreactive for peptides such as VIP, neuropeptide Y, or enkephalin contain a predominance of small agranular vesicles, typical of cholinergic nerves. The coexistence of variable proportions of two or more transmitters in the same profile also complicates interpretation. Furthermore, acetylcholinesterase staining identifies many nerves in addition to cholinergic nerves.

Richardson. In bird airways (especially duck), small agranular vesicles correlate with cholinergic excitation and large dense granules correlate with inhibition.

Skoogh. Are adrenergic nerves closely related to cholinergic ganglia in human airways?

Laitinen. Very few catecholamine positive fibers are seen within extrachondrial and subchondrial nerve plexuses, but several fluorescent fibers were identified in plexuses close to blood vessels. In some cholinergic ganglia fluorescent fibers were located around nerve cell bodies. Few adrenergic fibers innervate bronchial vessels.

Vanhoutte. A small number of adrenergic fibers does not imply weak sympathetic control. Thus, in portal-mesenteric veins, when partial denervation is performed, the remaining few nerve fibers take over full control of the vascular smooth muscle.

References

Barnes, P. J. (1984). The third nervous system in the lung: physiology and clinical perspectives. *Thorax* **39**:561-567.

Bartlett, D., Jeffery, D., Sant'Ambrogio, G., and Wise, J. C. M. (1976). Location of stretch receptors in the trachea and bronchi of the dog. *J. Physiol.* **258**: 419-420.

Baumgarten, H. G., Holstein, A. F., and Owman, C. (1970). Auerbach's plexus of mammals and man; electron-microscopic identification of three different types of neuronal processes in myentric ganglia of the large intestine from rhesus monkeys, guinea-pigs and man. *Z. Zell Mikrosk.* **106**:376-397.

Bensch, K. G., Gordon, G. B., and Miller, L. R. (1965). Studies on the bronchial counterpart of the Kultschitzky (Argentaffin) cell and innervation of bronchial glands. *J. Ultrastruct. Res.* **12**:668-686.

Bower, A. J., Parker, S., and Molony, V. (1978). An autoradiographic study of the afferent innervation of the trachea, syrinx and extrapulmonary primary bronchus of Gallus gallus domesticus. *J. Anat.* **126**:169-180.

Bradley, G. W., and Scheuermier, N. (1977). Tracheal stretch receptor properties in vitro. *J. Physiol.* **267**:48-49P.

Burnstock, G. (1972). Purinergic nerves. *Pharmacol. Rev.* **24**:509-581.

Cauna, N. (1966). Fine structure of the receptor organs and its probable functional significance. In *Tough, Heat and Pain.* Edited by A. V. S. de Reuck and J. Knight. London, Churchill, pp. 117-127.

Cauna, N., Hinderer, K. H., and Wentges, R. T. (1969). Sensory receptor organs of the human nasal respiratory mucosa. *Am. J. Anat.* **14**:295-300.

Daniel, E. E., Davis, C., Jones, T., and Kannan, M. S. (1980). Control of airway smooth muscle. In *Airway Reactivity. Mechanisms and Clinical Relevance.* Edited by F. E. Hargreave. Canada, Astra Pharmaceuticals Canada Ltd., pp. 80-109.

Das, R. M., Jeffery, P. K., and Widdicombe, J. G. (1978). The epithelial innervation of the lower respiratory tract of the cat. *J. Anat.* **126**:123-131.

Das, R. M., Jeffery, P. K., and Widdicombe, J. G. (1979). Experimental degeneration of intra-epithelial nerve fibres in cat airways. *J. Anat.* **128**:259-267.

de la Torre, J. C. (1980). An improved approach to histofluorescence using the SPG method for tissue monoamines. *J. Neurosci. Methods* **3**:1-5.

Dey, R. D., Shannon, W. A. Jr., and Said, S. (1981). Localisation of VIP-immunoreactive nerves in airways and pulmonary vessels of dogs, cats, and human subjects. *Cell Tissue Res.* **220**:231-238.

DiAugustine, R. P., and Sonstegard, K. S. (1984). Neuroendocrine-like (small granule) epithelial cells of the lung. *Environ. Health Perspectives* **55**:271-295.

Doidge, J. M., and Satchell, D. G. (1982). Adrenergic and non-adrenergic inhibitory nerves in mammalian airways. *J. Autonom. Nerv. Syst.* **5**:83-99.

Fillenz, M., and Woods, R. I. (1970). Sensory innervation of the airways. In *Breathing. Proceedings of the Hering Breuer Centenary Symposium.* Edited by R. Porter. London, Churchill, pp. 101-107.

Gaylor, J. B. (1934). The intrinsic nervous mechanism of the human lung. *Brain* **57**:143-160.

Gibbins, I. L., and Haller, C. J. (1979). Ultrastructural identification of non-adrenergic, noncholinergic nerves in the rat anococcygeus muscle. *Cell Tissue Res.* **200**:257-271.

Heino, M., Mönkare, S., Haahtela, T., and Laitinen, L. A. (1982). Electromicroscopic study of the airways in patients with farmer's lung. *Eur. J. Respir. Dis.* **63**:52-61.

Hökfelt, T. (1967). Ultrastructural studies on adrenergic nerve terminals in the albino rat iris after pharmacological and experimental treatment. *Acta Physiol. Scand.* **69**:125-126.

Hökfelt, T., and Jonsson, G. (1968). Studies on reaction and binding of monoamines after fixation and processing for electron microscopy with special reference to fixation with potassium permanganate. *Histochemie* **16**:45-67.

Hoyes, A. D., and Barber, P. (1981). Morphology and response to vagus nerve section of the intraepithelial axons of the rat trachea. A quantitative ultrastructural study. *J. Anat.* **132**:331-339.

Hung, K. S., Hertwech, M. S., Hardy, J. D., and Loosli, C. G. (1973). Ultrastructure of nerves and associated cells in bronchiolar epithelium of the mouse lung. *J. Ultrastruct. Res.* **43**:426-437.

Jabonero, V., and Sabadell, J. (1972). Die sensible Innervation der glatten Muskulatur der Luftwege. *Z. Mikrosk. Anat. Forsch.* **86**:213-243.

Jeffery, P. K. (1982). The innervation of the bronchial mucosa. In *Cellular Biology of the Lung.* Edited by C. Cuming and G. Bonsignore. New York, Plenum Press, pp. 1-25.

Jeffery, P. K., and Reid, L. (1973). Intra-epithelial nerves in normal rat airways: a quantitative electron microscopic study. *J. Anat.* **114**:35-45.

Johansson, O., and Lundberg, J. M. (1981). Ultrastructural localization of VIP-like immunoreactivity in large dense-core vesicles of 'cholinergic-type' nerve terminals in cat exocrine glands. *Neuroscience* **6**:847-862.

King, A. S., McLelland, J., Cook, R. D., King, D. A., and Walsh, C. (1974). The ultrastructure of afferent nerve endings in the avian lung. *Respir. Physiol.* **22**:21-40.

Krauhs, J. M. (1984). Morphology of presumptive slowly adapting receptors in dog trachea. *Anat. Rec.* **210**:73-85.

Lacey, M. (1978). Studies of pulmonary innervation in the rat using horse-radish peroxidase as a neuronal marker. *J. Physiol.* **277**:16-17P.

Laitinen, A. (1985). Ultrastructural organisation of intraepithelial nerves in the human airway tract. *Thorax* **40**:488-492.

Laitinen, A., Laitinen, L. A., Hervonen, A., and Partanen, M. (1982). Innervation of the human lower airway tract. *Eur. J. Respir. Dis.* **63** (Suppl. 124):83.

Laitinen, A., Laitinen, L. A., Heino, M., and Haahtela, T. (1985a). Intraepithelial nerves fibres in a normal subject and asthmatic patients. In *Progress in Respiration Research,* Vol. 19. Edited by H. Herzog. Basel, S. Karger, pp. 137-142.

Laitinen, A., Partanen, M., Hervonen, A., and Laitinen, L. A. (1985b). Electron microscopic study on the innervation of the human lower respiratory tract. Evidence of adrenergic nerves. *Eur. J. Respir. Dis.* **67**:209-215.

Laitinen, A., Partanen, M., Hervonen, A., Pelto-Huikko, M., and Laitinen, L. A. (1985c). VIP-like immunoreactive nerves in human respiratory tract. *Histochemistry* **82**:313-319.

Laitinen, L. A., Heino, M., Laitinen, A., Kava, T., and Haahtela, T. (1985d). Damage of the airway epithelium and bronchial reactivity in patients with asthma. *Am. Rev. Respir. Dis.* **131**:599-606.

Larsell, G., and Dow, R. S. (1933). The innervation of the human lung. *Am. J. Anat.* **52**:125-146.

Larsson, L. J. (1977). Ultrastructural localization of a new neuronal peptide (VIP). *Histochemistry* **54**:173-176.

Lauweryns, J. M., and Cocelaere, M. (1973). Intrapulmonary neuro-epithelial bodies: hypoxia sensitive neuro-(chemo) receptors. *Experientia* **29**:1384-1386.

Lauweryns, J. M., and Goddeeris, P. (1975). Neuroepithelial bodies in the human child and adult lung. *Am. Rev. Respir. Dis.* **111**:469-476.

Lauweryns, J. M., and Peuskens, J. C. (1972). Neuroepithelial bodies (neuroreceptor of secretory organs?) in human infant bronchial and bronchiolar epithelium. *Anat. Rec.* **172**:471-482.

Lauweryns, J. M., Peuskens, J. C., and Cokelaere, M. (1970). Argyrophil, fluorescent and granulated (peptide and amine-producing?) AFG cells in human infant bronchial epithelium: light and electron microscopic studies. *Life Sci.* **9**:1417-1429.

Lundberg, J. M., Hökfelt, T., Kewenter, J., Petersson, G., Ahlman, H., Towin, R., Dahlstrom, A., Nilsson, G., Terenius, L., Uvnas-Wallensten, K., and Said, S. I. (1979). Substance P-, VIP-, and enkephalin-like immunoreactivity in the human vagus nerve. *Gastroenterology* **77**:468-471.

Mann, S. P. (1971). The innervation of mammalian bronchial smooth muscle: the localisation of catecholamines and cholinesterases. *Histochem. J.* **3**:319-331.

McDonald, D. (1977). Structure-function relationships of chemoreceptive nerves in the carotid body. *Am. Rev. Respir. Dis.* **115**:193-207.

Nadel, J. A., and Barnes, P. J. (1984). Autonomic regulation of the airways. *Annu. Rev. Med.* **35**:451-467.

Orehek, J. (1981). Neurohumoral control of airway caliber. In *International Review of Physiology, Respiratory Physiology* III. Edited by J. G. Widdicombe. Baltimore, University Park Press, pp. 1-74.

Pack, R. J., and Richardson, P. S. (1984). The aminergic innervation of the human bronchus: a light and electron microscopic study. *J. Anat.* **138**:493-502.

Pack, R. J., Al-Ugaily, L. H., and Widdicombe, J. G. (1984). The innervation of the trachea and extrapulmonary bronchi of the mouse. *Cell Tissue Res.* **238**:61-68.

Partanen, M., Hervonen, A., Toivanen, M., Laitinen, A., and Laitinen, L. A. (1982a). The innervation of human lower respiratory tract as revealed by catecholamine histofluorescence and neuropeptide immunohistochemistry. In *International Conference on Bronchial Hyperreactivity. Conference Summary.* Oxford, Medicine Publishing Foundation, pp. 73-74.

Partanen, M., Laitinen, A., Hervonen, A., Toivanen, M., and Laitinen, L. A. (1982b). Catecholamine- and acetylcholinesterase-containing nerves in human lower respiratory tract. *Histochemistry* **76**:175-188.

Pearse, A. J. (1969). The cytochemistry and ultrastructure of polypeptide hormone-producing cells of the APUD series and the embryologic, physiologic and pathologic implications of the concept. *J. Histochem. Cytochem.* **17**:303-313.

Pearse, A. J. (1976). Neurotransmission and the APUD concept. In *Chromaffin, Enterochromaffin and Related Cells.* Edited by R. E. Coupland and T. Fujita. New York, Elsevier, pp. 147-154.

Pessacq, T. P. (1971). The innervation of the lung f newborn children. *Acta Anat.* **79**:93-101.

Reichlin, S. (1980). Peptides in neuroendocrine regulation. In *Peptides: Integrators of Cell and Tissue Function.* Edited by F. E. Bloom. New York, Raven Press, pp. 235-250.

Rhodin, J. A. G. (1966). The ciliated cell. Ultrastructure and function of the human tracheal mucosa. *Am. Rev. Respir. Dis.* **93**:1-15.

Richardson, J. B. (1979). Nerve supply to the lungs. *Am. Rev. Respir. Dis.* **119**: 785-802.

Richardson, J. B., and Beland, J. (1976). Noradrenergic inhibitory nervous system in human airways. *J. Appl. Physiol.* **41**:764-771.

Richardson, J. B., and Ferguson, C. C. (1979). Neuromusculator structure and function in the airways. *Fed. Proc.* **38**:202-208.

Richardson, K. C. (1966). Electron microscopic identification of autonomic nerve endings. *Nature* **210**:756.

Said, S. I., Giachetti, A., and Nicosia, S. (1980). VIP: possible functions as a neural peptide. In *Neural Peptides and Neuronal Communication.* Edited by E. Costa and M. Trabucchi. New York, Raven Press, pp. 75-82.

Said, S. I., Kitamura, S., Yoshida, T., Preskitt, J., and Holden, L. D. (1974). Humoral control of airways. *Ann. N.Y. Acad. Sci.* **221**:103-114.

Sant'Ambrogio, G. (1982). Information arising from the tracheobronchial tree of mammals. *Physiol. Rev.* **62**:531-569.

Sant'Ambrogio, G., Bartlett, D., and Mortola, J. (1977). Innervation of stretch receptors in the extrathoracic trachea. *Respir. Physiol.* **29**:93-99.

Simonsson, B. G., Svedmyr, M., Skoogh, B. E., Andersson, R., and Bergh, N. P. (1972). In vivo and in vitro studies on alpha-receptors in human airway. Potentiation with bacterial endotoxine. *Scand. J. Respir. Dis.* **53**:227-236.

Spencer, H., and Leof, D. (1964). The innervation of the human lung. *J. Anat.* **98**:599-609.

Tranzer, J. P., and Richards, J. G. (1976). Ultrastructural cytochemistry of biogenic amines in nervous tissue. Methodological improvements. *J. Histochem. Cytochem.* **24**:1178-1193.

Uddman, R., and Sundler, F. (1979). Vasoactive intestinal peptide nerves in human upper respiratory tract. *Otorhinolaryngology* **41**:221-226.

Von Düring, M. V., Andres, K. H., and Irvani, J. (1974). The fine structure of the pulmonary stretch receptor in the rat. *Z. Anat. Entwickl. Gesch.* **143**: 215-222.

Wharton, I., Polak, J. M., Probert, L., De Mey, J., McGregor, G. P., Bryant, M. G., and Bloom, S. K. (1981). Peptide-containing nerves in the ureter of the guinea-pig and cat. *Neuroscience* **6**:969-982.

Widdicombe, J. G. (1954). Receptors in the trachea and bronchi of the cat. *J. Physiol.* **123**:71-104.

Widdicombe, J. G. (1982). Pulmonary and respiratory tract receptors. *J. Exp. Biol.* **100**:41-57.

4

Adrenergic Regulation of Airway Function

PETER J. BARNES

The Cardiothoracic Institute
Brompton Hospital
London, United Kingdom

I. Introduction

Epinephrine has been used in the relief of airway obstruction since the beginning of the century, yet only recently has adrenergic control of human airways been studied in depth. This has been made possible by the development of precise assays for endogenous catecholamines, the use of radioligand binding assays to study adrenoceptors directly, and with the introduction of new adrenergic agents. Despite major advances in our understanding of adrenergic control, the role of adrenergic mechanisms in the pathogenesis of asthma and bronchial hyperresponsiveness remains controversial (Barnes, 1984, 1985; Nadel and Barnes, 1984).

Adrenergic control of airways concerns adrenergic innervation and circulating catecholamines (of which epinephrine is the most relevant), which act on β- and α-adrenergic receptors on the various target cells of the airway (Fig. 1).

II. Adrenergic Innervation

The sympathetic nerve supply to the lung originates from the upper six thoracic segments of spinal cord and postganglionic fibers synapse in the middle and in-

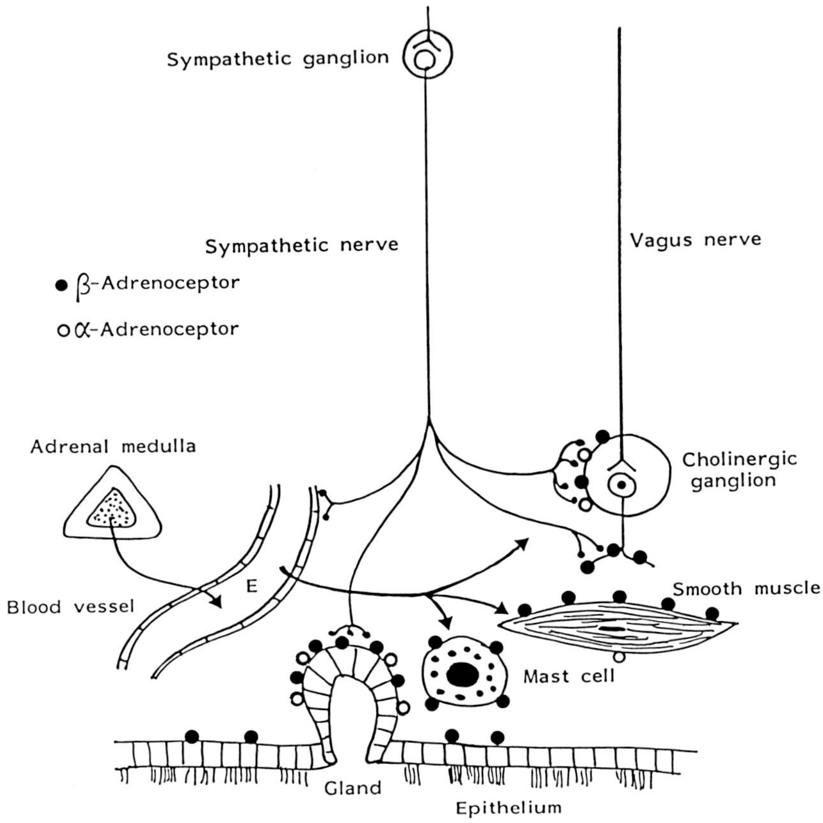

Figure 1 Adrenergic regulation of human airways. Sympathetic nerve and circulating epinephrine (E) are shown: these interact with β-receptors (●) and α-receptors (○) on target cells in the airway.

ferior cervical ganglia and the upper four thoracic ganglia. Postganglionic fibers run from these ganglia to the lung and enter at the hilum to intermingle with the cholinergic nerves, which form a dense plexus around airways and vessels (Richardson, 1979; Barnes, 1986a). The content of norepinephrine in human lung is rather low in comparison with other organs, such as heart and systemic vessels, indicating that few sympathetic nerves are likely to be present (Anton and Sayre, 1962). In contrast to the dense parasympathetic nerve supply to airways in all species, sympathetic innervation is generally sparse, but there is considerable variation between species (Richardson, 1979; Doidge and Satchell, 1982). Thus, in cat there is a rich sympathetic innervation (Silva and Ross,

1974), whereas in primates adrenergic innervation of airways is very sparse (El-Bermani, 1978). In human airways a sparse adrenergic innervation has been demonstrated by fluorescence histochemistry; adrenergic nerve fibers have been found in close association with submucosal glands (Partanen et al., 1982; Pack and Richardson, 1984) and bronchial vessels (Doidge and Satchell, 1982; Partanen et al., 1982), but very few, if any, adrenergic fibers have been demonstrated in smooth muscle of intrapulmonary airways (Doidge and Satchell, 1982; Partanen et al., 1982; Richardson and Beland, 1976). An immunocytochemical method using an antibody to dopamine β-hydroxylase, which is specific for adrenergic nerves, has recently confirmed sympathetic innervation of human submucosal glands and bronchial vessels, and the paucity of fibers in airway smooth muscle (Sheppard et al., 1983). Ultrastructural studies have confirmed the presence of adrenergic nerve profiles, which are characterized by small dense core granules in human airways, but they are greatly outnumbered by the cholinergic nerve type of profile (Laitinen et al., 1985). Adrenergic profiles are found in relation to glands (Pack and Richardson, 1982; Meyrick and Reid, 1970) and airway ganglia (Richardson and Ferguson, 1979), but very few are found in relation to airway smooth muscle (Laitinen et al., 1985).

Functional studies that have used electrical field stimulation to activate nerves selectively have demonstrated neurally mediated relaxation, which is blocked by β-antagonists, in isolated trachea but not bronchus of guinea pig (Doidge and Satchell, 1982; Grundstrom et al., 1981). This is consistent with the demonstration of adrenergic nerve fibers in tracheal but not bronchial smooth muscle of this species (O'Donnell et al., 1978). Cocaine, which blocks neuronal reuptake of norepinephrine, increases the sensitivity of guinea pig trachea but not lung strips to exogenous norepinephrine, again suggesting the presence of functional adrenergic nerves in smooth muscle of trachea but not intrapulmonary airways in this species (Zaagsma et al., 1983). Field stimulation in human airway obtained post mortem or at surgery (usually for carcinoma) causes a cholinergic contraction, followed by relaxation that is inhibited by tetrodotoxin but unaffected by propranolol (Davis et al., 1982; Taylor et al., 1984; Palmer et al., 1986a). This suggests that there is no functional sympathetic innervation of human airway smooth muscle, although there is a potent nonadrenergic inhibitory neural mechanism. Cocaine has no effect on norepinephrine responses in either human bronchi or lung strips, again suggesting a lack of direct sympathetic innervation to human airway smooth muscle (Zaagsma et al., 1983).

Although there appears to be no direct functional sympathetic innervation of human airway smooth muscle, it is possible that adrenergic nerves may influence bronchomotor tone indirectly. In dogs electrical stimulation of thoracic sympathetic nerves causes bronchodilatation, which is abolished by β-antagonists and unaffected by adrenalectomy. However, the magnitude of bronchodilatation is dependent on the degree of preexisting vagal tone (Cabezas et al., 1971). This suggests that sympathetic nerves may have a modulatory influence on cholinergic neurotransmission. Stimulation of sympathetic outflow to the lungs in guinea pigs produces bronchodilation (Ainsworth et al., 1981), and yet there is no evidence for direct sympathetic nerve supply of intrapulmonary airways, as discussed over (O'Donnell et al., 1978). This suggests either interaction with cholinergic tone, or overflow of norepinephrine from the adrenergic nerves that supply other structures, such as pulmonary vessels. Thus, sympathetic nerves might influence bronchomotor tone indirectly. Tyramine, which releases norepinephrine from sympathetic nerves, has profound cardiovascular effects when infused into normal individuals (Scriven et al., 1983), but has no bronchodilator effect in mild asthmatic subjects who readily bronchodilate with an infused β-agonist (Ind et al., 1983b). This suggests that sympathetic nerves do not influence resting bronchomotor tone in humans, but this does not preclude the possibility that sympathetic nerves may have an inhibitory effect when bronchomotor tone is increased. Indeed, the demonstration of adrenergic nerves within human airway ganglia suggests that sympathetic nerves could exert a modulatory effect on cholinergic ganglionic neurotransmission. Norepinephrine inhibits the firing of airway ganglion cells in cat and ferret via α-adrenoceptors (Baker et al., 1983), suggesting that such modulation of cholinergic neurotransmission is possible. In a group of patients who had upper dorsal sympathectomy for extensive sweating, a small decrease in lung volumes compared with preoperative assessment was noted. This change might be explained by a reduction in sympathetic bronchodilator tone or an impairment in diaphragmatic function because of concomitant phrenic nerve damage (Molho et al., 1977).

β-Adrenoceptor antagonists have no effect on resting bronchomotor tone in normal individuals, indicating an absence of any tonic sympathetic bronchodilator tone (Zaid and Beall, 1966; Tattersfield et al., 1973; Richardson and Sterling, 1969). However, patients with asthma and chronic obstructive pulmonary disease (COPD) may suffer profound bronchoconstriction with β-blockers, suggesting an increased adrenergic drive to the airways (Richardson and Sterling, 1969; McNeil and Ingram, 1966; van Herwaarden, 1983).

The possible role of sympathetic nerves in control of bronchial vessels has not been studied. The reduced vascularity of dog trachea after α-agonists suggests that sympathetic nerves may reduce blood flow (Laitinen et al., 1987). In animals, stimulation of sympathetic nerves stimulates secretion from submucosal glands, an effect which is almost abolished by α-adrenoceptor blockade (Borson et al., 1980, Peatfield and Richardson, 1982). Electrical field stimulation of resected human bronchi in Ussing chambers has demonstrated cholinergic nerve stimulation, but no detectable sympathetic neural effect (Baker et al., 1985), although α- and β-agonists stimulate mucus secretion in similar preparations (Phipps et al., 1982). The lack of apparent sympathetic effects may reflect the large variability in human airway responses. β-Antagonists have no significant effect on mucociliary clearance in humans, suggesting an absence of sympathetic tonic secretion, at least via β-receptors (Pavia et al., 1980).

III. Endogenous Catecholamines

Human airway smooth muscle is potently relaxed by β-agonists in vitro (Zaagsma et al., 1983; Davis et al., 1982; Goldie et al., 1982) and the absence of direct functional adrenergic innervation suggests that circulating catecholamines might be important in regulating human airway tone. Although epinephrine has been used in the treatment of asthma since 1900, it has only relatively recently been possible to determine accurately plasma concentrations of endogenous catecholamines and therefore to investigate the role of endogenous epinephrine in controlling airway tone (Barnes, 1983, 1986b). Norepinephrine in plasma is derived almost entirely from overspill of sympathetic nerve activity (Brown et al., 1981). Infusions of norepinephrine in normal subjects have no significant effects on cardiovascular (Silverberg et al., 1978) or airway function (Berkin et al., 1985; Larsson et al., 1986) at concentrations within the physiological range, suggesting that circulating norepinephrine probably does not function as a hormone in humans. By contrast, epinephrine has potent metabolic effects within its physiological range (FitzGerald et al., 1980) and is a potent bronchodilator in normal (Warren and Dalton, 1983) and asthmatic subjects (Barnes et al., 1982b). Epinephrine can protect against both histamine- and methacholine-induced bronchoconstriction in humans (Warren et al., 1984; Sands et al., 1985). Thus, epinephrine, secreted by the adrenal medulla, functions as a circulating hormone, whereas norepinephrine is a neurotransmitter.

Studies in animals have shown that β-blockers potentiate the bronchoconstrictor response to intravenous histamine (Drazen, 1978; Leff et al., 1982) and to antigen in sensitized animals (Piper et al., 1967). This can probably be explained by blocking the effects of circulating catecholamines since similar results are produced by surgical adrenalectomy (Leff et al., 1982; Collier and James, 1967). These animal studies suggest that circulating epinephrine has a protective effect against bronchoconstrictor influences.

A. Beta-Blockers and Airway Function

While β-blockers, such as propranolol, have no effect on bronchomotor tone or bronchial responsiveness in normal subjects (Zaid and Beall, 1966; Tattersfield et al., 1973; Richardson and Sterling, 1969), in asthmatic subjects these drugs may precipitate bronchoconstriction (McNeill, 1964; McNeill and Ingram, 1966;

Richardson and Sterling, 1969; van Herwarden, 1983) and increase bronchial responsiveness to methacholine in atopic subjects (Townley et al., 1976). It has been suggested that the mechanism of bronchoconstriction after propranolol is unrelated to β-blockade, since in animals (D)-propranolol, which has no significant β-blocking effect, is as potent as (L)-propranolol in causing bronchoconstriction. This implies that some nonspecific property may be responsible (Maclagan and Ney, 1979; Ney, 1983). In humans, however, since in asthmatic patients infusion of (D)-propranolol has little effect on airway function, whereas (DL)-propranolol causes bronchoconstriction in proportion to the degree of β-blockade (Ind et al., 1984). Furthermore, other β-blockers, such as pindolol and timolol, which do not share the local anesthetic properties of propranolol, also cause bronchospasm in asthmatic and COPD patients (Ruffin et al., 1979; van Herwarden, 1983). This suggests that the airways in asthmatics may be under increased adrenergic drive and, in the absence of functional sympathetic nerves, this might be provided by circulating epinephrine.

B. Catecholamines in Asthma

Plasma catecholamine levels are no higher in stable asthmatic subjects at rest than in age-matched normal subjects, nor is there any relationship between plasma catecholamine concentration and severity of bronchoconstriction, as judged by percent predicted lung function (Barnes et al., 1982c). Even in those subjects who develop bronchoconstrictor responses to infused propranolol, plasma concentrations of epinephrine are within the normal range (Ind et al., 1984). This suggests that the normal circulating concentrations of epinephrine may be sufficient to protect asthmatic patients against bronchoconstrictor influences. This is further supported by the close coincidence between circulating epinephrine concentrations and diurnal variation in airway function, with lowest values occurring at 4 a.m. (Barnes et al., 1980b). How epinephrine can exert this protective effect at the low concentrations found in plasma (< 0.5 nmol/l) is difficult to understand, since these concentrations of epinephrine could exert little effect on airway smooth muscle itself. It is possible that epinephrine may influence airway mast cells, since in vitro epinephrine has inhibitory effects against IgE-induced histamine release from human lung fragments (Assem and Schild, 1969; Butchers et al., 1980). Furthermore, cromolyn sodium prevents the bronchoconstriction induced by inhaled propranolol in asthmatic subjects (Koeter et al., 1982), although this could be unrelated to its mast cell stabilizing properties. Measurement of histamine (Ind et al., 1985a) and neutrophil chemotactic activity (Ind et al., 1984) in plasma during propranolol-induced bronchoconstriction has not provided any direct evidence for increased mediator release in vivo, although these techniques may not be sufficiently sensitive to detect airway mediator release. Another possibility is that epinephrine may be exerting an inhibitory effect on airway ganglia, and such an effect may be more likely if cholinergic neurotransmission were increased (Skoogh, 1983). Thus, β-blockers could enhance cholinergic tone, which would have a greater effect in asthmatic subjects because of the enhanced sensitivity of airway smooth muscle to acetylcholine. This idea is supported by the fact that anticholinergic drugs prevent and reverse β-blocker-induced bronchoconstriction (Grieco and Pierson, 1971; Ind et al., 1986).

There is some evidence that the secretion of epinephrine may be abnormal in asthma, and this would tend to exacerbate any bronchoconstrictor influences such as inflammatory mediators or vagal tone. Early studies in which circulating catecholamines and their metabolites were measured in asthmatic subjects suggested that their excretion was reduced in asthma and did not increase normally during stresses such as mental arithmetic (Mathé and Knapp, 1969) or during acute exacerbations (Morris et al., 1972). Exercise causes a rise in circulating catecholamine levels in normal subjects, but in asthmatics who perform an exercise test sufficient to induce bronchoconstriction the expected rise in norepinephrine is blunted and epinephrine concentrations fail to rise (compared with a threefold rise in normal subjects who perform the same task) (Barnes et al., 1981a; Warren et al., 1982). Similarly, the rise in plasma cyclic AMP, which is an indirect measurement of β-receptor stimulation by endogenous epinephrine (FitzGerald et al., 1980), is blunted during exercise in asthmatics compared with normal subjects (Barnes et al., 1981a; Hartley et al., 1981). However, if asthmatics perform more vigorous exercise they increase circulating catecholamines to the concentrations seen in normal subjects (Larsson et al., 1982), suggesting that there may be a defect in initiating epinephrine secretion in asthma. This would fit in with the clinical observation that asthmatics are able to "run through" their asthma, and may be prevented by a "warm-up" run, presumably as catecholamines become mobilized (Schnall and Landau, 1980). No rise in circulating catecholamine levels occurs during bronchoconstriction induced by hyperventilation (Barnes et al., 1981a), antigen (Ind et al., 1983a; Larsson et al., 1985), methacholine (Sands et al., 1985), or infused propranolol (Ind et al., 1984).

Most surprisingly, even in acute severe asthma of sufficient severity to require hospitalization, there is no elevation of plasma epinephrine levels, although plasma norepinephrine levels are elevated, probably reflecting increased respiratory muscle activity (Ind et al., 1985b). The failure of epinephrine to rise in response to bronchoconstriction may be explained by impaired secretion from the adrenal medulla, or increased clearance from the circulation. Clearance of epinephrine is no greater in asthmatic subjects than in normal controls, however, suggesting that impaired secretion from the adrenal medulla is responsible. Under some circumstances asthmatic subjects are able to secrete epinephrine normally, since both insulin-induced hypoglycemia and histamine infusion produce a normal increase in plasma epinephrine in both stable asthmatics (Ind et al., 1983a) and during recovery from acute asthma (Clarke et al., 1985).

Thus, the normally low circulating concentrations of endogenous epinephrine may provide a defense against bronchoconstrictor influences, such as inflammatory mediators and vagal reflexes, but under some circumstances plasma epinephrine levels fail to rise. This unexplained defect in catecholamine response may contribute to bronchial hyperresponsiveness. However, this is unlikely to be a primary defect in asthma, since neither adrenalectomy nor prolonged β-blockade converts normal subjects to asthmatic patients.

IV. Beta Adrenoceptors

A. Localization and Function

β-Agonists affect several aspects of lung function (Table 1) (Barnes et al., 1984). Radioligand binding studies have demonstrated a high density of β-receptors in lung of many species, including humans (Rugg et al., 1978; Barnes et al., 1980c; Engel, 1981). More recent autoradiographic techniques have revealed that β-receptors are localized to many different cell types within lung (Barnes et al., 1982a; Carstairs et al., 1984). β-Receptors are found in smooth muscle of all airways from trachea to terminal bronchioles. This is not surprising, since β-agonists are potent relaxants of human bronchi, bronchioles, and peripheral lung strips in vitro (Zaagsma et al., 1983; Davis et al., 1982; Goldie et al., 1982). The density of β-receptors increases with decreasing size of airway in animals and humans (Barnes and Basbaum, 1983; Carstairs et al., 1985).

Table 1 Airway Adrenoceptor Function

Cell type	Beta-receptor	Alpha-receptor
Smooth muscle	Relax	Contract
Mast cell	Inhibit secretion	Enhance secretion
Submucosal gland	Increase secretion (mucous)	Increase secretion (serous)
Epithelium	Increase ion transport	?
Cholinergic nerves	Inhibit	Inhibit
Clara cell	Increase secretion	?
Type 2 pneumocyte	Increase secretion	No effect
Bronchial vessels	Dilate Reduce permeability	Constrict

β-Agonists stimulate secretion of airway mucus in several species, but the effects of β-agonists in human airways have been variable. In one study β-agonists had a stimulatory effect (Phipps et al., 1982), whereas in another there was no significant effect on human bronchi in vitro (Shelhamer et al., 1980a). In animals β-agonists result in a more viscous secretion (Leikhauf et al., 1984), probably because of selective stimulation of mucous rather than serous cells of submucosal glands. Autoradiographic studies confirm a high density of β-receptors in airway glands, with greater labeling of mucous cells (Barnes and Basbaum, 1983). In addition, β-agonists stimulate chloride ion transport, and therefore water secretion, across human airway epithelium in vitro (Knowles et al., 1984) and a very high density of β-receptors is found on epithelial cells of all airways (Carstairs et al., 1984). Thus, β-agonists may increase mucus and water secretion into airways, which should result in increased mucociliary clearance, thereby reversing the slowing of clearance that occurs in asthma (Pavia et al., 1980). The effect of β-agonists on mucociliary clearance in vivo has been variable; some studies report increased clearance in normal and asthmatic subjects whereas others have shown little effect. A greater effect is apparent when clearance is already impaired (as in asthma). Recent studies in animal airways have demonstrated that isoprotenerol is a more effective relaxant in the presence of intact epithelial cells, suggesting that β-agonists may release an (unidentified) relaxant factor from epithelial cells (Flavahan et al., 1985; Barnes et al., 1985; Goldie et al., 1986).

Clara cells, which may secrete a lipid into the airway and are present in human bronchiolar epithelium, are also stimulated by β-agonists (Massaro et al., 1981). Their function is not certain, but their secretion may function as an "antiglue," preventing closure of small airways with deflation. Type 2 pneumocytes, which secrete surfactant, are also stimulated by β-agonists (Dobbs and Mason, 1979) and surfactant may enter airways and play an important role in their stabilization during deflation.

β-Agonists inhibit antigen-induced release of mast cell mediators from human lung fragments and isolated lung mast cells in vitro (Assem and Schild, 1969; Orange et al., 1971; Butchers et al., 1980; Peters et al., 1982), indicating inhibitory β-receptors on human lung mast cells. Whether this contributes to the bronchodilator effect of β-agonists in asthma is not certain, however. In vivo the infusion of epinephrine in asthmatic subjects lowers plasma histamine concentrations (Barnes et al., 1980b), and a β-agonist prevents the rise in plasma histamine after antigen challenge (Howarth et al., 1985), suggesting that therapeutic concentrations of β-agonists may inhibit mast cell mediator release.

Histamine-induced microvascular leakiness in airways of guinea-pigs is reduced by prior treatment with a β-agonist, suggesting that β-receptors also may regulate bronchial microvascular permeability (Persson et al., 1982). There is no evidence that β-agonists reverse airway edema, although they may be capable of preventing its development.

In animals, β-agonists also modulate cholinergic neurotransmission, either at the level of cholinergic ganglia or at postsynaptic nerve terminals (Skoogh, 1983; Vermiere and Vanhoutte, 1979). This may be an important site of action for β-agonists in asthma, although there is no direct proof in human airways. The mechanism by which β-blockers produce bronchoconstriction is still uncertain, but it is possible that endogenous epinephrine exerts a tonic braking effect on cholinergic neurotransmission, as discussed above. When this is removed by a β-blocker, there is an increase in acetylcholine released in the vicinity of airway smooth muscle cells. In normal individuals this would have no detectable effect on airway function, but in asthmatic patients who are hyperresponsive to acetylcholine this would cause bronchoconstriction. Similarly, in chronic bronchitic patients the effect of increased acetylcholine release would be greater because of the geometric effect of an already narrowed airway.

β-Agonists, therefore, have several possible beneficial actions on airway obstruction. In addition to relaxing airway smooth muscle, they also reduce release of mediators from mast cells, reduce cholinergic tone, possibly reduce plasma extravasation and mucosal edema, and increase clearance of airway mucus.

B. Beta-Receptor Subtypes

Although originally β-receptors of airway smooth muscle were classified as β-$_2$ receptors (Lands et al., 1967), later studies showed that, in several species, relaxation of tracheal smooth muscle was intermediate between a β-$_1$- and β-$_2$-mediated response (Furchgott et al., 1975); this suggested the presence of β-$_1$ in addition to β-$_2$ receptors. Using direct receptor binding techniques and selective β-antagonists the coexistence of β-$_1$ and β-$_2$ receptors was confirmed in animal and human lung (Rugg et al., 1978; Engel, 1981), with a ratio of β-$_1$ to β-$_2$ receptors of approximately 1:3 in human lung. In canine tracheal smooth muscle, while β-$_2$ receptors predominate, 20% of receptors are of the β-$_1$ subtype (Barnes et al., 1983c). Parallel functional studies of the same tissue in vitro show that relaxation to exogenous β-agonists is mediated by β-$_2$ receptors, whereas relaxation to sympathetic nerve stimulation is mediated by β-$_1$ receptors. These findings are consistent with the hypothesis that β-$_1$ receptors are regulated by sympathetic nerves ("innervated" β-receptors), whereas β-$_2$ receptors are regulated by circulating epinephrine ("hormonal" β-receptors) (Ariens and Simonis, 1983).

In human airway smooth muscle, which lacks significant sympathetic innervation, no β-$_1$ receptor-mediated effects would be expected. This has been confirmed in functional studies in vitro, in which relaxation of central and peripheral airways is mediated only by β-$_2$ receptors (Zaagsma et al., 1983; Goldie et al., 1984). Similarly, in vivo prenalterol, a β-$_1$-selective agonist, has no bronchodilator effect in asthmatic subjects, despite significant cardiac effects (Lofdahl and Svedmyr, 1982), and isoproterenol, which stimulates β-$_1$ and β-$_2$ receptors, gives no additional bronchodilator effect compared with a selective β-2 agonist (Barnes and Pride, 1983). Recent autoradiographic studies of human lung have confirmed that the β-receptors of human airway smooth muscle from bronchi to terminal bronchioles are entirely of the β-2 receptor subtype (Carstairs et al., 1985).

Human submucosal glands, which receive a sparse sympathetic nerve supply, have a small population (10%) of β-1 receptors determined by autoradiography (Carstairs et al., 1985), and functional studies show that mucus secretion is probably mediated by β-1 and β-2 receptors (Phipps et al., 1982). Epithelial β-receptors, which are not adrenergically innervated, are entirely of the β-2 subtype. Similarly, mast cells, which are not innervated, have only β-2 receptors from functional studies (Butchers et al., 1980). Remarkably, autoradiographic studies have shown that >90% of all β-receptors in lung are localized to alveolar walls (Barnes et al., 1982a; Carstairs et al., 1984). Type 2 pneumocytes, which have functional β-receptors, make up only 7% of the alveolar wall, so that alveolar β-receptors must also be located on capillary endothelial cells and/or type 1 pneumocytes. Approximately one-third of these alveolar receptors are of the β-1 subtype (Carstairs et al., 1985), which goes against the notion that β-receptors are always "neuronal." The functional significance of these alveolar β-receptors has not yet been established.

C. Beta-Receptor Function in Asthma

Because β-agonists reverse the bronchospasm in asthmatic airways, it was logical to suggest that there might be a defect in β-receptor function underlying asthma and bronchial hyperresponsiveness (Szentivanyi, 1968). A fundamental defect in β-receptor function in asthma seems unlikely, since chronic blockade of β-receptors does not produce asthma or bronchial hyperresponsiveness in normal individuals. However, there is still debate about whether there may be an impairment in β-receptor function in asthma secondary to the disease. A defect in β-receptors would not only apply to airway smooth muscle (tipping the balance in favor of cholinergic and possibly α-adrenergic constriction), but may also increase mast cell mediator release, increase the tendency to develop bronchial wall edema, and increase cholinergic tone.

Early studies showed that cardiovascular, metabolic, and leukocyte responses to β-agonists were impaired, and the density of β-receptors reduced in circulating leukocytes in asthmatic patients when compared with normal controls. However, similar changes could be demonstrated in normal and asthmatic subjects as a result of treatment with β-agonists, suggesting that the defect in β-receptor function may be explained by tolerance or subsensitivity resulting from prior therapy with β-agonists (see Barnes et al., 1984 for review). Studies of β-receptor function in untreated asthmatics are conflicting. Some studies show no significant differences compared with normal subjects (Galant et al., 1980; Tashkin et al., 1982) whereas others have described impaired cardiovascular or metabolic responses to β-agonists (Shelhamer et al., 1980b) or reduced β-receptor density on peripheral leukocytes (Brooks et al., 1979). The magnitude of these changes is small compared with the changes secondary to β-agonist therapy and, although these changes are too small to have clinical relevance, they are not easily explained. It was assumed that they may be secondary to elevated circulating epinephrine concentrations in asthma, but no such elevations have been reported, even in severe asthma, and the changes in epinephrine that could occur within the physiological range would, in any case, be insufficient to account for significant receptor down-regulation. It has been suggested that reduced β-receptor function might be explained by the presence of autoantibodies to β-2 receptors, which have been detected in the serum of some asthmatics (Venter et al., 1980), but this seems unlikely since these antibodies have been detected in only a small proportion of asthmatic patients and also occur in normal subjects. A reduction in leukocyte β-receptor density and responses to isoproterenol has been detected in asthmatic patients after antigen challenge, suggesting that any defect in β-receptors might be secondary to the disease (Meurs et al., 1982), possibly as a result of release of inflammatory mediators.

Studies of cardiovascular, metabolic, and leukocyte β-receptors may not reflect an abnormality of β-receptors in the airways, however. Because of methodologic problems, however, it has been difficult to determine whether airway β-receptor function is impaired in asthma. In asthmatics who develop nocturnal wheezing there is no impairment in airway responsiveness to either inhaled or infused epinephrine at night when bronchoconstriction is maximal, providing no evidence that reduced airway β-receptor function contributes to exacerbation of asthma at night (Barnes et al., 1982b). No significant difference in bronchodilator dose-responses to an inhaled β-agonist is found in mild asthmatics (Tattersfield et al., 1983), but more severe asthmatics appear to be less sensitive to β-agonists. The reduction in response is related to the severity of asthma, as judged by baseline lung function (Barnes and Pride, 1983). This could be explained by functional antagonism due to greater initial bronchoconstriction, rather than a defect in β-receptor function per se. In guinea pig airways in vitro the potency of isoproterenol decreases as the degree of initial contraction of airway smooth muscle is increased (Karlsson and Persson, 1981), and similar results may apply to human airways. Another reason for the apparent impairment in airway β-adrenergic responses may be that the dose of inhaled β-agonist delivered to the airway is less in the presence of preexisting airway obstruction (Dolovich et al., 1976). Some of the difficulties encountered in vivo may be overcome by studying β-receptors in isolated airways, but asthmatic airways are only rarely available. In three asthmatics who died during an attack, an apparent reduction in isoproterenol responsiveness was found (Paterson et al., 1982), although in another similar study no change in β-receptor responsiveness could be detected (Svedmyr et al., 1976). It may be difficult to interpret responses in airway tissue obtained at postmortem from patients who had been very ill and exposed to a variety of drugs.

Because airway β-receptor function has been difficult to study in asthma, various animal models have been used, although unfortunately none closely mimics human disease. In *Ascaris*-sensitive dogs airway smooth muscle cyclic AMP content is reduced compared with nonallergic controls, although the cyclic AMP response to isoproterenol is not impaired, which argues against a defect in β-receptor function (Rinard et al., 1979). In the Basenji greyhound, a crossbreed with bronchial hyperresponsiveness, impaired leukocyte β-receptor function has been demonstrated (Peters et al., 1981). In a guinea pig model of asthma, while there is a 20% reduction in pulmonary β-receptor density, there is no change in β-agonist-induced adenylate cyclase activation, suggesting no significant functional defect (Barnes et al., 1980a). However, since airway β-receptors, it would be difficult to detect changes in β-receptor function in the airways using these methods. Products of inflammation, such as oxygen radicals, may also impair airway β-receptor function (Engels et al., 1985), and the inflammatory phospholipid mediator platelet-activating factor reduces β-receptor density (Braquet et al., 1985). Thus, it is possible that some impairment in airway β-receptor response may occur as a result of the inflammatory reaction in asthma.

The question of whether β-receptor function is impaired in asthma has not yet been resolved, but such a defect is likely to be of little clinical significance, since asthmatic patients bronchodilate so readily to β-agonists. The apparent failure of asthmatics to respond to β-agonists during acute exacerbations might be explained by luminal plugging (with mucus and extravasated plasma) or bronchial edema. In one such patient who failed to respond to β-agonists and subsequently died, the airways responded normally to β-agonists in vitro (Svedmyr et al., 1976).

V. Alpha-Adrenoceptors

A. Localization and Function

There are relatively few α-adrenoceptors in lung (Barnes et al., 1979) and their role in regulation of airway function is disputed. α-Receptors, which mediate contraction of airway smooth muscle, have been demonstrated in many species, including humans (Simonsson et al., 1972; Kneussl and Richardson, 1978), although α-adrenergic responses may only be demonstrated under certain conditions. No α-adrenergic contraction can be demonstrated in canine airways in vitro, even in the presence of β-adrenergic blockade. However, with pretreatment with histamine or serotonin, a marked contractile response to α-agonists or sympathetic nerve stimulation is found (Simonsson et al., 1972; Barnes et al., 1983e), suggesting that these mediators have enhanced α-adrenergic responsiveness. This increased α-adrenergic response is not due to any change in either α-receptor density or affinity and is therefore likely to be due to some postreceptor mechanism, possibly involving opening of voltage-dependent calcium channels (Barnes et al., 1983e). Similar activation of canine tracheal α-adrenergic responses has also been demonstrated in vivo (Barnes et al., 1983e; Brown et al., 1983). In human airways, although no α-adrenergic contraction is found in normal airways, when airways are diseased (chronic bronchitis, bronchopneumonia) or are exposed to endotoxin, α-adrenergic contractile responses appear (Simonsson et al., 1972; Kneussl and Richardson, 1978), suggesting that disease may activate α-adrenergic responses. Human peripheral lung strips contract with norepinephrine, suggesting that small airways might have α-receptors (Black et al., 1981), although the contractile response is more likely to be due to α-receptors on other contractile elements such as pulmonary vessels or contractile interstitial (Kapanci) cells. Autoradiographic mapping of pulmonary α-receptors in ferret lung has demonstrated few α-receptors in large airways, but a high density in small bronchioles (Barnes et al., 1983a,b).

α-Agonists also stimulate secretion from submucosal glands of several species, including humans (Phipps et al., 1982; Shelhamer et al., 1980a). In animals, direct micropipette sampling of secretions from these glands shows that α-agonists produce a watery secretion (Leikhauf et al., 1984), probably explained by selective stimulation of serous cells. Autoradiographic studies have confirmed that α-receptors are localized to serous rather than mucous cells of submucosal glands (Barnes and Basbaum, 1983). It is likely that these α-receptors are activated by the adrenergic nerves that supply submucosal glands.

α-Agonists facilitate histamine release from human lung fragments in vitro, suggesting the presence of α-receptors on lung mast cells (Kaliner et al., 1972). In a pure preparation of well-differentiated canine mastocytoma cells, however, there is no evidence for α-receptors either by direct receptor binding or by functional studies (Phillips et al., 1985). While pulmonary vessels have a high density of α-receptors, the role of α-receptors in the bronchial circulation is not yet certain. It is possible that sympathetic control of bronchial blood flow in α-receptors may play a role in the conditioning of inspired air and this may be relevant to the development of exercise-induced asthma. α-Receptors may also be present in airway ganglia, since norepinephrine inhibits firing of neurons in airway ganglia via α-receptors (Baker et al., 1982) and presynaptic α-2 receptors may inhibit acetylcholine release from cholinergic nerve endings (Grundstrom et al., 1981b).

B. Alpha-Receptor Subtypes

α-Receptors, similarly to β-receptors, may be classified into subtypes, depending on the selectivity of specific antagonists. α_1-Receptors are the classic α-receptors that are postsynaptic, whereas α_2-receptors are presynaptic and inhibit the release of norepinephrine from synaptic nerve terminals. More recently, postsynaptic α_2-receptors have also been recognized. In canine trachea the contractile response to both exogenous norepinephrine and sympathetic nerve stimulation is mediated entirely by α_2-receptors, and direct binding studies have demonstrated the presence of α_2-receptors, with very few α_1-receptors (Barnes et al., 1983f). Similar results have been obtained in dogs in vivo (Brown et al., 1983). Whether this is true in human airways has not yet been determined, however.

C. Alpha-Receptor Function in Asthma

The demonstration that α-adrenergic responses may be activated by inflammatory mediators in vitro supports the idea that there may be enhanced α-adrenergic responses in asthma (Szentivanyi, 1968). Furthermore, in a guinea-pig model of asthma there is a marked increase in pulmonary α_1-receptor density in "asthmatic" animals (Barnes et al., 1980a), although whether this is present in airway smooth muscle is not certain. Similarly, in humans the density of α-receptors is much higher in lung taken from patients with airway obstruction than from normal lung (Barnes et al., 1980c). Asthmatic subjects bronchoconstrict with inhaled α-agonists (Simonsson et al., 1972; Snashall et al., 1978), even in the absence of β-blockade (Black et al., 1982), whereas normal subjects are unaffected. Moreover, the bronchoconstrictor effect of the α-agonist methoxamine is inhibited by the selective α_1-antagonist prazosin, suggesting that α_1-receptors are involved (Black et al., 1984). Since the bronchoconstrictor response to methoxamine is also inhibited by an anticholinergic drug, this suggests the involvement of cholinergic pathways (Black et al., 1984). Others have failed to demonstrate a bronchoconstrictor effect of α-agonists in asthmatic patients, however (Thomson et al., 1982). Enhanced α-adrenergic responsiveness is not confined to the airways, since exaggerated pupillary and cutaneous vascular responses to locally administered phenylephrine are found in atopic asthmatic subjects (Henderson et al., 1979) and exaggerated metabolic responses to the infused α_2-agonist clonidine have been reported in a few asthmatic subjects (Kallenbach et al., 1984). These studies support the hypothesis that α-adrenergic responses may be increased in asthma, but the bronchoconstrictor response to inhaled α-agonists in asthma may merely reflect nonspecific bronchial hyperresponsiveness. Proof that α-adrenergic mechanisms contribute to asthma is dependent upon the demonstration that specific α-adrenoceptor antagonists have a beneficial effect in asthma.

D. Alpha-Antagonists in Asthma

The effect of α-antagonists in asthma remains controversial. The nonselective α-antagonists, phentolamine, thymoxamine, and indoramin, have been shown to cause resting bronchodilatation (Campbell, 1982) and protect against bronchoconstriction induced by histamine (Kerr et al., 1970; Bianco et al., 1972), allergen (Patel and Kerr, 1975), exercise (Beil and de Koch, 1978; Walden et al., 1984), and cold air (Walden et al., 1984). However, these α-antagonists have other pharmacologic actions, such as antihistamine activity and direct effects on airway smooth muscle, and they may release circulating catecholamines. Prazosin is a potent and specific α-antagonists with a high selectivity for α_1 receptors. Prazosin has been reported to cause bronchodilation after oral administration (Marlin et al., 1982), but this could be explained by a baroreflex response to the fall in blood pressure. Inhaled prazosin has no bronchodilator effect in asthmatic subjects (Barnes et al., 1981b) and no effect on histamine-induced bronchoconstriction (Barnes et al., 1981c), although there is a partial protection against exercise-induced bronchoconstriction, suggesting the involvement of α_1 receptors in this response. However, it is difficult to understand how α_1 receptors, if present in airway smooth muscle, are activated endogenously, since neither circulating epinephrine nor norepinephrine cause bronchoconstriction (Berkin et al., 1985; Larsson et al., 1986), and there is no direct adrenergic innervation of airway smooth muscle. It is possible that norepinephrine might reach airway α-receptors by overflow from adrenergic nerves to other pulmonary structures, as in guinea pig (Ainsworth et al., 1981). However, infusion of norepinephrine in asthmatic subjects fails to cause bronchoconstriction, so that this possibility seems unlikely (Berkin et al., 1986). Another possibility is that α-receptors may regulate bronchial blood flow and if bronchial blood flow were to decrease during exercise, as part of a generalized sympathetic activation, this would facilitate the airway cooling that may lead to bronchoconstriction in asthmatics. An α-antagonist would prevent this and, by increasing bronchial blood flow and thus reducing airway cooling, may prevent exercise-induced asthma. This is supported by the effectiveness of phentolamine against exercise and cold air-induced asthma, although allergen-induced bronchoconstriction is unaffected (Walden et al., 1984). The role of α-receptors in the pathogenesis of asthma thus appears to be rather limited and α-antagonists have no useful part to play in the therapy of asthma.

VI. Conclusions

Adrenergic regulation of airway function is complex and still poorly understood. The role of sympathetic nerves in controlling airway tone in humans is still uncertain; it is possible that these nerves may have a modulatory effect on other neural pathways. Similarly, the physiological significance of circulating epinephrine is difficult to assess, but the fact that β-blockers exacerbate asthmatic bronchoconstriction suggests that the low circulating concentrations of epinephrine are protective against bronchoconstriction in asthma. If epinephrine plays this defensive role in asthma, it is surprising that there is no increase in its secretion during bronchoconstriction. Whether β-adrenoceptor function in asthma is abnormal is still disputed; it is possible that there is a small defect in β-receptor function (which could be due to various inflammatory mediators), but this is unlikely to be of clinical significance. Exaggerated α-adrenergic responses, which have been demonstrated in asthma, are probably a reflection of nonspecific bronchial hyperresponsiveness and of no significance in asthma, since specific α-antagonists have little effect in asthma.

The adrenergic nervous system does not function in isolation and there must be complex interactions with cholinergic mechanisms and with the various neuropeptides that have been identified in airways. Neuropeptide Y has been particularly associated with adrenergic nerves, but its role in regulating airway function is not yet known. With improvements in biochemical and pharmacologic techniques, some of these uncertainties about adrenergic control of airways should soon be resolved.

Discussion

Laitinen. Since adrenergic innervation of human airways is sparse, it is possible that a small response to tyramine could be missed if insensitive measurements, such as FEV1 and peak flow, are used.

Barnes. The subjects in the tyramine study were mild asthmatics, who readily bronchodilated with an infused β-agonist, so that it is unlikely that a small bronchodilator (or bronchoconstrictor) response would be missed.

Said. Synergy between VIP and norepinephrine has been demonstrated in the cerebral cortex. If this exists in the airways, removal of even subthreshold concentrations of epinephrine might explain why bronchoconstriction occurs with β-blockers.

Barnes. We have investigated the question of synergy between VIP and β-agonist in human airways. Infused VIP has no bronchodilator effect in normal subjects and does not enhance the bronchodilator dose-responses to an inhaled beta-agonist (Palmer et al., 1986b).

Lundberg. Can β-agonist-induced bronchoconstriction be explained by blockade of β-receptors on airway smooth muscle, since basal concentrations of endogenous epinephrine are so low and adrenergic nerves are so sparse?

Barnes. The low concentration of endogenous epinephrine (0.2-0.4 nmol/l) is unlikely to exert any direct effect on airway smooth muscle, but it is possible that there may be an inhibitory effect on acerylcholine release from cholinergic nerves. In addition, adrenergic nerves may exert an inhibitory effect on cholinergic nerves and ganglia. β-Agonists, by blocking the inhibitory effect of adrenergic nerves and/or epinephrine, would increase acetylcholine release. This would not have any effect on normal airways, but with bronchial hyperresponsiveness a bronchoconstrictor response would occur. Propranolol-induced bronchoconstriction can be prevented by cholinergic antagonists.

Widdicombe. Do the β_1-receptors you demonstrated in glands have any significance?

Barnes. β_1-Receptors make up only 10% of β-receptors in submucosal glands, so exogenous β-agonists would stimulate mucus secretion mainly via β_2-receptors. The β_1-receptors, however, may regulate secretion in response to adrenergic nerve stimulation and so functionally could be just as important as the more numerous β_2-receptors.

Nadel. Are β-receptors on airway epithelial cells polarized?

Barnes. Presumably epinephrine more readily reaches the basolateral membrane, but it is not yet possible to say whether the β-receptor density differs between basolateral and luminal surfaces.

References

Ainsworth, G. A., Garland, L. G., and Payne, A. N. (1981). Modulation of bronchoconstrictor responses to histamine in purebred guinea-pigs by sympathetic nerve stimulation. *Br. J. Pharmacol.* **77**:249-254.

Anton, A. H., and Sayre, D. F. (1962). A study of the factors affecting the aluminum oxide-trihydroxyindole procedure for the analysis of catecholamines. *J. Pharmacol. Exp. Ther.* **138**:360-375.

Ariens, E. J., and Simonis, A. M. (1983). Physiological and pharmacological aspects of adrenergic receptor classification. *Biochem. Pharmacol.* **32**:1539-1545.

Assem, E. S. K., and Schild, H. O. (1969). Beta adrenergic receptors concerned with the anaphylactic mechanisms. *Int. Arch. Allergy* **45**:62-69.

Baker, D. G., Basbaum, C. B., Herbert, D. A., and Mitchell, R. A. (1983). Transmission in airway ganglia of ferrets: inhibition by norepinephrine. *Neurosci. Lett.* **41**:139-143.

Baker, B., Peatfield, A. C., and Richardson, P. S. (1985). The nervous control of mucus secretion from human bronchus. *J. Physiol.* **365**:297-305.

Barnes, P. J. (1983). Endogenous plasma adrenaline in asthma. *Eur. J. Respir. Dis.* **64**:559-563.

Barnes, P. J. (1984). Adrenergic receptors of normal and asthmatic airways. *Eur. J. Respir. Dis.* **65**:72-79.

Barnes, P. J. (1985). Adrenoceptors in bronchial asthma. In *Pharmacology of*

Adrenoceptors. Edited by E. Szbadi, C. M. Bradshaw, and S. R. Nahorski. London, Macmillan, pp. 205-214.

Barnes, P. J. (1986a). Neural control of human airways in health and disease. State of the art. *Am. Rev. Respir. Dis.* **134**:1289-1314.

Barnes, P. J. (1986b). Endogenous catecholamines and asthma. *J. Allergy Clin. Immunol.* **77**:791-795.

Barnes, P. J., and Basbaum, C. B. (1983). Mapping of adrenergic receptors in the trachea by autoradiography. *Exp. Lung Res.* **5**:183-192.

Barnes, P. J., and Pride, N. B. (1983). Dose-response curves to inhaled beta-adrenoceptor agonists in normal and asthmatic subjects. *Br. J. Clin. Pharmacol.* **15**:677-682.

Barnes, P., Karliner, J., Hamilton, C., and Dollery, C. (1979). Demonstration of $alpha_1$-adrenoceptors in guinea pig lung using [^{3}H] prazosin. *Life Sci.* **25**: 1207-1214.

Barnes, P. J., Dollery, C. T., and MacDermot, J. (1980a). Increased pulmonary α-adrenergic and reduced β-adrenergic receptors in experimental asthma. *Nature* **285**:569-571.

Barnes, P., FitzGerald, G., Brown, M., and Dollery, C. (1980b). Nocturnal asthma and changes in circulating epinephrine, histamine and cortisol. *N. Engl. J. Med.* **303**:263-267.

Barnes, P. J., Karliner, J. S., and Dollery, C. T. (1980c). Human lung adrenoceptors studied by radioligand binding. *Clin. Sci.* **58**:457-461.

Barnes, P. J., Brown, M. J., Silverman, M., and Dollery, C. T. (1981a). Circulating catecholamines in exercise and hyperventilation-induced asthma. *Thorax* **36**:435-440.

Barnes, P. J., Ind, P. W., and Dollery, C. T. (1981b). Inhaled prozosin in asthma. *Thorax* **36**:378-381.

Barnes, P. J., Ind., P. W., and Dollery, C. T. (1984). Beta adrenoceptors in asthma and their response to agonists. In *Asthma: Physiology, Immunopharmacology and Treatment.* Edited by A. B. Kay, K. F. Austen, and L. M. Lichtenstein. London, New York, Academic Press, pp. 339-358.

Barnes, P. J., Wilson, N. M., and Vickers, H. (1981c). Prazosin, an $alpha_1$-adrenoceptor antagonist partially inhibits exercise-induced asthma. *J. Allergy Clin. Immunol.* **68**:411-419.

Barnes, P. J., Basbaum, C. B., Nadel, J. A., and Roberts, J. M. (1982a). Localization of β-adrenoceptors in mammalian lung by light microscopic autoradiography. *Nature* **299**:444-447.

Barnes, P. J., FitzGerald, G. A., and Dollery, C. T. (1982b). Circadian variation in adrenergic responses in asthmatic subjects. *Clin. Sci.* **62**:349-354.

Barnes, P. J., Ind, P. W., and Brown, M. J. (1982c). Plasma histamine and catecholamines in stable asthmatic subjects. *Clin. Sci.* **62**:661-665.

Barnes, P. J., Basbaum, C. B., Nadel, J. A., and Roberts, J. M. (1983b). Pulmonary α-adrenoceptors: autoradiographic localization using [3H] prazosin. *Eur. J. Pharmacol.* **88**:57-62.

Barnes, P. J., Nadel, J. A., Skoogh, B.-E., and Roberts, J. M. (1983c). Characterization of beta-adrenoceptor subtypes in canine airway smooth muscle by radioligand binding and physiologic responses. *J. Pharmacol. Exp. Ther.* **225**:456-461.

Barnes, P. J., Basbaum, C. B., and Nadel, J. A. (1983d). Autoradiographic localization of autonomic receptors in airway smooth muscle: marked differences between large and small airways. *Am. Rev. Respir. Dis.* **127**:758-762.

Barnes, P. J., Skoogh, B.-E., Brown, J. K., and Nadel, J. A. (1983e). Activation of alpha-adrenergic responses in tracheal smooth muscle: a post-receptor mechanism. *J. Appl. Physiol.* **54**:1469-1476.

Barnes, P. J., Skoogh, B.-E., Nadel, J. A., and Roberts, J. M. (1983f). Postsynaptic $alpha_2$-adrenoceptors predominate over $alpha_1$-adrenoceptors in canine tracheal smooth muscle and mediate neuronal and humoral alpha-adrenergic contraction. *Mol. Pharmacol.* **23**:570-575.

Barnes, P. J., Cuss, F. M. C., and Palmer, J. B. D. (1985). The effect of airway epithelium on smooth muscle contractility in bovine trachea. *Br. J. Pharmacol.* **86**:685-691.

Beil, M., and De Koch, M. A. (1978). Role of alpha-adrenergic receptors in exercise-induced bronchoconstriction. *Respiration* **35**:78-86.

Berkin, K. G., Inglis, G. C., Ball, S. G., and Thomson, N. C. (1985). Airway responses to low concentrations of adrenaline and noradrenaline in normal subjects. *Q. J. Exp. Physiol.* **70**:203-209.

Berkin, K. E., Inglis, G. C., Ball, S. G., and Thomson, N. C. (1986). Effect of low dose adrenaline and noradrenaline infusions on airway calibre in asthmatic patients. *Clin. Sci.* **70**:347-352.

Bianco, S., Griffin, J. P., Kamburoff, P. L., and Prime, F. J. (1972). The effect of thymoxomine on histamine induced bronchospasm in man. *Br. J. Dis. Chest* **66**:27-32.

Black, J. L., Salome, C. M., Yan, K., and Shaw, J. (1982). Comparison between airways response to an α-adrenoceptor agonist and histamine in asthmatic and non-asthmatic subjects. *Br. J. Clin. Pharmacol.* **14**:464-465.

Black, J. L., Salome, C., Yan, K., and Shaw, J. (1984). The action of prazosin and propylene glycol on methoxamine-induced bronchoconstriction in asthmatic subjects. *Br. J. Clin. Pharmacol.* **18**:349-353.

Black, J., Turner, A., and Shaw, J. (1981). Alpha-adrenoceptors in human peripheral lung. *Eur. J. Pharmacol.* **72**:83-86.

Borson, D. B., Chinn, R. A., Davis, B., and Nadel, J. A. (1980). Adrenergic and cholinergic nerves mediate fluid secretion from tracheal glands of ferrets. *J. Appl. Physiol.* **49**:1027-1031.

Braquet, P., Etienne, A., and Clostre, F. (1985). Down-regulation of β_2-adrenergic receptors by PAF-acether and its inhibition by the PAF-acether antagonist BN 52021. *Prostaglandins* **30**:721.

Brooks, S. M., McGowan, K., Bernstein, L., Altenau, P., and Peagler, J. (1979). Relationship between numbers of beta adrenergic receptors in lymphocytes and disease severity in asthma. *J. Allergy Clin. Immunol.* **63**:401-406.

Brown, M. J., Jenner, D. A., Allison, D. J., and Dollery, C. T. (1981). Variations in individual organ release of noradrenaline measured by an improved radioenzymatic technique; limitations of peripheral venous measurements in the assessment of sympathetic nervous activity. *Clin. Sci.* **61**:585-590.

Brown, J. K., Shields, R., Jones, C., and Gold, W. M. (1983). Augmentation of alpha-adrenergic responsiveness in trachealis muscle of living dogs. *J. Appl. Physiol.* **54**:1558-1566.

Butchers, P. R., Skidmore, I. F., Vardey, C. J., and Wheeldon, A. M. (1980). Characterization of the receptor mediating the anti-anaphylactic effects of beta-adrenoceptor agonists in human lung tissue in vitro. *Br. J. Pharmacol.* **71**:663-667.

Cabezas, G. A., Graf, P. D., and Nadel, J. A. (1971). Sympathetic versus parasympathetic nervous regulation of airways in dogs. *J. Appl. Physiol.* **31**:651-655.

Campbell, S. C. (1982). Effects of alpha-adrenergic blockade with phentolamine on airway function in asthma. *Ann. Allergy* **49**:135-138.

Carstairs, J. R., Nimmo, A. J., and Barnes, P. J. (1984). Autoradiographic localisation of beta-adrenoceptors in human lung. *Eur. J. Pharmacol.* **103**:189-190.

Carstairs, J. R., Nimmo, A. J., and Barnes, P. J. (1985). Autoradiographic visualization of beta-adrenoceptor subtypes in human lung. *Am. Rev. Respir. Dis.* **132**:541-547.

Clarke, B., Ind, P. W., Causson, R., and Barnes, P. J. (1985). Bronchodilator and catecholamine responses to induced hypoglycaemia in acute asthma. *Clin. Sci.* **69**:35.

Collier, H. O. J., and James, G. W. L. (1967). Humoral factors affecting pulmonary inflation during acute anaphylaxis in the guinea-pig in vivo. *Br. J. Pharmacol.* **30**:283-301.

Davis, C., Kannan, M. S., Jones, T. R., and Daniel, E. E. (1982). Control of human airway smooth muscle: in vitro studies. *J. Appl. Physiol.* **53**:1080-1087.

Dobbs, L. G., and Mason, R. J. (1979). Pulmonary alveolar type II cells isolated from rats: release of phosphatidylcholine in response to beta adrenergic stimulation. *J. Clin. Invest.* **63**:378-387.

Doidge, J. M., and Satchell, D. G. (1982). Adrenergic and non-adrenergic inhibitory nerves in mammalian airways. *J. Auton. Nerv. Syst.* **5**:83-99.

Dolovich, M. B., Sanchis, J., Rossman, C., and Newhouse, M. T. (1976). Aerosol penetrance: a sensitive index of peripheral airways obstruction. *J. Appl. Physiol.* **40**:468-471.

Drazen, J. M. (1978). Adrenergic influences on histamine-mediated bronchoconstriction in the guinea pig. *J. Appl. Physiol.* **44**:340-345.

El-Bermani, A. I. (1978). Pulmonary noradrenergic innervation of rat and monkey: a comparative study. *Thorax* **33**:167-174.

Engel, G. (1981). Subclasses of beta-adrenoceptor—a quantitative estimation of $beta_1$- and $beta_2$- adrenoceptors in guinea pig and human lung. *Postgrad. Med. J.* **57**:77-83.

Engels, F., Oosting, R. S., and Nijkamp, F. P. (1985). Pulmonary macrophages induce deterioration of guinea-pig tracheal β-adrenergic function through release of oxygen radicals. *Eur. J. Pharmacol.* **111**:143-144.

FitzGerald, G. A., Barnes, P., Hamilton, C. A., and Dollery, C. T. (1980). Circulating adrenaline and blood pressure: the metabolic effects and kinetics of infused adrenaline in man. *Eur. J. Clin. Invest.* **10**:401-406.

Flavahan, N. A., Aarhus, L. L., Rimele, T. J., and Vanhoutte, P. M. (1985). REspiratory epithelium inhibits bronchial smooth muscle tone. *J. Appl. Physiol.* **58**:834-838.

Furchgott, R. F., Wakade, T. D., Sorace, R. A., and Stollak, J. S. (1975). Occurrence of both beta, and $beta_2$ receptors in guinea pig tracheal smooth muscle and the variation of the beta1:beta2 ratio in different animals. *Fed. Proc.* **34**:794.

Galant, S. P., Durisetti, L., Underwood, S., Allred, S., and Insel, P. A. (1980). Beta-adrenergic receptors of polymorphonuclear particulates in bronchial asthma. *J. Clin. Invest.* **65**:577-585.

Goldie, R. G., Paterson, J. W., and Wale, J. L. (1982). Pharmacological responses of human and porcine lung parenchyma, bronchus and pulmonary artery. *Br. J. Pharmacol.* **76**:515-521.

Goldie, R. G., Paterson, J. W., Spina, D., and Wale, J. L. (1984). Classification of β-receptors in human isolated bronchus. *Br. J. Pharmacol.* **81**:611-615.

Goldie, R. G., Papadimitriou, J. M., Paterson, J. W., Rigby, P. J., Self, H. M., and Spina, D. (1986). Influence of epithelium on responsiveness of guinea-pig isolated trachea to contractile and relaxant agonists. *Br. J. Pharmacol.* **87**:5-14.

Grieco, M. H., and Pierson, R. N. (1971). Mechanism of bronchoconstriction due to beta-adrenergic blockade. *J. Allergy Clin. Immunol.* **48**:143-152.

Grundstrom, N., Andersson, R. G. G., and Wikberg, J. E. S. (1981a). Pharmacological characterization of the autonomous innervation of guinea pig tracheobronchial smooth muscle. *Acta Pharmacol. Toxicol.* **49**:150-157.

Grundstrom, N., Andersson, R. G. G., and Wikberg, J. E. S. (1981b). Prejunctional alpha$_2$-adrenoceptors inhibit contraction of tracheal smooth muscle by inhibiting cholinergic neurotransmission. *Life Sci.* **28**:2981-2986.

Hartley, J. P. R., Davies, C. J., Money, R. D. H., Nogrady, S. G., and Winson, M. D. (1981). Plasma cyclic nucleotide levels in exercise-induced asthma. *Thorax* **36**:823-827.

Henderson, W. R., Shelhamer, J. H., Reingold, D. B., Evans, R., and Kaliner, M. (1979). Alpha-adrenergic hyper-responsiveness in asthma. Analysis of vascular and pupillary responses. *N. Engl. J. Med.* **300**:642-647.

Howarth, P. H., Durham, S. R., Lee, T. H., Kay, A. B., Church, M. K., and Holgate, S. T. (1985). Influence of albuterol, cromolyn sodium and ipratropium bromide on the airway and circulating mediator responses to allergen bronchial provocation in asthma. *Am. Rev. Respir. Dis.* **132**:986-992.

Ind, P. W., Brown, M. J., and Barnes, P. J., (1983a). Sympathoadrenal responses in asthma. *Thorax* **38**:702.

Ind, P. W., Scriven, A. J. I., and Dollery, C. T. (1983b). Use of tyramine to probe pulmonary noradrenaline release in asthma. *Clin. Sci.* **64**:9.

Ind, P. W., Barnes, P. J., Durham, S. R., and Kay, A. B. (1984). Propranolol-induced bronchoconstriction in asthma: beta-receptor blockade and mediator release. *Am. Rev. Respir. Dis.* **129**:10.

Ind, P. W., Barnes, P. J., Brown, M. J., and Dollery, C. T. (1985a). Plasma histamine concentration during propranolol induced bronchoconstriction. *Thorax* **40**:903-909.

Ind, P. W., Causon, R. C., Brown, M. J., and Barnes, P. J. (1985b). Circulating catecholamines in acute asthma. *Br. Med. J.* **290**:267-279.

Ind, P. W., Dixon, C. M. S., Fuller, R. W., and Barnes, P. J., (1986). Anticholinergic blockade of propranolol-induced bronchoconstriction. *Thorax* **41**:718.

Kaliner, M., Orange, R. P., and Austen, K. F. (1972). Immunological release of histamine and slow reacting substance of anaphylaxis from human lung. IV. Enhancement by cholinergic and alpha-adrenergic stimulation. *J. Exp. Med.* **136**:556-567.

Kallenbach, J. M., Joffe, B. I., Seftel, H. C., and Zwi, S. (1984). Comparison of the metabolic responses to alpha-adrenergic stimulation in asthmatics and non-asthmatics after clonidine. *S. Afr. Med. J.* **65**:131-134.

Karlsson, J.-A., and Persson, C. G. A. (1981). Influence of tracheal contraction on relaxant effects in vitro of theophylline and isoprenaline. *Br. J. Pharmacol.* **74**:73-79.

Kerr, J. W., Govindaraj, M., and Patel, K. R. (1970). Effect of alpha-receptor blocking drugs and disodium cromoglycate on histamine hypersensitivity in bronchial asthma. *Br. Med. J.* **2**:139-141.

Kneussl, M. P., and Richardson, J. B. (1978). Alpha-adrenergic receptors in human and canine tracheal and bronchial smooth muscle. *J. Appl. Physiol.* **45**:307-311.

Knowles, M., Murray, G., Shallal, J., Askin, F., Ranga, V., Gatzy, J., and Boucher, R. (1984). Bioelectric properties and ion from oxron excised human bronchi. *J. Appl. Physiol.* **56**:868-877.

Koeter, G. H., Meurs, H., Kauffman, H. F., and De Vries, K. (1982). The role of the adrenergic system in allergy and bronchial hyperreactivity. *Eur. J. Respir. Dis.* **121**:72-78.

Laitinen, A., Partanen, M., Hervonen, A., and Laitinen, L. A. (1985). Electron microscopic study on the innervation of human lower respiratory tract. Evidence of adrenergic nerves. *Eur. J. Respir. Dis.* **67**:209-215.

Laitinen, L. A., Laitinen, A., and Widdicombe, J. G. (1987). Effects of inflammatory and other mediators on airway vascular beds. *Am. Rev. Respir. Dis.* (in press).

Lands, A. M., Arnold, A., McAuliff, J. P., Luduena, F. P., and Brown, T. G. (1967). Differentiation of receptor systems activated by sympathomimetic amines. *Nature* **214**:597-598.

Larsson, K., Grunneberg, R., and Hjemdahl, P. (1985). Bronchodilatation and inhibition of allergen-induced bronchoconstriction by circulatory epinephrine in asthmatic subjects. *J. Allergy Clin. Immunol.*

Larsson, K., Hjemdahl, P., and Martinsson, A. (1982). Sympathoadrenal reactivity in exercise-induced asthma. *Chest* **82**:561-567.

Larsson, K., Martinsson, A., and Hjemdahl, P. (1986). Influence of circulating α-adrenoceptor agonists on pulmonary function and cardiovascular variables in patients with exercise induced asthma and healthy subjects. *Thorax* **41**:552-558.

Leff, A. R., Munoz, N. M., and Hendrix, S. G. (1982). Sympathetic inhibition of histamine-induced contraction of canine trachealis in vivo. *J. Appl. Physiol.* **53**:21-29.

Leikhauf, G. D., Ueki, I. F., and Nadel, J. A. (1984). Selective autonomic regulation of the viscoelastic properties of submucosal gland secretions from cat trachea. *J. Appl. Physiol.* **56**:426-430.

Lofdahl, C.-G., and Svedmyr, N. (1982). Effects of prenalterol in asthmatic patients. *Eur. J. Clin. Pharmacol.* **23**:297-303.

MacLagan, J., and Ney, U. M. (1979). Investigation of the mechanism of propranolol-induced bronchoconstriction. *Br. J. Pharmacol.* **66**:409-418.

Marlin, G. E., Thompson, P. J., Reddell, H. K., Chow, C. M., and Cheng, S. (1982). Bronchodilator activity of prazosin in patients with allergic rhinitis and asthma. *Br. J. Clin. Pharmacol.* **13**:445-448.

Massaro, G. D., Fischman, C. M., Chiang, M. J., Amado, C., and Massaro, D. (1981). Regulation of secretion in Clara cells. Studies using the isolated perfused lung. *J. Clin. Invest.* **67**:345-351.

Mathé, A. A., and Knapp, P. (1969). Decreased plasma free fatty acids and urinary epinephrine in bronchial asthma. *N. Engl. J. Med.* **281**:234-238.

McNeill, R. S. (1964). Effect of a beta-adrenergic blocking agent propranolol, on asthmatics. *Lancet* **2**:1101-1102.

McNeill, R. S., and Ingram, C. G. (1966). Effect of propranolol on ventilatory function. *An. J. Cardiol.* **18**:473-475.

Meurs, H., Koeter, G. H., De Vries, K., and Kauffman, H. F. (1982). The beta-adrenergic system and allergic bronchial asthma: changes in lymphocyte beta-adrenergic receptor number and adenylate cyclase activity after an allergen-induced attack. *J. Allergy Clin. Immunol.* **70**:272-280.

Meyrick, B., and Reid, L. (1970). Ultrastructure of cells in human bronchial submucosal glands. *J. Anat.* **107**:281-299.

Molho, M., Kurchin, A., Ohry, A., Bass, A., and Adar, R. (1977). Pulmonary functional abnormalities after upper dorsal sympathectomy. *Am. Rev. Respir. Dis.* **116**:879-883.

Morris, H. G., Deroche, G., and Earle, M. R. (1972). Urinary excretion of epinephrine and norepinephrine in asthmatic children. *J. Allergy Clin. Immunol.* **50**:138-145.

Nadel, J. A., and Barnes, P. J., (1984). Autonomic regulation of the airways. *Annu. Rev. Med.* **35**:451-467.

Ney, U. M. (1983). Propranolol-induced airway hyperreactivity in guinea-pigs. *Br. J. Pharmacol.* **79**:1003-1009.

O'Donnell, S. R., Saar, N., and Wood, L. J. (1978). The density of adrenergic nerves at various levels in the guinea-pig lung. *Clin. Exp. Pharmacol. Physiol.* **5**:325-332.

Orange, R. P., Austen, W. G., and Austen, K. F. (1971). Immunological release of histamine and slow-reacting substance of anaphylaxis from human lung. I. Modulation by agents influencing cellular levels of cyclic 3′,5′-adenosine monophosphate. *J. Exp. Med.* **134**:136-148.

Pack, R. J., and Richardson, P. S. (1984). The adrenergic innervation of the human bronchus: a light and electron microscopic study. *J. Anat.* **138**:493-502.

Palmer, J. B., Cuss, F. M. C., and Barnes, P. J. (1986a). VIP and PHM and their role in nonadrenergic inhibitory responses in isolated human airways. *J. Appl. Physiol.* **61**:1322-1328.

Palmer, J. B., Cuss, F. M. C., Warren, J. B., and Barnes, P. J. (1986b). The effect of infused vasoactive intestinal peptide on airway function in normal subjects. *Thorax* **41**:663-666.

Partanen, M., Laitinen, A., Hervonen, A., Toivanen, M., and Laitinen, L. A. (1982). Catecholamine and acetylcholinesterase-containing nerves in human lower respiratory tract. *Histochemistry* **76**:175-188.

Patel, K. R., and Kerr, I. W. (1975). Effect of alpha-receptor blocking drug, thymoxamine, on allergen-induced bronchoconstriction in extrinsic asthma. *Clin. Allergy* **5**:311-316.

Paterson, J. W., Lulich, K. M., and Goldie, R. G. (1982). The role of β-adrenoceptors in bronchial hyperreactivity. In *Bronchial Hyperreactivity*. Edited by J. Morley. London, Academic Press, pp. 19-38.

Pavia, D., Bateman, J. R. M., and Clarke, S. W. (1980). Deposition and clearance of inhaled particles. *Bull. Eur. Physiopathol. Respir.* **16**:335-366.

Peatfield, A. C., and Richardson, P. S. (1982). The control of mucus secretion into the lumen of the cat by α- and β-adrenoceptors, and their relative inducement during sympathetic nerve stimulation. *Eur. J. Pharmacol.* **81**: 617-626.

Persson, C. G. A., Ejefalt, I., Grega, G. J., and Svensjo, E. (1982). The role of β-receptor agonists in the inhibition of pulmonary oedema. *Ann. N. Y. Acad. Sci.* **384**:544-556.

Peters, J. E., Chan, S. C., Hanifin, J. M., and Hirshman, C. A. (1981). The Basenji-greyhound dog model of asthma: defective leukocyte nucleotide response. *Clin. Res.* **29**:171.

Peters, S. P., Schulman, E. S., Schleimer, R. P., Macglashan, D. W., Newball, H. H., and Lichtenstein, L. M. (1982). Dispersed human lung mast cells. Pharmacologic aspects and comparison with human lung tissue fragments. *Am. Rev. Respir. Dis.* **126**:1034-1039.

Phillips, M. J., Barnes, P. J., and Gold, W. M. (1985). Characterization of purified dog mastocytoma cells: autonomic membrane receptors and pharmacologic modulation of histamine release. *Am. Rev. Respir. Dis.* **132**:1019-1026.

Phipps, R. J., Williams, I. P., Richardson, P. S., Pell, J., Pack, R. J., and Wright, N. (1982). Sympathetic drugs stimulate the output of secretory glycoprotein from human bronchi in vitro. *Clin. Sci.* **63**:23-28.

Piper, P. J., Collier, H. O. J., and Vane, J. R. (1967). Release of catecholamines in the guinea-pig by substances involved in anaphylaxis. *Nature* **213**:838-840.

Richardson, J. B. (1979). Nerve supply to the lungs. *Am. Rev. Respir. Dis.* **119**: 785-802.

Richardson, J., and Beland, J. (1976). Nonadrenergic inhibitory nervous system in human airways. *J. Appl. Physiol.* **41**:764-771.

Richardson, J. B., and Ferguson, C. C. (1979). Neuromuscular structure and function in the airways. *Fed. Proc.* **38**:202-208.

Richardson, P. S., and Sterling, G. M. (1969). Effects of beta-adrenergic receptor blockade on airway conductance and lung volume in normal and asthmatic subjects. *Br. Med. J.* **3**:143-145.

Rinard, G. A., Rubinfield, A. R., Brunton, L. L., and Mayer, S. A. (1979). Depressed cyclic AMP levels in airway smooth muscle for asthmatic dogs. *Proc. Natl. Acad. Sci.* **76**:1472-1476.

Ruffin, R. E., Frith, M. B., and Anderton, R. C. (1979). Selectivity of beta-adrenoceptor antagonist drugs assessed by histamine bronchial provocation. *Clin. Pharmacol. Ther.* **25**:536-540.

Rugg, E. L., Barnett, D. B., and Nahorski, S. R. (1978). Coexistence of beta 1 and beta 2 adrenoceptors in mammalian lung: evidence from direct binding studies. *Mol. Pharmacol.* **14**:996-1005.

Sands, M. F., Douglas, F. L., Green, J., Banner, A. S., Robertson, G. L., and Leff, A. R. (1985). Homeostatic regulation of bronchomotor tone by sympathetic activation during bronchoconstriction in normal and asthmatic humans. *Am. Rev. Respir. Dis.* **132**:993-998.

Schnall, R. P., and Landau, L. I. (1980). Protective effects of repeated short sprints in exercise-induced asthma. *Thorax* **35**:828-832.

Scriven, A. J. I., Dollery, C. T., Murphy, M. B., Macquin, I., and Brown, M. J. (1983). Comparison of changes in plasma noradrenaline concentration and blood pressure induced by tyramine and cold stress. *Clin. Pharmacol. Ther.* **33**:710-716.

Shelhamer, J., Marom, Z., and Kaliner, M. (1980a). Immunologic and neuropharmacologic stimulation of mucous glycoprotein release from human airways in vitro. *J. Clin. Invest.* **66**:1400-1408.

Shellhamer, J. H., Metcalfe, D. D., Smith, L. J., and Kaliner, M. (1980b). Abnormal beta-adrenergic responsiveness in allergic subjects: Analysis of isoproterenol-induced cardiovascular and plasma cyclic adenosine monophosphate responses. *J. Allergy Clin. Immunol.* **66**:52-60.

Sheppard, M. N., Kurian, S. S., Henzen Logmans, S. C., Michetti, F., Cocchia, D., Cole, P., Rush, R. A., Marangos, P. J., Bloom, S. R., and Polak, J. M. (1983). Neuron-specific enolase and S-100. New Markers for delineating the innervation of the respiratory tract in man and other animals. *Thorax* **38**:333-340.

Silva, D. G., and Ross, G. (1974). Ultrastructural and fluorescence histochemical studies on the innervation of the tracheo-bronchial muscle of normal cats treated with 6-hydroxydopamine. *J. Ultrastruct. Res.* **47**:310-328.

Silverberg, A. B., Shah, S. D., Haymond, M. W., and Cryer, P. E. (1978). Norepinephrine: hormone and neurotransmitter in man. *Am. J. Physiol.* **234**:252-256.

Simonsson, B. G., Svedmyr, N., Skoogh, B. E., Anderson, R., and Bergh, N. P. (1972). In vivo and in vitro studies on alpha-adrenoceptors in human airways; potentiation with bacterial endotoxin. *Scand. J. Respir. Dis.* **53**:227-236.

Skoogh, B.-E. (1983). Transmission through airway ganglia. *Eur. J. Respir. Dis.* **64** (Suppl 131):159-170.

Snashall, R., Boother, F. A., and Sterling, G. M. (1978). The effect of alpha-adrenergic stimulation on the airways of normal and asthmatic man. *Clin. Sci.* **54**:283-289.

Svedmyr, N. A., Larsson, A. L., and Thiringer, G. K. (1976). Development of "resistance" in beta adrenergic receptors of asthmatic patients. *Chest* **69**: 479-483.

Szentivanyi, A. (1968). The beta adrenergic theory of the atopic abnormality in bronchial asthma. *J. Allergy* **42**:203-232.

Tashkin, D. P., Conolly, M. E., Deutsch, R. I., Hui, K. K., Littner, M., Scarpace, P., and Abrass, I. (1982). Subsensitization of beta-adrenoceptors in airways and lymphocytes of healthy and asthmatic subjects. *Am. Rev. Respir. Dis.* **125**:185-193.

Tattersfield, A. E., Leaver, D. G., and Pride, N. B. (1973). Effect of beta adrenergic blockade and stimulation on normal airways. *J. Appl. Physiol.* **35**: 613-619.

Tattersfield, A. E., Holgate, S. T., Harvey, J. E., and Gribbin, H. R. (1983). Is asthma due to partial beta-blockade of airways? *Agents Actions* **13**:265-271.

Taylor, S. M., Paré, P. D., and Schellenberg, R. (1984). Cholinergic and non-adrenergic mechanisms in human and guinea pig airways. *J. Appl. Physiol.* **56**:958-965.

Thomson, N. C., Daniel, E. E., and Hargreave, F. E. (1982). Role of smooth muscle alpha-1-receptors in non-specific bronchial responsiveness in asthma. *Am. Rev. Respir. Dis.* **126**:521-525.

Townley, R. G., McGeady, S., and Bewtra, A. (1976). The effect of beta-adrenergic blockade on bronchial sensitivity to acetyl-beta-methacholine in normal and allergic rhinitis subjects. *J. Allergy Clin. Immunol.* **57**:358-366.

van Herwaarden, C. L. A. (1983). β-Adrenoceptor blockade and pulmonary function in patients suffering from chronic obstructive lung disease. *J. Cardiovasc. Pharmacol.* **5**:46-50.

Venter, J. C., Fraser, C. M., and Harrison, L. C. (1980). Autoantibodies to β_2-adrenergic receptors: a possible cause of adrenergic hyporesponsiveness in allergic rhinitis and asthma. *Science* **207**:1361-1363.

Vermiere, P. A., and Vanhoutte, P. M. (1979). Inhibitory effects of catecholamines in isolated canine bronchial smooth muscle. *J. Appl. Physiol.* **46**: 787-791.

Walden, S. M., Bleeker, E. R., Chahal, K., Britt, E. J., Mason, P., and Permutt, S. (1984). Effect of alpha-adrenergic blockade on exercise-induced asthma and conditioned dry air. *Am. Rev. Respir. Dis.* **130**:357-362.

Warren, J. B., and Dalton, N. (1983). A comparison of the bronchodilator and vasopressor effects of exercise levels of adrenaline in man. *Clin. Sci.* **64**: 475-479.

Warren, J. B., Keynes, R. J., Brown, M. J., Jenner, D. A., and McNicol, M. W. (1982). Blunted sympathoadrenal response to exercise in asthmatic subjects. *Br. J. Dis. Chest* **76**:147-150.

Warren, J. B., Dalton, N., Turner, C., and Clark, T. J. H. (1984). Protective effect of circulating epinephrine within the physiological range on the airway response to inhaled histamine in non-asthmatic subjects. *J. Allergy Clin. Immunol.* **74**:683-686.

Zaagsma, J., van der Heijden, P. J. C. M., van der Schaar, M. W. G., and Blank, C. M. C. (1983). Comparison of functional β-adrenoceptor heterogeneity in central and peripheral airway smooth muscle of guinea pig and man. *J. Recept. Res.* **3**:89-106.

Zaid, G., and Beall, G. N. (1966). Bronchial response to beta-adrenergic blockade. *N. Engl. J. Med.* **275**:580-584.

5

Autonomic Function in Patients with Airway Obstruction

PAMELA B. DAVIS

Case Western Reserve University
School of Medicine
Cleveland, Ohio

There is marked individual variability in human physiological processes. Under normal conditions, even substantial variation from the norm is of no consequence because of homeostatic adjustments, complex interrelated compensatory systems, or the enormous reserve in most biologic systems. However, under stress, variations from the norm may become clinically important and determine which person thrives and which person cannot. For example, persons with glucose 6-phosphate dehydrogenase deficiency usually have no problems. But, under conditions of oxidant stress, massive hemolysis, illness, and even death may occur in the glucose-6-phosphate-dehydrogenase-deficient individual in response to the same environmental stress that is inconsequential to others. Inborn variations can also prove advantageous: persons heterozygous for hemoglobin S resist the acquisition of malaria.

Some persons are vulnerable to obstructive pulmonary disorders. Only 20% of heavy smokers develop chronic obstructive pulmonary disease (Weiss, 1984): they may be genetically predisposed or they may acquire vulnerability to this disease later in life. Persons with asthma respond to environmental irritant such as smog, fog, or frigid air with bronchoconstriction and illness, whereas most people do not. Inborn or acquired physiological variations in asthmatics may predispose them to respond abnormally to these stimuli.

Of the several hypotheses about the vulnerability to airways disease, one has considerable appeal: that variations in autonomic responses can render individuals vulnerable to airway reactivity, a cardinal feature of asthma and a component of other obstructive lung diseases, which may in turn lead to development and progression of obstructive pulmonary disease. This hypothesis arose from observations that the key mechanisms of reversible airways obstruction are regulated in part by autonomic systems. A particular constellation of autonomic abnormalities (increased alpha-adrenergic and cholinergic responses and reduced beta-adrenergic responses) might increase smooth muscle constriction, increase mucus secretion, and augment the inflammatory response, that is, increase reversible airways obstruction. This very combination of autonomic aberrations has been identified in patients with asthma and patients with cystic fibrosis (CF), and the autonomic abnormalities are correlated with airway reactivity in these populations.

This chapter will list only briefly the autonomic influences on mechanisms of reversible airways obstruction (they are discussed in greater detail elsewhere), and discuss the evidence for autonomic dysfunction in patients with obstructive airways diseases. Finally, the functional significance of autonomic abnormalities will be discussed, and directions for research suggested.

I. Autonomic Influences on Mechanisms of Reversible Airway Obstruction

A. Bronchial Smooth Muscle Constriction

Bronchial smooth muscle constriction is a major cause of reversible airways obstruction. Vagal (parasympathetic, muscarinic cholinergic) neurons mediate the constriction of bronchial smooth muscle in humans (Nadel, 1977), but cholinergic stimuli applied through nonneural pathways are also effective (e.g., inhaled methacholine) (Tiffeneau, 1955). Bronchial smooth muscle is relaxed by beta$_2$-adrenergic stimulation (Scheid et al., 1979). When there is preexisting bronchoconstriction and/or when the homeostatic beta-adrenergic adjustment mechanisms are blocked, alpha-adrenergic stimulation may cause further bronchoconstriction (Mathe et al., 1981), though the exact anatomic location, pharmacologic class, or physiological importance of these alpha-adrenergic receptors has not been established in humans.

B. Accumulation of Secretions

Airflow may be obstructed by the accumulation in the lumen of fluid transported into the lumen, mucus secretions, and inflammatory exudate (cells and serum). Epithelial electrolyte transport (and therefore movement of water) may help maintain the proper depth of perciliary fluid (critical for mucociliary transport), and may regulate viscosity and composition of the transported secretions. Acetylcholine decreases net sodium absorption and increases chloride secretion in human bronchi in an electroneutral manner (possibly simply through gland secretion), whereas electrogenic flux of chloride into the trachea and bronchi is stimulated by beta-adrenergic and other cAMP-mediated systems (Nadel, 1977). Surface secretory cells contribute only a small portion of the total mucous glycoprotein in the airways, but these goblet cells occur in distal airways where even small amounts of secretion may obstruct. It is not clear how goblet cell secretion is regulated in humans. The tracheobronchial glands contribute most of the mucous glycoprotein in the airways and secrete in response to vagal stimulation. In culture, human glands secrete in response to alpha-adrenergic and cholinergic agents (Shelhamer et al., 1980a). Inflammation causes increase in gland size: enlarged glands are more sensitive to cholinergic stimulation and less sensitive to anticholinergic inhibition (Sturgess and Reid, 1972). Removal of airway secretions is accomplished by cough and by mucociliary clearance, which is stimulated by beta-adrenergic agents, and possibly tonically regulated by the cholinergic systems.

C. Inflammation

Inflammation leads to increase in size, wider distribution, and greater cholinergic sensitivity of mucus-secreting cells, and thus may contribute to airflow obstruction by increasing secretion volume. However, inflammation itself can cause obstruction to airflow. Edema and engorgement of blood vessels narrow the airway lumen (the airway swells inward) and the tissue destruction that accompanies inflammation causes epithelial desquamation. Many steps in the initiation and maintenance of inflammation are regulated, in part, by autonomic systems. One important source of inflammatory mediators is the mast cell. Once mediator release is initiated (e.g., by bridging of IgE molecules on the mast cell surface), alpha-adrenergic and cholinergic agents enhance it (Kaliner et al., 1972) and beta-adrenergic agents inhibit it (Orange et al., 1971).

The inflammatory response may also be regulated by autonomic systems. Some cardinal features of inflammation (e.g., erythema, edema, and heat) depend on increased blood flow and increased vascular permeability. Alpha-adrenergic stimulation causes vasoconstriction (reducing vascular engorgement) and beta-adrenergic stimulation results in vasodilation (increasing vascular engorgement), but also reduces microvascular permeability, thereby reducing fluid leak into the tissues.

Maintenance of inflammation depends on recruitment of inflammatory and/or phagocytic cells. Margination and adherence of neutrophils and thus possibly neutrophil accumulation, is reduced by beta-adrenergic agents. Release of lytic enzymes and other factors from neutrophils (and therefore perhaps tissue destruction, driving further inflammation) is enhanced by alpha-adrenergic and cholinergic agents and reduced by beta-adrenergic agonists (Zurier et al., 1974).

II. Autonomic Dysfunction in Airways Disease

Because there is prominent autonomic regulation of several of the processes that produce airways obstruction, it is tempting to speculate that derangement of autonomic function predisposes to airways disease. Specifically, failure of beta-adrenergic responses could result in impaired bronchial smooth muscle relaxation, less well-hydrated mucus, poor mucociliary clearance, and removal of the usual attenuation mechanisms from mast cell degranulation and neutrophil lysosomal enzyme release (Ignarro et al., 1974). Increased response to cholinergic stimuli could result in increased bronchial smooth muscle constriction, enhanced mediator release from mast cells, and increased secretion by tracheobronchial glands. Increased alpha-adrenergic responses could result in increased bronchoconstriction, enhanced release of inflammatory mediators from mast cells, and increased mucus secretion. Persons with increased alpha-adrenergic and cholinergic responses and decreased beta-adrenergic responses might be at particular risk for obstructive airways disease. In addition, if autonomic dysfunction worsens with increasing pulmonary obstruction, this could contribute to progression of disease.

For these reasons, considerable effort has been devoted to assessing autonomic function in persons with obstructive airways diseases. Because of the eloquent enunciation of the "beta-adrenergic theory of asthma" by Szentivanyi (1968), much of this effort has been directed at the study of beta-adrenergic function in asthma. More recently other branches of the autonomic nervous system have been examined, and patients with other obstructive airways diseases have been tested. There is, however, considerable difficulty in studying autonomic function in patients with airways disease. Drugs used to treat airways obstruction often affect autonomic functions. For example, beta-adrenergic agonists cause desensitization of beta-adrenergic receptor systems (Stiles et al., 1984), theophylline derivatives promote adrenal catecholamine release, with resulting adrenergic down-regulation (Goodman and Gilman, 1975), and corticosteroids increase beta-adrenergic responses (Davies and Lefkowitz, 1980). Drug effects can persist for weeks (Morris et al., 1977), so special care must be taken to separate the effects of drugs from the properties of the disease state. Secondary concomitants of airways disease may also affect autonomic function. Some infections (e.g., viral or *Hemophilus* infections) cause reduced beta-adrenergic responses (Busse, 1977; Schreurs and Nijkamp, 1982). Hypoxia or stress from dyspnea might cause adrenal catecholamine release and down-regulation of beta-adrenergic systems. Although these potential secondary effects on autonomic responses in disease make it difficult to determine whether abnormal responses are primary or secondary, they do not exclude the postulate that development or exacerbation of abnormal autonomic responses is a mechanism of disease progression, or part of the disease itself.

Another problem in the study of autonomic dysfunction in lung disease is that the human lung is relatively inaccessible and difficult to test. The secondary effects of disease are most prominent in the affected tissue. Excised tissue is difficult to obtain, and is usually available under uncontrolled circumstances (surgery or autopsy). Studies in vivo are complicated by uncertain drug delivery to target sites by either aerosol or parenteral route, and responses to drugs in vivo are difficult to interpret unambiguously because of complex local and central reflexes and homeostatic adjustments. Standard pulmonary outcome measures such as flow or resistance are indirect measures of autonomic response and may be confounded by subclinical disease. For these reasons, and because the basic components of autonomic receptor systems are conserved from tissue to tissue and even across species, extrapulmonary model systems have been studied. However, extrapulmonary responses must ultimately be related to pulmonary responses if they are to be meaningful in the pathogenesis of airways disease.

In spite of all these difficulties, a considerable body of information has accumulated on autonomic function in patients with airways disease. Much of the evidence points are to an association of autonomic dysfunction with airway reactivity, which in turn may be a risk factor for development and progression of obstructive airways disease.

A. Alpha-Adrenergic Function

Asthma

Allergic asthmatics with near-normal pulmonary function who have taken no medications for at least a month require a lower concentration of topical phenylephrine to produce mydriasis than do healthy controls (Henderson et al., 1979; Kaliner et al., 1982; Davis et al., 1985). Neither patients with allergic rhinitis nor asymptomatic atopic subjects differ from controls, so atopy, per se, is not associated with increased alpha-adrenergic response (Table 1). These results have been confirmed in two separate laboratories with different measuring equipment and different norms. The pupillary response is probably largely $alpha_1$-adrenergic in character, for the pupil responds to phenylephrine but not to clonidine (Hodapp et al., 1981); however, specific inhibitor studies have not been done. Asthmatics also have increased $alpha_1$-adrenergic sensitivity in the peripheral blood vessels (Henderson et al., 1979): pupillary and vascular alpha-adrenergic sensitivity are positively correlated.

The biochemical basis of this $alpha_1$-adrenergic sensitivity is unknown. No

Table 1 Pupillary Sensitivity to Cholinergic and Alpha-Adrenergic Agents

Subjects	PC_{1mm} phenylephrine[a] (mean ± SD)	PC_{1mm} carbachol[a] (mean ± SD)
Nonatopic healthy (n = 73)	1.52 ± 0.67%	0.35 ± 0.19%
Atopic healthy (n = 6)	1.86 ± 0.81%	0.41 ± 0.14%
Allergic asthmatic (n = 19)	1.11 ± 0.68%[b]	0.23 ± 0.12%[b]
CF heterozygote (n = 45)	1.00 ± 0.50%[b]	0.26 ± 0.15%[b]

[a]PC_{1mm} was calculated as follows: measurements of pupil size were made at baseline and following topical administration of each succeeding drug dose (for phenylephrine 0.1, 0.5, 1.0, 1.5, 2.0, 2.5%; for carbachol 0.01, 0.05, 0.10, 0.25, 0.5, 0.75%). From the relation of pupil size to concentration, the concentration for 1 mm change in pupil size was determined (Davis, 1986b).
[b]Significantly different from healthy controls, $p < 0.05$.

human in vitro alpha$_1$-adrenergic model system is currently available. Platelet-free lymphocytes and granulocytes display no change in cAMP levels in response to alpha agonists and antagonists, no change in intracellular Ca^{2+} (monitored by Quin 2) in response to alpha agonists and antagonists, and no change in lysosomal enzyme release (by granulocytes) (Davis, 1986a). Binding sites for [^{3}H]-prazosin (an alpha$_1$-adrenergic ligand) or [^{3}H] dihydroergocryptine (a nonselective alpha ligand) cannot be detected on these cells (Davis, 1986a; Casale and Kaliner, 1984).

Platelets contain a "pure" alpha$_2$-adrenergic system in which occupation of receptor by agonist inhibits cAMP production and increases intracellular calcium (Hoffman and Lefkowitz, 1980). The ability of alpha$_2$-adrenergic agonists to inhibit platelet adenylate cyclase is normal in asthmatics (Davis et al., 1985); Davis and Lieberman, 1982), even those with increased pupillary alpha$_1$-adrenergic responses, and alpha$_2$-adrenergic receptors are present in normal concentration and have normal binding affinity for antagonists in platelets from asthmatics (Davis et al., 1985).

Thus, in asthmatics, two separate extrapulmonary alpha$_1$-adrenergic model systems display increased responsiveness, but at least one alpha$_2$-adrenergic system functions normally. In the lung, both alpha$_1$- and alpha$_2$-adrenergic systems have been identified. For normals and most asthmatics, treatment with either an alpha$_1$-adrenergic antagonist or a nonselective antagonist has no effect on baseline pulmonary function, though a subpopulation of asthmatics may respond to such therapy (Barnes et al., 1981; Campbell and Dyson, 1977; Black et al., 1978). Alpha-adrenergic agonists, such as phenylephrine or methoxamine in the presence of beta-adrenergic blockade, produce bronchoconstriction in asthmatics, but not normal subjects (Anthracite et al., 1971; Patel and Kerr, 1973; Snashall et al., 1978). Pretreatment of asthmatics with nonselective alpha-adrenergic blockers has been found by most investigators to attenuate exercise-induced bronchoconstriction in asthmatics (Bianco et al., 1974; Beil and de Kock, 1978). In some studies, but not all, attenuation of histamine-induced bronchoconstriction by alpha-adrenergic blockers was observed, but because of the intrinsic antihistaminic properties of some alpha blockers, these studies are difficult to interpret (Kerr et al., 1970; Gaddie et al., 1972; Bianco et al., 1972). Nevertheless, the weight of the evidence is that alpha-adrenergic receptor systems exist in the airway, play some role in the regulation of airway caliber, and may participate in the pathogenesis of exercise-induced bronchoconstriction at least. Moreover, the influence of the alpha-adrenergic system on airway caliber is greater in asthmatics than in normals.

Cystic Fibrosis

Patients with CF also require less phenylephrine to produce pupillary dilation than controls, displaying alpha-adrenergic sensitivity to a degree comparable to that of asthmatics (Davis et al., 1980) which cannot be explained by drugs, stage of disease, or organ involvement. Moreover, parents of patients with CF also require lower concentrations of phenylephrine for pupillary dilation than controls (Table 1) (Davis et al., 1980); Davis 1984). The PC_{1mm} (phenylephrine) or the concentration of phenylephrine required to produce a 1 mm dilation of the pupil in the light, is significantly lower than normal in CF heterozygotes. Preliminary analysis of the distribution of pupillary alpha-adrenergic responses in healthy subjects and CF parents shows that, while the data from healthy controls are best described as a single population distributed about a mean, there is a bimodal distribution of alpha-adrenergic responses of CF heterozygotes. Half the CF parents have PC_{1mm} (phenylephrine) normally distributed about the normal mean, and half have striking alpha-adrenergic sensitivity (Byard and Davis, 1986). More detailed family analysis and path analysis will be required to understand this observation. It is not yet clear, for example, whether autonomic sensitivity is limited to only some CF families, or to only one parent in a family.

Alpha$_2$-adrenergic inhibition of cAMP production in platelets occurs normally in CF patients and their parents (Davis et al., 1984a). Alpha$_2$-adrenergic receptor numbers and binding properties are normal in platelets from CF patients (Davis et al., 1984a). It is surprising that pulmonary alpha-adrenergic responses have not been studied in CF patients, although therapeutic administration of phenylephrine by aerosol is common in CF.

Emphysema/Chronic Bronchitis

Few studies have been done to investigate alpha-adrenergic function in this disease.

B. Cholinergic Systems

Asthma

Asthmatics who have not taken medication for a month and who have near-normal pulmonary function require a lower concentration of carbachol for miosis than controls (Kaliner et al., 1982; Smith et al., 1980; Davis, 1986). Kaliner and co-workers found that atopy (in the absence of asthma) was also associated with a small degree of increased pupillary cholinergic response (Kaliner et al., 1982, Smith et al., 1980), but we could not differentiate atopic and nonatopic controls with respect to cholinergic pupillary sensitivity (Davis, 1986). Thus, cholinergic sensitivity may be associated with atopy as well as asthma, but the effect of atopy per se is probably small. The volume response of sweat to injected methacholine is greater in asthmatics and other allergic subjects than in nonatopic normals (Kaliner, 1976). Our preliminary studies of heart rate variability show that asthmatics have increased heart rate variability at respiratory frequencies (8-24 cpm), a phenomenon mediated almost entirely by muscarinic influence. Thus, enhanced cholinergic sensitivity may be a concomitant of asthma. Its biochemical basis and subclassification as M_1 or M_2 are unknown.

The airways of asthmatics are exquisitely sensitive to inhaled methacholine (Tiffeneau, 1955). Although this might, at first glance, appear to indicate cholinergic hypersensitivity of the bronchi, more detailed analysis of the carbamylcholine bronchial response suggests that it is an index of nonspecific airways reactivity and not of cholinergic sensitivity per se (Orehek et al., 1977). The airways of normal subjects do react to carbachol at very high dosages. Bronchial smooth muscle removed from asthmatics undergoing lung resection shows no greater cholinergic sensitivity than normal muscle (Cerrina et al., 1985). Thus, it is difficult at present to implicate the cholinergic receptor system directly and not its effector mechanisms in the pathogenesis of airways obstruction. However, vagal tone may be increased in asthmatics, and cholinergic influences more profound in the asthmatics' lungs than in others.

In most asthmatics, administration of anticholinergic agents produces significant bronchodilation, suggesting that increased cholinergic tone helps to maintain airways obstruction in these patients (Cropp, 1975; Cavanaugh and Cooper, 1976). Pretreatment with cholinergic blockers inhibits the bronchoconstrictive response to methacholine (Sheppard et al., 1983). However, the effect of atropine on antigen-induced bronchoconstriction is small (Fish et al., 1977). Some, but not all, laboratories find that atropine attenuates cold air or exercise-induced bronchoconstriction (Sheppard et al., 1983; Breslin et al., 1980; Simonsson et al., 1967). These data, taken together, suggest a role for muscarinic receptor systems in the development and maintenance of airways obstruction in asthma.

Cystic Fibrosis

The pupils of CF patients in good to excellent condition who took no autonomic-active medications for at least a month prior to testing require a lower concentration of carbachol for constriction than the pupils of age-matched controls (Davis et al., 1980). This abnormality could not be related to atopy. However, the most marked cholinergic sensitivity was observed in patients who had had episodes of intestinal obstruction. Parents of CF patients also have increased pupillary cholinergic sensitivity (Davis et al., 1980; Davis, 1984). Again, there appear to be two populations of heterozygotes, one normal and one with marked cholinergic sensitivity (Byard and Davis, 1986). In CF patients themselves, we have recently identified other muscarinic responses that are increased: respiratory and total heart rate variability in the supine position.

Barbero's laboratory found that both the sweat and salivary glands of CF patients had increased volume responses to cholinergic agents (Sibinga and Barbero, 1961; Marmer et al., 1966). More recent studies in isolated sweat glands have cast doubt upon the interpretation of these results (Sato and Sato, 1984; Harper and Quinton, 1984). However, cholinergic responsiveness of the sweat gland varies with heat acclimatization and fitness of the subject, so group differences between the sick and the well are hard to interpret. Direct assessments of cholinergic innervation of sweat glands were reported years ago and did not show abnormal total cholinesterase activity or distribution about the sweat glands or cholinergic-stimulated incorporation of radioactive phosphate into the skin phospholipids in CF patients (Holzel et al., 1962; Hokin et al., 1963). In another exocrine system, no differences were found between CF and normal rectal mucosa with respect to the secretory response to cholinergic agents assessed histologically or autoradiographically (Neutra et al., 1977). So not all systems tested in CF show cholinergic hyperresponsiveness.

The airways of CF patients may have increased cholinergic responses. In vitro, tracheal explants from CF patients secrete excess mucus in response to cholinergic agents, but this may simply reflect the hypertrophy and hyperplasia of the mucus-secreting apparatus (Sturgess and Reid, 1972). About half of all patients with CF bronchoconstrict in response to inhaled methacholine (compared to nearly all asthmatics and less than 5% of normals) (Mitchell et al., 1978), though as noted above, a positive methacholine challenge test may be an index of nonspecific airway reactivity and not cholinergic sensitivity. Cholinergic blockers are effective bronchodilators in CF (Larsen et al., 1979). All these lines of evidence suggest that either increased cholinergic tone or increased muscarinic sensitivity may occur in the CF lung as well as at some extrapulmonary sites.

Emphysema/Chronic Bronchitis

Little has been done to evaluate extrapulmonary cholinergic systems in patients with chronic obstructive pulmonary disease. In the lung, however, substantial cholinergic influences can be demonstrated. Atropine or other cholinergic blockers are effective bronchodilators for some COPD patients (Passamonte and Martinez, 1984). Moreover, the prevalence of bronchial reactivity to methacholine is high, but the $PC_{20}FEV_1$ is well-correlated with resting airway caliber, so it may be a result or concomitant of disease progression rather than a primary factor in the development of disease (Ramsdale et al., 1984). Also, cigarette smoking may induce or potentiate methacholine bronchial reactivity, and most patients with COPD smoke (Malo et al., 1982; Gerrard et al., 1980). When COPD patients are tested for nonspecific bronchial reactivity with inhalation of frigid air, only a few respond and this response is not related to the methacholine response (Arnup et al., 1983). These factors, as well as the lack of information on extrapulmonary cholinergic responses in COPD, make the increased bronchial methacholine responsiveness of these patients difficult to interpret. One possible interpretation is that the methacholine challenge test in COPD reflects the degree of airways inflammation. Another explanation might be that, unlike in asthma, in COPD the methacholine challenge response does result from increased muscarinic sensitivity. A third possible explanation is that mechanical factors of baseline airways obstruction account for the apparent increase in airway reactivity to methacholine.

C. Beta-Adrenergic Responses

Asthma

Despite years of investigation of beta-adrenergic responses in asthmatic subjects, controversy remains over the existence of a beta-adrenergic defect in asthmatics, and if it exists, its origin. Early studies are difficult to interpret because of inattention to the medication history of the patient and are not discussed here. However, studies in which only drug-free asthmatics with mild disease were included may be biased. Asthmatics who are well enough to withstand protracted withdrawal of therapy might be those least likely to display physiological abnormalities; or they may have different physiology from those who are more severely affected. Therefore, results from this population may not be readily generalized to all asthmatics. Nevertheless, it appears that even in such a highly selected population, definite beta-adrenergic defects can be detected.

The cardiovascular system of unmedicated mild asthmatic subjects is less sensitive to the effects of beta-adrenergic agents than the cardiovascular systems of age-matched healthy controls. Infusion of low doses of isoproterenol, which produce relatively little tachycardia, produces widening of the pulse pressure due to a drop in diastolic pressure (beta$_2$-adrenergically mediated peripheral vasodilation) and increase in systolic pressure (inotropic effect of isoproterenol). In asthmatics, a higher dose of infused isoproterenol is required to increase pulse pressure than in controls (Shelhamer et al., 1980b; Davis et al., 1986). Shelhamer et al. (1980b) found that in asthmatics, the diastolic drop was especially blunted compared to normals, so the pulse pressure response deficit in asthmatics probably reflects impairment of the beta$_2$-adrenergic responses to a greater extent than the beta$_1$-adrenergic system. The decreased pulse pressure response to isoproterenol occurs in patients with allergic rhinitis (Shelhamer et al., 1980) and asymptomatic persons with positive allergic skin tests (Kaliner et al., 1982; David et al., 1986) as well, suggesting that diminished responses in this system are a concomitant of allergy as well as allergic asthma.

Drug-free allergic asthmatics required a higher dose of isoproterenol to increase pulse pressure by a target amount than normal controls. Even at this higher dose and at the same target increase in pulse pressure, asthmatics did not demonstrate the increase in baroreceptor heart rate variability that characterized normal subjects (Davis et al., 1986). The increase in heart rate variability produced in normals by isoproterenol probably results from either peripheral or cardiac interference by isoproterenol with baroreceptor control of blood pressure (Simpson and Davis, 1985). These results suggest decreased responsiveness of several cardiovascular beta-adrenergic regulatory systems in asthma. Alternatively, the failure of low-frequency heart rate variability to increase during isoproterenol infusion in asthmatics could result from diminished vagal (cholinergic) responses to baroreceptor stimulation rather than deficit in the response of the beta-adrenergic system. This postulate is, however, inconsistent with other data that indicate that asthmatics have increased cholinergic responses and, possibly, increased vagal tone (see above).

Metabolic beta-adrenergic responses are also blunted in asthmatics. The eosinopenic response and the plasma cAMP response to epinephrine are impaired (Shelhamer et al., 1980b; Apold and Aksnes, 1977; Makino et al., 1970).

Because of their accessibility, leukocytes have been widely used as models for beta-adrenergic systems in humans. Lymphocytes and granulocytes bear beta$_2$-adrenergic receptors that, when occupied, result in increased intracellular cAMP content. In granulocytes, this causes reduced lysosomal enzyme release, cellular adherence, and margination. In lymphocytes, beta-adrenergic stimulation results in impaired mitogenic response. However, leukocytes also display substantial day-to-day variability in the normal beta-adrenergic responses of these cells and marked sensitivity to circulating catecholamine levels (Aarons et al., 1980;

Fraser et al., 1981), making them less attractive as model systems. The catecholamine content of plasma in asthmatics is not increased, however, and, surprisingly, there is little change in catecholamines in the blood following experimentally induced bronchoconstriction (Ind et al., 1984; Barnes et al., 1981a) or even during spontaneous asthma attacks. Indeed, some have suggested from these data that failure of release of adrenergic neurotransmitters to compensate for bronchoconstrictive stimuli may contribute to the development of an asthma attack (Ind et al., 1984; Barnes et al., 1981a). Nevertheless, the possibility that changes in endogenous catecholamines could affect beta-adrenergic response in asthmatic leukocytes has not been excluded. There is some controversy over the leukocyte receptors and responses in asthma. Inhibition of lysosomal enzyme release from granulocytes by isoproterenol is reduced in cells from asthmatics but also from subjects with other atopic conditions (Busse and Lee, 1976; Busse, 1977). However, in most (but not all) studies of asthmatics in which medications were withheld for at least 2 weeks prior to testing, normal lymphocyte and granulocyte cAMP responses to beta-adrenergic agents were found (Lee et al., 1977; Tashkin et al., 1982, Conolly and Greenacre, 1976; Makino et al., 1977). Our own findings agree with these observations (Davis et al., 1986) (Figs. 1 and 2).

Since the number of beta-adrenergic receptors on lymphocytes and granulocytes is in excess of the number required to be occupied for maximal functional response (Davis et al., 1983; Galant and Allred, 1981), abnormal beta-adrenergic receptor number might occur even with normal cAMP response to isoproterenol. If enough "spare" receptors are present, even large changes in receptor number would not affect the maximal cAMP production and would shift the agonist-response relation only slightly. However, studies using current methodology in cells or membranes from drug-free asthmatics have found granulocyte beta-adrenergic receptor number to be normal (Davis et al., 1986; Galant et al., 1980; Sano et al., 1981). Lymphocyte beta-adrenergic receptor number was found to be normal by some (Davis et al., 1986; Tashkin et al., 1982) and reduced by others (Sano et al., 1981).

Our own studies suggest that some of the controversy in the literature over the beta-adrenergic status of patients with asthma may result from differences in test systems and outcome measures used to assess beta-adrenergic responses (Davis et al., 1986). In our study, the same asthmatic subjects whose pulse pressure and heart rate variability responses to isoproterenol were significantly impaired had normal leukocyte response to isoproterenol. Beta-adrenergic receptor number was normal as well. The explanation for this differential response may be that the beta$_2$-adrenergic systems of lymphocytes and granulocytes are poor models either for the beta$_2$-adrenergic response in the lung, or for the mixed beta$_1$- and beta$_2$-adrenergic response of the cardiovascular system to isoproterenol, or for the complex homeostatic adjustments of heart rate variability to

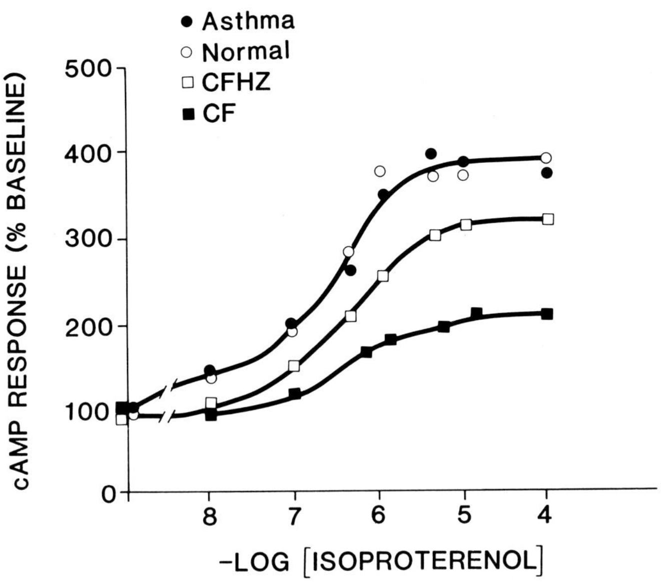

Figure 1 Isoproterenol-stimulated cAMP production by lymphocytes from unmedicated patients with CF, asthmatics, obligate heterozygotes for CF, and healthy controls. CF homo- and heterozygotes differ from the others.

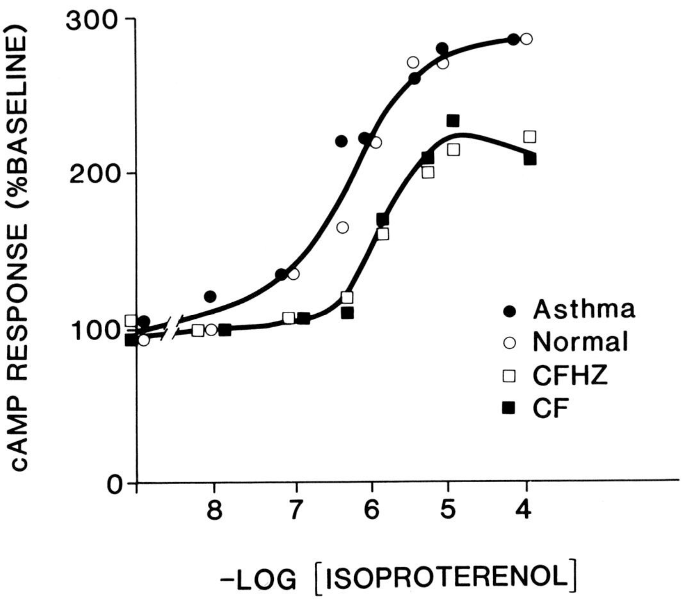

Figure 2 Isoproterenol-stimulated cAMP production by granulocytes from unmedicated patients with CF, asthmatics, obligate heterozygotes for CF, and healthy controls. CF homo- and heterozygotes differ from the others.

beta-adrenergic challenge. It is also possible that a beta-adrenergic defect in asthma (as seen in the cardiovascular system) results from a lesion distal to the generation of cAMP. Others have suggested that the controversy may be due to the existence of beta-adrenergic abnormalities in subjects with exercise-induced asthma but not other types of asthma (Larsson, 1985). However, since most studies show that bronchoconstriction is induced by respiratory heat loss in all asthmatics (Deal et al., 1980), one is concerned that differentiating a subgroup of "exercise-induced asthmatics" is artificial.

Evaluation of beta-adrenergic function in the intact lung of living asthmatics is difficult, because the potential for improvement of flows with a beta-adrenergic agent may depend upon the initial degree of obstruction, and so adequate controls may not be available. Clearly, beta-adrenergic responses are not absent, since these agents are useful therapeutically. Desensitization of lung beta-adrenergic receptors may occur at a slower rate or to a lesser extent than desensitization of receptors at other sites, such as the leukocyte (Lee et al., 1977). Thus, if the putative beta-adrenergic defect in asthma arises from especially rapid desensitization of beta-adrenergic receptors, nonpulmonary beta-adrenergic systems might display more profound defects than the pulmonary. However, this is difficult to assess experimentally. Smooth muscle isolated from bronchi of unmedicated asthmatics undergoing lung resection displays reduced beta-adrenergic responses (Cerrina et al., 1985).

The biochemical basis of the beta-adrenergic defect in asthma is unknown. An antibody to the beta-adrenergic receptor, found in many asthmatics, might produce beta-adrenergic resistance, which might in turn perturb other autonomic systems (Venter et al., 1980). This idea has considerable appeal, though the question of causation or association has not yet been settled. As noted above, the number of beta-adrenergic receptors on leukocytes is most likely normal in unmedicated asthmatics, and adenylate cyclase seems to function normally as well. Whether there exists a lesion distal to the generation of cAMP, or whether the beta-adrenergic receptor from the asthmatic is subject to abnormal regulation by agonist (more prone to desensitization and/or slower to recover) (Morris et al., 1977; Tashkin et al., 1982) remains to be tested unambiguously.

Cystic Fibrosis

Beta-adrenergic responses are abnormal in CF. The dosage of infused isoproterenol required to increase the pulse pressure by $\geqslant 22$ mmHg is higher in CF patients than in healthy controls (Davis et al., 1980). The cAMP response to isoproterenol is reduced in CF lymphocytes (Davis et al., 1978, 1983) and granulocytes (Davis et al., 1978, 1983; Galant et al., 1981). The inhibition of zymosan-stimulated lysosomal enzyme release by isoproterenol is reduced in CF granulocytes (Lemanske et al., 1981). The volume response of CF sweat glands to isoproterenol is blunted (Sato and Sato, 1984): normal changes in nasal biopotentials in response to isoproterenol fail to occur in CF patients (Knowles et al., 1983a). However, whether these defects in regulation of ion transport phenomena in CF represent defects in the beta-adrenergic regulation or in the effector system is not yet clear. The beta-adrenergic defect is unrelated to the severity of the disease, malnutrition, organ involvement, or atopy, and is not associated with elevated levels of circulating catecholamines (Davis et al., 1970, 1980b, 1983; Galant et al., 1981; Lake et al., 1979). Cultured CF skin fibroblasts do not necessarily display defective beta-adrenergic responses (Davis et al., 1980b; Roscher et al., 1980; Buchwald and Mapleson, 1977), but the reproducibility of beta-adrenergic responses is poor in this system (Davis et al., 1980b), and firm conclusions cannot be drawn.

Parents of patients with CF also display abnormal beta-adrenergic responses in lymphocytes (Davis, 1984; Davis et al., 1978, 1983), granulocytes (Davis et al., 1978, 1983; Galant et al., 1981), and the sweat gland (Sato and Sato, 1984), suggesting that there may be a heritable component of the beta-adrenergic defect in CF. However, analysis of lymphocyte beta-adrenergic responses in CF heterozygotes suggests heterogeneity, with only half the CF parents showing significant dysfunction, and the remainder normal (Byard and Davis, 1986).

The biochemical basis of the CF beta-adrenergic defect is uncertain. It is unlikely that a circulating substance accounts for the beta-adrenergic dysfunction in CF, since normal leukocytes exposed to CF serum do not develop reduced beta-adrenergic responses (Davis, 1980), and only one of seven patients with CF had detectable levels of antibody that reacts with the beta-adrenergic receptor (Venter et al., 1980). Moreover, cultured nasal and tracheal cells appear to retain phenotypic expression of the abnormal functional beta-adrenergic response, suggesting that the defect is intrinsic to the cells. Galant and coworkers (1981) found reduced numbers of beta-adrenergic receptors in granulocytes, but Davis et al. (1983) found receptor numbers to be normal on granulocytes and on lymphocytes. Although both lymphocytes and granulocytes from CF patients have reduced cAMP response to beta-adrenergic agents (Davis et al., 1978, 1983; Galant et al., 1981), sweat glands and nasal epithelial cells have normal cAMP responses to beta-adrenergic agents (Sato and Sato, 1984; Knowles et al., 1983). Most studies agree that the adenylate cyclase itself is normal in CF samples.

Leukocyte cAMP responses distinguish the beta-adrenergic lesions in asthma and CF since, unlike asthmatics, patients with CF have significantly reduced lymphocyte and granulocyte cAMP responses to isoproterenol. Thus the characteristics of beta-adrenergic dysfunction in these two disorders, and probably the mechanisms, are different, although the functional manifestations are similar in many respects.

It has been difficult to evaluate beta-adrenergic responses in the CF lung because changes in flow can be confounded by shifts in mucus, changes in lung volume, or preexisting bronchoconstriction. However, Mitchell et al. (1978) found that methacholine-induced bronchoconstriction was reversed to a lesser extent in CF than it was in asthma. This would suggest some blunting of the beta-adrenergic response in the CF lung.

Emphysema/Chronic Bronchitis

Granulocyte beta-adrenergic responses are reduced in patients with COPD, but the degree of reduction is proportional to the degree of impairment of the FEV_1 (Lemanske et al., 1980). Pulmonary beta-adrenergic responses are difficult to assess, since adequate controls with lung mechanics impairment comparable to those of COPD patients may not exist.

III. Functional Significance of Autonomic Dysfunction

A. Autonomic Dysfunction and Airway Reactivity

In the foregoing section we have presented evidence that increased alpha-adrenergic responses, increased cholinergic responses, and decreased beta-adrenergic responses occur in patients with the obstructive airways diseases, asthma, and CF. Beta-adrenergic dysfunction may occur in chronic bronchitis/emphysema as well. The combination of all three abnormalities in the same person might be the most deleterious pattern. Indeed, the studies of Kaliner et al. (1982) and our own studies (Davis, 1986b; Davis et al., 1986) suggest that this constellation does tend to occur together. Pupillary alpha-adrenergic and cholinergic responses were positively correlated in studies from both laboratories, that is, the subjects whose pupils were the most sensitive to phenylephrine were also sensitive to carbachol. In the studies of Kaliner et al. (1982), pupillary alpha-adrenergic sensitivity was inversely related to cardiovascular beta-adrenergic sensitivity, that is, those whose pupils were sensitive to phenylephrine tended to have cardiovascular systems resistant to isoproterenol. Table 2 shows the concordance between studies from two different laboratories. These data provide experimental support for grouping the autonomic abnormalities together, as shown in Figure 3.

For pupillary alpha-adrenergic and cholinergic sensitivity and cardiovascular beta-adrenergic sensitivity, the degree of autonomic aberration correlates with bronchial reactivity ($PC_{20}FEV_1$ for methacholine, or the concentration of inhaled methacholine required to cause a 20% drop in FEV_1) (Table 2). That is, those with the greatest alpha-adrenergic sensitivity, greatest cholinergic sensitivity, or the least beta-adrenergic reactivity have the most reactive airways. The same general result was obtained in two separate laboratories using different experimental protocols, different subjects, and different measuring equipment

Table 2 Correlation of Autonomic and Airway Reactivity

	R_s (number of subjects)			
	Pupils–alpha	Pupils–cholinergic	Pulse pressure–beta	$PC_{20}FEV_1$
Pupils–alpha	–	0.44 (118)[b]	-0.21 (22)	0.35 (39)[b]
Pupils–cholinergic	0.44[b]	–	-0.04 (22)	0.45 (39)[b]
Pulse pressure–beta	-0.56[b]	NS	–	-0.46 (22)[b]
$PC_{20}FEV_1$	0.49[b]	NS	-0.62[b]	–

Upper triangle shows results from Davis et al. (1986b,c) lower triangle from Kaliner et al. (1982) (number of subjects studied by Kaliner et al. was 47-111 for the different tests but numbers for correlations were not reported). For upper triangle, pupillary responses were expressed as PC_{1mm} (see Table 1). For lower triangle, pupillary responses were expressed as dosage administered to achieve ⩾1 mm constriction or ⩾0.5 mm dilation. "Pulse pressure–beta" refers to dosage of infused isoproterenol required to achieve a ⩾22 mmHg increase in pulse pressure.
[a]R_s = Spearman rank correlation coefficient.
[b]$p<0.05$.

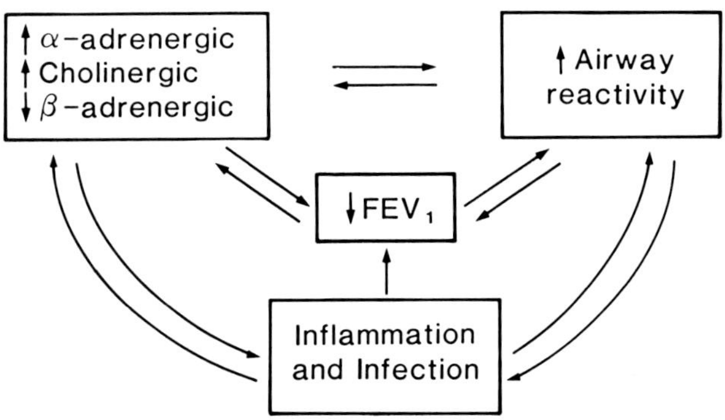

Figure 3 Scheme showing correlation of autonomic dysfunction and airway reactivity.

(Table 2). The subjects used to derive these correlations were healthy atopic and nonatopic controls, subjects with allergic rhinitis, and mild asthmatics, all of whom had taken no medication in 30 days and had normal baseline pulmonary function. Other laboratories have also demonstrated significant negative correlation between metabolic (plasma cAMP or eosinopenic) beta-adrenergic responses and nonspecific airway reactivity in asthmatics and controls (Apold and Aksnes, 1977; Makino et al., 1970). However, since asthma is defined, in part, by airway reactivity, it may not be surprising that physiological aberrations in asthmatics correlate with airway reactivity in the combined subject group. In our studies, however, when asthmatics are considered separately, those with the greatest airway reactivity also had the most profound cholinergic (Davis, 1986b) and beta-adrenergic dysfunction (Davis et al., 1986). Therefore, the observed correlations probably do not result simply from combining data from different subject groups.

If this correlation holds, other patient groups with the same pattern of abnormal autonomic reactivity should also have increased airway reactivity. Indeed, patients with CF have high prevalence of airway reactivity, but this finding is hard to interpret in the face of the resting airways obstruction, profound inflammation, and mucus impactions in CF (Holzel et al., 1962; Lemanske et al., 1980; Van Asperen et al., 1981; Haluzka and Schislichi, 1975; Day and Mearns, 1973). A better test of the association of autonomic and airway reactivity would be in subjects without apparent disease. Obligate heterozygotes for CF, selected for their genotype and *not* by disease, have the critical combination of autonomic aberrations. Parents of CF patients, who took no medications for at least 30 days, had no history of lung disease, and had normal pulmonary function, have a high prevalence of airway reactivity (30% had $PC_{20}FEV_1$ less than 3 mg/ml methacholine, compared to less than 4% of controls) that cannot be explained by atopy, cigarette smoking, age, or history of drug use (Davis, 1984). Moreover, $PC_{20}FEV_1$ among these CF heterozygotes correlates with production of cAMP by lymphocytes in response to beta-adrenergic agents (Davis, 1984). Because these results were obtained in a highly select population, we were concerned that they might not apply to all CF heterozygotes. However, we found a higher prevalence of wheezing among 314 unselected CF heterozygotes than among 162 unselected control parents of children with congenital heart disease (Davis et al., 1984). This difference was not explained by age, sex, or cigarette habits. Although it is possible that the CF heterozygotes are more attuned to respiratory symptoms because of their child's disease, respiratory symptoms other than wheeze were not more prevalent in CF parents, so generalized overreporting of lung symptoms by CF parents seems unlikely. Moreover, among those who had never smoked, CF heterozygotes who reported wheeze had significantly poorer FEV_1 and $FEF_{25\text{-}75\%}$ than those who denied wheezing, providing some objective validation of the subjective complaint (Fig. 4). The prevalence of wheezing in the population in this

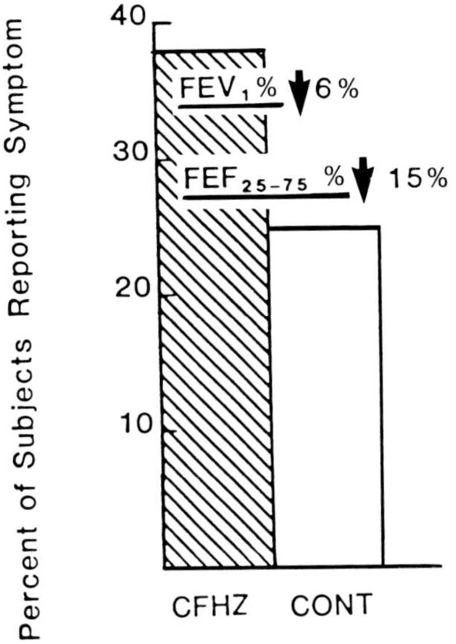

Figure 4 Among patients who had never smoked, more CF parents reported wheezing. CF heterozygotes who reported wheeze had significantly poorer FEV_1 and $FEF_{25\text{-}75\%}$ than controls who reported wheezing.

study cannot be directly linked with abnormal autonomic reactivity, since no measures of autonomic function were made. A causal relationship cannot be inferred. Nevertheless, this study shows that a population with high prevalence of autonomic dysfunction also has high prevalence of airway reactivity and its associated symptoms. Taken together, these data provide experimental support for the association of autonomic and airway reactivity shown in Figure 3.

Additional evidence for the importance of autonomic responsiveness in airway reactivity comes from the effects of manipulation of autonomic systems on airway reactivity. In asthmatics, beta-adrenergic agonists reduce airway reactivity (Boushey et al., 1980). Viral infection results in reduced beta-adrenergic responses and a coordinated increase in airway reactivity (Busse, 1977; Buckner et al., 1981; Empey et al., 1976). For some test stimuli, atropine (a cholinergic blocker) reduces airway reactivity (Sheppard et al., 1983; Simonsson et al., 1967). In subjects with airway reactivity or preexisting airways obstruction, beta-adrenergic blockade worsens airways obstruction (Grieco and Pierson, 1971).

In animal models there is also a relation between autonomic responses and airway reactivity. Basenji greyhounds, with highly reactive airways but normal resting pulmonary function, who have never received medication, have reduced beta-adrenergic responses (Hirschman, 1983). Moreover, the bronchoconstrictive response to *Ascaris* antigen in greyhounds correlates with beta-adrenergic responses of isolated bronchial smooth muscle in vitro (Rinard et al., 1985a). An excellent predictor of in vivo methacholine bronchial reactivity in these dogs is the imbalance between in vitro responses of smooth muscle to methacholine and isoproterenol. The combination of increased cholinergic response *and* reduced beta-adrenergic response is a better predictor of in vivo airway reactivity than either autonomic aberration alone (Rinard et al., 1985b). Dogs with experimentally induced asthma display increased alpha-adrenergic receptor sites and decreased beta-adrenergic receptors. Studies on other animals also reinforce this link. Rats bred for cholinergic sensitivity develop airway reactivity. Guinea pigs whose airways are reactive to histamine or methacholine in vivo have reduced sensitivity of airway smooth muscle to beta agents in vitro (Douglas et al., 1977).

However, association does not necessarily imply causation. Although it makes sense that autonomic dysfunction might produce airway reactivity, it might also be that airway reactivity somehow causes a change in the "set point" of the autonomic nervous system. Alternatively, a factor quite separate from the airway or the autonomic nervous system might perturb both in a coordinated fashion. For example, inflammation and/or infection may be associated with both increased airway reactivity and autonomic dysfunction, or airways obstruction itself may predispose to increased airway reactivity as well as altered autonomic responses (Fig. 3). However, mounting evidence on the time course of development of airway reactivity and inflammation following inhaled irritant exposure, and studies of induced airway reactivity in leukocyte-depleted animals, indicate that leukocyte accumulation may follow and not cause airway reactivity.

Autonomic dysfunction alone cannot account for the lung disease of either asthma or CF. Some patients with CF have no apparent autonomic dysfunction (Davis et al., 1980a, 1978), so autonomic abnormalities are not necessary for CF to occur. Conversely, some asymptomatic CF heterozygotes have autonomic dysfunction as great as that of patients (Davis, 1984), so autonomic abnormalities are not sufficient for the CF disease state to develop. Moreover, allergic asthmatic subjects have a similar pattern of abnormal autonomic responses to CF (Kaliner et al., 1982). Although asthma and CF share such features as obstructive airways disease, mucus hypersecretion, airway reactivity, a high prevalence of atopy, and involvement of the upper airway, they are clinically quite distinct. However, our recent data suggest that although the functional abnormalities in CF and asthma are the same, their biochemical bases probably differ, at least in the beta-adrenergic system. Though autonomic dysfunction of appropriate pattern may be associated with airway reactivity, airway reactivity to methacholine, even of substantial degree, does not necessarily define disease.

B. Extrapulmonary Implications

Cystic fibrosis is a systemic disorder that affects the airways, and so it is not surprising that there is derangement of physiological processes outside of the lung. In fact, CF has been described as a "generalized exocrinopathy" or a "generalized epitheliopathy." Autonomic dysfunction in CF could contribute to the abnormalities, not only in the lungs, but also in salivary glands, pancreas, the gut, and the sweat glands. The presence of autonomic regulatory systems in most organs affected by CF makes the hypothesis that autonomic dysfunction contributes to the disease attractive (Davis and Kaliner, 1983). Indeed, lesions resembling those seen in CF can be created in animals by the administration of autonomic-active agents. However, the variety of agents that are effective (isoproterenol, reserpine, atropine, pilocarpine) and the high dosages in which they are administered make it difficult to ascribe CF-like lesions unambiguously to a particular perturbation of the autonomic nervous system. Even if such an association could be made, creation of lesions in animals by one mechanism does not necessarily mean that the human lesion arises in the same way. However, if there is general autonomic dysfunction in CF, nonexocrine systems traditionally considered to be under autonomic control should also function abnormally in CF. In CF patients in good to excellent condition with normal plasma catecholamine levels, blood pressure is significantly lower than in age-matched controls (Lake et al., 1979; Lieberman and Rodbard, 1975), the increase in pulse from supine to standing posture is reduced (Lake et al., 1979), and pupillary dilation in darkness or in response to pain is less (Davis et al., 1980a; Rubin et al., 1966). Respiratory heart rate variability is increased, and the postural change in low-frequency (baroreceptor-mediated) heart rate variability is reduced in CF patients. Therefore, widespread autonomic imbalance exists in the absence of pharmacologic perturbation in CF, and this suggests that autonomic imbalance is pervasive, and not limited to exocrine glands. Cardiovascular responses have not been evaluated in CF heterozygotes, but pupillary dilation in darkness is reduced in this population as well (Davis, 1984).

Asthma, on the other hand, has usually not been considered a systemic disorder, except for secondary effects of stress or hypoxia, or perhaps manifestation of the atopic state (in affected patients) in other organs. However, demonstration of autonomic dysfunction at extrapulmonary sites upon pharmacologic stimulation suggests that perhaps subtle physiological abnormalities exist outside the lung as well. We have found that the pupillary excursion between constriction in light and dilation in darkness is reduced in asthmatics (Davis, 1986b). There is some suggestion that premature birth may be a risk for pregnant mothers with increased airway reactivity; it has been suggested that irritability of both bronchial and uterine smooth muscle, for whatever reason, might occur together (Bertrand et al., 1985). Since autonomic dysfunction in asthma extends beyond the lung itself, subtle abnormalities in many organ systems may be expected. However, thus far it is difficult to distinguish the possibilities that autonomic dysfunction is generalized in asthma, or that an abnormal ability of the smooth muscle system to respond is present.

IV. Directions for Future Research

The notion that autonomic dysfunction may be a preexisting (congenital or acquired) risk factor for development of airway reactivity and/or obstructive airways disease has some appeal. If true, this hypothesis has both theoretical and practical implications. Such a risk factor could conceivably be identified early in life and, because of the extensive available autonomic-active pharmacopeia, might be modifiable. However, proof of a causal relationship between autonomic dysfunction and airway reactivity will be necessary before such hypothesis can be accepted. If quick noninvasive unambiguous assessments of autonomic function could be devised, subjects with autonomic dysfunction could be identified early in life and evaluated to determine the fate of their airways. Less demanding and lengthy approaches to the problem of assigning causal relationships may be possible, however, by using drugs that change airway reactivity and determining autonomic reactivity and vice versa, or identifying new subject populations in whom contamination of results by drugs or disease does not occur. The CF heterozygote population may be especially useful in this regard.

Since the results in CF suggest that there is a heritable component of autonomic response (although it may not track with the CF gene itself), another interesting question is the heritability of autonomic dysfunction. Studies in CF families may be confounded by difficulties in interpreting results of tests of autonomic function in severely ill, medicated patients. Families of asthmatics offer an alternative. Asthma runs in families, and increased airway reactivity occurs frequently in the families of asthmatic patients (Godfrey and Konig, 1975; Konig and Godfrey, 1973a,b). Families of allergic asthmatic children could be examined for autonomic function and airway reactivity, and the nature of their inheritance determined by path analysis. Information about the nature of inheritance of autonomic traits might allow us to identify persons at high risk for autonomic dysfunction and/or airways disease by their relation to an identified patient.

It would be useful to know whether altering autonomic systems affects the development and/or progression of obstructive airways disease. While it is already clear that blocking homeostatic adjustment mechanisms (e.g., by beta-adrenergic blockade) can exacerbate preexisting airways disease, it is not clear that stimulating beta-adrenergic receptors or blocking cholinergic transmission will prevent or delay development or progression of airways disease. A multicenter trial, now in progress, of the effects of cholinergic blockade on the course of chronic obstructive pulmonary disease will address this question. However, the issue remains for asthma and CF, and even for asymptomatic individuals with marked autonomic dysfunction.

It is critical to assess the function of autonomic receptor systems in the tissues of interest (human bronchial smooth muscle, blood vessels, airway epithelial cells, secretory cells, the nerves themselves, ganglia, and bronchial mast cells) in healthy and diseased subjects. If autonomic dysfunction has meaning for lung disease, it must occur in the lung itself. Inaccessibility and complexity of tissue have limited such studies so far. Tissue is available only at surgery or autopsy, which procedures are performed for cause under uncontrolled conditions, and may yield damaged tissues. Techniques of separating some of these cell types and maintaining them in culture, remote from the effects of drugs and disease, and with opportunity to recover, may help to solve this problem. In fact, tracheal epithelial cells recovered from brush biopsy specimens during fiberoptic bronchoscopy may be suitable for culture, permitting sampling of epithelial cells from healthy persons as well as patients in varying stages of disease. However, it would be optimal to have all of the potential regulatory and effector cells (smooth muscle, mucous and serous cells, epithelial cells, and blood vessel as well) isolated for examination of their regulatory systems.

Finally, little is known of the nonclassic autonomic regulators in airways disease. Purinergic, peptidergic, and other systems may contribute to the development of airways obstruction. Indeed, Heinz-Erian and co-workers (1985) have proposed that CF may be a disorder associated with functional deficit of the action of VIP. Much more needs to be known about the normal regulatory functions and importance of these systems as well as their role in the pathophysiology of disease.

Discussion

Wanner. In the CF heterozygotes who have autonomic abnormalities, are there any clinical effects?

Davis. They are asymptomatic, but in a questionnaire CF heterozygotes admit to asthma twice as frequently as controls, although with the small numbers of subjects this does not reach statistical significance.

Kaliner. In CF heterozygotes is there any correlation between wheezing and autonomic abnormalities?

Davis. Increased airway responsiveness was correlated with a reduced cyclic AMP response to isoproterenol in lymphocytes.

Barnes. Is there any relationship between the degree of autonomic abnormality and the degree of bronchial responsiveness in asthmatic patients?

Davis. Pupillary cholinergic responsiveness ($r = 0.45$, $p < 0.05$) and pupillary alpha-adrenergic responsiveness ($r = 0.35$, $p < 0.05$) are significantly related to airway reactivity. Whether both change concomitantly, spontaneously, or with therapy has not been studied.

Vanhoutte. If this generalized augmented responsiveness of alpha-receptors and cholinergic receptors were to occur at a presynaptic level, this would tend to offset changes in bronchial smooth muscle responsiveness.

Davis. A reduced function of beta-receptors in cholinergic nerves would enhance bronchoconstriction. The interaction of different components of the autonomic nervous system at a presynaptic level may account for the pattern of autonomic dysfunction (i.e., that abnormalities of different components of the autonomic system tend to occur together).

References

Aarons, R. D., Nies, A. S., Gal, J., et al. (1980). Elevation of beta-adrenergic receptor density in human lymphocytes after propranolol administration. *J. Clin. Invest.* **65**:949-957.

Anthracite, R. L., Vachon, L., and Knapp, P. H. (1971). Alpha adrenergic receptors in the human lung. *Psychosom. Med.* **33**:481-488.

Apold, J., and Aksnes, L. (1977). Correlation between increased bronchial responsiveness to histamine and diminished plasma cyclic adenosine monophosphate response after epinephrine in asthmatic children. *J. Allergy Clin. Immunol.* **59**:343-347.

Arnup, M. E., et al. (1983). Effects of cold air hyperpnea in patients with chronic obstructive lung disease. *Am. Rev. Respir. Dis.* **128**:236-239.

Barnes, P. J., Brown, M. J., Silverman, M., and Dollery, C. T. (1981a). Circulatory catecholamines in exercise and hyperventilation-induced asthma. *Thorax* **36**:435-440.

Barnes, P. J., Ind, P. W., and Dollery, C. T. (1981b). Inhaled prazosin in asthma. *Thorax* **36**:378-381.

Beil, M., and de Kock, M. A. (1978). Role of alpha-adrenergic receptors in exercise induced bronchoconstriction. *Respiration* **35**:78-86.

Bertrand, J., Riley, S. P., Popkin, J., and Coates, A. L. (1985). The long-term pulmonary sequelae of prematurity: the role of familial airway hyperreactivity and the respiratory distress syndrome. *N. Engl. J. Med.* **312**:742-745.

Bianco, S., Griffin, J. P., Kamburoff, P. L., and Prime, F. J. (1972). The effect of thymoxamine on histamine induced bronchospasm in man. *Br. J. Dis Chest* **66**:27-32.

Bianco, S., Griffin, J. P., Jamburoff, P. H., and Prime, F. J. (1974). Prevention of exercise induced asthma by indoramin. *Br. Med. J.* **4**:18-20.

Black, J. L., Temple, D. M., and Anderson, S. D. (1978). Longterm trial of an alpha-adrenoreceptor blocking drugs (Indoramin) in asthma. *Scand. J. Respir. Dis.* **59**:307-312.

Boushey, H. A., et al. (1980). Bronchial hyperreactivity. *Am. Rev. Respir. Dis.* **121**:389-413.

Breslin, F. J., McFadden, E. R., Jr., Ingram, R. H., Jr., and Deal, E. D., Jr. (1980). Effects of atropine on respiratory heat loss in asthma. *J. Appl. Physiol.* **48**: 619-623.

Buchwald, M., and Mapleson, J. L. (1977). Adenosine 3′:5′ cyclic AMP in fibroblasts from patients with cystic fibrosis and its relationship to secretion. *Mod. Probl. Paediatr.* **19**:165-174.

Buckner, C. K., Clayton, D. E., Ain Shoka, A. A., Busse, W. W., Dick, E. C., Dick, E. C., and Shult, P. (1981). Para-influenza 3 infection blocks the ability of a beta-adrenergic receptor agonist to inhibit antigen-induced contraction of guinea pig isolated airway smooth muscle. *J. Clin. Invest.* **67**:376-384.

Busse, W. W. (1977). Decreased granulocyte response to isoproterenol in asthma during upper respiratory infection. *Am. Rev. Respir. Dis.* **115**:783-791.

Busse, W. W., and Lee, T. P. (1976). Decreased adrenergic responses on lymphocytes and granulocytes in atopic eczema. *J Allergy Clin. Immunol.* **58**:586-596.

Byard, P. J., and Davis, P. B. (1986). Heterogeneity in autonomic responses among obligate heterozygotes in cystic fibrosis (abstr.). Abstracts 7th Intl. Cong. Hum. Genet., p. 736.

Campbell, I. A., and Dyson, A. J. (1977). Indoramin, an alpha-adrenoreceptor antagonist for airway obstruction. *Br. J. Dis. Chest* **71**:105-108.

Casale, T. B., and Kaliner, M. (1984). Demonstration that circulating human blood cells have no detectable alpha-adrenergic receptors by radioligand binding analysis. *J. Allergy Clin. Immunol.* **74**:812.

Cavanaugh, M. J., and Cooper, D. M. (1976). Inhaled atropine sulfate: dose-response characteristics. *Am. Rev. Respir. Dis.* **114**:517-524.

Cerrina, J., Ladurie, M. L., Labat, C., Bayol, A., Raffestin, B., Benveniste, J., and Brink, C. (1985). The effects of contractile and relaxant agonists on bronchial muscle (BM) derived from asthmatic and non-asthmatic patients. *Am. Rev. Respir. Dis.* **131**:A275.

Conolly, M. E., and Greenacre, J. K. (1976). The lymphocyte beta-adrenoceptor in normal subjects and patients with bronchial asthma. *J. Clin. Invest.* **58**: 1307-1316.

Cropp, G. J. A. (1975). The role of the parasympathetic nervous system in the maintenance of chronic airway obstruction in asthmatic children. *Am. Rev. Respir. Dis.* **112**:599-605.

Davies, A. O., and Lefkowitz, R. J. (1980). Corticosteroid-induced differential regulation of beta-adrenergic receptors in circulating human polymorphonuclear leukocytes and mononuclear leukocytes. *J. Clin. Endocrinol. Metab.* **51**:599-603.

Davis, P. B. (1980). Plasma factors do not account for the leukocyte beta-adrenergic defect in cystic fibrosis. *IRCS Med. Sci.* **8**:413.

Davis, P. B. (1984). Autonomic and airway reactivity in obligate heterozygotes for cystic fibrosis. *Am. Rev. Respir. Dis.* **127**:911-914.

Davis, P. B. (1986a). Alpha-adrenergic receptors in circulating cells. *J. Allergy Clin. Immunol.* 77:769.

Davis, P. B. (1986b). Pupillary responses and airway reactivity in asthma. *J. Allergy Clin. Immunol.* **77**:667-672.

Davis, P. B., and Kaliner, M. (1983). Autonomic nervous system abnormalities in cystic fibrosis. *J. Chron. Dis.* **36**:269-278.

Davis, P. B., and Lieberman, P. (1982). Normal alpha$_2$-adrenergic responses in platelets from subjects with asthma. *J. Allergy Clin. Immunol.* **69**:35.

Davis, P. B., Braunstein, M., and Jay, C. (1978). Decreased adenosine 3′:5′ cyclic monophosphate response to isoproterenol in cystic fibrosis leukocytes. *Pediatr. Res.* **12**:703-707.

Davis, P. B., Shelhamer, J., and Kaliner, M. (1980a). Abnormal adrenergic and cholinergic sensitivity in cystic fibrosis. *N. Engl. J. Med.* **302**:1453-1456.

Davis, P. B., Laundon, S. C., and Ulane, M. M. (1980b). Hormone-stimulated cyclic AMP production by skin fibroblasts cultured from healthy persons and patients with cystic fibrosis. *Pediatr. Res.* **14**:863-868.

Davis, P. B., Dieckman, L., Boat, T. F., et al. (1983). Beta-adrenergic receptors in lymphocytes and granulocytes from patients with cystic fibrosis. *J. Clin. Invest.* **71**:1787-1795.

Davis, P. B., Dieckman, L., Boat, T. F., et al. (1984a). The alpha$_2$-adrenergic system of the platelet in cystic fibrosis. *Am. J. Med. Sci.* **288**:104-108.

Davis, P. B., et al. (1984b). Chest symptoms in obligate heterozygotes for cystic fibrosis. *Clin. Res.* **32**:767A.

Davis, P. B., Paget, G. L., and Turi, V. (1985). Alpha-adrenergic responses in asthma. *J. Lab. Clin. Med.* **105**:164-169.

Davis, P. B., Simpson, D. M., Paget, G. L., and Turi, V. (1986). Beta-adrenergic responses in drug-free asthmatic subjects. *J. Allergy Clin. Immunol.* **77**: 871-879.

Day, G., and Mearns, M. R. (1973). Bronchial lability in cystic fibrosis. *Arch. Dis. Child.* **48**:355-359.

Deal, E. C., McFadden, E. R., Jr., Ingram, R. H., et al. (1980). Airway responsiveness to cold air and hyperpnea in normal subjects and in those with hay fever and asthma. *Am. Rev. Respir. Dis.* **121**:621-628.

Douglas, V. S., Ridgway, P., and Brink, C. (1977). Airway responses of the guinea pig in vivo and in vitro. *J. Pharmacol. Exp. Ther.* **202**:116-124.

Empey, D. W., Laitinen, L. A., Jacobs, L., et al. (1976). Mechanisms of bronchial hyperreactivity in normal subjects after upper respiratory infection. *Am. Rev. Respir. Dis.* **113**:131-139.

Fish, J. E., Rosenthal, R. R., Summer, W. R., Menkes, A., Norman, P. S., and

Permutt, S. (1977). The effect of atropine on acute antigen-mediated airway constriction in subjects with allergic asthma. *Am. Rev. Respir. Dis.* **115**:371-379.

Fraser, J., Nadeau, J., Robertson, D., et al. (1981). Regulation of human leukocyte beta receptors by endogenous catecholamine. Relationship of leukocyte beta receptor density to the cardiac sensitivity to isoproterenol. *J. Clin. Invest.* **67**:1777-1784.

Gaddie, J., Legges, J. S., Petrie, G., and Palmer, K. N. (1972). The effect of an alpha-adrenergic receptor blocking drug on histamine sensitivity in bronchial asthma. *Br. J. Dis. Chest.* **66**:141-146.

Galant, S. P., and Allred, S. (1981). Binding and functional characteristics of beta-adrenergic receptors in the intact neutrophil. *J. Lab. Clin. Med.* **98**: 227-237.

Galant, S. P., Duriseti, L., Underwood, S., et al. (1980). Beta-adrenergic receptors of polymorphonuclear particulates in bronchial asthma. *J. Clin. Invest.* **65**:577-585.

Galant, S. P., Norton, L., Herbst, J., and Wood, C. (1981). Impaired beta-adrenergic receptor binding and function in cystic fibrosis neutrophils. *J. Clin. Invest.* **68**:253-258.

Gerrard, J. W. et al. (1980). Increased nonspecific bronchial reactivity in cigarette smokers with normal lung function. *Am. Rev. Respir. Dis.* **122**:577-581.

Godfrey, S., and Konig, P. (1975). Exercise induced bronchial lability in wheezy children and their families. *Pediatrics* **56** (Suppl.):851-856.

Goodman, L. S., and Gilman, A. (1975). *The Pharmacological Basis of Therapeutics.* New York, Macmillan, p. 367.

Grieco, M. T., and Pierson, R. N. (1971). Mechanism of bronchoconstriction due to beta-adrenergic blockade. *J. Allergy Clin. Immunol.* **48**:143-152.

Haluzka, J., and Scislichi, A. (1975). Bronchial lability in children suffering from diseases of the bronchi. *Respiration* **32**:217-226.

Harper, S., and Quinton, P. M. (1984). Adrenergic and cholinergic stimulation of sweat glands in cystic fibrosis. *CF Club Abstracts,* **25**:169.

Heinz-Erian, P., Dey, R. D., Paul, S., Flux, M., and Said, S. I. (1985). Deficient vasoactive intestinal peptide innervation in sweat glands of cystic fibrosis pattients. *Science* **229**:1407-1408.

Henderson, W. R., Shelhamer, J. H., Reingold, D. B., et al. (1979). Alpha-adrenergic hyperresponsiveness in asthma. *N. Engl. J. Med.* **300**:642.

Hirschman, C. A. (1983). Bronchial inhalation challenge testing in dog models of asthma. In *Provocative Challenge Procedures; Bronchial Oral and Exercise.* Vol. II. Edited by S. L. Spector. Boca Raton, Florida, CRC Press, pp. 13-32.

Hodapp, E., Kolker, A. E., Kass, M. A., Goldberg, I., Becker, B., and Gordon, M.

(1981). The effect of topical clonidine on intraocular pressure. *Arch. Ophthalmol.* **99**:1208.

Hoffman, B. B., and Lefkowitz, R. J. (1980). Alpha-adrenergic receptor subtypes. *N. Engl. J. Med.* **302**:1390.

Hokin, L. E., Hokin, M. R., and Lobeck, C. C. (1963). Effects of acetylcholine on incorporation of P into phospholipids in slices of skin from children with and without cystic fibrosis of pancreas. *J. Clin. Invest.* **42**:1232-1237.

Holzel, A., Schwarz, V., Torkington, P., and Williams, G. E. G. (1962). Mucoviscidosis and the autonomic nervous system. *Lancet* **1**:822-823.

Ignarro, L. J., Lint, T. F., and George, W. J. (1974). Hormonal control of lysosomal enzyme release from human neutrophils. *J. Exp. Med.* **139**:1395-1414.

Ind, P. W., Carson, R. C., and Barnes, P. J. (1984). Plasma catecholamine in acute severe asthma and antigen-induced bronchoconstriction. *Clin. Sci.* **67**:34-35.

Kaliner, M. (1976). The cholinergic nervous system and immediate hypersensitivity. I. Eccrine sweat responses in allergic patients. *J. Allergy Clin. Immunol.* **58**:308-315.

Kaliner, M., Orange, R. P., and Austen, K. F. (1972). Immunological release of histamine and slow reacting substance of anaphylaxis from human lung. IV. Enhancement by cholinergic and alpha-adrenergic stimulation. *J. Exp. Med.* **136**:556-567.

Kaliner, M., Shelhamer, J., Smith, L., Davis, P. B., et al. (1982). NIH Conference. Autonomic abnormalities and allergy. *Ann. Intern. Med.* **96**:349-357.

Kerr, J. W., Govindoraj, M., and Patel, K. R. (1970). Effect of alpha-receptor blocking drugs and disodium cromoglycate on histamine hypersensitivity in bronchial asthma. *Br. Med. J.* **2**:139-141.

Knowles, M. R., Gatzy, J., and Boucher, R. (1983a). Modulation of nasal epithelial ion permeability in normal and CF subjects in vivo. *Clin. Res.* **31**:858A.

Knowles, M., Stutts, M., Spock, A., Fischer, J., Gatzy, J., and Boucher, R. (1983b). Abnormal ion permeation through cystic fibrosis respiratory epithelium. *Science* **221**:1067-1070.

Konig, P., and Godfrey, S. (1973a). Prevalence of exercise-induced bronchial lability in families of children with asthma. *Arch. Dis. Child.* **48**:513-516.

Konig, P., and Godfrey, S. (1973b). Exercise-induced bronchial lability and atopic status of families of infants with wheezy bronchitis. *Arch. Dis. Child.* **48**:942-946.

Lake, C. R., Davis, P. B., Ziegler, M., and Kopin, I. (1979). Electrolytes and norepinephrine levels in blood of patients with cystic fibrosis. *Clin. Chim. Acta* **92**:141-146.

Larsen, G. L., Barron, R. J., Cotton, E. K., and Brooks, J. G. (1979). A comparative study of inhaled atropine sulfate and isoproterenol hydrochloride in cystic fibrosis. *Am. Rev. Respir. Dis.* **119**:399-407.

Larsson, K. (1985). Striders of sympatho-adrenal reactivity and adrenoceptor function in bronchial asthma. *Eur. J. Respir. Dis.* (Suppl.) **141**:21-53.

Lee, T. P., Busse, W. W., and Reed, C. E. (1977). Effect of beta-adrenergic agonists, prostaglandin, and cortisol on lymphocyte levels of cyclic adenosine monophosphate and glycogen. *J. Allergy Clin. Immunol.* **59**:408-413.

Lemanske, R. F., Anderson, C., Braun, S., Skatrud, J., and Busse, W. W. (1980). Impaired in vitro beta-adrenergic granulocyte response in chronic obstructive pulmonary disease. *Am. Rev. Respir. Dis.* **122**:213-219.

Lemanske, R. F., Mischler, E. H., Farrell, P. M., Anderson, C., and Busse, W. E. (1981). Analysis of granulocyte beta-adrenergic response in cystic fibrosis: correlation of decreased responsiveness with disease severity. *Am. Rev. Respir. Dis.* **123**:622-626.

Lieberman, J., and Rodbard, S. (1975). Low blood pressure in young adults with cystic fibrosis. An effect of chronic salt loss in sweat? *Ann. Intern. Med.* **82**:806-808.

Makino, S., Oulette, J. J., Reed, C. E., et al. (1970). Correlation between increased bronchial response to acetylcholine and diminished metabolic and eosinopenic responses to epinephrine in asthma. *J. Allergy Clin. Immunol.* **46**:178-186.

Makino, S., Ikemori, K., Kashima, T., et al. (1977). Comparison of cyclic adenosine monophosphate response of lymphocytes in normal and asthmatic subjects to norepinephrine and salbutamol. *J. Allergy Clin. Immunol.* **59**:348-352.

Malo, J. L., et al. (1982). Bronchial responsiveness to inhaled methacholine in young asymptomatic smokers. *J. Appl. Physiol.* **52**:1404-1470.

Marmar, J., Barbero, G. J., and Sibinga, M. S. (1966). The pattern of parotid gland secretion in cystic fibrosis of the pancreas. *Gastroenterology* **50**:551-556.

Mathe, A. A., Astrom, A., and Persson, N. A. (1981). Some bronchoconstricting and bronchodilating responses of human isolated bronchi: evidence for the existence of alpha-adenoreceptors. *J. Pharm. Pharmacol.* **23**:905.

Mitchell, I., et al. (1978). Bronchial hypersensitivity in cystic fibrosis and asthma. *J. Pediatr.* **93**:744-748.

Morris, H. G., Rusnak, S. A., Selner, J. C., et al. (1977). Adrenergic desensitization in leukocytes of normal and asthmatic subjects. *J. Cyclic Nucl. Res.* **3**:439-446.

Nadel, J. A. (1977). Autonomic control of airway smooth muscle and airway secretions. *Am. Rev. Respir. Dis.* **115**:117-126.

Neutra, M. R., Grand, R. J., and Trier, J. S. (1977). Glycoprotein synthesis, transport, and secretion by epithelial cells of human rectal mucosa: normal and cystic fibrosis. *Lab. Invest.* **36**:535-546.

Orange, R. P., Kaliner, M. A., La Raia, P. J., et al. (1971). Immunological release of histamine and slow reacting substance of anaphylaxis from human lung II. Influence of cellular levels of cyclic AMP. *Fed. Proc.* **30**: 1725-1729.

Orehek, J., Gayrard, P., Smith, A. P., Grimaud, C., and Chapkin, J. (1977). Airway response to carbachol in normal and asthmatic subjects. *Am. Rev. Respir. Dis.* **115**:937-942.

Passamonte, P. M., and Martinez, A. J. (1984). Effect of inhaled atropine or metaproterenol in patients with chronic airway obstruction and therapeutic serum theophylline levels. *Chest* **85**:610-615.

Patel, K. R., and Kerr, J. W. (1973). The airways response to phenylephrine after blockade of alpha and beta receptors in extrinsic bronchial asthma. *Clin. Allergy* **3**:439-448.

Ramsdale, E. H., Morris, M. M., Roberts, R. S., and Hargreave, F. E. (1984). Bronchial responsiveness to methacholine in chronic bronchitis: relationship to airflow obstruction and cold air responsiveness. *Thorax* **39**:912-918.

Rinard, G. A., Puckett, A. M., Jensen, A. D., Minneman, K. L., Torphy, T. J., and Mayer, S. E. (1985a). Pulmonary hyperreactivity of greyhound dogs to methacholine is related to beta-adrenergic-cholinergic sensitivity imbalance of airway smooth muscle. *Am. Rev. Respir. Dis.* **131**:A340.

Rinard, G. A., Torphy, T. J., Jensen, A. D., Puckett, A. M., Minneman, K. L., and Mayer, S. E. (1985b). Pulmonary reactivity to ascaris in inversely related to tracheal smooth muscle beta receptor density and isoproterenol sensitivity, responsiveness and cyclic AMP dependent protein kinase in greyhound dogs. *Am. Rev. Respir. Dis.* **131**:A340.

Roscher, A. A., Schmid, A. J., Hadorn, B., and Weismann, U. (1980). Enhanced adenosine 3′:5′-monophosphate response to beta-adrenergic stimulation in cystic fibrosis fibroblasts after removal of conditioned medium. *Pediatr. Res.* **14**:261-265.

Rubin, L. S., Barbero, G. J., and Chernick, W. S. (1966). Pupillary dysfunction as a concomitant of cystic fibrosis. *Pediatrics* **38**:865-873.

Sano, Y., Begley, M., Watt, G., et al. (1981). Disease and sex difference in leukocyte beta-adrenergic receptors. *Am. Rev. Respir. Dis.* **123**:55.

Sato, K., and Sato, F. (1984). Defective beta-adrenergic response of cystic fibrosis sweat glands in vivo and in vitro. *J. Clin. Invest.* **73**:1763-1771.

Scheid, C. R., Honeyman, T. W., and Fay, F. S. (1979). Mechanism of beta-adrenergic relaxation of smooth muscle. *Nature* **277**:32-36.

Schreurs, A. J. M., and Nijkamp, F. P. (1982). Hemophilus influenza induced loss of lung-adrenoceptor binding sites and modulation by changes in peripheral catecholaminergic input. *Eur. J. Pharmacol.* **47**:95-102.

Shelhamer, J., Marom, Z., and Kaliner, M. (1980a). Immunologic and neuropharmacologic stimulation of mucous glycoprotein release from human airways in vitro. *J. Clin. Invest.* **66**:1400-1408.

Shelhamer, J. H., Metcalf, D. D., Smith, L. J., et al. (1980b). Abnormal beta-adrenergic responsiveness in allergic subjects: analysis of isoproterenol-induced cardiovascular and plasma cAMP responses. *J. Allergy Clin. Immunol.* **66**:52-60.

Sheppard, D., Epstein, J., Holtzman, M. J., Nadel, J. A., and Boushey, H. A. (1983). Effect of route of atropine delivery on bronchospasm from cold air and methacholine. *J. Appl. Physiol.* **54**(1):130-133.

Sibinga, M. S., and Barbero, G. J. (1961). Studies in physiology of sweating in cystic fibrosis I. Experimental sweat gland fatigue. *Pediatrics* **27**:912-920.

Simonsson, B. G., Jacobs, F. M., and Nadel, J. A. (1967). Role of autonomic nervous system and the cough reflex in the increased responsiveness of airways in patients with obstructive airway disease. *J. Clin. Invest.* **46**: 1812-1818.

Simpson, D. S., and Davis, P. B. (1985). Isoproterenol infusion recruits compensatory vagal activity. *Clin. Res.* **33**:288A.

Smith, L. J., Shelhamer, J. H., and Kaliner, M. (1980). Cholinergic nervous system and immediate hypersensitivity. *J. Allergy Clin. Immunol.* **66**:374-378.

Snashall, P. D., Boother, F. A., and Sterling, G. M. (1978). The effect of alpha-adrenoceptor stimulation on the airways of normal and asthmatic man. *Clin. Sci. Mol. Med.* **54**:283-289.

Stiles, G. L., Caron, M. G., and Lefkowitz, R. J. (1984). Beta-adrenergic receptors: biochemical mechanisms of physiological regulation. *Physiol. Rev.* **64**:661-743.

Sturgess, J., and Reid, L. (1972). An organ culture study of the effect of drugs on the secretory activity of the human bronchial submucosal gland. *Clin. Sci.* **43**:533-543.

Szentivanyi, A. (1968). The beta-adrenergic theory of the atopic abnormality in bronchial asthma. *J. Allergy* **42**:203-209.

Tashkin, D. P., Conolly, M. E., Deutsch, R. I., et al. (1982). Subsensitization of beta-adrenoceptors in airways and lymphocytes of healthy and asthmatic subjects. *Am. Rev. Respir. Dis.* **125**:185-193.

Tiffeneau, R. (1955). L'hyperexacetabilitie acetylcholinique de poumon: critère physio-pharmacodynamique de la maladie asthmatique. *Presse Med.* **63**:227-233.

Van Asperen, P., et al. (1981). Bronchial reactivity in cystic fibrosis with normal pulmonary function. *Am. J. Dis. Child.* **135**:815-819.

Venter, J. C., Fraser, C. M., and Harrison, L. C. (1980). Auto-antibodies to $beta_2$-adrenergic receptors: a possible cause of adrenergic hyporesponsiveness in allergic rhinitis and asthma. *Science* **207**:1361-1363.

Weiss, S. T. (1984). Increased levels of airways responsiveness as a risk factor for development of chronic obstructive lung disease. *Chest* **86**:3-4.

Zurier, R. B., Weissman, C., Hoffstein, S., Kammerman, S., and Tai, H. A. (1974). Mechanism of lysosomal enzyme release from human leukocytes. II. Effects of cAMP and cGMP, autonomic agonists and agents which affect microtubular function. *J. Clin. Invest.* **53**:279-309.

6

Adrenergic Agonists in Asthma

JEAN BOUSQUET, ANNE-MARIE CLAUZEL, and FRANÇOIS-BERNARD MICHEL

Centre Hospitalier Universitaire
Montpellier, France

Beta-2 agonists are widely used and in many countries they represent the most common treatment for asthma. Their action is the result of sympathomimetic effects on lung tissues. Initially, they were used as purely bronchodilating agents but, based on their ability to decrease the release of inflammatory mediators from mast cells, they also tend to be prescribed as prophylactic drugs.

Side effects were important with initial products that differed only slightly from endogenous catecholamines. The introduction of less specific beta$_2$-agonists was apparently associated with the rise in asthma deaths in certain countries in the 1960s (Inman and Adelstein, 1969; Campbell, 1976). After the demonstration that bronchial adrenoceptors were mainly of the beta-2 subtype (Lands et al., 1967), more recently synthesized drugs are beta-2-selective and the rate of side effects has decreased. One unresolved problem remains tachyphylaxis, initially reported by Herxheimer (1946); however, its real importance is not yet fully determined.

I. Basic Pharmacology

A. Adrenoceptors of the Airways

All the tissues involved in the pathophysiology of asthma are well supplied with adrenoceptors even though they do not appear, at least in humans, to possess any sympathetic nerve endings. In 1967, Lands et al. proposed the division of beta receptors into beta-1 and beta-2, each mediating different activities. They found different receptors in different organs; beta-1 was present in the heart, adipose tissue, and small intestine, whereas beta-2 receptors were found in the airways, peripheral vascular tissue, and skeletal muscle. However, recent studies indicate that beta-1 receptors are also found in the airways but their exact role still remains to be elucidated. Adrenoceptors increase from the proximal to the distal airways. In the trachea, 70-80% of them are from the beta-1 subtype whereas in the periphery of the lung beta-2 adrenoceptors predominate. The number of alpha adrenoceptors is equal to that of beta adrenoceptors (Barnes et al., 1982).

In humans, beta adrenoceptors of the airways are localized in bronchial smooth muscle, blood vessels, mucous glands, epithelial cells, and pneumocytes II. They are also distributed to blood vessels, mucous glands, and to a wide variety of cells involved in the allergic and nonallergic inflammation of the bronchi such as mast cells and macrophages.

In asthma, it was suggested in 1968 by Szentivanyi that there was a relative beta-blockade or a relative increase of the alpha/beta receptor ratio. This relative beta-blockade may be involved in the interpatient variable effects of the drugs.

B. Beta-2 Agonist Drugs

Beta-1 receptors do not appear to contribute largely to bronchodilation in asthmatics, according to studies performed with selective beta-1 blockers (metoprolol) and beta-1 agonists (prenalterol) (Lofdahl et al., 1984). These studies have been confirmed by in vitro experiments on isolated human bronchi (Zaagsma et al., 1983) and indicate that the more selective the beta-2 agonist, the better its activity in asthma.

Adrenoceptor agonists are chemically derived from the naturally occurring catecholamines. The studies of Lands et al. (1967) showing that beta-2 receptors were specific to the airways led to the synthesis of beta-2 selective bronchodilators and focused the attention of chemists on the value of the N-substitution for enhancing beta-2 selectivity. Moreover, the initial compounds were rapidly metabolized by catechol-O-methyl transferase (COMT) and monoamine oxidase (MAO) into relatively inert metabolites. Newly synthesized drugs are more resistant or totally insensitive to these enzymes and the duration of action of the drugs has been increased. However, the activities of the drugs vary with their structure in terms of spasmolytic, anti-inflammatory, or antiallergic activities.

Table 1 Beta-Adrenergic Agonists Commonly Used in Asthma

Name	Structural formula	Adrenergic selectivity	Duration (hr)	Dosage: Inhaled (μg)	Dosage: Oral (mg)
Catecholamines					
Adrenaline (epinephrine)	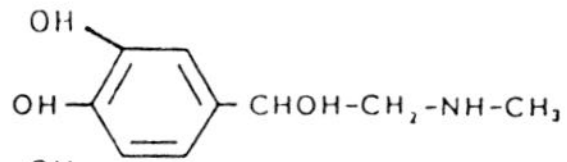	$\alpha\ \beta_1\ \beta_2$	<1	250	—
Isoprenaline (isoproterenol)	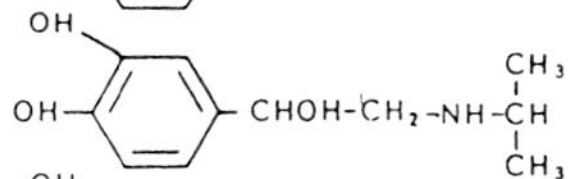	$\beta_2 \cong \beta_2$	1-2	80-160	—
Isoetharine	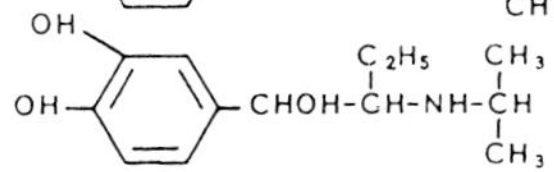	$\beta_2 > \beta_1$	1-2	350	10
Rimiterol	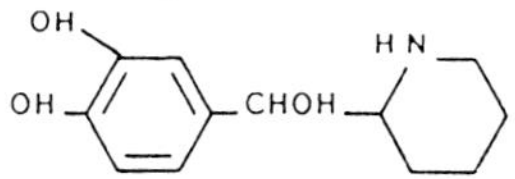	$\beta_2 > \beta_1$	1-2	200	10
Resorcinols					
Orciprenaline (metaproterenol)	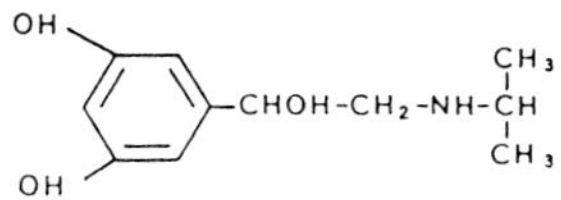	$\beta_2 > \beta_1$	1-3	750	20
Fenoterol	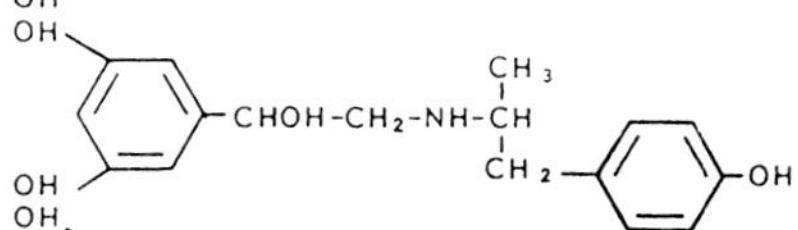	$\beta_2 >> \beta_1$	4-8	200	2.5
Terbutaline	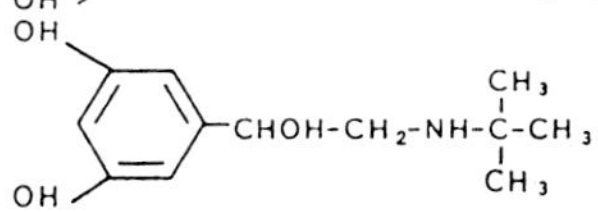	$\beta_2 >> \beta_1$	4-6	250	2.5, 5

(continued)

Table 1 (continued)

Name	Structural formula	Adrenergic selectivity	Duration (hr)	Dosage: Inhaled (μg)	Dosage: Oral (mg)
Resorcinols (continued)					
Reproterol	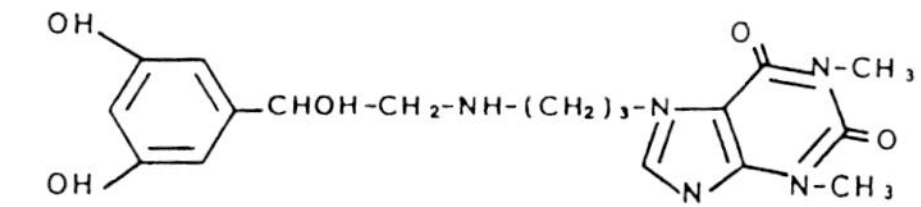	$\beta_2>\beta_1$	3-6	500	20
Salbutamol (albuterol)	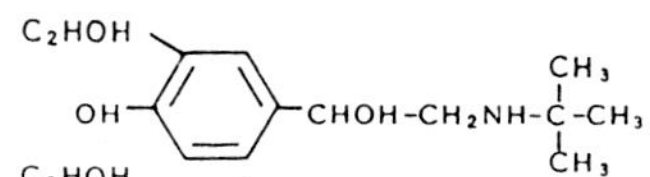	$\beta_2>>\beta_1$	4-6	200	2, 4
Pirbuterol	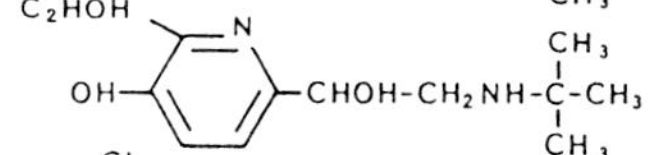	$\beta_2>>\beta_1$	4-6	200	10, 15
Clenbuterol	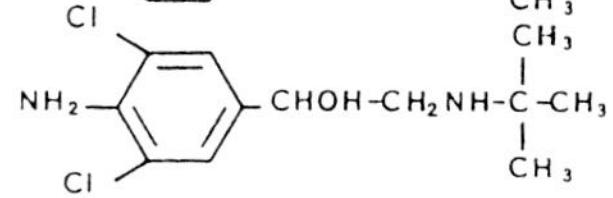	$\beta_2>>\beta_1$	>12	–	10, 20 μg
Tolubuterol	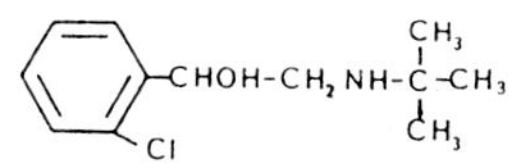	$\beta_2>>\beta_1$	6-9	400	1

Procaterol	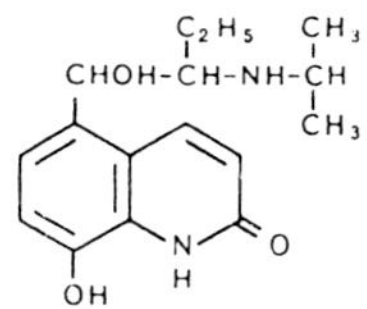	$\beta_2 >> \beta_1$	6-8	—	50
Bitolterol	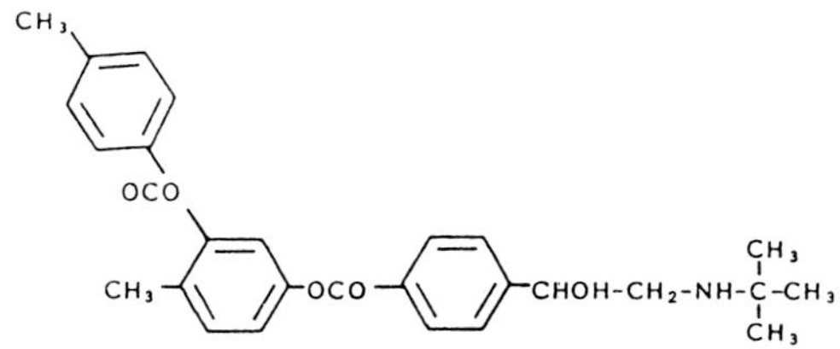	$\beta_2 >> \beta_1$	4-6	4	
Trimetoquinol	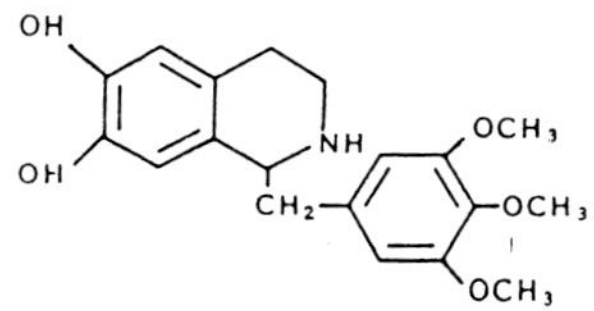	$\beta_2 > \beta_1$	2	—	3

Two approaches to improving chemically the potency of beta-2 agonists were applied and are summarized here (Table 1).

Replacement of the 3-hydroxyl group (salbutamol, soterenol, carbuterol), movement of the 4-hydroxyl to 5-position to form a resorcinol (orciprenaline, terbutaline, fenoterol), or replacement of the 3,4-dihydroxygroups with 3,5-dichloro-4-amino substituents (clenbuterol) has given compounds metabolic stability and long duration of action. Fortuitously, modifications designed to reduce O-methylation have also reduced O-sulfation therefore promoting oral activity and general metabolic stability.

Substitutions of the alpha-carbon result in blockage of oxidation by MAO.

Drugs with large substitutions of the amine head show greater beta-2 selectivity and are also more resistant to inactivation by MAO.

The aromatic nucleus can be modified (pirbuterol, procaterol).

Some of the most common beta-2 agonists used are (Paterson et al., 1979) salbutamol (Cullum et al., 1969), metaproterenol (Hurst, 1973), fenoterol (Heel et al., 1978, Minette et al., 1976; O'Donnell, 1970), clenbuterol (del Bono et al., 1977), bitolterol (Shargel and Dorrbecker, 1976; Orgel et al., 1985), tolubuterol (Patel, 1985).

II. Pharmacologic Properties of Beta-2 Agonists

Beta-2 agonists in the airways cause a bronchodilation but they have wider effects since they can efficiently block the activation of mast cells and may therefore be effective as antiallergic drugs. Macrophage beta-receptors are involved in the regulation of the inflammatory process by modulating histamine and leukotriene release.

A. Bronchodilation

Most normal subjects experience bronchodilation in response to beta-2 agonists but FEV_1 does not change significantly (Barnes et al., 1981; Holgate et al., 1977; Watanabe et al., 1974). The effect of beta-2 agonists is greater in patients with asthma and a significant improvement in FEV_1 is commonly observed. The mechanisms by which beta-2 agonists operate combine a direct action of the drug on the smooth muscle beta-receptors, a decreased mucosal edema, and an enhanced mucociliary function. The exact role of beta-2 agonists on the mucociliary function is reviewed by Wanner (see Chap. 18). These drugs stimulate the mucociliary transport in patients with chronic bronchitis and asthma but the clinical significance of such an effect must be evaluated. Although the doubling of transport in a normal individual may represent a significant increase, the same increment may only induce a slight effect in asthmatic patients (Mossberg et al., 1976; Wanner and Ahmed, 1983). Moreover, the pulmonary function improvement occurs within minutes after the administration of an inhaled drug and it appears therefore that the bronchorelaxing effects may be predominant (Tattersfield, 1983).

B. Antiallergic Properties of Beta-2 Agonists

A number of in vivo and in vitro studies have shown that beta-2 agonists have antiallergic properties as well as bronchodilating activities. The use of a range of agonists and both selective and nonselective antagonists has shown that the human mast cell carries predominantly beta-2 receptors. Beta-2 agonists were widely studied with human cells in vitro. They inhibit or decrease histamine release from human chopped lung, nasal polyps, basophils, and isolated human lung mast cells when these cells are triggered by a variety of stimuli such as allergen or anti-IgE (Assem and Schild, 1969; Mita and Shida, 1983; Marone et al., 1984; Petersson, 1984). Their effects on allergen-induced skin tests is variable but when they are injected with allergens some drugs, such as terbutaline or KWD 2131, were shown to decrease the wheal and flare reaction (Bousquet et al., 1987; Gronneberg et al., 1980; Imbeau et al., 1978). The inhibition of the immediate allergic reaction in the nose by beta-2 agonists was observed with fenoterol, salbutamol, KWD 2131, terbutaline (Borum and Mygind, 1980), or clenbuterol (Bousquet et al., 1986) (Fig. 1). The effects of beta-2 agonists in preventing the allergic reaction in the airways is more difficult to prove since they are also potent bronchodilating agents (Hegardt and Arner, 1981). In a recent study, Howarth et al. (1985) have shown that albuterol was able to block both the release of mediators and immediate-type bronchoconstriction during allergen challenge. Others have also shown that terbutaline blocked both exercise-induced asthma and the rise in plasma histamine that accompanies the bronchoconstriction. Animal studies have confirmed these findings (Fügner, 1977). It therefore seems probable that beta-2 agonists are capable of inhibiting the release of mediators from mast cells in the skin, lung, or nose. However, the exact role of beta-2 agonists in the bronchial allergic inflammation remains to be clarified since these drugs do not appear to prevent the late phase reaction that is one of the key feature of the asthmatic inflammation (Fig. 2).

A few long-term studies have been performed. A 12-month follow-up study of asthmatic patients showed that the peak flows of patients regularly treated with fenoterol were significantly higher than those who received either prednisone or cromoglycate. This important study shows that long-term treatment with beta-2 agonists is effective (van As, 1975). However, it appears unlikely that beta-2

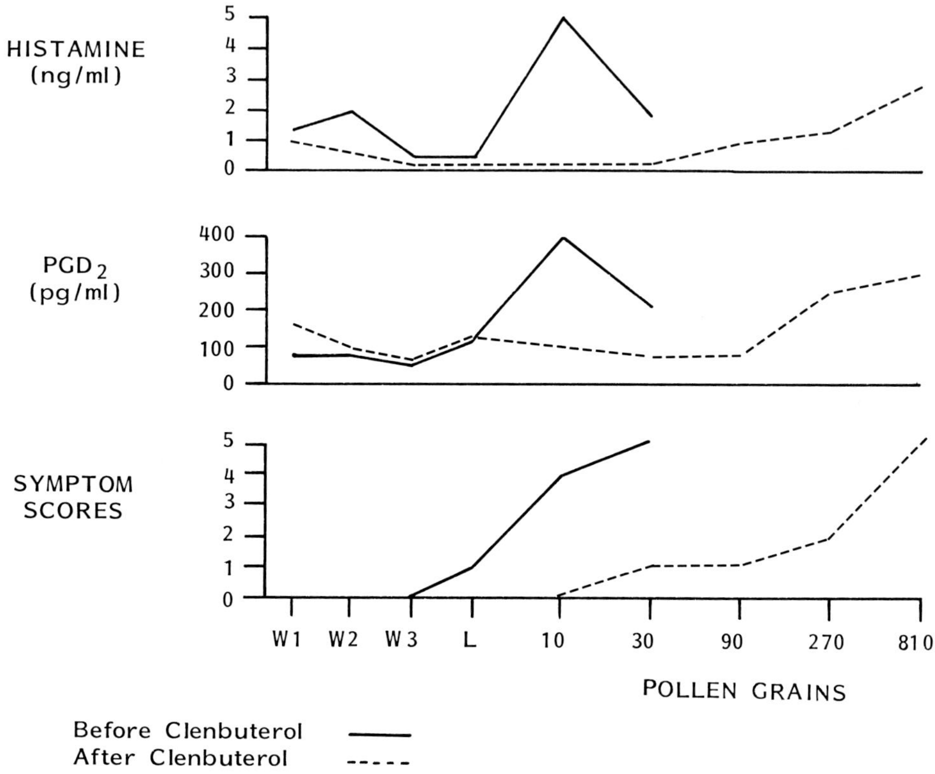

Figure 1 Antiallergic activity of clenbuterol. Histamine in nasal secretions was titrated by radioimmunoassay using monoclonal antiacetylated histamine. PGD_2 in nasal secretions was titrated by enzyme immunoassay. Symptom scores combined nasal blockade, pruritus, rhinorrhea, sneezing. W1, W2, W3, nasal lavage before provocation; L, lactose (From Bousquet et al., 1986).

agonists block bronchial inflammation since nonspecific bronchial hyperreactivity was found to be either unchanged (Peel and Gobson, 1980; Kraan et al., 1985) or slightly decreased (Salome et al., 1983). These findings suggest that although symptoms are controlled, the course of the disease leading to a slow alteration of the bronchi may not stop in asthmatic patients routinely treated with beta-2 agonists alone and warrants further studies to fully determine the antiallergic activity of these drugs.

C. Cardiovascular Effects

Beta-2-selective agonists have much less cardiac effects than poorly selective ones. However, they are potent vasodilators and have some cardiac effects representing

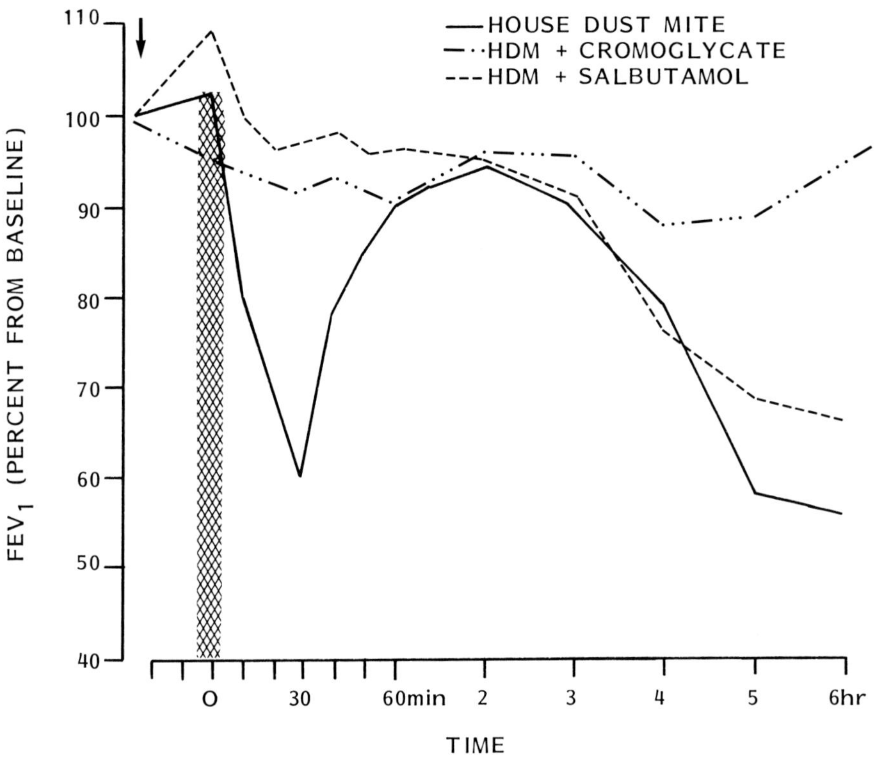

Figure 2 Inhibition of bronchial challenge with a standardized mite extract by cromoglycate or salbutamol. The arrow indicates the time of inhalation of the drug.

side effects. They also augment the right ventricular performance and can be used in some patients with chronic obstructive pulmonary disease (COPD) (Brent et al., 1982; Slutsky et al., 1981).

D. Metabolic Actions

Intravenous and oral beta-2 agonists can induce several dose-related metabolic changes in normal and asthmatic subjects, including an increase in levels of glucose, insulin, and nonesterified fatty acids, and a fall in levels of serum potassium, phosphate, calcium, and magnesium. These effects are dosage-related and are more rarely observed with inhaled drugs (Haalboom et al., 1985; Harvey et al., 1981; Phillips et al., 1980; Smith and Kendall, 1984).

III. Clinical Pharmacology

A. Beta-2 Agonist Metabolism and Bioavailability

Beta-2 agonists are usually given by the inhaled route but their fate is complex since 90% of the drug is swallowed. Beta-2 agonists with a catecholamine-like structure are metabolized to 3-hydroxy inert metabolites by COMT and MAO, and therefore are rapidly inactivated. The newly synthetized drugs are metabolized into sulfo- or glucuroconjugates (McIlleny and Gholy, 1979; Nilsson et al., 1972). These processes are dependent on the number of hydroxyl groups on the benzene ring. Drugs with a high number, such as fenoterol, are more rapidly metabolized than those that do not have any group (clenbuterol) (Bres et al., 1985).

Most beta-agonists are only active when their structure remains intact, except for bitolterol, which is a prodrug (Orgel et al., 1985; Shargel and Dorrbecker, 1976), and tolubuterol, which is metabolized to at least three active metabolites (Kubo et al., 1980).

The metabolism varies according to the administration route. When drugs are taken orally, the active plasma fraction is least with fenoterol, and progressively larger with terbutaline, salbutamol, pirbuterol and clenbuterol, which is the most stable drug. The oral route may be recommended for the latter three drugs, and for tolubuterol. Inhaled and parenteral routes are more appropriate for drugs with a lower digestive stability, such as terbutaline. Inhaled drugs are metabolized by both digestive and pulmonary tissues to inactive metabolites (Laros et al., 1977).

B. Pharmacokinetics

Plasma concentrations of beta-2 agonists are very low and require a highly sophisticated technique—gas chromatography with ion capture or mass spectrometry—to be accurately measured (Evans et al., 1971; Leferink et al., 1982a; Falkner and McIlheny, 1976). Techniques using labeled molecules do not seem to be appropriate since they measure both the unchanged drugs and their inactive metabolites. Since only a few studies have been performed in humans it is difficult to compare their results. However, it appears that beta-2 agonists have a large distribution volume and a short half-life, ranging from 30 min for isoprenaline to 6 hr or more for the newest compounds. Absorption of oral forms vary according to the molecule. Salbutamol and tolubuterol are rapidly absorbed, terbutaline exhibits large interpatient variations, and pirbuterol behaves like a slow-releasing drug in most patients exhibiting two peaks of plasma concentration (Fig. 3) (van den Berg et al., 1980; Clauzel et al., 1985; Leferink et al., 1982b; McFadden, 1981). Long-term treatment does not appear to modify significantly the pharmacokinetics of beta-2 agonists (Clauzel et al., 1984).

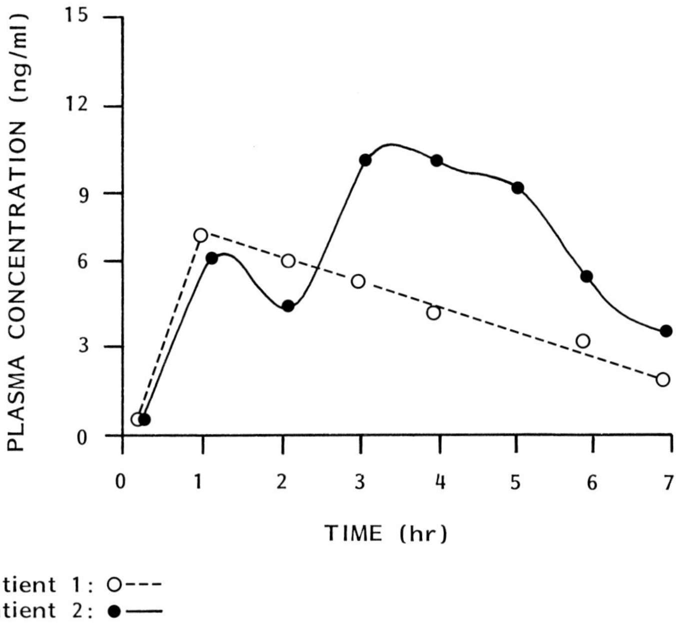

Figure 3 Plasma concentrations of pirbuterol demonstrating the large interpatient variability (one or two peaks) (From Clauzel et al., 1984).

C. Relationship Between Pharmacokinetic and Pharmacoclinical Data

The relationship between plasma concentrations and pulmonary effects is often related and this was observed for salbutamol, terbutaline, pirbuterol and tolubuterol (Clauzel et al., 1985; Leferink et al., 1982b) (Figs. 4 and 5).

The correlations between plasma concentrations and the pulmonary function improvement may help to identify poor and good responders to beta-agonists. When beta-2 agonists are given for a long period of time, early variations in the dose-response curve may indicate a subsequent tolerance to the drug (Clauzel et al., 1985).

IV. Side Effects and Complications of Beta-2 Agonists

Beta-2 agonists are very effective bronchodilating drugs and in many countries represent the first line treatment of asthma. The first compounds used (epinephrine, ephedrine, and isoprenaline) were shown to induce a wide array of side effects. In the early 1960s in Great Britain and some other countries, the mortality

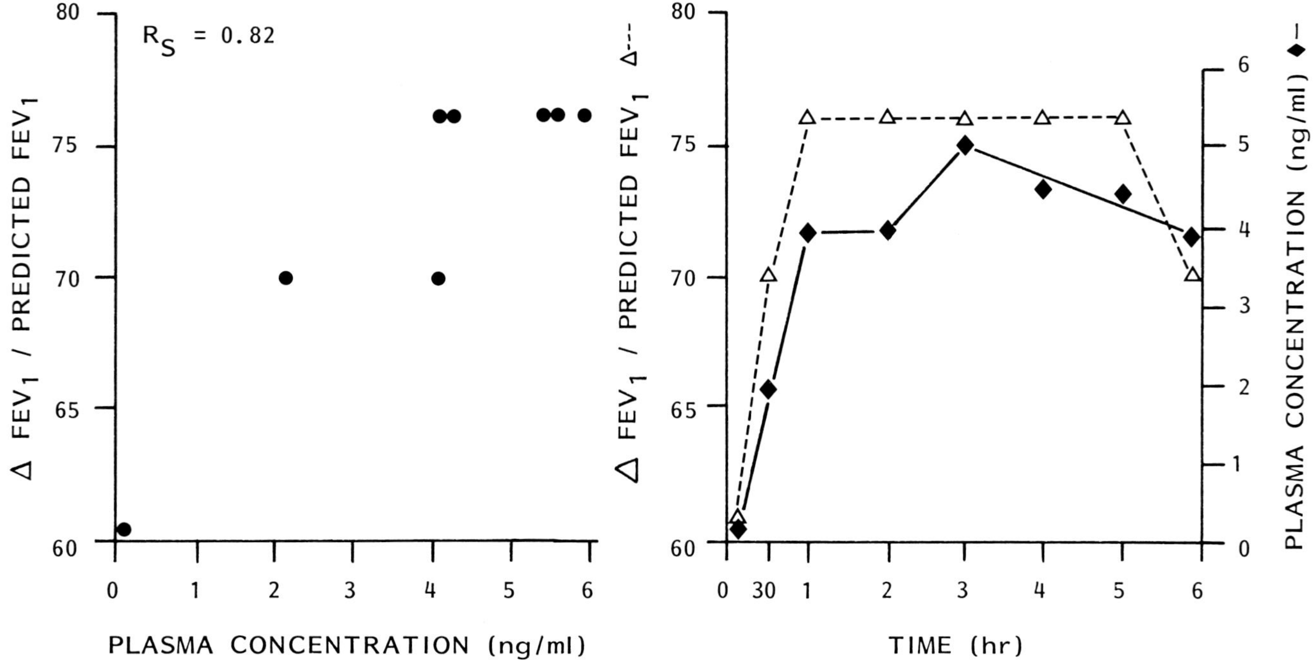

Figure 4 Correlation between plasma concentrations and improvement in FEV_1 with an oral dose of pirbuterol (10 mg) (from Clauzel et al., 1984).

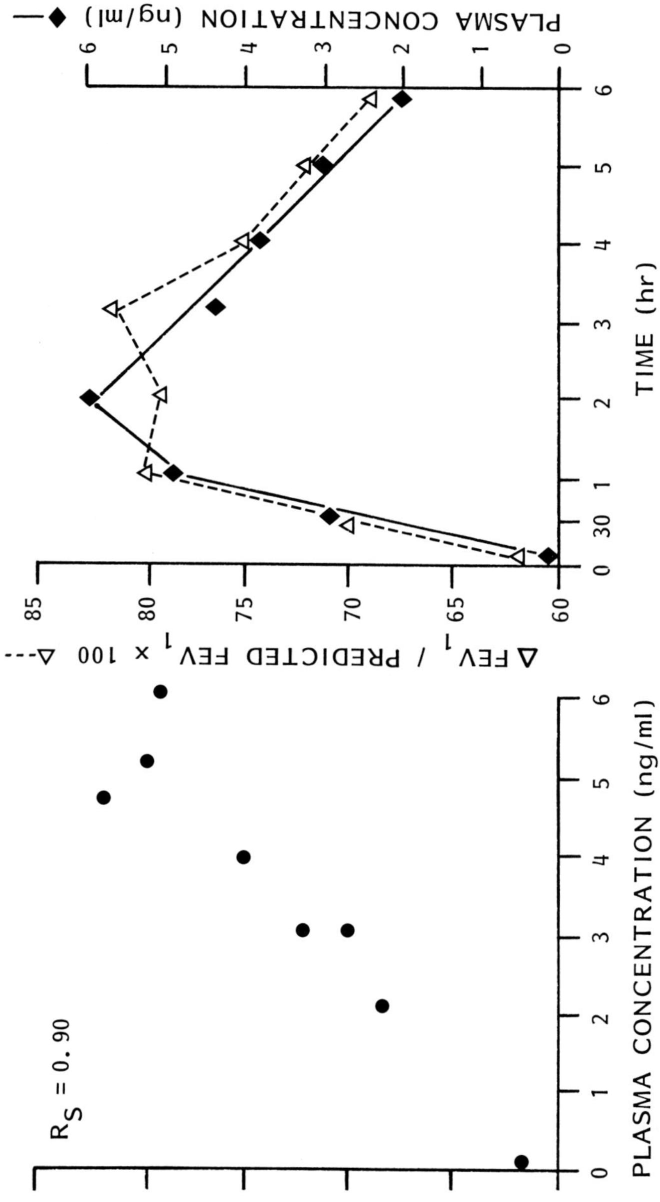

Figure 5 Correlation between plasma concentrations and improvement in FEV_1 with tolubuterol (oral dose of 1 mg) (from Clauzel et al., 1985).

rate of asthmatics rose sharply and there was concern that beta agonists might be implicated, particularly the more concentrated preparation of isoprenaline (Campbell, 1976; Harris, 1971; Inman and Adelstein, 1969). However, there is no clear evidence that any of the deaths were due to abuse of beta agonists. The aerosols might have had a direct cardiac effect or have induced tolerance (Tattersfield, 1983).

A. Aggravation of Hypoxemia

Inhalation of therapeutic doses of beta-2 agonists has been shown to decrease arterial PO_2. The decrease rarely exceeds 20 mmHg and does not last more than 30 min, but in occasional patients this side effect may be serious (Harris et al., 1977).

B. Hypokalemia

This metabolic side effect of beta-2 agonists appears to be of some clinical significance. It is seen after large oral and parenteral doses (Haalboom et al., 1985).

C. Cardiac Effects

The cardiac effects of nonselective beta-2 agonists are well documented. Beta-2 adrenoceptors have been identified in the human myocardium and can mediate tachycardia. Tachycardia may also be a consequence of the fall in systemic vascular resistances, leading to a vagal reflex (Teule and Majid, 1980). Some patients with severe asthma may be more prone to arrhythmia since they may exhibit hypokalemia and decreased arterial oxygen tension. Beta-2 agonists may aggravate the hypoxemia and hypokalemia, resulting in tachycardia. Although poorly selective beta-2 drugs induce more cardiac side effects, all newer beta-2 selective compounds can be arrhythmogenic in susceptible individuals (Banner et al., 1979).

Some exceptional patients may experience cardiac ischemia with beta-2 agonists (Kurland et al., 1979) and asthma deaths have been attributed to beta-2 agonist induced myocardial infarction.

D. Muscle Tremor

The most common side effect is tremor, which is related to a direct effect of the drug on striated muscle beta-2 adrenoceptors. Since beta-2 agonists act both on bronchial and skeletal muscle, it would be most desirable to find a drug that could have separate effects in the bronchi and skeletal muscle, but it appears that beta-2 receptors on both muscles are identical (Lofdahl and Svedmyr, 1984). After a few weeks of continuous administration, tremor usually decreases in most patients (Larsson and Svedmyr, 1977b).

E. Tachyphylaxis

It has been suggested that patients who tend to overuse beta-2 agonist inhalers might become resistant to their bronchodilating effect. This phenomenon has been described as tachyphylaxis, tolerance, subsensitivity, resistance, or impaired responsiveness.

The questions that are raised concern (1) the possible preexisting tolerance of cells from asthmatic patients, (2) which cells are desensitized and to what level, (3) whether this phenomenon occurs in normal subjects and/or in patients taking beta-2 agonists at recommended dosage and/or in those who persistently use higher dosages than those recommended, and (4) its clinical relevance.

Pharmacology

At the molecular level, the phenomenon of desensitization is probably better understood for the beta-adrenoceptor-adenylate cyclase-cyclic AMP system than for any other example of transmembrane signal. The receptor-specific desensitization is a two-stage process. Initially, a readily reversible "uncoupling" of the receptor from the cyclase occurs. This results in a lack of activation of the cyclase. Later, after more prolonged exposure to agonists, a loss of receptor number occurs that is reversed more slowly. During this stage, receptors appear to be internalized. There is also evidence that receptor-drug affinity decreases. The immediate consequence of desensitization is a reduction in the ability of the cell to respond to a given stimulus by synthesizing cyclic AMP (Harden, 1983; Skidmore, 1984; Stiles et al., 1984).

Preexisting Tolerance

Studies have shown that some asthmatics exhibit a beta-2 agonist hyporesponsiveness before treatment (Shelhamer et al., 1983). Beta-blockers are known to induce severe asthmatic reactions. These findings suggest that there is an instability of the alpha/beta-adrenoceptor equilibrium. However, this impairment has also been reported in nonasthmatic atopic and normal individuals, which shows that this relative beta-blockage is neither specific nor constitutive of asthma (Djurup, 1981; Shelhamer et al., 1983; Zaagsma et al., 1983).

Acquired Tolerance or Tachyphylaxis

When treatment is initiated, it is usual to observe a transient and small hyporesponsiveness of the airways to beta-2 agonists that clears in a few days. The most important problem remains the possible induction of tolerance after long-term treatment. In vitro and in vivo studies have been performed and if it is widely accepted that some degree of tachyphylaxis develops after long-term treatment, there is no consensus on its exact relevance in asthmatic patients (Jenne, 1982).

In vitro studies on lymphocytes and leukocytes of normal and asthmatic patients show that incubation of these cells with beta-2 agonists rapidly reduces the number of beta-receptors present on their surface (Conolly and Greenacre, 1976). A reduction in beta-receptor numbers has also been shown to occur in lymphocytes of asthmatic patients taking therapeutic dosages of oral terbutaline (Tashkin et al., 1982). Incubation in isoproterenol of bronchial smooth muscle from nonasthmatic subjects cause a decrease in sensitivity to the relaxing effects of this drug (Avner and Jenne, 1981; Guillot et al., 1984).

Many prospective studies have been performed to investigate the airway response of normal subjects and asthmatic patients after a period of regular treatment with inhaled or oral beta-2 agonist treatment. It appears that asthmatic patients are less prone to tachyphylaxis than are normal individuals. Most asthmatic patients do not develop resistance to the effects of beta-agonists after using recommended dosages of inhaled or oral beta-2 agonists (Angelici et al., 1984; Harvey and Tattersfield, 1982; Holgate et al., 1977; Larsson et al., 1977; Nelson, 1982). However, there is evidence that very large dosages can lead to tolerance, and this may be relevant to the larger dosages of drugs recommended for use by nebulizer (Bhatia and Davies, 1975; Conolly et al., 1982; Nelson et al., 1977). Long-term treatment may also lead to some degree of tolerance, even with inhaled drugs (Weber et al., 1982). Tolerance was also observed with exercise challenge (Gibson et al., 1978). Beta-2 agonists administered systemically reduce the bronchial response in all parts of the bronchial tree while those given by inhalation cause desensitization only in the larger airways, where, for the most part they are deposited (Conolly et al., 1982). Transient loss of bronchial responsiveness may eventually occur during treatment, induced by several factors among which are hypersecretion, inflammation, influenza infection (Busse, 1977), or when concomitant drugs such as antidepressants are being used (Banerjee et al., 1977) (Figs. 6, 7).

Prevention of beta-2 adrenoceptor tachyphylaxis has been demonstrated with corticosteroids or ketotifen. Thus, these drugs can be administered in combination with beta-2 agonists when long-term treatment is being planned, in order to prevent the development of resistance (Brodde et al., 1985; Arnaud and Charpin, 1982; Coffey et al., 1973; Davies and Lefkowitz, 1983; Tashkin et al., 1982) (Fig. 8).

F. Side Effects of Inhaled Beta-2 Agonists

Metered-dose inhalers (MDI) contain beta-2 agonists with hydrocarbon propellants and, in some instances, preservatives such as metabisulfite (Simon, 1985). Hydrocarbon propellants have been shown to cause cardiac arrhythmias in animals and it has been suggested that the combination of these propellants with beta-2 agonists may enhance the cardiac side effects of the drug (Aviado, 1975;

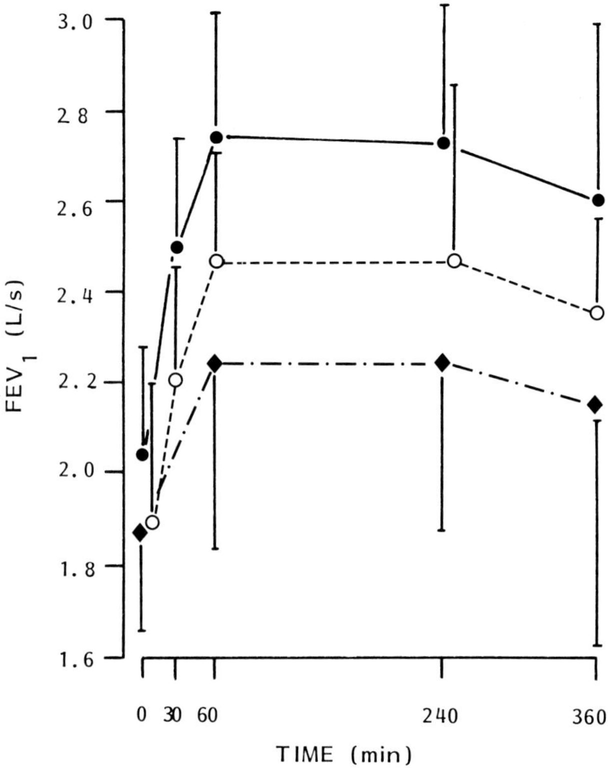

Figure 6 Improvement in FEV_1 after an oral dose of 10 mg of pirbuterol in 9 patients before treatment (●—), and after 3 (○ ---) and 29 days (♦— • —) of oral treatment with pirbuterol (30 mg daily). There was no significant difference between the three curves (From Clauzel et al., 1985).

Collier et al., 1980). Metabisulfite contained in some MDI was found to induce some degree of bronchial obstruction in sensitive asthmatics. Finally, bacterial and mold contamination of MDI may occur (Levesque and Johnson, 1984).

Psychological dependence on aerosols may occur. Several reports have focused attention on the abuse of inhalers and suggested that the addiction to aerosol treatment could be compared to "the asthmatic alternative to glue sniffing" (Pratt, 1982; Thompson et al., 1983).

G. Side Effects of Ingested and Inhaled Beta-2 Agonists

Tremor, palpitation, and metabolic effects are more marked when beta-2 agonists are taken orally or when they are injected since these side effects are dos-

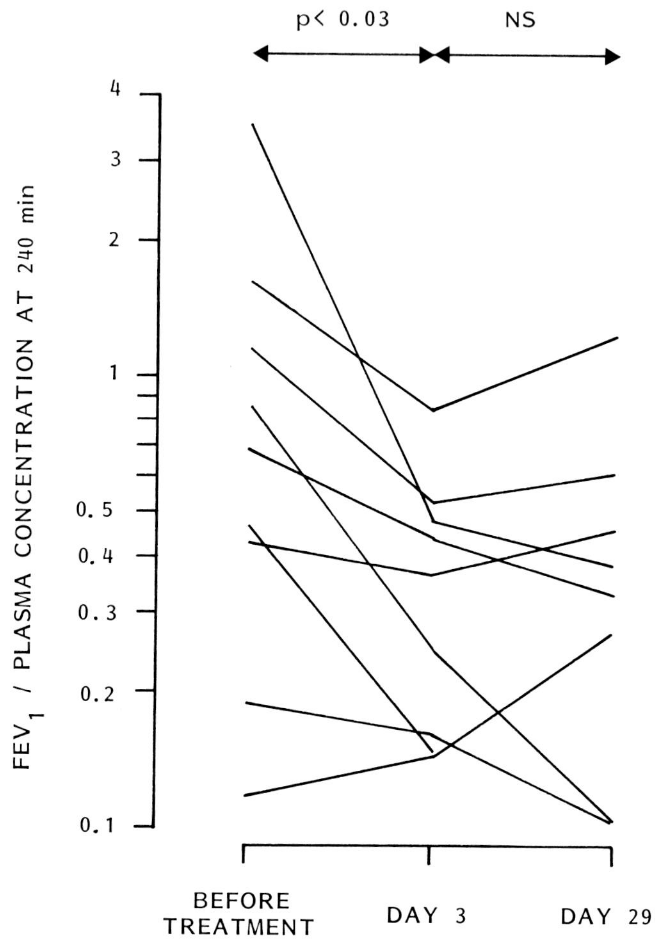

Figure 7 Evolution of the ratio of improvement in FEV_1 to plasma concentration of pirbuterol in the same nine patients as Figure 6. Three days after the onset of treatment there was a significant tolerance of the product that persisted at 29 days (statistical analysis by Wilcoxon W test) (From Clauzel et al., 1985).

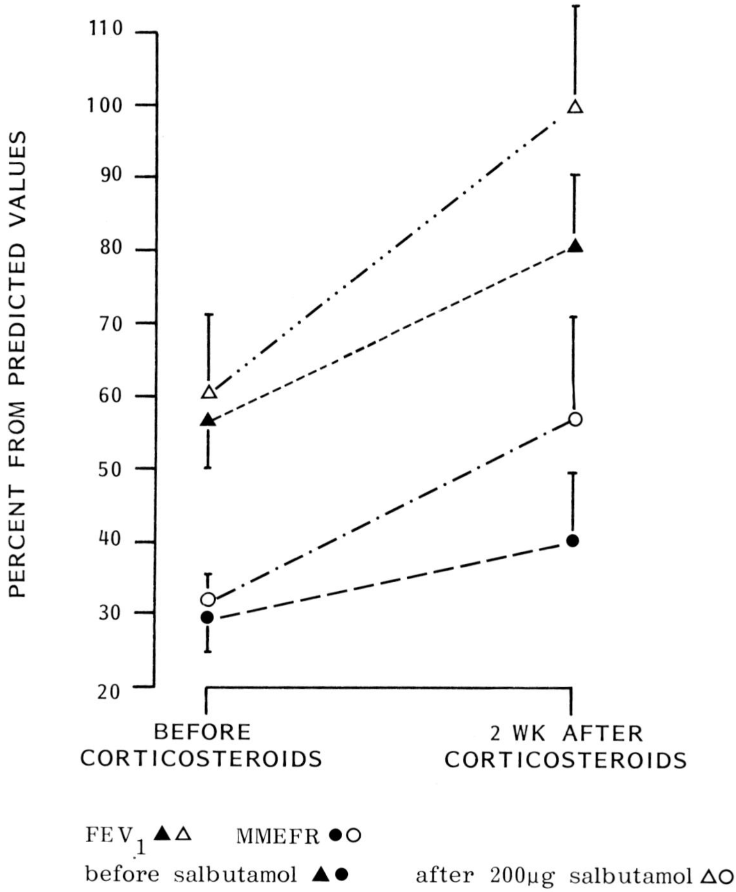

Figure 8 Restoration of the response to salbutamol in 10 poorly responsive patients after 2 weeks of prednisone (120 mg daily).

age-related. They decline with continued administration (Larsson and Svedmyr, 1977a,b).

V. Clinical Applications

A. Choice of Beta-2 Agonists

Most beta-2 agonists available commercially are listed in Table 1. Owing to their pharmacokinetics, it is possible to choose different drugs or administration routes according to the severity and type of asthma. Acute attacks are better treated

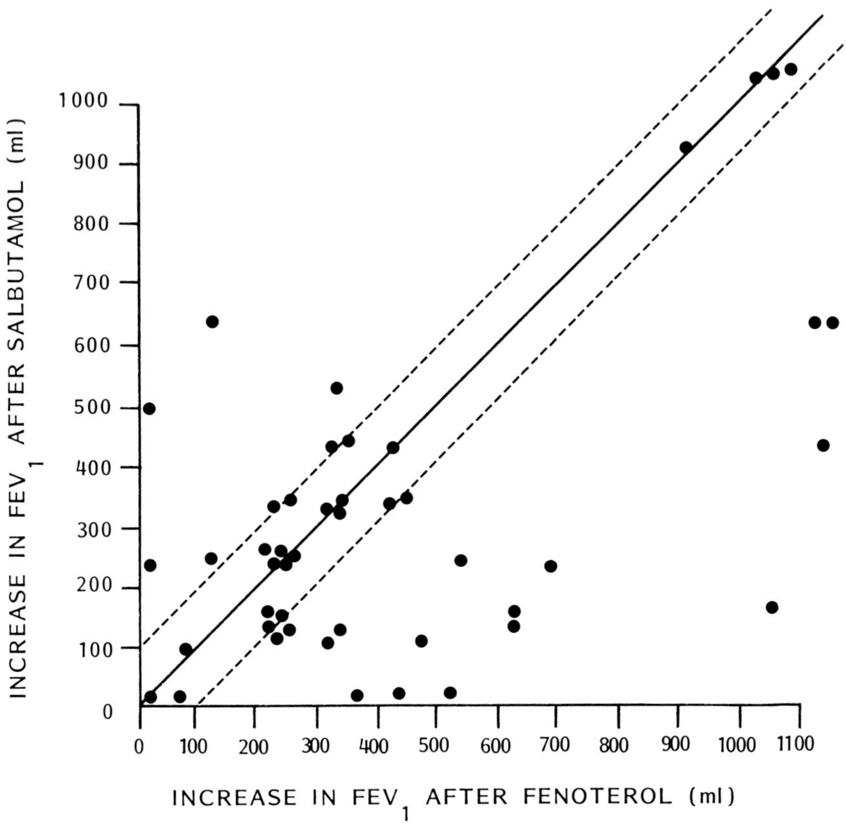

Figure 9 Increase in FEV_1 after inhalation of 400 μg salbutamol and 400 μg fenoterol showing large interpatient variation (From Clauzel, 1986).

with inhaled drugs, whereas persistent bronchial obstruction may be better relieved by other routes. Although Poppa (1984) showed that there is some equivalence between different beta-2 agonists, it appears that patients do not respond equally to all drugs (Clauzel et al., 1986; Madsen et al., 1979) (Fig. 9), suggesting therefore that drugs, routes of administration, and dosages should be assessed for each severe asthmatic who requires long-term treatment.

B. Choice of Routes of Administration (Table 2)

Inhalation

Inhalation is usually the preferred route of administration for beta-2 agonists, since the pharmacologic effect occurs rapidly and provides a better ratio of bronchodilation to plasma drug level and a lower incidence of untoward side reactions than when used by oral or parenteral routes. Low dosages are conveniently given by MDI whereas higher dosages can be administered by nebulizer (Newhouse and Ruffin, 1978).

Metered Dose Inhalers

Metered dose inhalers have gained wide acceptance for the convenient, rapid, and effective administration of bronchodilators. Ten to 15% of the active drug delivered by MDI is deposited into the airways (Newman et al., 1981b). The apparent simplicity of MDI administration is misleading and reports indicate that many patients do not use MDI correctly (Coady et al., 1976; Orehek et al., 1976; Paterson and Crompton, 1976). The response of asthmatic patients to MDI depends largely on the technique of inhalation. It has been shown that inhaling a bronchodilator drug at the end of a full inspiration causes a relatively greater bronchodilation than inhaling the same dosage at the beginning of inspiration (Riley et al., 1976). Increased penetration of aerosol particles into the deep lung is more likely with slow inspiration, since an increased flow rate augments the impaction of particles in the mouth and central airways (Pavia et al., 1977). Deep expiration may cause either bronchial collapse or bronchoconstriction in some asthmatic patients (Orehek et al., 1980) and respiratory maneuvers required by MDI may lead to their ineffectiveness. There is a strict dependance of timing and coordination between the patient's respiratory maneuvers and the actuation of the aerosol, so young children and some uncompliant older patients cannot use such devices. Newman et al. (1981c) proposed the following technique for inhalation using MDI:

1. Shake the canister thoroughly.
2. Place the mouthpiece 4 cm in front of the open mouth, or use a spacer between the actuator and mouth.
3. Breathe out steadily to functional residual capacity.
4. Discharge the inhaler while taking a slow deep breath.
5. Hold the breath at full inspiration for 10 sec.

Heimer et al. (1980) proposed the inhalation of three consecutive puffs of beta-2 agonist at 5 or 10 min intervals rather than three consecutive inhalations, since they found that there was a better penetration of the bronchodilator aerosol after some bronchodilation had been achieved.

Spacers used as an auxiliary delivery system can overcome some of the problems encountered with MDI (Tobin et al., 1983; Lee and Evans, 1984). They promote deposition of aerosols on the lower airways and do not require any compliance of the patient or deep respiratory maneuvers since the patients breathe at tidal volume. Their effectiveness is dependent on their size and shape. Spacer

Table 2 Relative Advantages and Drawbacks of the Different Routes of Administration of Beta-Adrenoceptor Agonists

Route of administration	Advantages	Drawbacks	
MDI	In situ administration	Related to patients	
	Rapidity of action	Lack of coordination (coordination not required with spacers)	
	Low doses	Abuses	
	Tachyphylaxis relatively rare at regular dosage	Related to asthma	
		Severe bronchial obstruction	Only the large airways are reached
		Hypersecretion	
		Related to aerosols	
		Propellants	
		Preservatives	
Nebulizers	In situ administration	Related to asthma	
	Rapidity of action	Severe bronchial obstruction	Only the large airways are reached
	Large dosages	Hypersecretion	
		Large doses	
		Possible tachyphylaxis	
		Other side effects increased	

Oral	Defined dosages	Large doses and systemic administration
	Distribution to small airways	Possible tachyphylaxis
	Long lasting effect	Muscle tremor, cardiac, metabolic side effects
	Large dosages	Delayed onset (older compounds)
Parenteral	Defined dosages	Large doses and systemic administration
	Distribution to small airways	Tachyphylaxis rare (short-term treatment)
	Rapidity of action	Muscle tremor, cardiac, and metabolic side effects
	Large dosages	Short-lasting effect

devices were shown in some studies (Lindren et al., 1980; Newman et al., 1981a) to increase the bronchodilating effects of MDI but others (Eriksson et al., 1980; Gomm et al., 1980) did not find such beneficial effects.

The MDI have other pitfalls. The active drug is combined with propellants and preservatives that may induce side effects by themselves. Moreover, MDI aerosols increase the automedication and abusive use of the drugs. In very severe bronchial obstruction, the drug cannot penetrate into the airways.

An alternative to MDI is represented by the dry powder inhaler in which a capsule of salbutamol or fenoterol is inserted into the inhaler and actuated by inspiration. This method is particularly convenient in young children who find using a spray difficult (Croner et al., 1981; Duncan et al., 1977; Grimwood et al., 1981).

Nebulizers

Beta-2 agonists can also be inhaled from a nebulizer driven by air or oxygen (Editorial, 1984) or during intermittent positive pressure breathing. They are particularly adequate when patients cannot coordinate the use of metered dose aerosols or in acute severe asthma, since some studies have shown that they were more effective than MDI (Cayton et al., 1981; Crompton et al., 1979; Grimwood et al., 1981; Pierce et al., 1981). In chronic asthma the advantages of nebulizers do not appear to be so important (Anderson et al., 1982). In some studies, nebulizers have been found to be as effective as the parenteral route. The dosages of beta-2 agonists recommended for nebulizers are 20-50 times higher than those for MDI but only 10% of the drug is effectively inhaled: most of the drug is lost to the atmosphere or left in the device and a little amount is swallowed (Lewis et al., 1982).

Other Routes

In a recent Danish study it was suggested that beta-2 agonists may be administered in the nose and that drugs administered through this route have a similar effect to those inhaled (Groth et al., 1984).

Oral Route

Noncatecholamines may be administered as oral drugs in the form of tablets (Formgren, 1975) or syrup particularly formulated for children (Pierson et al., 1985). The dosages required are much higher than for the inhaled route, so blood levels are higher. These agents are distributed to every tissue in the body. These two characteristics lead to increased side effects (Larsson and Svedmyr, 1977a). However, Formgren (1975) followed up adults who had been treated with terbutaline for 3 years and did not observe any indication of resistance when the drug was given at regular dosages. Moreover, oral drugs also have advantages. There is less self-medication and abuses of the drug. They reach all parts of the respiratory tract, expecially small bronchi even when there is a severe bronchial obstruction (Fairshter et al., 1981). The duration of bronchodilation is usually longer than that induced by aerosols and can reach 8-10 hr with the newest drugs. A rapid onset of bronchodilation is also observed with the newly synthesized compounds and may be as short as 30 min.

Parenteral Route

Beta-2 agonists can be administered by infusion or subcutaneous routes and these cholines are particularly suitable in emergency cases. The potential side effects are considerably greater with parenteral drugs and the more severe metabolic problems with them have been described. The fall in potassium is particularly relevant to asthmatic patients. At present, there is no general consensus as to whether it would be better for patients with severe asthma to use beta-2 agonists delivered by nebulizers or injected, but the latter route appears to be superior when bronchial obstruction is severe (Williams and Seaton, 1977) since the drugs are distributed to the whole respiratory tract (Tashkin et al., 1982).

C. Choice of Protocol for Administration: Dose/Effect Curves, Effect/Time Curves

In patients requiring long-term treatment, it is necessary to choose the optimum dosage and the interval between the administration of the drugs. Dose-response curves may help to determine the response of each individual patient to the adrenergic treatment, and their variations during long-term treatment is of great interest for assessing tachyphylaxis. Both inhaled and oral drugs can be studied and although this is time-consuming, the performance of these curves should be done carefully.

D. Drug Interactions

In chronic asthma, symptoms are not always effectively controlled by recommended dosages of a single type of drug and increasing the dosage of any single drug may increase its side effects. Combinations of drugs have therefore been proposed for decades but some associations appear now to be less safe than was previously supposed.

Theophylline

Theophylline and its derivatives are often associated with beta-2 agonists. The demonstration that beta-2 agonists and methylxanthines may act through related biochemical and cellular pathways has logically encouraged their association. An additive effect is obtained in terms of bronchodilation when both drugs are used at full therapeutic dosages (Nicklas et al., 1984; Rossing et al., 1981; Wolfe et al.,

1978). Theophylline also increases the antiallergic properties of beta-2 agonists (Mita and Shida, 1983; Marone et al., 1984). Moreover, it appears that a reduction in the dosages of both drugs induces the same degree of bronchodilation as the full dosage with a single drug. However, the side effects of these drugs may be additive. It has been recently suggested in New Zealand that the increased use of combined treatments with oral sustained release theophylline and inhaled beta-2 agonists might be responsible for an increased incidence of cardiac arrest in patients with asthma (Wilson et al., 1981). These suggestions are supported by animal studies showing that the myocardial toxicity of isoproterenol was significantly enhanced when it was administered with therapeutic dosages of theophylline, although more selective beta-2 agonists such as terbutaline or bitolterol were shown to be less cardiotoxic (Whitehurst et al., 1983). In humans, the cardiotoxicity of this combination is not well characterized but continuous electrocardiographic monitoring in patients receiving both theophylline and biltolterol did not reveal the presence of cardiac arrhythmias (Kemp et al., 1984). When the drugs are being used at lower dosages, it appears that beta-adrenergic tachyphylaxis (van den Berg et al., 1982) and side effects of both drugs are reduced (Wolfe et al., 1978) while retaining the bronchodilating activity. Some investigators have therefore suggested therapeutic advantages in combining both drugs in lower dosages, especially in patients experiencing severe side effects from a therapeutic dosage of either drug, but there are no data documenting the absence of cardiovascular toxicity.

Anticholinergic Drugs

Many studies have tried to determine the benefits of the combination of anticholinergics and beta-2 agonists. Studies reviewed by Shenfield (1982) and Rudolf (1984) indicated that (1) there was an increased duration of bronchodilator response with the combination and (2) there was some degree of additive, though not synergistic, bronchodilation with the combination. The incidence of side effects was not increased with the combination or with either drug alone. It was therefore concluded that patients who do not tolerate regular dosages of beta-2 agonists may use this combination by using lower dosages of the adrenergic drug.

Corticosteroids

Glucorticosteroids were shown to reverse the partial tolerance induced by long-term treatment with beta-2 agonists (Arnaud and Charpin, 1982; Coffey et al., 1973; Davies and Lefkowitz, 1983). Moreover, they increase the effects of adrenergic agents on bronchial smooth muscle and mucociliary clearance.

In chronic asthmatics, the association between salbutamol and beclomethasone was found to add to the effects of both drugs. However, the short-term effects of beclomethasone are less profound than its long-term ones, especially in patients who had some degree of irreversible bronchoconstriction when treated with beta-2 agonists. It does not seem that the chronology of administration of either drug is important (Clark and Anderson, 1978). Dahl and Johansson (1982) confirmed this observation since they found that the combination of inhaled budenoside and terbutaline results in an additive effect in bronchodilation.

Other Combinations

Alpha-blockers are not very potent bronchodilating drugs when used alone, but in combination with beta-2 agonists their effects are potentiated (Marlin et al., 1983).

Ketotifen, similarly to corticosteroids, was shown to decrease tolerance of beta-2 adrenoceptors (Bretz et al., 1983; Brodde et al., 1985) (Fig. 10).

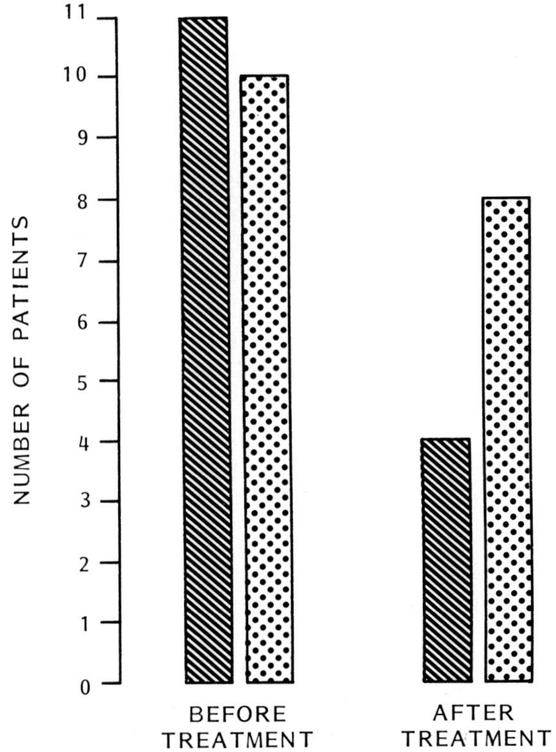

Figure 10 Corticoid-sparing effect of cromolyn ( ) and ketotifen ( ) in asthmatic patients.

E. Variations with Age

Salbutamol delivered as a nebulized solution was shown to be effective in reducing bronchospasm in children over 20 months but it was poorly active in infants (Lenney and Milner, 1978). In pertussis, Peltola and Michelsson (1982) noticed, however, that oral salbutamol was active in infants. On the other hand, aging decreases hormone responsiveness in several receptor systems including the beta-adrenergic system and it was shown that the response to salbutamol declined in patients over 40 years of age (Feldman et al., 1984; Ullah et al., 1981).

F. Variations with Diseases

An interaction between asthma and thyroid diseases has been recognized; when thyrotoxicosis occurs in asthmatic patients, beta-2 agonist and corticosteroid requirements increase (Harrison and Tattersfield, 1984).

G. Assessment of Bronchial Effects Induced by Beta-2 Agonists

Bronchodilation is commonly assessed with flow measurements that are dependent on the airway caliber and the rheologic properties of the airflow, so that the spasm is not the only parameter explored. When pulmonary function tests are compared, FEV_1 and flow/volume loops are less accurate and sensitive than measurement of airway resistance but this latter test is less reproducible. In general, bronchodilation may be monitored by FEV_1 measurements and by determining flow at 50% of vital capacity (VC). The area under the flow/volume loop takes into account the whole variation of flow and volume and may be useful. Twenty percent improvement of FEV_1 from initial values is used as evidence of bronchodilation but it may be more accurate to express the results as a percentage of the optimal achievable value, that is the predicted values when age, sex, and weight are matched.

In practice, the improvement of patients under long-term treatment with beta-2 agonists should be serially investigated by simple methods based on the patient's subjective improvement, physical examination, and serial measures of peak flows twice daily.

VI. The Future of Beta-2 Agonists

Beta-2 agonists are widely used, and often represent the first line drug, since they are highly potent drugs with few side effects at regular dosages. They were initially used as bronchodilating agents but since they may have antiallergic properties they tend to be prophylactic drugs. However, they do not seem to act as anti-inflammatory agents, and when used alone in chronic asthma they may lead to a false impression of security.

New compounds that will be synthetized in the future may have an improved beta-2 selectivity, but it is not known whether this will be an advantage since beta-1 receptors are present in the airways and cardiac or skeletal muscle side effects are mediated essentially through beta-2 receptor activities. The duration of action of the drugs may be increased since the treatment of patients with so-called morning dipping is still difficult. Finally, the pharmacokinetics of these drugs should be better established.

Discussion

Barnes. There are now both animal and human studies showing that beta-agonists have no effect on bronchial hyperresponsiveness, and may even lead to an increase.

Bousquet. Beta-2 agonists do not seem to affect the course of airway inflammation in asthma.

Laitinen. What are the differences in the use of beta-agonists between countries. There is a trend in Britain, Scandinavia, and France to treat the inflammation of the airways, in addition to bronchospasm, even as a first-line treatment.

Kaliner. In the United States the trend is also towards earlier and more aggressive use of corticosteroids, although theophylline compounds are still a major early approach. I predict that inhaled corticosteroids will become a major first-line drug in the subject who regularly experiences asthma, while beta-2 agonists will be used for intermittent asthma.

Lefkowitz. The observation that some patients develop tachyphylaxis when treated with beta-2 agonists yet others does not seem very important.

References

Anderson, P. B., Goud, A., and Peake, M. D. (1982). Comparison of salbutamol given by intermittent positive-pressure breathing and pressure-packed aerosol in chronic asthma. *Thorax* **37**:612-616.

Angelici, E., Delfino, M., Carlone, S., Serra, P., Fineberg, N. S., and Farber, M. O. (1984). Tolerance to inhaled fenoterol. *Am. Rev. Respir. Dis.* **129**:1014-1016.

Arnaud, A., and Charpin, J. (1982). Interaction between corticosteroids and beta-2 agonists in acute asthma. *Eur. J. Respir. Dis.* **122**:126-131.

As (van), A. (1975). Beta-adrenergic stimulant bronchodilators. In *New Directions in Asthma.* Edited by M. Stein. Park Ridge, Il, The American College of Chest Physicians, pp. 415-432.

Assem, E. S. K., and Schild, H. O. (1969). Inhibition by sympathomimetic amines of histamine release induced by antigen in passively sensitized human lung. *Nature* **224**:1028-1029.

Aviado, D. M. (1975). The toxicity of aerosols. *J. Clin. Pharm.* **15**:86-104.

Avner, B. P., and Jenne, J. H. (1981). Desensitization of isolated human bronchial smooth muscle to beta-receptor agonists. *J. Allergy Clin. Immunol.* **68**:51-57.

Banner, A. S., Sunderrajan, E. V., Agarwal, M. K., and Addington, W. W. (1979). Arrhythmogenic effects of orally administered bronchodilators. *Arch. Intern. Med.* **139**:434-437.

Banerjee, D. P., Kung, L. S., Riggi, S. J., and Chandra, S. K. (1977). Development of beta-adrenergic receptor subsensitivity by antidepressants. *Nature* **268**:455-456.

Barnes, P. J., Gribbin, H. R., Osmanliev, D., and Pride, N. B. (1981). Partial flow-volume curves to measure bronchodilator dose response curves in normal humans. *J. Appl. Physiol.* **50**:1193-1197.

Barnes, P. J., Basbaum, C. B., Nadel, J. A., and Roberts, J. M. (1982). Localization of beta-adrenoceptors in mammalian lung by light microscopic autoradiography. *Nature* **299**:444-447.

Berg (van der), W., Leferink, J. G., Kreukniet, J., and Bruynzeel, P. L. B. (1980). Correlation between terbutaline serum levels, cAMP plasma levels and FEV_1 in normals and asthmatics after subcutaneous administration. *Ann. Allergy* **44**:235-239.

Berg, (van der), W., Leferink, J. G., Fokkens, J. K., Kreukniet, J., Maes, R. A. A., and Bruynzeel, P. L. B. (1982). Clinical implications of drug-induced desensitization of beta receptor after continuous oral use of terbutaline. *J. Allergy Clin. Immunol.* **69**:410-417.

Bhatia, S. P., and Davies, H. S. (1975). Evaluation of tolerance after continuous and prolonged oral administration of salbutamol to asthmatic patients. *Br. J. Pharmacol.* **2**:463-466.

Bono (del) N., D'Aula, S., and Vibelli, C. (1977). Dose-response of patients with reversible bronchospasm to oral clenbuterol: four doses compared. *Bull. Ther. Res.* **22**:376-384.

Borum, P., and Mygind, N. (1980). Inhibition of immediate allergic reaction in the nose by the beta-2 adrenostimulant fenoterol. *J. Allergy Clin. Immunol.* **66**:25-32.

Bousquet, J. (1988). In vivo methods for study of allergy. I. Skin tests. In *Allergy, Principles and Practice,* third edition. Edited by E. Middleton Jr. et al. St. Louis, C. V. Mosby, in press.

Bousquet, J., Fabre, J., Lebel, B., et al. (1986). Anti-allergic properties of clenbuterol. *J. Allergy Clin. Immunol.,* in press.

Brent, B. N., Mahler, D., Berger, H. J., Matthay, R. A., Pytlik, L., and Zaret, B. L. (1982). Augmentation of right ventricular performance in chronic obstructive pulmonary disease by terbutaline: a combined radionucleotide and hemodynamic study. *Am. J. Cardiol.* **50**:313-319.

Bres, J., Clauzel, A. M., Pistre, M. C., Rachmat, H., and Bressolle, F. (1985). Métabolisme des substances béta-adrenergiques. Implications thérapeutiques. *Bull. Eur. Physiopathol. Respir.* **21**:19S-34S.

Bretz, U., Martin, U., Mazzoni, L., and Ney, U. M. (1983). Beta-adrenergic tachyphylaxis in the rat and its reversal and prevention by ketotifen. *Eur. J. Pharmacol.* **86**:321-328.

Brodde, O. E., Brinkmann, M., Schemuth, R., O'Hara, N., and Daul, A. (1985). Terbutaline-induced desensitization of human lymphocyte beta-2-adrenoceptors. Accelerated restoration of beta-adrenoceptor responsiveness by prednisone and ketotifene. *J. Clin. Invest.* **76**:1096-1101.

Busse, W. W. (1977). Decreased granulocyte response to isoproterenol in asthma during upper respiratory infection. *Am. Rev. Respir. Dis.* **115**: 783-791.

Campbell, A. H. (1976). Mortality from asthma and bronchodilator aerosols. *Med. J. Aust.* **1**:386-391.

Cayton, R. M., Webber, B., and Paterson, J. W. (1981). A comparison of salbutamol given by pressure-packed aerosol or nebulization via IPPB in acute asthma. *Br. J. Dis. Chest.* **72**:222-224.

Clark, R. A., and Anderson, P. B. (1978). Combined therapy with salbutamol and beclomethasone inhalers in chronic asthma. *Lancet* **2**:70-72, 1978.

Clauzel, A. M. (1987). Beta-2-agonists in asthma. In *Highlights in Asthmology.* Edited by F. B. Michel, J. Bousquet, and P. Godard. Heidelberg, Springer Verlag, in press.

Clauzel, A. M., Calvayrac, P., Bres, J., and Michel, F. B. (1984). Pirbuterol: relation between pharmacokinetics and bronchodilation. *Am. Rev. Respir. Dis.* **129**:87.

Clauzel, A. M., Bres, J., Bousquet, J., and Michel, F. B. (1985). An attempt to predict beta-adrenergic tachyphylaxis. *J. Allergy Clin. Immunol.* **75**:180.

Coady, T. J., Steward, C. J., and Davies, H. J. (1976). Synchronization of bronchodilator release. *Practitioner* **217**:273-279.

Coffey, R. G., Logsdon, P. J., and Middleton, E. Jr. (1973). Leukocyte adenyl cyclase and ATPase in asthma: effect of corticosteroid therapy. *Chest* **63**: 25-27.

Collier, J. G., Dobbs, R. J., and Williams, I. (1980). Salbutamol aerosol causes a tachycardia due to inhaled rather than the swallowed fraction. *Br. J. Clin. Pharmacol.* **9**:273-274.

Conolly, M. E., and Greenacre, J. K. (1976). The lymphocyte beta-adrenoceptor in normal subjects and patients with bronchial asthma. *J. Clin. Invest.* **58**:1307-1316.

Conolly, M. E., Tashkin, D. P., and Hui, K. K. (1982). Selective subsensitization of beta-adrenergic receptors in central airways of asthmatics and normal subjects during long-term therapy with inhaled salbutamol. *J. Allergy Clin. Immunol.* **70**:423-431.

Crompton, G. (1979). Comparison of salbutamol given intravenously and by intermittent positive-pressure breathing in life-threatening asthma. *Br. J. Med.* **278**:848.

Croner, S., Hedenskog, S., Kjellman, N. I., and Odelram, H. (1981). Salbutamol powder or spray inhalation in childhood asthma. *Allergy* **35**:589-592.

Cullum, V. A., Farmer, J. B., Jack, D., and Levy, G. P. (1969). Salbutamol: a new, selective beta-adrenoceptive receptor stimulant. *Br. J. Pharmacol.* **35**: 371-376.

Dahl, R., and Johansson, S. A. (1982). Effect on lung function of budenoside by inhalation, terbutaline s.c. and placebo given simultaneously or as single treatments. *Eur. J. Respir. Dis.* Suppl **122**:132-137.

Davies, A. O., and Lefkowitz, R. J. (1983). In vitro desensitization of beta-adrenergic receptor in human neutrophils. Attenuation by corticosteroids. *J. Clin. Invest.* **71**:565-571.

Djurup, R. (1981). Adrenoceptors: molecular nature and role in atopic diseases. *Allergy* **36**:289-307.

Duncan, D., Paterson, I. C., Harris, D., and Crompton, G. K. (1977). Comparison of the bronchodilator effects of salbutamol inhaled as a dry powder and by conventional pressurized aerosol. *Br. J. Clin. Pharmacol.* **4**:669-671.

Editorial (1984). The nebulizer epidemic. *Lancet* **2**:789-790.

Eriksson, N. E., Haglind, K., and Hidinger, K. G. (1980). A new inhalation technique for freon aerosols: terbutaline aerosol with a tube extension in a two-day cross over comparison with salbutamol aerosol. *Allergy* **35**:620.

Evans, M. E., Richards, A. J., Walker, S. R., and Paterson, K. W. (1971). The fate of 3H-salbutamol in asthmatic patients. *Biochem. J.* **125**:27-28.

Fairshter, R. D., Novey, H. S., and Wilson, A. F. (1981). Site and duration of bronchodilatation in asthmatic patients after oral administration of terbutaline. *Chest* **79**:50-59.

Falkner, F. C., and McIlheny, N. M. (1976). Selected ion monitoring assay for the bronchodilator pirbuterol. *Biomass. Spectrom.* **3**:207-211.

Feldman, R. D., Limbird, L. E., Nadeau, J., Robertson, D., and Wood, J. J. (1984). Alterations in leukocyte beta-receptor affinity with ageing. *N. Engl. J. Med.* **310**:815-819.

Formgren, H. (1975). The therapeutic value of oral long-term treatment with terbutaline in asthma. A follow-up study of its efficacy and side effects. *Scand. J. Respir. Dis.* **56**:321-328.

Fügner, A. (1977). Inhibition of antigen-induced histamine release by beta-adrenergic stimulants in vivo. *Int. Arch. Allergy Appl. Immunol.* **54**: 78-87.

Gibson, G. J., Greenaire, J. K., Konig, P., Conolly, M. E., and Pride, N. B.

(1978). Use of exercise challenge to investigate possible tolerance to beta-adrenoceptor stimulation in asthma. *Br. J. Dis. Chest* **72**:199-206.

Gomm, S. A., Keaney, N. P., Winsey, N. P., and Stretton, T. B. (1980). Effect of an extension tube on the bronchodilator efficacy of terbutaline delivered from a metered dose inhaler. *Thorax* **35**:552-557.

Grimwood, K., Johnson-Barrett, J., and Taylor, B. (1981). Salbutamol: tablets, inhalational powder, or nebulizer? *Br. Med. J.* **282**:105-106.

Gronneberg, R., Strandberg, K., and Hagermark, O. (1980). Effect in man of oral terbutaline on cutaneous reactions induced by allergen and cold stimulation. *Allergy* **35**:143-147.

Groth, S., Dirksen, H., and Mygind, N. (1984). Intranasal fenoterol in asthmatic subjects: an alternative route of administration. *J. Allergy Clin. Immunol.* **74**:536-539.

Guillot, C., Fornaris, M., Badier, M., and Orehek, J. (1984). Spontaneous and provoked resistance to isoproterenol in isolated human bronchi. *J. Allergy Clin. Immunol.* **74**:713-718.

Haalboom, J. R. E., Deenstra, M., and Struyvenberg, A. (1985). Hypokalaemia induced by inhalation of fenoterol. *Lancet* **2**:1125-1127.

Harden, T. K. (1983). Agonist induced desensitization of the beta-adrenergic receptor linked adenylate cyclase. *Pharmacol. Rev.* **35**:5-41.

Harris, L. (1971). Are bronchodilator aerosol inhalation responsible for an increase in asthma mortality? *Ann. Allergy* **29**:250-255.

Harris, L. (1972). Comparison of the effect on blood gases, ventilation and perfusion of isoproterenol-phenylephrine and salbutamol in chronic bronchitis with asthma. *J. Allergy Clin. Immunol.* **49**:63-71.

Harrison, R. N., and Tattersfield, A. E. (1984). Airway response to inhaled salbutamol in hyperthyroid and hypothyroid patients before and after treatment. *Thorax* **39**:34-39.

Harvey, J. E., Baldwin, C. J., Wood, P. J., Alberti, K. G. M. M., and Tattersfield, A. E. (1981). Airway and metabolic responsiveness to intravenous salbutamol in asthma: effect of regular inhaled salbutamol. *Clin. Sci.* **60**:579-585.

Harvey, J. E., and Tattersfield, A. E. (1982). Airway response to salbutamol inhalations in normal, atopic and asthmatic subjects. *Thorax* **37**:280-287.

Heel, R. C., Brogden, R. N., Speight, T. M., and Avery, G. S. (1978). Fenoterol: a review of its pharmacological properties and therapeutic efficacy in asthma. *Drugs* **15**:3-32.

Hegardt, B., and Arner, B. (1981). Evaluation of the inhibition of allergen-induced intracutaneous reactions by a new beta-agonist, KWD 2131, and by terbutaline. *Eur. J. Respir. Dis.* **62**:352-359.

Heimer, D., Shim, D., and Williams, M. H. Jr. (1980). The effect of sequential inhalations of metaproterenol in asthma. *J. Allergy Clin. immunol.* **66**: 75-77.

Herxheimer, H. (1946). Dosage of ephedrine in bronchial asthma and emphysema. *Br. Med. J.* **2**:350-852.

Holgate, S. T., Baldwin, C. J., and Tattersfield, A. E. (1977). Beta-adrenergic agonist resistance in normal human airways. *Lancet* **2**:375-377.

Howarth, P. H., Durham, S. P., Lee, T. H., Kay, A. B., Church, M. K., and Holgate, S. T. (1985). Influence of albuterol, cromolyn sodium and ipratropium bromide on the airway and circulating mediator responses to allergen bronchial provocation is asthma. *Am. Rev. Respir. Dis.* **132**: 986-992.

Hurst, A. (1973). Metaproterenol, a potent and safe bronchodilator. *Ann. Allergy* **31**:460-466.

Imbeau, S. A., Harruff, R., Hirscher, M., and Reed, C. E. (1978). Terbutaline's effects on the allergy skin test. *J. Allergy Clin. Immunol.* **62**:193-106.

Inman, W. H. W., and Adelstein, A. M. (1969). Rise and fall of asthma mortality in England and Wales in relation to use of pressurized aerosols. *Lancet* **2**: 279-285.

Jenne, J. W. (1982). Whither beta-adrenergic tachyphylaxis. *J. Allergy Clin. Immunol.* **70**:413-416.

Kemp, J. P., Chervinsky, P., Orgel, H. A., Metlzer, E. O., Noyes, J. H., and Mingo, T. S. (1984). Concomitant bitolterol mesylate aerosol and theophylline for asthma therapy, with 24 hr electrocardiographic monitoring. *J. Allergy Clin. Immunol.* **73**:32-43.

Kraan, J., Koeter, G. H., Mark, Th. W. v. d., Sluiter, H. J., and de Vries, K. (1985). Changes in bronchial hyperreactivity induced by 4 weeks of treatment with antiasthmatic drugs in patients with allergic asthma: a comparison between budenoside and terbutaline. *J. Allergy Clin. Immunol.* **76**:628-636.

Kubo, S., Matsubara, J., Kasamatsu, S., et al. (1980). Pharmacological studies of 1-(2-chloro-4-hydroxyphenyl)-2-t-butylaminoethanol (HOKU 81) a new bronchodilator. *Drug Res.* **30**:1272-1278.

Kurland, G., Williams, J., and Lewiston, N. J., (1979). Fatal myocardial toxicity during continuous infusion intravenous isoproterenol therapy of asthma. *J. Allergy Clin. Immunol.* **63**:407-411.

Lands, A. M., Arnold, A., McAuliff, J. P., et al. (1967). Differentiation of receptor systems activated by sympathomimetic amines. *Nature* **214**:597-598.

Laros, C. D., Van Urk, P., and Rominger, K. L. (1977). Absorption, distribution and excretion of tritium labelled beta-2 stimulator, fenoterol hypobromid, following aerosol administration and instillation into the trachea. *Respiration* **34**:131-140.

Larsson, S., and Svedmyr, N. (1977a). Bronchodilating effect and side effects of beta-2-adrenoceptor stimulants by different modes of administration (Tablets, metered aerosol and combination therapy). *Am. Rev. Respir. Dis.* **116**:861-869.

Larsson, S., and Svedmyr, N. (1977b). Cumulative dose-response curves for comparison of oral bronchodilating drugs: a study of salbutamol and fenoterol. *Ann. Allergy* **39**:362-368.

Larsson, S., Svedmyr, N., and Thiringer, G. (1977). Lack of bronchial adrenoceptor resistance in asthmatics during long term treatment with terbutaline. *J. Allergy Clin. Immunol.* **59**:131-140.

Lee, H., and Evans, H. E. (1984). Aerosol bag for administration of bronchodilators to young asthmatic children. *Pediatrics* **73**:230-232.

Leferink, J. G., Dankers, J., and Maes, R. R. A. (1982a). A time saving method for the determination of beta-2 sympathomimetics (terbutaline salbutamol and fenoterol). Preliminary results. *J. Chromatogr.* **229**:217-221.

Leferink, J. G., Van Der Berg, W., Wagemakhe-Engej, I., Kreukniet, J., and Maes, R. A. A. (1982b). Pharmacokinetics of terbutaline, a sympathomimetic, in healthy volunteers and asthmatic patients. *Drug Res.* **32**:159-164.

Lenney, W., and Milner, A. D. (1978). At what age do bronchodilators work? *Arch. Dis. Child.* **53**:532-535.

Levesque, K. A., and Johnson, C. E. (1984). Bacterial contamination of pressurized inhalers. *Drug. Intell. Clin. Pharm.* **18**:735-737.

Lewis, R. A., Cushley, M. J., Fleming, S. J., and Tattersfield, A. E. (1982). Is a nebulizer less efficient than a mettered dose inhaler and do pear-shaped extension tubes work? *Am. Rev. Respir. Dis.* **125**:94.

Lindren, S. B., Formgren, H., and Moren, F. (1980). Improved aerosol therapy of asthma: effect of actuator tube size on drug availability. *Eur. J. Respir. Dis.* **61**:56-64.

Lofdahl, C.-G., and Svedmyr, N. (1984). Selectivity of beta-adrenergic stimulating and blocking agents. *Eur. J. Respir. Dis. Suppl.* **136** 65:101-113.

McFadden, E. R. (1981). Beta-2-receptor agonists: metabolism and pharmacology. *J. Allergy Clin. Immunol.* **68**:91-97.

McIlheny, N. M., and Choly, M. D. S. (1979). Biotransformation of pirbuterol by the rat, dog and human. *Fed. Proc.* **38**:442-443.

Madsen, B. W., Tandon, M. K., and Paterson, J. H. (1979). Cross-over study of the efficacy of four beta-2-sympathomimetic bronchodilator aerosols. *Br. J. Pharmacol.* **8**:75-82.

Marlin, G. E., Jenkins, C. R., and Breslin, A. B. X. (1983). The protective effect of inhaled prazosin and salbutamol on histamine-induced bronchoconstriction. *Aust. N. Z. Med. J.* **13**:556.

Marone, G., Ambrosio, G., Bonaduce, D., Genovese, A., Triggiani, M., and Condorelli, M. (1984). Inhibition of IgE-mediated histamine release from human basophils and mast cells by fenoterol. *Int. Arch. Allergy Appl. Immunol.* 356-361.

Minette, A., Marcq, M., and Gepts, L. (1976). Carbuterol, Fenoterol, orciprenaline, salbutamol and terbutaline per os in reversible obstructive chronic bronchitis. *Bull. Europ. Physiopathol. Respir.* **12**:545-553.

Mita, H., and Shida, T. (1983). Anti-allergic activity of formoterol, a new beta-adrenoceptor stimulant and salbutamol in human leucocytes and human lung tissue. *Allergy* **38**:547-553.

Mossberg, B., Stranberg, K., Philipson, K., and Camner, P. (1976). Tracheobronchial clearance in asthma: Response to beta-adrenceptor stimulation. *Scand. J. Respir. Dis.* **57**:119-128.

Nelson, H. S. (1982). Beta-adrenergic agonists. *Chest* Suppl 33S-38S.

Nelson, H. S., Raine, D. J., and Doner, H. C. (1977). Subsensitivity to the bronchodilator action of albuterol produced by chronic administration. *Am. Rev. Respir. Dis.* **116**:871-877.

Newhouse, M. T., and Ruffin, R. E. (1978). Deposition and fate of aerosolized drugs. *Chest* **73**:936-943.

Newman, S. P., Moren, F., Pavia, D., et al. (1981a). Deposition of pressurized suspension aerosols inhaled through extension devices. *Am. Rev. Respir. Dis.* **124**:317-320.

Newman, S. P., Pavia, D., and Clarke, S. W. (1981b). Simple instructions for using pressurized aerosol bronchodilators. *J. R. Soc. Med.* **73**:776-782.

Newman, S. P., Pavia, D., Moren, F., Shealan, N. F., and Clarke, S. W. (1981c). Deposition of pressurized aerosols in the human respiratory tract. *Thorax* **36**:52-55.

Nicklas, R. A., Whitehurst, V. E., Donohoe, R. F., and Balazs, T. (1984). Concimitant use of beta adrenergic agonists and methylxanthines. *J. Allergy Clin. Immunol.* **73**:20-23.

Nilsson, R. T., Persson, K., and Tegner, K. (1972). The metabolism of terbutaline in man. *Xenobiotica* **2**:363-375.

O'Donnell, S. R. (1970). A selective beta-adrenreceptor stimulant (Th 1165a) related to orciprenaline. *Eur. J. Pharmacol.* **12**:35-43.

Orehek, J., Gayrard, P., Grimaud, C. H., and Charpin, J. (1976). Patient error in use of bronchodilator aerosols. *Br. Med. J.* **1**:76.

Orehek, J., Charpin, D., Velardocchio, J. M., and Grimaud, C. (1980). Bronchomotor effect of bronchoconstriction-induced deep inspirations in asthmatics. *Am. Rev. Respir. Dis.* **121**:297-305.

Orgel, H. A., Kemp, J. P., Tinkelman, D. G., and Webb, D. R. Jr. (1985). Bitolterol and albuterol metered-dose aerosols: comparison of two long-acting beta-2-adrenergic bronchodilators for treatment of asthma. *J. Allergy Clin. Immunol.* **75**:55-62.

Patel, K. R. (1985). Tulobuterol in the management of obstructive airways disease in adults. *Clin. Ther.* **7**:452-467.

Paterson, I. C., and Crompton, G. K. (1976). Use of pressurized aerosols by asthmatic patients. *Br. Med. J.* **1**:76.

Paterson, J. W., Woolcock, A. J., and Shenfield, G. M. (1979). Bronchodilator drugs. *Am. Rev. Respir. Dis.* **120**:1149-1188.

Pavia, D., Thompson, M. L., Clarke, S. W., and Shannon, H. S. (1977). Effect of lung function and mode of inhalation on penetration of aerosol into the human lung. *Thorax* **32**:194-199.

Peel, E. T., and Gibson, G. J. (1980). Effects of long-term inhaled salbutamol therapy on the provocation of asthma by histamine. *Am. Rev. Respir. Dis.* **121**:973-978.

Peltola, H., and Michelsson, K. (1982). Efficacy of salbutamol in treatment of infant pertussis demonstrated by sound spectrum analysis. *Lancet* **1**:310-312.

Petersson, B. A. (1984). Sustained inhibition of antigen-induced histamine release from human lung by beta-2-adrenoceptor agonist terbutaline. *Allergy* **39**:351-357.

Phillips, P. J., Vedig, A. E., Jones, P. L., et al. (1980). Metabolic responses and cardiac side effects to selective beta-2-adrenoceptor agonists, salbutamol and rimiterol. *Br. J. Clin. Pharmacol.* **9**:483-493.

Pierce, R. J., Payne, C. R., Williams, S. J., Denison, D. M., and Clark, T. J. H. (1981). Comparison of intravenous and inhaled terbutaline in the treatment of asthma. *Chest* **79**:506-510.

Pierson, W. E., Shapiro, G. G., Furukawa, C., and Bierman, C. W. (1985). Albuterol syrup on the treatment of asthma. *J. Allergy Clin. Immunol.* **76**: 228-233.

Poppa, V. (1984). Clinical pharmacology of adrenergic drugs. *J. Asthma* **21**: 183-207.

Pratt, H. F. (1982). Abuse of salbutamol inhalers in young people. *Clin. Allergy* **12**:203-209.

Riley, D. J., Weitz, B. W., and Edelman, N. M. (1976). The responses of asthmatic subjects to isoproterenol inhaled at differing lung volumes. *Am. Rev. Respir. Dis.* **114**:509-516.

Rossing, T. H., Fanta, C. H., and McFadden, E. R. (1981). A controlled trial of the use of single versus combined-drug therapy in the treatment of acute episodes of asthma. *Am. Rev. Respir. Dis.* **123**:190-194.

Rudolf, M. (1984). Combination therapy—a review of clinical studies. *Postgrad. Med. J.* **60** (suppl 1):9-12.

Salome, C. M., Schoeffel, R. E., Yan, K., and Woolcock, A. J. (1983). Effect of aerosol fenoterol on the severity of bronchial hyperreactivity in patients with asthma. *Thorax* **38**:854-858.

Shargel, L., and Dorrbecker, S. A. (1976). Physiological distribution and metabolism of 3H-bitolterol in man and dog. *Drug Metab. Disp.* **4**:72-78.

Shelhamer, J. H., Marom, Z., and Kaliner, M. (1983). Abnormal beta-adrenergic responsiveness in allergic subjects. II. The role of beta-2-adrenergic hyporeactivity. *J. Allergy Clin. Immunol.* **71**:57-61.

Shenfield, G. M. (1982). Combination bronchodilator therapy. *Drugs* **24**:414-439.

Simon, R. A. (1984). Adverse reactions to drug additives. *J. Allergy Clin. Immunol.* **74**:623-630.

Skidmore, I. F. (1984). Drugs acting at adrenoceptors. In *Development of Anti-Asthma Drugs.* Edited by D. R. Buckle and H. Smith. London, Butterworths, pp. 185-203.

Slutsky, R., Hooper, W., Gerber, K., Ashburn, W., Curtis, G., and Karliner, J. (1981). Left ventricular size and function after sub-cutaneous administration of terbutaline. Assessment by cardiac blood pool imaging. *Chest* **79**:401-405, 1981.

Sly, R. M., Anderson, J. A., Bierman, C. W., et al. (1985). Adverse effects and complications of treatment with beta-adrenergic agonist drugs. *J. Allergy Clin. Immunol.* **75**:443-449.

Smith, S. R., and Kendall, M. J. (1984). Metabolic responses to beta-2-stimulants. *J. R. Coll. Physicians Lond.* **13**:190-194.

Stiles, G. L., Caron, M. G., and Lefkowitz, R. J. (1984). Beta-adrenergic receptors: biochemical mechanisms of physiological regulation. *Physiol. Rev.* **64**:661-743.

Szentivanyi, A. (1968). The beta-adrenergic theory of the atopic abnormality in bronchial asthma. *J. Allergy* **42**:203-232.

Tashkin, D. P., Conolly, M. E., Deutsch, R. I., et al. (1982). Subsensitization of beta-adrenoceptors in airways and lymphocytes of healthy and asthmatic subjects. *Am. Rev. Respir. Dis.* **125**:185-193.

Tattersfield, A. E. (1983). Autonomic bronchodilators. In *Asthma.* Edited by T. J. H. Clark and S. Godfrey. London, Chapman and Hall, pp. 301-335.

Teule, G. J. J., and Majid, P. A. (1980). Haemodynamic effects of terbutaline in chronic obstructive airway disease. *Thorax* **35**:536-543.

Thompson, P. J., Dhillon, P., and Cole, P. (1983). Addiction to aerosol treatement: the asthmatic alternative to glue sniffing. *Br. Med. J.* **287**:1515-1516.

Tobin, M. J., Jenouri, G., Danta, I., Kim, C., Watson, H., and Sackner, M. A. (1982). Response to bronchodilator drug administration by a new reservoir aerosol delivery system and a review of other auxilliary delivery systems. *Am. Rev. Respir. Dis.* **126**:670-675.

Ullah, M. I., Newman, G. B., and Saunders, K. B. (1981). Influence of age on response to ipratropium and salbutamol. *Thorax* **36**:523-529.

Wanner, A., and Ahmed (1983). Immunopharmacology of the mucociliary clearance. In *Immunopharmacology of the Lung. Lung Biology in Health and Disease.* Vol. 19. Edited by H. H. Newball. New York, Marcel Dekker, pp. 369-400.

Watanabe, S., Renzetti, A. D., Begin, R., and Bigler, A. H. (1974). Airway responsiveness to a bronchodilator aerosol. I. Normal subjects. *Am. Rev. Respir. Dis.* **109**:530-537.

Weber, R. W., Smith, J. A., and Nelson, H. S. (1982). Aerosolized terbutaline in asthmatics: development of subsensitivity with long-term administration. *J. Allergy Clin. Immunol.* **70**:417-422.

Whitehurst, V. E., Joseph, X., Hohmann, J. R., Pledger, G., and Balazs, T. (1983). Cardiotoxic effects in rats and rabbits treated with terbutaline alone and in combination with aminophylline. *J. Am. Coll. Toxicol.* **2**:147-153.

Williams, S., and Seaton, A. (1977). Intravenous or inhaled salbutamol in acute asthma. *Thorax* **32**:555-558.

Wilson, J. D., Sutherland, D. C., and Thomas, A. C. (1981). Has the change to beta-agonists combined with oral theophylline increased cases of fatal asthma? *Lancet* **1**:1235-1237.

Wolfe, J. D., Tashkin, D. P., Calvarese, B., and Simmons, M. (1978). Bronchodilator effect of terbutaline and aminophylline alone and in combination in asthmatic patients. *N. Engl. J. Med.* **298**:363-367.

Zaagsma, J., Van Den Heijden, P. J. C. M., Van Der Schaar, N. W., and Bank, C. M. C. (1983). Comparison of functional beta-receptor heterogeneity in central and peripheral airway smooth muscle of guinea pig and man. *J. Receptor Res.* **3**:89-106.

7

Cholinergic Neuroeffector Mechanisms in Airway Smooth Muscle

RONALD F. COBURN

University of Pennsylvania School of Medicine
Philadelphia, Pennsylvania

I plan to review information related to two aspects of cholinergic neurotransmission to airway smooth muscle that are of current interest and under investigation in my laboratories: neurotransmission in airway peripheral ganglia and coupling mechanisms involved in cholinergic activation of airway smooth muscle. Figure 1 illustrates various steps involved in the activation of airway smooth muscle via neural input, and highlights the two areas that will be discussed here. Both of these areas are in their infancy and our state of knowledge at this time reflects this. Both areas deserve study to determine if they play roles in various hypersensitivity states seen clinically.

I. Ganglionic Neurotransmission

A. Properties of Neurons

In the last decades our understanding of neural control of airway smooth muscle has advanced in several steps. Prior to 1972, neural control was seen as mediated via the vagal parasympathetic cholinergic system and the sympathetic adrenergic system (Cabazas et al., 1971; Widdecombe, 1967). There was little or no consideration of neural integration of inputs at the level of the airway peripheral para-

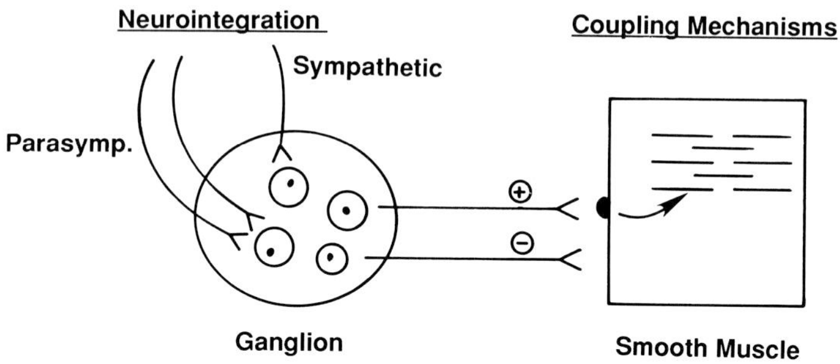

Figure 1 Neurointegration at the level of airway peripheral ganglia and smooth muscle coupling mechanisms involved in cholinergic activation of airway smooth muscle. These two areas are reviewed in this chapter.

sympathetic ganglia. After about 1970, field stimulation experiments indicated the presence of a strong nonadrenergic inhibitory nerve system in airway smooth muscle of most species, including human (Altiere et al., 1985; Coburn and Tomita, 1973; Richardson, 1979; Richardson and Beland, 1976; see chapter by Dr. L. Diamond in this volume). The paucity of catecholamine fluorescence in airway smooth muscle in some species (Coburn and Tomita, 1973; O'Donnell and Soar, 1973) led to the concept that direct sympathetic innervation to airway smooth muscle might be of minor importance. Evidence showed that preganglionic nonadrenergic inhibitory neurons may run in the vagus and synapse in peripheral airway ganglia (Chesrown et al., 1980; Yip et al., 1981). Catecholamine-containing neuron terminals were observed encircling cell bodies in airway peripheral ganglia, suggesting adrenergic input may be mediated at this level (Wacobowitz et al., 1973). Workers in this area are now debating whether evidence that a noncholinergic, nonadrenergic excitatory transmitter (apparently substance P), which is released from sensory neurons under experimental conditions, has physiological importance (Anderson and Grundstrom, 1983).

The anatomy of peripheral airway ganglia was actually described very early by workers such as Fisher (1964), Honjin (1954), and Elfman (1943). More recently, Dr. John Richardson's electron microscopic (EM) studies of parabronchial ganglia in humans focused the attention of many investigators on the possible role of these structures in integration of neural inputs to airway muscle and other innervated cells (Richardson, 1949).

There have been a number of approaches to the study of integration of neural inputs to airway smooth muscle. Yip et al. (1981) developed an in vivo approach in which effects of field stimulation of trachaelis muscle were compared with effects of preganglionic nerve stimulation. Data obtained on the guinea pig suggested that peripheral airway ganglia filter inhibitory input to trachealis muscle. Recently, a similar approach that studied excitatory preganglionic neural input in anesthetized ferrets has shown that peripheral ganglia can filter excitatory input as well (Skoogh, 1983). The use of nicotinic agonists, such as dimethyl-4-phenylpiperazinium, has also proven to be an effective way of stimulating neural input to smooth muscle at the level of the autonomic ganglia, and is useful in studying different types of neural input (Leff and Munox, 1981).

Three different preparations suitable for studying electrophysiological properties of neurons in airway peripheral ganglia have been developed; in vitro preparations that study paratracheal peripheral ganglia in the ferret (Baker et al., 1983; Cameron and Coburn, 1984) and rabbit (Fowler and Weinreich, 1986) and an in vivo preparation for study of the cat peripheral paratracheal ganglia (Mitchell et al., 1984). The preparations in use in our laboratory will be described in greatest detail in this section. For electrophysiological study of the ferret paratracheal ganglia, the trachea is dissected with care to preserve neural structures located on its posterior surface in close aposition to trachealis muscle. Trachea cartilages are cut longitudinally and the preparation placed posterior surface up in an organ bath that allows dark field and/or bright field illumination of the ganglion-nerve plexus. Studies using silver impregnation (Coburn, 1984a) and acetylcholinesterase staining (Baker et al., 1986) have indicated the complexity of this plexus. The latter approach has identified two layers of structures. Our studies have been performed on deep ganglia connected by interganglionic nerve trunks (IGNT). Beautiful freeze-fracture sections showing the anatomy of the guinea pig paratracheal ganglia have recently been published (Baluk et al., 1985).

Somal microelectrode penetrations of ganglion cells in ferret paratracheal ganglia have revealed two different types of neurons, classified on the basis of responses to intracellular current injection and the characteristics of postsynaptic potentials evoked via preganglionic electrical stimulation. These approaches revealed a cell type (Fig. 2) characterized during cathodal current injection by the appearance of a single action potential followed by a very large, long-duration after-hyperpolarization (Cameron and Coburn, 1984). These action potentials are inhibited by tetrodotoxin. Current-voltage relationships show that most of these cells exhibit outward rectification. Single preganglionic nerve stimulations always evoke a fast EPSP and, rarely, evidence of a fast IPSP. The fast EPSP is graded, inhibited by hexamethonium, and frequently evokes a single action potential. This cell type, which we have termed AH cells because of the prominent after-hyperpolarization, seems very similar to type II AH cells described in the myenteric plexus (Wood, 1985).

The morphology of neurons in ferret paratracheal ganglia has been studied using horseradish peroxidase (HRP) (Baker et al., 1986; Kalia and Coburn, 1986) and lucifier yellow (Baker et al., 1986). Figure 3 shows an example of an AH

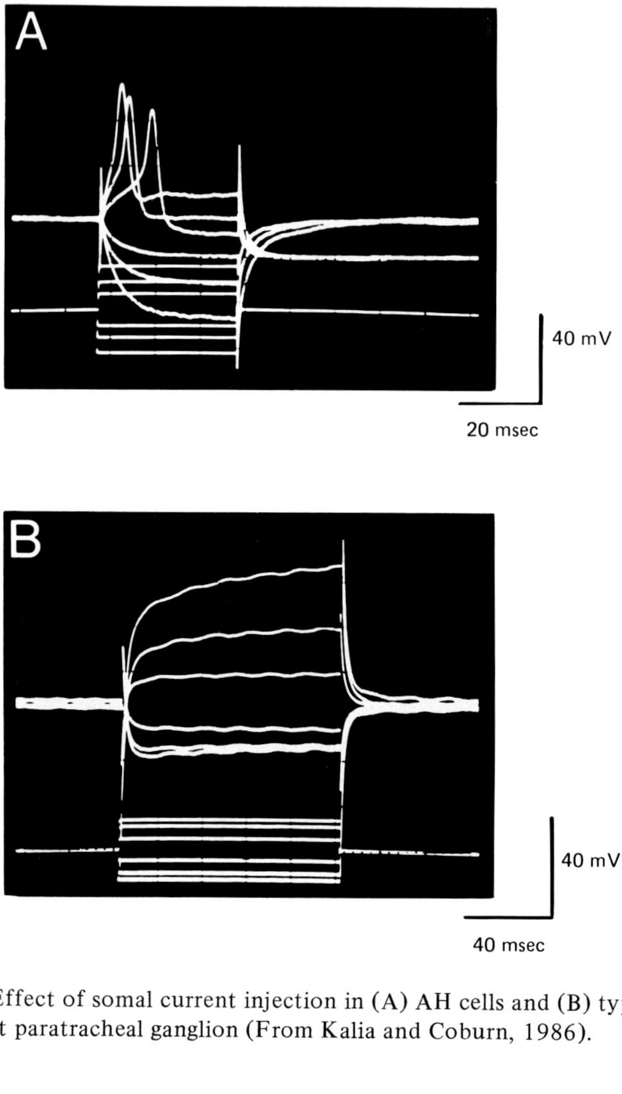

Figure 2 Effect of somal current injection in (A) AH cells and (B) type B cells in the ferret paratracheal ganglion (From Kalia and Coburn, 1986).

cell. They are all multipolar cells and provide single to multiple axons, some of which run bidirectionally in the IGNT and appear to come into close contact with neighboring ganglia. Axons are observed running into smooth muscle. These cells show multiple processes within the ganglia that may be dendrites. The evidence these cells innervate smooth muscle includes the presence of axons within smooth muscle and the finding that AH cell somal current injection evokes

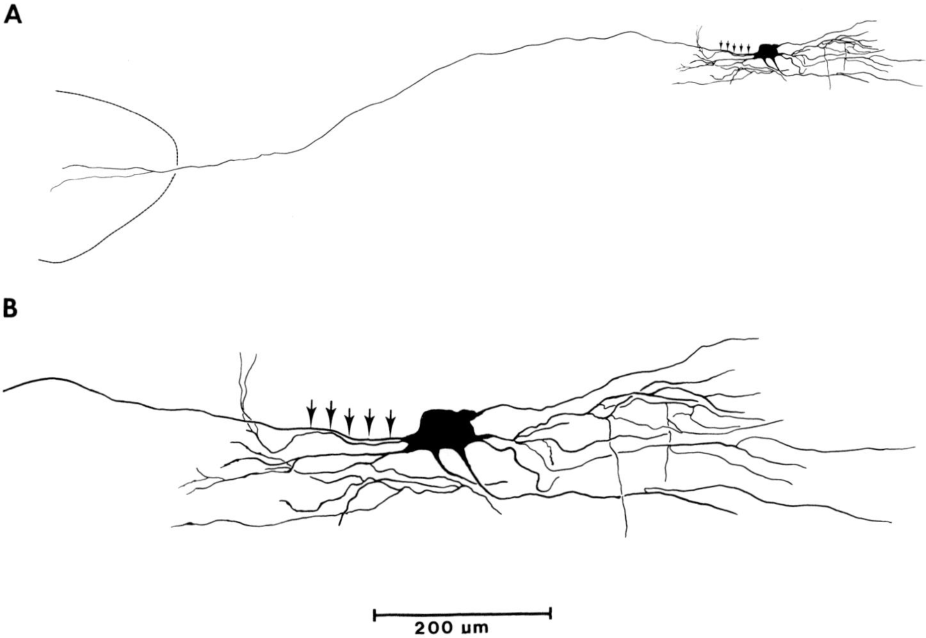

Figure 3 Morphology of an AH cell in the ferret paratracheal ganglion. The cell was filled by somal injection and electrophoresis. (From Kalia and Coburn 1986).

excitatory junction potentials in smooth muscle cells (Coburn, unpublished data).

The second type of cell in this structure is characterized by a lack of evoked action potentials when cathodal current in injected into the soma (Fig. 2B). Sixty to 70% of the penetrations are of this type. Voltage-current studies often show anomalous rectification. This cell shows, on multiple preganglionic nerve stimulation, an apparent slow excitatory synaptic potential (Fig. 4). Typically the resting membrane potential in these cells is larger than seen in AH cells. HRP studies have indicated that at least some of these cells are neurons with morphology very similar to that seen with AH cells.

The above classification may be crude and it is likely in the future that there will be further subclassifications of neurons in the ferret paratracheal peripheral ganglia.

Morphologic characteristics of neurons in the paratracheal nerve ganglion

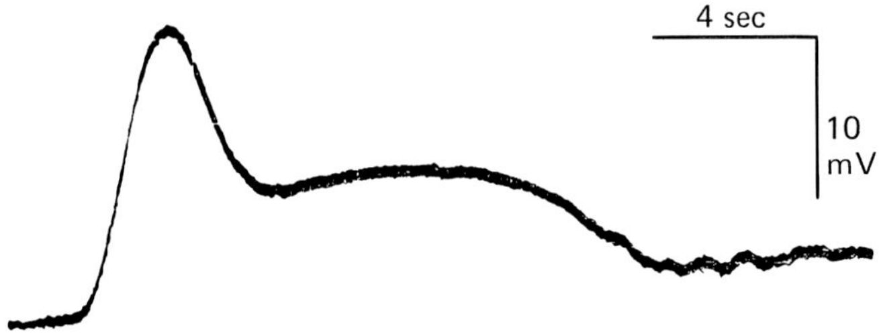

Figure 4 Slow excitatory postsynaptic potential evoked in type B cell of the ferret paratracheal ganglia. This was measured using an intracellular microelectrode placed in the cell body. Stimulation was 1 sec 5 Hz of the interganglionic nerve trunk. (The stimulus artifact is not on the tracing) (From Cameron and Coburn, 1984).

plexus have also been performed using EM (Cameron and Coburn, 1984). We were unable to identify two cell types on the basis of size or other morphologic characteristics, but the number of cells studied was small.

In other species, the characteristics of neurons in the paratracheal ganglia are different from those observed in the ferret. In the rabbit (Fowler and Weinreich, 1986), two cell types have been identified, one of which appears to be similar to the AH cell in the ferret. The other type cell also shows evoked action potentials, but action-potential-producing channels do not inactivate with sustained depolarizing current and multiple action potentials are evoked. The nature of postsynaptic potentials in this preparation has yet to be studied.

The cat paratracheal ganglia shows three populations of neurons that have been classified on the basis of spontaneous action potentials in an in vivo preparation: cells that show inspiratory spikes inhibited by lung inflation; cells that fire during expiration; and cells that fire randomly (Mitchell et al., 1984). Rabbit and cat paratracheal ganglia seem more similar to other peripheral parasympathetic ganglia (Blackman et al., 1969; King and Szurszewski, 1984), with the finding of cells that show repetitive action potentials during prolonged cathodal current injection, than is the ferret paratracheal ganglia.

There is a real need for studies of how various neural inputs are integrated by airway peripheral ganglia. Available evidence, largely from the ferret, suggests these ganglia may have complex integrative functions and not function merely as relay stations. This evidence includes the ability of these ganglia to filter inputs (Skoogh, 1983; Yit et al., 1981); the presence of multiple postsynaptic potentials, including a slow EPSP, which is known in other neurons to control neuronal excitability (Hartzell, 1981; Wood and Mayer, 1978); the presence of several different neuropeptides that presumably serve as neurotransmitters or modulators (Uddman et al., 1978; Hakanson et al., 1983); evidence that sympathetic adrenergic nerve fibers synapse in airway peripheral ganglia (Jacobowitz et al., 1973).

Our ability to study integration of "inputs" to airway periphal ganglia depends on our developing preparations that allow us to study this phenomenoa. The approach of comparing field stimulation evoked changes in airway muscle tension, and preganglionic nerve stimulation evoked changes in muscle tension, shows promise for studying neurointegration and has already documented strong inhibitory effects of exogenous norepinephrine on neurotransmission of excitatory signals through the ferret paratracheal ganglia (Skoogh, 1983). However, field stimulation and nerve stimulation may generate different patterns of neurotransmitter release and give differences in tension response not due to "filtering." The mechanisms of neurointegration of inputs can, perhaps, be best studied using in vitro peripheral ganglion preparations. Figure 5 illustrates one approach using the ferret paratracheal ganglia. Preganglionic nerves are stimulated at a known frequency and electrical events monitored in postsynaptic neurons, in this case AH cell somal recordings. Figure 5 illustrates an intrinsic mechanism of integration of neural inputs to smooth muscle cells, the effect of after-hyperpolarization providing a relative refractory period for triggering of subsequent action potentials by evoked ESPSs. The effect of the after-hyperpolarization on neurotransmission has also been directly demonstrated by showing that short cathodal pulses that evoke action potentials fail to do so during the after-hyperpolarization. We have learned some characteristics of the after-hyperpolarization seen in this cell (Cameron and Coburn, 1982). It is not seen with depolarizations that do not evoke action potentials, nor is it activated by EPSPs that do not evoke action potentials. There is evidence that after-hyperploarizations are due to activation of a K-conductance by increases in cytoplasmic [Ca]. The evidence for this includes inhibition of the after-hyperpolarization by increases in [Mg]/[Ca] in the bathing solution, and inhibition by displacing the resting membrane potential to -90 mV, the presumed equilibrium potential for K. It is known that the K channel involved is not inhibited by TEA and 4-amino pyridine. There is some evidence that the amplitude and duration of the after-hyperpolarization may be related to the amplitude of evoked action potentials; this is expected if inward calcium current occurs via a potential-dependent calcium channel.

Wood (1985) has suggested that the after-hyperpolarization that follows action potentials in type II AH cells in the myenteric plexus may be under control of neurotransmitters or mediators. This hypothesis suggests that neurointegration of inputs to this cell could be controlled by mediators or transmitters acting on the after-hyperpolarization mechanism.

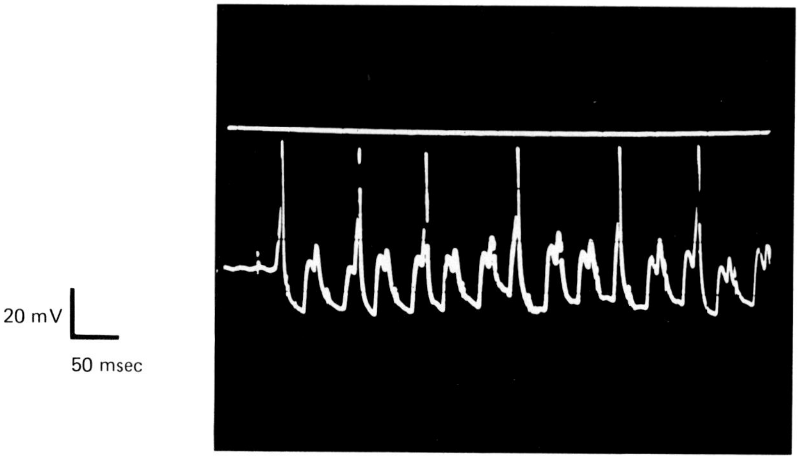

Figure 5 Neurointegration in airway peripheral ganglia. Data collected using the ferret paratracheal ganglion preparation. The interganglionic nerve trunk was stimulated at 30 Hz. Microelectrodes were placed in a AH cell body. This figure shows effects of postaction potential after-hyperpolarizations on EPSP evoked action potentials.

There may be many extrinsic mechanisms for controlling integration of inputs in airway peripheral ganglia. Baker et al. (1983) studied effects of norepinephrine on neurotransmission in the in vitro ferret ganglion by determining effects of this agent on EPSPs evoked by single-pulse preganglionic stimulation. It was found that norepinephrine added to the organ bath was associated with decrease in the amplitude of evoked EPSPs. Although the norepinephrine effect was not reversible following removal of norepinephrine from the perfusing fluid, evoked EPSPs did increase following administration of phentolamine, giving fairly convincing pharmacologic evidence that this agent may alter the size of EPSP, and exert an effect on release of acetylcholine from presynaptic neurons. Figure 6 shows similar data obtained in our laboratory, which confirm the basic finding of Baker et al. As indicated above, Skoog (1983) has

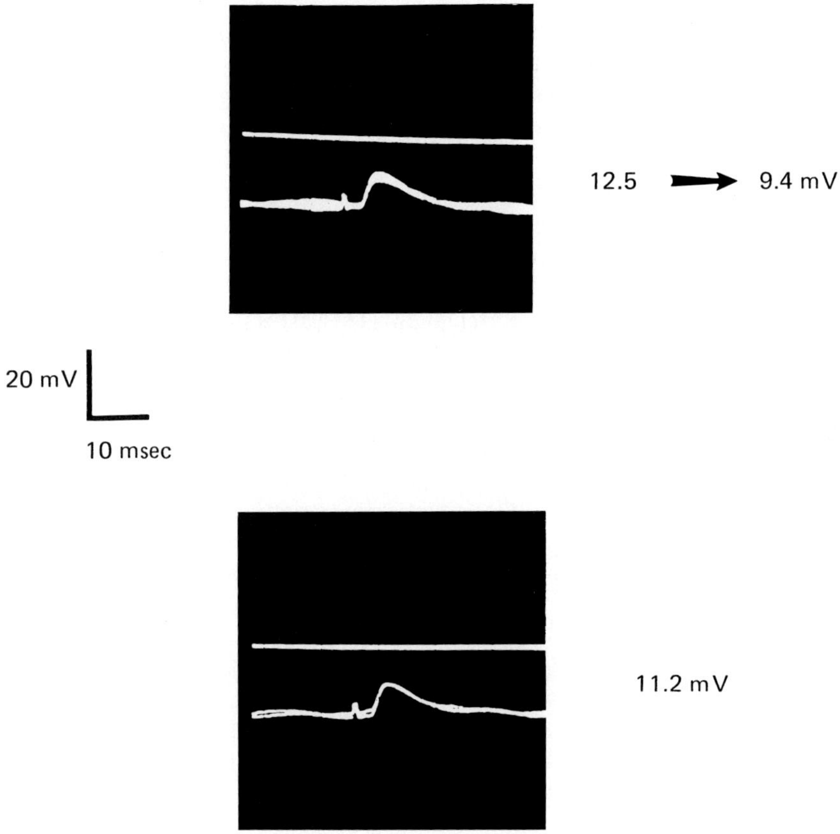

Figure 6 Effect of norepinephrine on the amplitude of evoked EPSPs in ferret paratracheal AH cells. The EPSPs were evoked every 1 min by a single pulse stimulation, with the stimulating electrode over the interganglionic nerve trunk 2 cm from the penetrated AH cell. Upper tracing shows effects of injecting 10^{-6} M NOR: EPSP decreased from 12.5 to 9.4 mV in 3 min. The lower tracing shows recovery following removal of NOR; tracing recorded 30 min after NOR removal. The input resistance of the AH cell did not change, which suggests that the effect is mediated presynaptically. However, NOR usually caused a small depolarization. The straight lines indicate zero potential.

convincingly shown that exogenous norepinephrine inhibits excitatory neurotransmission to airway smooth muscle in the ferret peripheral ganglia. There may be a host of neurotransmitters and mediators that are able to influence neurotransmission via a preganglionic mechanism, as has already been shown to influence neurotransmission at the myoneural junction of many different tissues, as well as postsynaptic mechanisms.

Although some concepts are already in place about how sympathetic adrenergic input might alter excitatory neural input to smooth muscle, our knowledge of how nonadrenergic inhibitory inputs are processed by airway peripheral ganglia is even less complete. In the guinea pig, the evidence is strong that vagal preganglionic nonadrenergic inhibitory neurons synapse in airway peripheral ganglia, since transmission to smooth muscle is inhibited by hexamethonium (Yip et al., 1981).

Several possibilities require evaluation. The first is that AH nerve terminals in airway smooth muscle contain both acetylcholine and inhibitory transmitters (cotransmitters) (Burnstock, 1976). However, to our knowledge there is no example in mammalian tissues in which the major excitatory and inhibitory neurotransmitters controlling a single cell type are found in the same neuron. The evidence that AH cell terminals release ACh includes correlation between excitation of AH cells and excitatory junction potentials in smooth muscle cells (Coburn, 1984), and the finding that somal injection of cathodal current into a single AH cells can evoked excitatory junction potentials in a single smooth muscle cell (unpublished data).

A secondary possibility is that there is a population of neurons that mediates excitatory input to smooth muscle and a second population that mediates inhibitory inputs to smooth muscle. A better understanding of the function of the various cells types found in airway peripheral ganglia should give insight into this possibility. Immunocytochemistry studies to determine the nature of neurotransmitters in nerve terminals in airway smooth muscle may be able to answer the question of whether there are two populations of neurons or a single population.

We are particularly interested in the function of neurons that do not show evoked action potentials with somal recordings, and whether these neurons could be "inhibitory" neurons. These neurons are of additional interest due to the presence of an apparent slow EPSP evoked by preganglionic nerve stimulation. The significance of a slow EPSP is that this is a mechanism in many different neural systems, with altering neuronal excitability, over a relatively long time period. This area is studied in other peripheral ganglia preparations (Wood and Mayer, 1978).

B. Role of the Ganglion-Nerve Plexus in Coordinating Neural Input to Smooth Muscle

Our comments above have related to the basic properties of neurons in airway peripheral ganglia and their potential roles in integrating neural inputs to smooth muscle. We now want to comment on data indicating that the peripheral ganglia and their plexus may also have a major function in the coordination of input, as

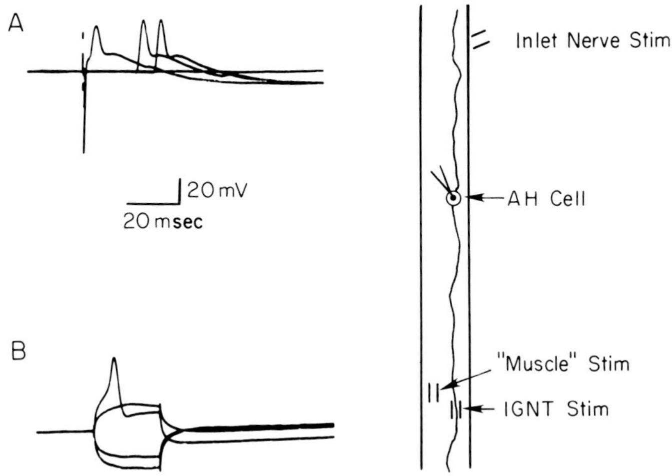

Figure 7 Approach used for electrical mapping of the ferret paratracheal nerve-ganglion smooth muscle preparation. A microelectrode was placed in the soma of a AH cell (right panel). Single-pulse electrical stimulations were performed over the inlet nerve, over the IGNT, and over muscle, as indicated. Panel B identifies the AH cells studied, using long-pulse intracellular current injection. Panel A shows evoked EPSPs and action potentials with stimulation at the three different locations; the first EPSP was evoked with inlet nerve stimulation, the second by stimulation over the IGNT, and the third by stimulation over muscle (From Coburn, 1984a).

well as integrating inputs, to airway smooth muscle cells. This area developed as a result of our attempts to map neural inputs in the in vitro ferret preparation (Coburn, 1984b). It was found that point stimulation of single nerves entering the plexus, or stimulation at a single point over an IGNT, evoked excitatory junction potentials in muscle cells and fast EPSPs in AH ganglion cells located throughout the preparation, regardless of the location of the stimulating electrode. Evoked excitatory junction potentials were nearly simultaneous in widely separated muscle cells, suggesting that excitation is coordinated. Figure 7 illustrates data obtained in one of these experiments, and the approach used in these studies. We were able to deduce some of the properties of the nerve-ganglion plexus in coordinating signals by analyzing conduction velocities of signals originating from a stimulation of the IGNT or nerves entering the plexus ("inlet nerves") (Fig. 8). Most neurons activated by "inlet" nerve stimulation had a high apparent conduction velocity, but the apparent conduction velocity decreased with increasing distance between the point of stimulation and the penetrated AH cell. Neurons

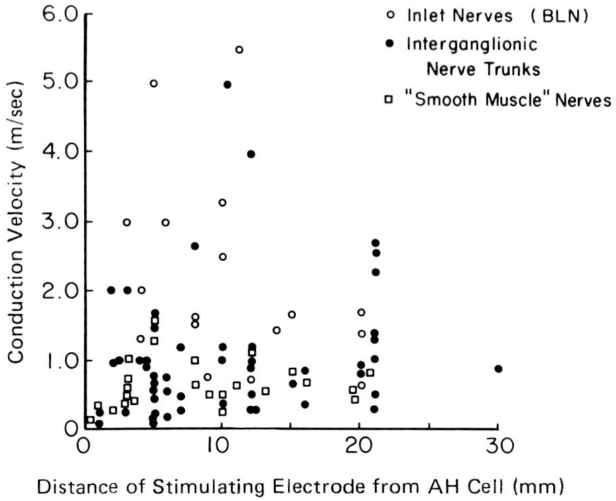

Figure 8 Apparent conduction velocities between points of electrical stimulation and the penetrated AH cell. These data are discussed in the text (From Coburn, 1984a).

activated by IGNT electrical stimulation showed a small fraction of fast conducting neurons and mostly slowly conducting neurons. Single-pulse stimulation of the IGNT frequently evoked multiple EPSOs showing different conduction velocities. This approach had led to the concept that the anatomy of the plexus is such that there is an interlacing arrangement of myelinated, fast-conducting preganglionic neurons that enter the plexus at several different locations via branches of the laryngeal nerves. Each branch contains neurons that synapse on several AH cells; the electrical signal is then carried to all ganglia in the preparation via nonmyelinated, slowly conducting postganglionic neurons. This extrapolation of electrophysiological data to anatomy is supported by the HRP neuron images, described above, in which neurons with cell bodies in one ganglion send axons into neighboring ganglia; and histologic sections of the IGNT, which show that only a small fraction of neurons in this structure are myelinated (Cameron and Coburn, 1984). The conduction velocity of the electrical signals between stimulating electrode and smooth muscle cells was such that coordination must occur via neurons rather than via conduction in a muscle syncytium (Prosser and Sperelakis, 1956).

The concept that autonomic innervation is specialized to ensure widespread effects of released neurotransmitters seems established and the nature of the synapse at the myoneural junction is an important factor in the coordination of contractions of the thousands of cells present in smooth muscle (Barr, 1963; Bennett and Merrillees, 1966; Hillarp, 1959). Studies of sympathetic neurons have shown that their morphology is consistent with the interlacing innervation that coordinates input to effector cells. The concept that autonomic nerve plexus may be constructed to coordinate neural input to different cells in effector tissues was apparently first postulated in 1904 by Langely (1904). The multiple nerves that carry signals into the peripheral airway ganglia have allowed us to test the importance of the plexus in this regard. The ferret paratracheal nerve-ganglion preparation has the advantage that we are able to study simultaneously electrophysiological characteristics of both smooth muscle cells and ganglion cells.

C. Airway Smooth Muscle Innervation and Hypersensitivity

An important question is whether clinical hypersensitivity states could relate to altered ganglionic neurotransmission (Nadel and Barnes, 1984). There are suggestions that this hypothesis is worthy of testing: (1) the finding in the myenteric plexus that inflammatory mediators such as histamine and serotonin increase the excitability of ganglion cells (Nemeth et al., 1984; Wood and Mayer, 1978); and (2) the presence of mast cells in close proximity to peripheral airway ganglia. However, Holtzman et al., 1980) already have published evidence that ganglionic neurotransmission is not abnormal in an experimental atopic hypersensitivity model.

Preparations and approaches are available for looking at different points in the neuronal apparatus providing input to airway smooth muscle, examining neurotransmission effects of various mediators, or studying preparations obtained from animals with induced airway smooth muscle hypersensitivity (Nadel and Barnes, 1984).

II. Phosphoinositide Coupling Mechanisms in Airway Smooth Muscle

This section reviews current concepts in the mushrooming field of inositol phospholipid transduction mechanisms, and gives evidence that inositol phospholipid metabolism may be involved in coupling mechanisms in airway smooth muscle.

A. Background

That phosphatidylinositol metabolism is a segment of a transduction mechanism linking receptor occupancy to physiological response is supported by observations made in many tissues that a wide range of neurotransmitters and other agents induce a specific hydrolysis of inositol phospholipids during the time when a physiological response is occurring, and that this response is generally associated with an increase in cytosolic free [Ca] (Berridge et al., 1983). Prior to 1979, the most commonly accepted schema for phosphoinositide turnover was that receptor occupancy activated a specific phospholipase C, which was thought to catalyze conversion of phosphatidylinositol (PI) in the plasma membrane to diacylglycerol (DAG) and inositol phosphate (IP). More recently, direct analysis of phosphoinositides and inositol phosphates led to a hypothesis that the rate-limiting step is hydrolysis of phosphatidylinositol bisphosphate (PIP_2) yielding inositol trisphosphate (IP_3) and DAG (that receptor occupancy activates a specific PIP_2 phosphodiesterase (Berridge et al., 1983; Heslop et al., 1986; Ishizuka et al., 1984).

Biophysical and biochemical evidence from different areas of research have led to the concept, now generally accepted, that inositol phospholipid metabolism generates the second messengers, IP_3 and DAG, which activate cellular effector mechanisms (Berridge, 1984). IP_3 has been shown to release calcium from non-mitochondrial, ATP-dependent, intracellular stores in a variety of different tissues (Berridge et al., 1984; Goldman et al., 1986; Joseph et al., 1984; Somlyo et al., 1985; Streb et al., 1983, Suematsu et al., 1984). Studies performed on isolated liver cells show convincingly that decreases in PIP_2 and increases in IP_3 precede increases in cytosolic free [Ca] (Joseph et al., 1984).

At approximately the same time, evidence was obtained that DAG can function as a powerful second messenger (Nishizuka, 1984). Unsaturated DAG in micromolar concentration was shown to activate a newly discovered enzyme, Ca-phospholipid-dependent kinase (C-kinase) and initiate protein phosphorylation that may control or modulate effector mechanisms (Nishizuka, 1984). There is now evidence of C-kinase-mediated phosphorylation of the myosin light chain, but at a site distinct from that catalyzed by myosin light chain kinase (Naka et al., 1983). The tying together of an extensive literature reporting diverse effects of various phorbol esters on various cells, and experiments showing a mechanism of action of phorbol esters is activation of C-kinase, has led to an approach in which study of phorbol ester effects gives an indication of the spectra of cellular mechanisms that may be under the control of the phosphoinositide transduction system and be mediated by increases in DAG (Nishizuka, 1984).

Figure 9 is a simplified diagram of the phosphoinositide cycle that appears to generate second messengers in many different cell types. This diagram does not point out areas of uncertainty and controversy. For example, some data support the existence of a nonspecific activating phosphodiesterase so that hydrolysis of PI, PIP, and PIP_2 may occur (Ishizuka et al., 1984; Wilson et al., 1985). The implications are that since IP_2 and IP may not exert biological effects, hydrolysis of PI or PIP would produce only one of the two known messengers, DAG, provided by phosphoinositide metabolism. Thus, hydrolysis of PI and PIP could alter the pattern of response of receptor activation of the PI transduction system.

Recent evidence suggests that there may be more than one rate-controlling site for PI metabolism and that PI kinase and PIP kinase may modulate or control

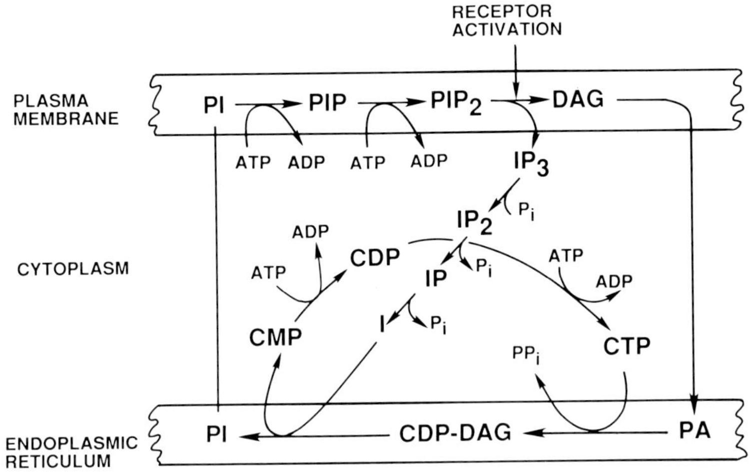

Figure 9 The phosphoinositide cycle.

this system (DeChaffoy de Courcelles et al., 1984; Enyedi et al., 1983; Farkas et al., 1984; Halenda and Feinstein, 1984). Inositol phosphate chemistry appears to be very complex and is poorly understood (Michell, 1986). IP_3 exists in two isomers, $I(1,3,4)P_3$ and $I(2,4,5)P_3$, but PIP_2 does not have the 1,3,4 configuration. IP_4, IP_5, and IP_6 have been found in trace amounts (Batty et al., 1985; Heslop et al., 1986; Irvine et al., 1985; Michell, 1986).

There may be other second messengers generated by the PI transduction system: phosphatidic acid (Salmon and Honeyman, 1980), an inositol phosphate, other than $I(1,4,5)P_3$, perhaps a cyclic 4,5 triphosphate (Wilson et al., 1985). Changes in the plasma membrane concentration of PIP_2 may exert effects in plasma membrane proteins (Joseph et al., 1984).

Recent information suggests that there are GTP binding proteins that regulate phosphoinositide activity initiated by receptor occupancy (Blackmore et al., 1985; Cockcroft and Gomperts, 1985; Litosch and Fain, 1985).

Inositol phospholipid metabolism can be activated in various cell types by multiple agonists. Berridge et al. (1983) has classified coupling mechanisms that produce intracellular messengers in terms of those that activate adenylate cyclase and those that activate phosphodiesterase. However, it seems clear these mechanisms are not entirely independent, since there is considerable evidence that these two different transducing mechanisms communicate with each other. This includes the observation that acetylcholine treatment effects generation of cAMP (Butcher, 1978); the finding that cAMP protein kinase exerts stimulatory effects on PI kinase in the plasma membrane (Enyedi et al., 1983; Farkas et al., 1984);

and the finding that PA inhibits adenylate cyclase (Proll et al., 1985). Undoubtedly more examples will be uncovered as effects of phosphoinositide generated signals are further studied.

Watson and Lapetina (1985) have recently shown that phorbol esters and DAG inhibit formation of inositol phosphates in human platelets, suggesting an additional mechanism whereby a cascade of biochemical events initiated by DAG can modulate formation of the other known second messenger formed by this system. This finding has been repeated in other cells, including cultured vascular smooth muscle cells (Brock et al., 1985), astrocytes (Orellana et al., 1985), and hippocampal slices (Labarcas et al., 1984). There is also a literature suggesting that phorbol esters may alter receptor agonist affinity or uncouple receptors from inositol phospholipid metabolism, but data vary in different cell types (Garte and Belman, 1981; Labarca et al., 1984; Leeb-Lundberg et al., 1986; Nemeth et al., 1984). Phorbol esters may also exert control on inositol phospholipid metabolism at the level of PI-4-P kinase (DeChaffoy de Courcelles et al., 1984). There is evidence that the second messenger, Ca, can modulate or control phosphoinositide metabolism (Akhtar and Abdel-Latif, 1978; Egawa et al., 1981). There is now convincing data that second messengers generated by inositol phospholipid metabolism can exert effects independent of increases in cytosolic free [Ca] and that there may be synergism between effects of Ca and C-kinase-mediated actions (Rink et al., 1983; Yamanishi et al., 1983).

B. Airway Smooth Muscle Studies

Our interest in coupling mechanisms in airway smooth muscle stems from previous studies of membrane-potential-dependent and -independent mechanisms for activation of canine trachealis muscle (Coburn, 1979; Coburn and Yamaguchi, 1977). Membrane-potential-independent mechanisms have been termed pharmacomechanical coupling. There is considerable evidence that contractions of canine trachealis muscle evoked by high acetylcholine concentration (ACh) utilize pharmacomechanical coupling mechanisms. ACh contractions occur in K-depolarized preparations (Coburn, 1979); increasing [ACh] 10^{-6}-10^{-5} M results in a contraction that occurs without a further membrane depolarization (Farley and Miles, 1977). Membrane potential-tension relationships are shifted to the left with ACh compared to that seen with graded K, so that more tension is developed for a given Em change (Coburn, 1979). Airway smooth muscle is known to be refractory to Ca antagonist agents (Golenhofen et al., 1973) at high ACh (Coburn, 1979; Eberlin et al., 1982; Farley and Miles, 1978), suggesting that Em-dependent Ca channels are not involved in delivery of calcium to the myofibrils. ACh contractions seem to be insensitive to decreases in external Ca (Farley and Miles, 1978). Current "clamp" displacement of Em does not cause appropriate tension responses during ACh stimulation. But a similar "clamp" displacement causes appropriate tension responses during 5HT or K contractions (Coburn, 1979). The coupling mechanisms used during pharmacomechanical coupling type of contractions are not understood. Likewise, events by which receptor occupancy can signal ionic channels resulting in changes in Em are not well understood in smooth muscle.

There are considerable data in the literature, based on measurement of ^{32}P incorporation in PI (Akhtar and Abdel-Latif, 1978; Baron and Coburn, 1984; DeScarneti and Lapetina, 1974; Egawa et al., 1981), that PI metabolism is activated during cholinergic muscarinic contractions and contractions evoked by many other agents. It seems likely that the inositol phospholipid transduction system is activated and provides second messengers during these contractions. Key studies include the observation (Alexander et al., 1985; Eberlin et al., 1982) that angiotensin-evoked contractions of cultured vascular smooth muscle cells were associated with increases in IP_3, and increase in cytosolic free calcium, and that phorbol esters that inhibit contractions also inhibit increases in IP_3 and increases in cytoplasmic free calcium concentration; data establishing that IP_3 releases Ca from internal stores in skinned muscle fibers (Somlyo et al., 1985; Suematsu et al., 1984). Thus, the basic studies obtained on nonmuscle cells, cited above, can be duplicated in smooth muscle and evidence obtained to date indicates that IP_3 generation is important in intracellular Ca release in smooth muscle.

Several studies have attempted to establish time relationships between smooth muscle contractions and activation of PI metabolism, and IP_3 generation. Aktar and Abdel-Latiffe (1984) have shown significant increases in $[IP_3]$ in rabbit iris smooth muscle 15 sec after addition of ACh to their organ bath fluid. Salmon and Honeyman (1980) showed correlation between ^{32}P uptake into phosphatidic acid and development of ACh contractions in isolated frog stomach cells, with measurements made in seconds. We have recently observed increases in $[IP_3]$ within 5 sec after the start of field-stimulation-evoked contractions of canine trachealis muscle (Fig. 10). A tentative conclusion is that IP_3 generation may be involved during development of contractions of smooth muscle cells, but whether IP_3 is involved in maintenance of the tonic phase of contraction in slow smooth muscle is another question. Our data, so far, suggest that $[IP_3]$ decreases during the tonic phase of canine trachealis muscle contraction.

The phorbol ester approach to studying possible roles of DAG-activated C-kinase has also been applied to smooth muscle. It has been shown that 4-phorbol-12-myristate-13-acetate (PMA) induces slowly developing Ca-dependent contractions in vascular smooth muscle (Rasmussen et al., 1984) and inhibition of alpha-adrenergic-mediated contractions of rat aorta (Danthuluri and Deth, 1984). As indicated above, phorbol esters inhibit angiotensin-induced contractions in cultured aortic cells, which appears to be a result of inhibition of IP_3 formation with resultant inhibition of increases in free cytosolic Ca (Brock et al., 1985). Menkes et al. (1985) have shown that TPA inhibits ACh-induced contractions

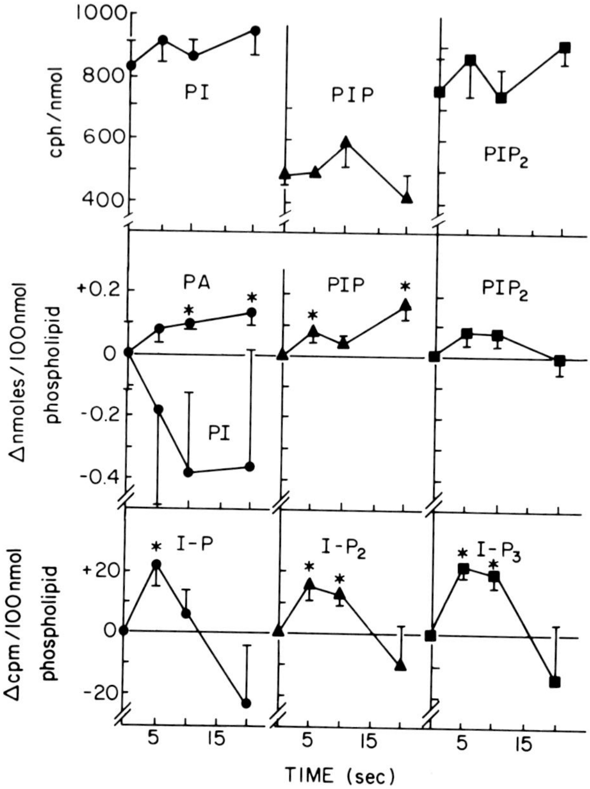

Figure 10 Total pool sizes of phosphatidylinositol (PI), phosphatidylinositol-4-phosphate (PIP), phosphatidylinositol bisphosphate (PIP_2), phosphatidic acid (PA), and inositol phosphates radioactivity during a field stimulation-evoked contraction of a single strip of canine trachealis muscle. The strip was incubated with [^{3}H] myoinositol for 30 min in the presence of carbamoylcholine, and was washed and incubated for 1 hr in the absence of the drug, prior to mounting and field stimulation. Top panel illustrates the specific activity of the phosphoinositides and indicates that the preparation was not labeled to equilibrium (Unpublished data, Baron and Coburn).

in canine trachealis muscle, a finding that could be due to inhibition of inositol phosphate generations of IP_3, but this is not yet proven.

Our studies on airway smooth muscle aim at elucidating pharmacomechanical and electromechanical coupling mechanisms and determining if phosphoinositide metabolism generates messengers involved in these coupling mechanisms. Our methodology is different from other laboratories in that we stress measure-

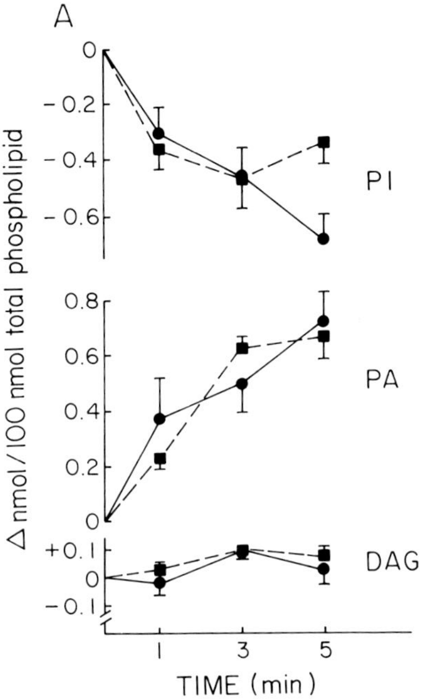

Figure 11 Changes in total pool size of phosphatidylinositol (PI), phosphatidic acid (PA), and diacylglycerol (DAG) during development of a contraction evoked by 5.5 μm carbamylcholine. (The fast phase of the contractions occurred in 0-1 min, slow phase in 1-3 min, and tonic phase in 3-5 min. Broken lines are data taken from single strips of canine trachealis muscle held isometrically; solid lines are data taken using multiple strips studied in a test tube (From Baron et al., 1984).

ments of total pool sizes, and specific radioactivity, of the various phosphoinositides in single strips of airway smooth muscle under known mechanical conditions. This technology depends on charring densitometry and radioscan approaches. Charring densitometry, as performed in our laboratory, has an advantage over high-performance liquid chromatography (HPLC) in that it is not influenced by changes in unsaturation of the various lipids (Baron and Coburn, 1984). It has such high sensitivity that we can study one muscle strip. Figure 11 shows data obtained during a pharmacomechanical coupling-type contraction of canine trachealis muscle, where decreases in PI and increases in PA and DAG paralleled the development of tension (Baron et al., 1984). These data suggest that phosphoinositide metabolism is activated during a pharmacomechanical coupling-type of contraction. It was also shown that PI metabolism is not activated during K-induced contractions of this muscle; therefore, PI metabolism is seen as Em-independent and could be involved in Em-independent mechanisms of contraction.

Figure 10 shows changes in phosphoinositides and inositol phosphates during contractions evoked by field stimulation (as discussed above). Field stimulation allows us to activate airway smooth muscle cells nearly simultaneously and removes the confusion originating from the diffusion times of administered exogenous agonists. Although field stimulation might cause effects on lipid metabo-

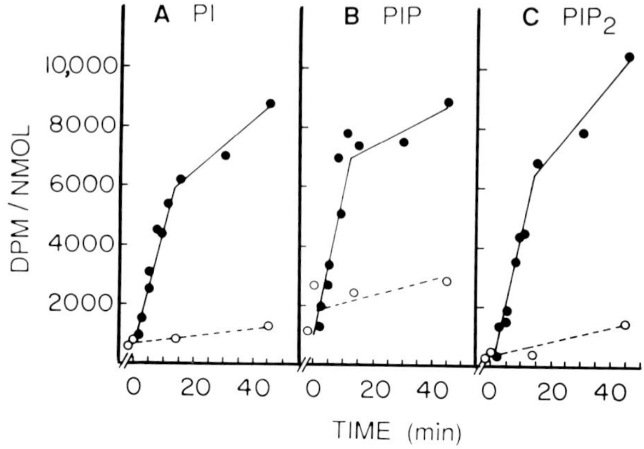

Figure 12 Method for studying phosphoinositide metabolism in smooth muscle is described in the text (Unpublished data, Baron and Coburn).

lism due to mechanisms unrelated to ACh release, atropine completely inhibits field stimulation contractions and evoked increases in IP_3.

Figure 12 illustrates data obtained in studies designed to help us understand the nature and control of phosphoinositide metabolism in canine trachealis muscle. This approach labels unstimulated canine trachealis muscle strips with $[^3H]$-myoinositol. Only a small fraction of label enters phosphoinositides under this condition, but the specific activity of myoinositol, presumably in the cytoplasm, reaches very high levels. Following activation of the tissue with carbamylcholine, the rate of incorporation of isotope into inositol phospholipids increases 20-45 times. This figure shows that the rate of increase in specific activities of PI, PIP, and PIP_2 are remarkably similar over a 10-20 min period, suggesting that similar fractions of total pools of each of these compounds are coupled to receptor proteins. Combination of isotopic flux data and total pool size data are allowing us to study control of inositol phospholipid transducing mechanisms in airway smooth muscle.

Acknowledgment

Some of the studies reviewed here were supported by grants HL19737 and HL31997 from the Heart, Lung Blood Institute, National Institutes of Health, Bethesda, MD.

Discussion

Barnes. What is the evidence for afferent input to airway ganglion cells?

Coburn. Only the finding that a localized stimulus well away from vagal nerve fibers will evoke an EPSP on AH cells.

Widdicombe. It is important to know the area of airway being stimulated. Most airway nerves are outside smooth muscle, so if the stimulus spreads to submucosa it may be acting on nerves there.

Coburn. Studies of the current density in saline suggest that the stimulated area would not be large, due to high electrical resistance in tissue.

Skoogh. Does atropine block the synaptic potential in type B cells, and the hyperpolarization in AH cells?

Coburn. Atropine did block the B cells but had no effect after hyperpolarization in AH cells.

Burnstock. When you stimulate single AH cells in ferret airway ganglia and record from smooth muscle cells, what sort of responses do you see?

Coburn. We have evoked excitatory junction potentials, but have never seen inhibitory junction potentials (although it is difficult to demonstrate nonadrenergic inhibitory nerve effects in ferret trachea).

Burnstock. Cultured enteric ganglia are useful for studying neural interactions and we have recently been able to culture tracheal ganglia of ferret and mouse. It may be possible to study ganglion cells with patch-clamp methods, which allow measurements of the effects of locally applied neurotransmitters and peptides on the characteristics of EPSPs and IPSPs.

References

Akhtar, R. A., and Abdel-Latif, A. A. (1978). Calcium ion requirement for acetylcholine-stimulated breakdown of triphosphoinositide in rabbit iris smooth muscle. *J. Pharmacol. Exp. Ther.* **204**:655-668.

Akhtar, R. A., and Abdel-Latif, A. A. (1984). Carbachol causes rapid phosphodiesteratic cleavage of phosphatidylinositol 4,5-bisphosphate and accumulation of inositol phosphates in rabbit iris smooth muscle. *Biochem. J.* **224**:291-300.

Alexander, R. W., Brock, T. A., Gimbrone, M. A. Jr., and Rittenhouse, S. E.

(1985). Angiotensin increases inositol trisphosphate and calcium in vascular smooth muscle. *Hypertension* **7**:447-451.

Altiere, R. J., Szarek, J. L., and Diamond, L. (1985). Neurally mediated nonadrenergic relaxation in cat airways occurs independent of cholinergic mechanisms. *J. Pharmacol. Exp. Ther.* **234**:590-597.

Andersson, R. G. G., and Grundstrom, N. (1983). The excitatory non-cholinergic, non-adrenergic nervous system of the guinea-pig airways. *Eur. J. Respir. Dis.* Suppl. **131**:141-157.

Baker, D. G., Basbaum, C. B., Herbert, D. A., and Mitchell, R. A. (1983). Transmission of airway ganglia of ferrets: inhibition by norepinephrine. *Neurosci. Letts.* **41**:139-143.

Baker, D. G., McDonald, D. M., and Mitchell, R. A. (1986). The architecture of nerves and ganglia of the ferret trachea as revealed by acetylcholinesterase histochemistry. *J. Comp. Neurol.* **246**:513-526.

Baluk, P., Fumiwara, T., and Matsuda, S. (1985). The fine structure of the ganglia of the guinea pig trachea. *Cell Tissue Res.* **239**:51-60.

Baron, C. B., and Coburn, R. F. (1984). Comparison of two copper reagents for detection of saturated and unsaturated neutral lipids by charring densitometry. *J. Liquid. Chromatogr.* **7**:2793-2801.

Baron, C. B., Cunningham, M., Strauss, J. F. III, and Coburn, R. F. (1984). Pharmacomechanical coupling in smooth muscle may involve phosphatidylinositol metabolism. *Proc. Natl. Acad. Sci. USA* **81**:6899-6903.

Barr, L. (1963). Propagation in vertebrate visceral smooth muscle. *J. Theoret. Biol.* **4**:73-85.

Batty, I. R., Nahorski, S. R., and Irvine, R. F. (1985). Rapid formation of inositol 1,3,4,5-tetrakisphosphate following muscarinic receptor stimulation of rat cerebral cortical slices. *Biochem. J.* **232**:211-215.

Bennett, M. R., and Merrillees, N. C. R. (1966). An analysis of the transmission of excitation from autonomic nerves to smooth muscle. *J. Physiol. London* **185**:520-535.

Berridge, M. J. (1984). Inositol trisphosphate and diacylglycerol as second messengers. *Biochem. J.* **220**:345-360.

Berridge, M. J., Dawson, R. M. C., Downes, C. P., Heslop, J. P., and Irvine, R. F. (1983). Changes in the levels of inositol phosphates after agonist-dependent hydrolysis of membrane phosphoinositides. *Biochem. J.* **212**:473-482.

Berridge, M. J., Heslop, J. P., Irvine, R. F., and Brown, K. D. (1984). Inositol trisphosphate formation and calcium mobilization in Swiss 3T3 cells in response to platelet-derived growth factor. *Biochem. J.* **222**:195-201.

Blackman, J. G., Crowcroft, P. J., Devine, C. E., Holman, M. E., and Yonemura

K. (1969). Transmission from preganglionic fibres in the hypogastric nerve to peripheral ganglia of male guinea-pigs. *J. Physiol. Lond.* **201**:723-743.

Blackmore, P. F., Bocckino, S. B., Waynick, L. E., and Exton, J. H. (1985). Role of a guanine nucleotide-binding regulatory protein in the hydrolysis of hepatocyte phosphatidylinositol 4,5-bisphosphate by calcium-mobilizing hormones and the control of cell calcium. *J. Biol. Chem.* **260**:14477-14483.

Brock, T. A., Rittenhouse, S. E., Powers, C. W., Ekstein, L. S., Gimbrone, M. A. Jr., and Alexander, R. W. (1985). Phorbol ester and OAG inhibit angiotensin activation of phospholipase C in cultured vascular smooth muscle cells. *J. Biol. Chem.* **260**:14158-14162.

Burgess, G. M., McKinney, J. S., Irvine, R. F., and Putney, J. W. Jr. (1985). Inositol 1,4,5-trisphosphate and inositol 1,3,4-trisphosphate formation in Ca^{2+}-mobilizing hormone-activated cells. *Biochem. J.* **232**:237-243.

Burnstock, G. (1976). Do some cells release more than one transmitter? *Neuroscience* **1**:239-248.

Butcher, R. W. (1978). Decreased cAMP levels in human diploid cells exposed to cholinergic stimuli. *J. Cyclic Nucleotide Res.* **4**:411-421.

Cabezas, G. A., Graf, P. D., and Nadel, J. A. (1971). Sympathetic versus parasympathetic nervous regulation of airways in dogs. *J. Appl. Physiol.* **31**:651-665.

Cameron, A. R., and Coburn, R. F. (1982). Calcium dependence of the after hyperpolarization of type AH cells of the ferret paratracheal ganglion. *Fed. Proc.* **41**:1356.

Cameron, A. R., and Coburn, R. F. (1984). Electrical and anatomic characteristics of cells of ferret paratracheal ganglion. *Am. J. Physiol.* **246**:C450-C458.

Chesrown, S. E., Venugopalan, C. S., Gold, W. M., and Drazen, J. M. (1980). In vivo demonstration of nonadrenergic inhibitory innervation of the guinea pig trachea. *J. Clin. Invest.* **65**:314-320.

Coburn, R. F., and Tomita, T. (1973). Evidence for nonadrenergic inhibitory nerves in the guinea pig trachealis muscle. *Am. J. Physiol.* **224**:1072-1080.

Coburn, R. F., and Yamaguchi, T. (1977). Membrane potential-dependent and -independent tension in the canine tracheal muscle. *J. Pharmacol. Exp. Ther.* **201**:276-284.

Coburn, R. F. (1979). Electromechanical coupling in canine trachealis muscle: acetylcholine contractions. *Am. J. Physiol.* **236**:C177-C184.

Coburn, R. F. (1984a). The anatomy of the ferret paratracheal parasympathetic nerve-ganglion plexus. *Exp. Lung Res.* **7**:1-9.

Coburn, R. F. (1984b). Neural coordination of excitation of ferret trachealis muscle. *Am. J. Physiol.* **246**:C459-C466.

Cockcroft, S., and Gomperts, B. D. (1985). Role of guanine nucleotide binding protein in the activation of polyphosphoinositide phosphodiesterase. *Nature* **314**:534-536.

Danthuluri, N. R., and Deth, R. C. (1984). Phorbol ester-induced contraction of arterial smooth muscle and inhibition of alpha adrenergic response. *Biochem. Biophys. Res. Commun.* **125**:1103-1109.

De Chaffoy de Courcelles, D., Roevens, P., and Van Belle, H. (1984). 1-oleoyl-2-acetyl-glycerol (OAG) stimulates the formation of phosphatidylinositol 4-phosphate in intact human platelets. *Biochem. Biophys. Res. Commun.* **123**:589-595.

De Scarnati, O. C., and Lapetina, E. G. (1974). Adrenergic stimulation of phosphatidylinositol labelling in rat vas deferens. *Biochim. Biophys. Acta* **360**: 298-305.

Eberlin, L. B., Cherniack, A. D., and Deal, E. C. Jr. (1982). Reversal of tracheal and pulmonary parenchymal smooth muscle contraction by verapamil. *Am. Rev. Respir. Dis. Suppl.* **125**:225-233.

Egawa, K., Sacktor, B., and Takenawa, T. (1981). Ca-dependent and Ca-independent degradation of phosphatidylinositol in rabbit vas deferens. *Biochem. J.* **194**:129-136.

Elfman, A. G. (1943). The afferent and parasympathetic innervations of the lung and trachea of the dog. *Am. J. Anat.* **72**:1-28.

Enyedi, A., Farago, A., Sarkadi, B., Szasz, I., and Gardos, G. (1983). Cyclic AMP-dependent protein kinase stimulates the formation of polyphosphoinositides in the plasma membranes of different blood cells. *FEBS Letts.* **161**:158-162.

Farkas, G., Enyedi, A., Sarkadi, B., Gardos, G., Nagy, Z., and Farago, A. (1984). Cyclic AMP-dependent protein kinase stimulates the phosphorylation of phosphatidylinositol to phosphatidylinositol-4-monophosphate in a plasma membrane preparation from pig granulocytes. *Biochem. Biophys. Res. Commun.* **125**:871-876.

Farley, J. M., and Miles, P. R. (1977). Role of depolarization in acetylcholine-induced contractions of dog trachealis muscle. *J. Pharmacol. Exp. Ther.* **201**:199-205.

Farley, J. M., and Miles, P. R. (1978). Sources of calcium for acetylcholine-induced contraction of dog tracheal smooth muscle. *J. Pharmacol. Exp.*

Ther. **207**:340-346.

Fisher, A. W. (1964). The intrinsic innervation of the trachea. *J. Anat.* **98**: 117-124.

Fowler, J. C., and Weinreich, D. (1986). Electrophysiological membrane properties of paratracheal ganglion neurons of the rabbit. *Neuro. Sci.* (Abstr.) **11**:1182.

Garte, S. J., and Belman, S. (1981). Tumour promoter uncouples B-adrenergic receptor from adenyl cyclase in mouse epidermis. *Nature* **284**:171-173.

Goldman, Y. E., Reid, G. P., Somlyo, A. P., Somlyo, A. V., Trentham, D. R., and Water, J. W. (1986). Activation of skinned vascular smooth muscle by photolysis of 'caged inositol trisphosphate' to inositol 1,4,5-trisphosphate. *J. Physiol. London* **377**:100 P.

Golenhofen, K., Hermstein, M., and Lammel, E. (1973). Membrane potential and contraction of vascular smooth muscle (portal vein) during application of noradrenaline and high potassium, and selective inhibitory effects of verapamil. *Microvasc. Res.* **5**:73-80.

Hakanson, R., Sundler, F., Moghimzadeh, E., and Leander, S. (1983). Peptide-containing nerve fibres in the airways: distribution and functional implications. *Europ. J. Respir. Dis.* Suppl **131**:115-139.

Halenda, S. P., and Feinstein, M. B. (1984). Phorbol myristate acetate stimulates formation of phosphatidylinositol 4-phosphate and phosphatidylinositol 4,5-bisphosphate in human platelets. *Biochem. Biophys. Res. Commun.* **124**:507-513.

Hartzell, H. C. (1981). Mechanisms of slow postsynaptic potentials. *Nature London* **291**:539-544.

Heslop, J. P., Irvine, R. F., Tashijian, A. T., and Berridge, M. J. (1986). Inositol tetrakis and pentakis phosphates $INGH_4$ cells. *J. Exp. Biol.* In press.

Hillarp, N. A. (1959). The construction and functional organization of the autonomic innervation apparatus. *Acta Physiol. Scand. Suppl.* **157**: 1-38.

Honjin, R. (1954). On the ganglia and nerves of the lower respiratory tract of the mouse. *J. Morphol.* **95**:263-288.

Hokfelt, T., Johansson, O., Ljungdahl, A., Lundberg, J. M., and Schultzberg, M. (1980). Peptidergic neurones. *Nature* **284**:515-521.

Jacobowitz, D., Kent, K. M., Fleisch, J. H., and Cooper, T. (1973). Histofluorescent study of catecholamine-containing elements in cholinergic ganglion from the calf and dog lung. *Proc. Soc. Exp. Biol. Med.* **144**: 464-466.

Holtzman, M. J., Sheller, J. R., Dimeo, M., Nadel, J. A., and Boushey, H. A. (1980). Effect of ganglionic blockade on bronchial reactivity in atopic subjects. *Am. Rev. Respir. Dis.* **122**:17-25.

Irvine, R. F., Anggard, E. D., Letcher, A. J., and Downes, C. P. (1985). Metabolism of inositol 1,4,5-trisphosphate and inositol 1,3,4-trisphosphate in rat parotid glands. *Biochem. J.* **229**:505-511.

Ishizuke, Y., Imai, A., and Nozawa, Y. (1984). Polyphosphoinositide turnover in rat mast cells stimulated by antigen: rapid and preferential breakdown of phosphatidylinositol 4-phosphate. *Biochem. Biophys. Res. Commun.* **123**:875-881.

Joseph, S. K., Thomas, A. P., Williams, R. F., Irvine, R. F., and Williamson, J. R. (1984). Myo-inositol 1,4,5-trisphosphate: a second messenger for the hormonal mobilization of intracellular Ca in liver. *J. Biol. Chem.* **259**:3077-3081.

Kaibuchi, K., Takai, Y., Ogawa, Y., Kimura, S., and Nishizuka, Y. (1982). Inhibitory action of adenosine 3′,5′-monophosphate on phosphatidylinositol turnover: difference in tissue response. *Biochem. Biophys. Res. Commun.* **104**:105-112.

Kalia, M., and Coburn, R. F. (1986). The morphology of spiking and non-spiking neurons in the ferret paratracheal ganglia. *J. Comp. Neurol.* **254**:341-367.

King, B. F., and Szurszewski, J. H. (1984). Intracellular recordings from vagally innervated intramural neurons in opossum stomach. *Am. J. Physiol.* **246**: G209-G212.

Labarca, R., Janowsky, A., Patel, J., and Paul, S. M. (1984). Phorbol esters inhibit agonist-induced inositol-1-phosphate accumulation in rat hippocampal slices. *Biochem. Biophys. Res. Commun.* **123**:703-709.

Langely, J. N. (1904). On the question of commissural fibres between nerve-cells having the same function and situated in the same plexuses. *J. Physiol. London* **31**:244-259.

Leeb-Lundberg, L. M., Cotecchia, S., Lomasney, J. W., DeBernardis, J. F., Lefkowitz, R. J., and Caron, M. G. (1986). Phorbol esters promote alfa$_1$-adrenergic receptor phosphorylation and receptor uncoupling from inositol phospholipid metabolism. *Proc. Natl. Acad. Sci. USA* **82**:5651-5655.

Leff, A. R., and Munox, N. M. (1981). Selective autonomic stimulation of canine trachealis with dimethylphenylpiperazinium. *J. Appl. Physiol.* **51**: 428-437.

Limas, C. J., and Limas, C. (1985). Phorbol ester and diacylglycerol-mediated desensitization of cardiac B-adrenergic receptors. *Circ. Res.* **57**:443-449.

Litosch, I., and Fain, J. N. (1985). 5-methyltryptamine stimulates phospholipase C-mediated breakdown of exogenous phosphoinositides by blowfly salivary gland membranes. *J. Biol. Chem.* **260**:16052-16055.

Menke, H., Baraan, J. M., and Snyder, S. H. (1985). Protein kinase C regulates smooth muscle tension in guinea pig trachea and ileum. *Eur. J. Pharmacol.* **122**:19-28.

Michell, B. (1986). Inositol phosphates: profusion and confusion. *Nature* **319**: 176-177.

Mitchell, R. A., Baker, D. G., Basbaum, C. G., and Herbert, D. A. (1984). In vivo recording from tracheal parasympathetic ganglia. *Physiologist* **26**: A-37.

Nadel, J. A., and Barnes, P. J. (1984). Autonomic regulation of the airways. *Annu. Rev. Med.* **35**:451-467.

Naka, M., Kishukawa, M., and Adelstein, R. S. (1983). Phorbal ester induced activation of human platelets is associated with protein kinase C phosphorylation of myosin light chains. *Nature* **308**:692-698.

Nemeth, P. R., Ort, C. A., and Wood, J. D. (1984). Intracellular study of effects of histamine on electrical behaviour of myenteric neurones in guinea-pig small intestine. *J. Physiol. Lond* **355**:411-425.

Nishizuka, Y. (1984). The role of protein kinase C in cell surface signal transduction and tumour promotion. *Nature* **308**:693-698.

O'Donnell, S. R., and Saar, N. (1973). Histochemical localization of adrenergic nerves in the guinea-pig trachea. *Br. J. Pharmacol.* **47**:707-710.

Orellana, S. A., Solski, P. A., and Brown, J. H. (1985). Phorbol ester inhibits phosphoinositide hydrolysis and calcium mobilization in cultured astrocytoma cells. *J. Biol. Chem.* **260**:5236-5239.

Proll, M. A., Clark, R. B., and Butcher, R. W. (1985). Phosphatidate and monooleylphosphatidate inhibition of fibroblast adenylate cyclase is mediated by inhibitory coupling protein, N_1. *Mol. Pharmacol.* **28**:331-337.

Prosser, C. L., and Sperelakis, N. (1956). Transmission in ganglion-free circular muscle from the cat intestine. *Am. J. Physiol.* **187**:536-545.

Rasmussen, H., Forder, J., Kojima, I., and Scriabine A. (1984). TPA-induced contraction of isolated rabbit vascular smooth muscle. *Biochem. Biophys. Res. Commun.* **122**:776-784.

Richardson, J. B. (1979). Nerve supply to the lungs. *Am. Rev. Respir. Dis.* **119**:785-802.

Richardson, J., and Beland, J. (1976). Nonadrenergic inhibitory nerves in human airways. *J. Appl. Physiol.* **41**:764-771.

Rink, T. J., Sanchez, A., and Hallam, T. J. (1983). Diacylglycerol and phorbol ester stimulate secretion without raising cytoplasmic free calcium in human platelets. *Nature* **305**:317-319.

Salmon, D. M., and Honeyman, T. W. (1980). Proposed mechanism of cholinergic action in smooth muscle. *Nature* **284**:344-345.

Sekar, M. C., and Roufogalis, M. D. (1984). Muscarinic-receptor stimulation enhances polyphosphoinositide breakdown in guinea-pig ileum smooth muscle. *Biochem. J.* **223**:527-531.

Skoogh, B. E. (1983). Transmission through airway ganglia. *Eur. J. Respir. Dis.* Suppl. **131**:159-170.

Somlyo, A. V., Bond, M., Somlyo, A. P., and Scarpa, A. (1985). Inositol trisphosphate-induced calcium release and contraction in vascular smooth muscle. *Proc. Nat. Acad. Sci. USA* **82**:5231-5235.

Streb, H., Irvine, R. F., Berridge, M. J., and Schulz, I. (1983). Release of Ca from a nonmitochondrial Intracellular store in pancreatic acinar cells by inositol-1,4,5-trisphosphate. *Nature* **306**:67-69.

Suematsu, E., Hirata, M., Hashimoto, T., and Kuriyama, H. (1984). Inositol 1,4,5,-trisphosphate releases Ca^{2+} from intracellular store sites in skinned single cells of porcine coronary artery. *Biochem. Biophys. Res. Commun.* **120**:481-485.

Tomita, T. (1967). Current spread in the smooth muscle of the guinea-pig vas deferens. *J. Physiol. London* **189**:1634-176.

Uddman, R., Alumets, J., Densert, O., Hakanson, R., and Sundler, F. (1978). Occurrence and distribution of VIP nerves in the nasal mucosa and tracheobronchial wall. *Acta Otolaryngol.* **86**:443-448.

Villalobos-Molina, R., Hong, E., and Garcia-Sainz, J. A. (1982). Correlation between phosphatidylinositol labeling and contraction in rabbit aorta: effect of alfa-1 adrenergic activation. *J. Pharmacol. Exp. Ther.* **222**:258-261.

Watson, S. P., and Lapetina, E. G. (1985). 1,2,-Diacylglycerol and phorbol ester inhibit agonist-induced formation of inositol phosphates in human platelets: Possible implications for negative feedback regulation of inositol phospholipid hydrolysis. *Proc. Natl. Acad. Sci. USA* **82**:2623-2626.

Widdecomb, J. G. (1963). Regulation of tracheobronchial smooth muscle. *Physiol. Rev.* **43**:1-37.

Wilson, D. B., Neufeld, E. J., and Majerus, P. W. (1985). Phosphoinositide interconversion in thrombin-stimulated human platelets. *J. Biol. Chem.* **260**:1046-1051.

Wilson, D. B., Connolly, T. M., Bross, T. E., Majerus, P. W., Sherman, W. R., Tyoer, A. N., Rubin, L. J., and Brown, J. W. (1985). Isolation and characterization of the inositol cyclic phosphate products of polyphosphoinositide cleavage by phospholipase C. *J. Biol. Chem.* **260**:13496-13501.

Wood, J. D., and Mayer, C. J. (1978). Slow synaptic excitation mediated by serotonin in Auerbach's plexus. *Nature* **276**:836-837.

Wood, J. D. (1984). Enteric neurons. *Am. J. Physiol.* **247**:G585-98.

Yamanishi, J., Takai, Y., Kaibuchi, K., Sano, K., Castagna, M., and Nishizuka, Y. (1983). Synergistic functions of phorbol ester and calcium in serotonin release from human platelets. *Biochem. Biophys. Res. Commun.* **112**:778-786.

Yip, P., Palombini, B., and Coburn, R. F. (1981). Inhibitory innervation to the guinea pig trachealis muscle. *J. Appl. Physiol.* **50**:374-382.

8

Vagal Reflexes in the Airways

JOHN G. WIDDICOMBE

St. George's Hospital Medical School
London, United Kingdom

The vagus nerves supply the respiratory tract from the larynx down to the smallest airways and alveoli. Their supply is double: they conduct sensory and/or afferent information from nerve receptors in the walls of the different airways (Table 1); these afferent networks also feed locally into other parts of the respiratory tract, where they have motor actions and may affect airway caliber and function. The vagus also has direct motor control of zones in the respiratory tract from the larynx down to the smaller airways. The respiratory tract cranial to the larynx is supplied by motor fibers in nerves other than the vagus. Thus there are vagovagal reflexes to the larynx and tracheobronchial tree, vagal afferent reflexes from these sites back to the same regions and to other parts of the respiratory tract, and reflexes that feed in from the whole respiratory tract and elsewhere down to the vagal motor supply of the larynx and lower respiratory tract. The exact tissues supplied in each part of the respiratory tract will depend on the anatomical structures there, which are very different for different areas (Table 1).

This highly complex system is made even more complicated by two further factors. The same anatomical zones are also supplied by motor and sensory fibers via the sympathetic nervous system, so that both sympathetic and parasympa-

Table 1 Nervous Receptors and Effector Tissues in the Airways

	Receptors	Effector tissues
Nose	Irritant Pressure/flow	Blood vessels Glands Skeletal muscle
Pharynx	Rapidly adapting Pressure	Blood vessels Glands Skeletal muscle
Larynx	Pressure Cold/flow Drive Hyposmolar Irritant C-fiber	Blood vessels Glands Skeletal muscle
Trachea/bronchi	Slowly adapting stretch Rapidly adapting irritant C-fiber bronchial Neuroepithelial	Blood vessels Glands Smooth muscle
Alveoli	C-fiber pulmonary	As above

pathetic systems interact in reflex control mechanisms. In addition the vagal supply to many of the relevant tissues is not a simple cholinergic motor pathway alone, but involves nonadrenergic noncholinergic (NANC) pathways either as nerves separate from the cholinergic ones or, more likely, combined with them with a system of cotransmission (Table 2). Table 3 lists the main sites of airway bronchoconstrictor and bronchodilator reflexes, and also shows the associated changes in mucus secretion and laryngeal caliber.

If one were to consider individual specific reflexes consisting of a receptor system and a single motor system, the list of individual reflexes resulting from a combination of the afferent and motor pathways summarized in Tables 1 and 2 would be formidably long; indeed many of these individual reflexes have been identified and each could justify detailed description. In this chapter some reflexes will be only briefly described. There are other recent reviews of

Table 2 Motor Pathways to Airways

Vagal cholinergic	Smooth muscle
	Laryngeal muscles
	Glands
	? Blood vessels
Sympathetic	? Smooth muscle
	Glands
	Blood vessels
Vagal noncholinergic	Smooth muscle
	Glands
	? Blood vessels
Axon reflex	Smooth muscle
	? Glands
	Blood vessels

Table 3 Airway Reflexes

Input	Bronchial muscle	Mucus	Larynx
Bronchoconstrictor			
Larynx	+	+	+
Cough receptors	+	+	+
Irritant receptors	+	+	+
C-fiber receptors	+	+	+
Chemoreceptors	+	+	+
Cold	+	?	+
Bronchodilator			
Nose	-(+)	+	+
Nasopharynx	-	+	-
Pulmonary stretch	-	?	-
Pain	-	?	?

+ positive effect; – negative effect; ? not known.

airway innervation and its reflex activation (Nadel, 1980; Nadel and Barnes, 1984; Widdicombe, 1964, 1986, 1987).

I. Vagal Reflexes Affecting the Nose

The nose is an important part of the respiratory tract, although in humans its role is sometimes neglected since we are not obligatory nose-breathers (unlike many other mammals) and nasal patency is not essential for life (Negus, 1929). However, breathing through the mouth due to nasal blockage can have important physiological effects, either beneficial in that total airways resistance is lowered when the mouth is open, as in exercise, or harmful, in that the filtering and air conditioning roles of the nose are eliminated and the lungs are therefore more exposed to danger (Proctor and Andersen, 1982).

A. Motor Systems

The three main motor systems in the nose that may be affected by vagal reflexes are the vascular bed, the mucus secretory glands, and the skeletal muscles of the nares and palate. The extensive work published on the innervation of the nose is beyond the scope of this chapter (see Eccles, 1982), but recent studies have established not only the importance of adrenergic and cholinergic motor systems to secretory tissue and vasculature, but also the presence of motor neuropeptides such as vasoactive intestinal peptide (VIP) (Nadel and Barnes, 1984; Barnes, 1984). On the sensory side, substance P is present (see Lundberg's chapter in this volume), and other neuropeptides have been identified and may turn out to be important. The role of this innervation in nasonasal axon and central reflexes affecting the nasal vasculature and secretion has been studied (Eccles, 1982). There has been rather less work on the control of nasal patency by changes in the contraction of the skeletal muscles of the nares and palate (Widdicombe, 1986).

B. Vagal Reflexes from the Nose

The role of the nose in affecting the lower respiratory tract supplied by the vagus has been extensively reviewed (Korpas and Tomori, 1979; Eccles, 1982; Daly, 1986; Widdicombe, 1986). Irritation causes either a bronchoconstriction or a bronchodilatation, the latter probably being more common in experimental animals and the former more common in asthmatic humans. The fact that either response may be obtained may reflect on the complexity of the sensory innervation of the nose. What is more consistent is the laryngeal constriction that occurs on irritation of the nose, whether or not there is sneezing. In humans, nasal irritation or application of cold to the nose usually causes an increase in airways resistance, associated with changes in respiration and in cardiac vascular variables.

A further response to nasal irritation is secretion of mucus not only in the nose but also in the lower respiratory tract, the latter being mainly a vagal reflex (Phipps, 1981; Richardson and Phipps, 1976; Widdicombe and Wells, 1982).

C. Vagal Reflexes to the Nose

This is a neglected subject, although the reverse mechanism, reflexes originating in the nose and affecting the lower respiratory tract, has received more attention (see above). However, stimulation of the central end of a vagus nerve can cause reflex nasal vasodilatation and congestion (Eccles, 1982), and recently the effects of various afferent inputs to the nose have been identified. Thus stimulation of vagal fibers in the superior laryngeal nerve (SLN) changes nasal vascular resistance in dogs (K. Dylewska and J. G. Widdicombe, unpublished data). One interesting aspect of the larynx-to-nose reflex is that it is asymmetrical; the ipsilateral side shows a dilatation whereas the contralateral side constricts. This is one of the few asymmetrical reflexes to the respiratory tract that has been studied, the best known example being the "crutch" reflex, whereby unilateral mechanical stimulation of the skin of the chest and axilla causes ipsilateral nasal congestion (Eccles, 1982). The functional advantage of such asymmetry is unknown.

Stimulation of lung C-fiber receptors in dogs causes nasal vasodilatation as part of the general cardiovascular response from these endings (M. Lung and J. G. Widdicombe, 1987), and the same may be true of rapidly adapting (irritant) lung receptors. Pulmonary stretch receptors have not been shown to influence the nasal vasculature; in humans a deep breath will increase nasal patency but this has not been established as a reflex from the lungs (Syabbalo et al., 1986a). It has also been shown that inputs from carotid sinus baroreceptors and carotid body chemoreceptors change nasal vascular resistance, although these reflexes seem to be less powerful than those from the same sensory zones to other vascular beds (K. Dylewska and J. G. Widdicombe, unpublished data).

The mechanisms described above have been studied almost entirely in experimental animals, but there is some evidence that they may also exist in humans. For example, inhalation of histamine aerosol into the lungs, which is known to stimulate lung afferent endings, causes nasal congestion in normal and atopic human subjects (Bundgaard et al., 1986). By analogy with animal work, it seems likely that this works by a vagonasal reflex. The significance of such a mechanism can only be speculated.

II. Vagal Pharyngeal Reflexes

A. Laryngopharyngeal Reflex

There has recently been considerable interest in the reflex control of the pharyngeal muscles, in particular the dilator muscles of the pharynx such as the genioglossus. The importance of these mechanisms is that their deficiency or ineffectiveness may lead to snoring and sleep apneas, conditions known to cause not only distress but a hazard to health (Phillipson and Bowes, 1986; Widdicombe, 1986). Although the main mechanisms influencing pharyngeal dilator muscle contraction, and therefore the patency of the pharynx, certainly include non-vagal mechanisms such as reflexes from the nose and from the pharynx itself (in the glossopharyngeal nerve), vagal reflexes from the larynx are an important component of the total upper airway response. Indeed, some studies suggest that this may be the most active pathway.

Thus pressure changes in the upper respiratory tract including the larynx lead to reflex changes in pharyngeal patency, and in experimental animals these are greatly reduced or even abolished by cutting the SLNs (Widdicombe, 1986). It is postulated that an important component of the control of oropharyngeal patency is this input from the larynx, although the actual nervous receptors in the larynx have not been identified. The pressure receptors described by Mathew et al. (1984) seem the most likely candidates. As discussed below, the receptor physiology of the larynx is formidably complex. Since the same receptors influence respiration and can, in particular, cause apnea, laryngeal inputs may be involved in phenomena such as sleep apneas, including those in young infants that may lead to the sudden infant death syndrome (SIDS) (Bryan et al., 1986). It should be emphasized that the vagal (laryngeal-SLN) component of these conditions is only one of several, and in humans the relative importance of different nervous inputs has not been identified.

B. Vagal Reflexes from the Nasopharynx

Mechanical and chemical irritation of the nasopharyngeal mucosa causes the aspiration reflex, repeated inspiratory efforts, and associated vagal reflexes (Tomori and Widdicombe, 1969; Korpas and Tomori, 1979; Widdicombe, 1986). These include bronchodilatation, laryngeal abduction, and mucus secretion in the lower respiratory tract. The afferent pathways for these changes have not been clearly identified, but may involve rapidly adapting receptors in the pharyngeal mucosa. They have not been studied extensively in humans.

III. Vagal Laryngeal Reflexes

The larynx is the first part of the respiratory tract, if one is traveling caudally, that has both an afferent and motor supply via the vagus nerves.

A. Afferent Innervation of the Larynx

This has been studied mainly by single-fiber recording from the SLN, and several different types of receptor have been identified (Widdicombe, 1964, 1986). The histologic nature of the end-organs attached to these nerves has not been determined. The afferent pathways are summarized in Table 1. The stimuli that activate these pathways include the classic interventions with irritant chemical and mechanical excitations, as well as several physiological mechanical events such as pressure and flow. Of recent current interest has been the study of afferent pathways that respond to low osmolarity, in particular low concentrations of permeant diffusible anions such as chloride (Boggs and Bartlett, 1982). This last stimulus may be relevant to SIDS.

B. Motor Pathways

With such a complex afferent innervation of the larynx it is not surprising that the motor effects of laryngeal stimulation are manifold (Bartlett, 1986). As already mentioned, they include changes in the nasal vasculature and patency, and in the patency of the oropharynx due to changes in contraction of the pharyngeal dilator muscles. However, some of the most powerful laryngeal reflexes affect laryngeal caliber itself, as part of the defensive system of the upper respiratory tract (Korpas and Tomori, 1979; Szereda-Przestaszewska and Widdicombe, 1973; Widdicombe, 1986). Thus mechanical or chemical irritation of the larynx leads to its prompt closure, and the threshold for this reflex is probably lower than that for other laryngeal motor actions. At the same time, laryngeal irritation causes pronounced cardiovascular effects, usually hypertension and bradycardia, as well as lower airway mucus secretion (Phipps, 1981). Recent studies have shown that stimulation of the SLN leads to a dilatation of the tracheal vessels (Widdicombe et al., 1986; Laitinen et al., 1987), and the response is asymmetrical, being stronger on the ipsilateral side. A more powerful laryngeal-pulmonary reflex is the bronchoconstriction seen on irritation of the larynx (Nadel, 1980; Widdicombe, 1986). The afferent mechanism of this reflex has not been worked out, but the motor system is the vagal cholinergic pathway. An important recent study has shown that if this cholinergic constrictor pathway is blocked by atropine, the mechanism is reversed with the laryngeal irritation causing a bronchodilatation (Szarek et al., 1986). This is presumably a manifestation of the NANC inhibitory system to the airways with a neuropeptide mediator, possibly VIP. It seems to be the first clear example of a reflex control of the vagal NANC system to the airways.

Laryngeal-vagal reflexes have been little studied in humans, although it is plausible that many of the respiratory and airway responses due to inhaled aerosols of mediators and irritants are due to activation of laryngeal reflexes, since in experimental animals these are highly sensitive, provided they have not been bypassed by tracheostomy. Recent studies have shown that inhalation of aerosols such as histamine and citric acid can cause both coughing and bronchoconstriction (Sheppard et al., 1983), but that the afferent mechanisms for these two presumed reflexes are different since they can be set up by different stimuli in human subjects. On the motor side it has been shown that in conditions such as chronic bronchitis and asthma, or on provocation of bronchoconstriction with aerosols of mediators such as histamine, laryngeal constriction in expiration is enhanced and presumably contributes to the total expiratory resistive load of breathing (Collett et al., 1983; Higenbottam and Payne, 1982). By analogy with animal experiments, it seems likely that this process is based upon vagal reflexes affecting the larynx.

IV. Tracheobronchial Tree

This region is rightly regarded as the dominating site for vagal reflexes affecting the airways, both because it is the structure from which the afferent end-organs affecting airway caliber and respiration have been most studied analytically, and because changes in caliber in the tracheobronchial tree are most definitely associated with common conditions such as asthma and chronic bronchitis. However, as indicated above, the role of these lower airways must be integrated into a more general pattern of airway response from nares to alveoli.

A. Afferent End-Organs

Four types of afferent end-organ have been identified in the lower airway walls, and these and some of their motor actions are listed in Table 3 (Widdicombe, 1964, 1987; Sant'Ambrogio, 1982; Pack and Widdicombe, 1984; Coleridge and Coleridge, 1986).

Slowly Adapting Stretch Receptors

Although these are probably the most studied of the airway nerve-endings, there is little indication that they have an important role in disease. Physiological and histologic evidence shows that the receptors lie in the airway smooth muscle, especially of the trachea and larger bronchi. They have been delineated by three-dimensional electron microscopy (Krauhs, 1984). Although their detailed attachments to the smooth muscle are not certain, they are sensitized by smooth muscle contraction and are stimulated by stretch of the airway wall. They can be inhibited by high carbon dioxide tensions. Thus in general their role is to signal the degree of stretch of the lungs, but their activity may be tuned by various mechanical and chemical factors (Coleridge and Coleridge, 1986; Sant'Ambrogio, 1982).

Their reflex role has been studied chiefly on pattern of breathing, where they inhibit inspiratory activity and prolong expiratory duration. Thus they play a major reflex role in modifying the pattern of breathing, which is primarily set by the respiratory rhythm generator in the brainstem. Their reflex actions in relation to airway caliber have been studied in detail only in one respect, namely relaxation of tracheobronchial smooth muscle. A deep breath will not only mechanically stretch the airways but will also reflexly inhibit smooth muscle constrictor tone (Widdicombe, 1963, 1987; Nadel, 1980; Coleridge and Coleridge, 1986). The importance of this reflex in pathophysiology has not been studied, although presumably it can be correlated with the fact that asthmatics tend to find increasing their functional residual capacity is beneficial in relieving airway obstruction. Far less is known of the role of pulmonary stretch receptors on other aspects of airway caliber. They seem to set laryngeal caliber at a partially opened level (Pressman and Kelmen, 1965; Wyke, 1978), but little is known about their action if any on airway mucus secretion or airway vascular beds.

Lung Irritant Receptors: Cough

Receptors in the larynx that cause coughing have been mentioned above. Those for the lower respiratory tract almost certainly consist of free nerve endings in and under the epithelium of the larger airways, with concentrations at sites of bifurcations such as the tracheal carina (Widdicombe, 1964, 1987; Sant'Ambrogio, 1982; Coleridge and Coleridge, 1986). These nerves have been shown by degeneration experiments to be afferent (Das et al., 1979; Hoyes and Barber, 1983), and their pattern of distribution corresponds closely to that of the sensitivity of the cough reflex. Indirect evidence suggests that those deeper in the lungs do not usually cause coughing, but hyperpnea and hyperventilation instead. Stimulation of the receptors by mechanical events such as inflation or deflation of the lungs causes rapidly adapting discharges in corresponding vagal myelinated nerve fibers, and the receptors are often referred to as rapidly adapting stretch receptors (Coleridge and Coleridge, 1986). In addition to their sensitivity to mechanical stimuli, the irritant receptors can be activated by inhalation of various irritant gases such as cigarette smoke, sulfur dioxide, and ammonia, and by a wide range of mediators such as histamine and prostaglandin F_{2a}. They are also sensitized in a number of lung pathologic conditions including pulmonary congestion and edema, pneumothorax, microembolism, and anaphylaxis.

The evidence for the reflex actions of these receptors is partly based on correlation between the stimuli that excite them and the reflex responses of coughing and hyperpnea, which can be abolished by bilateral vagotomy. In addition, it is significant that at least two species, mice and ferrets, lack the histologic appearance of epithelial nerves in their airways and have no cough in response to mechanical stimulation of the tracheobronchial tree (Korpas and Widdicombe, 1983; Pack et al., 1984). On the other hand rats, which have some epithelial nerves in their tracheas, have no cough reflex from that site but do respond with hyperpnea to tracheal irritation (Korpas and Tomori, 1979). Recent studies in rabbits have established that the irritant receptors are responsible for the occasional deep augmented breaths shown by mammalian species (Davies and Roumy, 1984), and that at least in the anesthetized rabbit they exert a continuous drive to respiration by shortening expiratory time.

With regard to their action on the airways, the stimuli that excite the irritant receptors also cause laryngeal constriction, bronchoconstriction, and tracheal mucus secretion (Widdicombe, 1963, 1964; Colleridge and Coleridge, 1986). However, before it can be concluded that the irritant receptors mediate these reflexes, the role of other pathways must be eliminated. This is difficult, since the same stimuli usually also excite C-fiber receptors in the airways and lungs that cause similar reflexes. As mentioned above, the dissociation between reflex coughing and reflex bronchoconstriction in response to some inhaled irritant and mediator stimuli in humans may also suggest that these reflexes do not have a common afferent pathway but that more than one type of nerve end-organ is involved.

C-Fiber Receptors

Receptors attached to vagal C-fibers are found throughout the tracheobronchial tree and in the alveolar wall, and probably also in the laryngeal mucosa (Sant' Ambrogio, 1982; Coleridge and Coleridge, 1986). They are usually classified anatomically into bronchial and pulmonary groups based on the branch of the blood circulation that supplies them. The receptors have not been unequivocally identified histologically, although nonmyelinated nerve fibers have been seen in the alveolar wall (Meyrick and Reid, 1976) and in the bronchial mucosa, although it cannot be established that these are not fibers passing through to other sites. Their sensory nature does not seem to have been established by degeneration studies.

The C-fibers are activated by almost the same group of stimuli as those that affect lung irritant receptors, although in general the C-fibers are less sensitive to mechanical stimuli such as lung volume changes (Coleridge and Coleridge, 1984, 1986). However, they are stimulated by inhaled irritants such as sulfur dioxide, and many mediators associated with inflammatory conditions such as prostaglandins, histamine, and bradykinin.

The reflex responses to stimulation of C-fiber receptors include apnea followed by rapid shallow breathing, bradycardia, and hypotension. Coughing has never been reported. In terms of airway responses, there is a powerful laryngeal constriction and also bronchoconstriction and tracheal mucus secretion, which features are also seen as responses to irritant receptor stimulation (Widdicombe, 1963, 1964; Stransky et al., 1973; Coleridge and Coleridge, 1986).

Since laryngeal constriction, bronchoconstriction, and mucus secretion are thought to be common features of stimulation of both C-fiber and irritant receptors in the airways, the question arises as to whether the two mechanisms can be differentiated. The distinction depends upon two types of experiment. One is the search for specific stimuli that affect only one group of receptors. In this respect some foreign chemicals such as capsaicin and phenylbiguanide in minimal dosages are thought to affect C-fiber receptors and not irritant receptors (Coleridge and Coleridge, 1986), although larger dosages stimulate both groups. Experiments with these agents strongly support the role of C-fibers in reflex bronchoconstrictions. No chemical stimuli specific to irritant receptors have been studied to the same extent, although possibly prostaglandin F_{2a} might fit this category. The second differential method is to block the vagus nerves in such a way that only one of the two reflexes is left intact. This method has been extensively used for many decades, but the types of differential blockade used—vagal cooling or electric currents—are not always sufficiently specific to allow firm conclusions to be drawn. In terms of whole-body pathophysiology, most of the lung inflammatory and immunologic conditions such as bronchitis and asthma will probably activate both groups of nervous receptors, which would interact to cause augmented airway responses.

Axon Reflexes

A further aspect of vagal control of airway caliber concerns axon reflexes within the airway walls. Rapidly adapting irritant receptors have a relatively large distribution of their nerve terminals, up to 1 cm^2 in the dog, and branches extend both into the epithelium and deeper into airway smooth muscle (Sant'Ambrogio, 1982). Other studies have shown that axon reflex activation by drugs such as capsaicin can release neuropeptides such as substance P with local responses in the vasculature and smooth muscle (Lundberg and Saria, 1983); at least this seems to apply to the larger bronchi of the guinea pig. The role of axon reflexes in lung neuropathology is discussed elsewhere in this volume (see chapters by Lundberg and Persson), but it should be pointed out that activation of the axon reflex must also include activation of the central nervous reflex mediated by the vagal afferent pathway.

Other Airway Responses from Lung Receptors

Although the main focus in research on the reflex control of airway caliber has been on the reflexes from the tracheobronchial tree described above, they may also have other important actions. For example, stimulation of lung C-fiber receptors causes not only vasodilatation in the nose (M. Lung and J. G. Widdicombe, 1987) but also dilatation of the vasculature of the trachea (G. Sahin, S. Webber, and J. G. Widdicombe, unpublished findings), together with mucus secretion (Phipps, 1981). Whether pulmonary stretch and irritant receptors have similar actions does not seem to have been determined. Peripheral and central chemoreceptor activation has been well established as a cause of bronchoconstriction, and it seems likely that the same stimuli also affect the vascular beds of the nose and tracheobronchial tree. Baroreceptor stimulation also causes nasal vasodilatation and tracheobronchial vascular changes, although the latter are probably weak compared with other baroreceptor reflexes. A baroreceptor reflex relaxation of lower airway smooth muscle has also been established.

V. Conclusions

It is clear that the role of vagal reflexes on airway caliber is highly complex, both because a number of primary reflexes feed into many effector tissues that influence airway caliber, such as the nasal vasculature, intrinsic laryngeal muscles, tracheobronchial muscles and vasculature, and submucosal glands, and also because in addition to primary reflexes that can be identified secondary responses may take place involving blood chemical changes and baroreceptor reflexes. Nearly all the animal studies of these reflexes have been analytical, in the sense that individual components of the mechanisms have been worked out. Fitting all the components into a single pattern is far more difficult and has been scarcely attempted. The relevance of such an integrative analysis in the anesthetized animal may be small when compared with what happens in unanesthetized humans, especially if the latter have respiratory pathology. Nonetheless, in spite of the uncertainty of the quantitation of these reflexes, their existence and powerful nature have been well established and there can be little doubt that they are important in human airways control.

Discussion

Bousquet. Can nasal stimulation cause bronchoconstriction, since pollen-induced asthma is poorly understood?

Widdicombe. Allergen challenge to the nose can cause bronchoconstriction. In animals, nasobronchial reflexes can be either a bronchoconstrictor or bronchodilator, so there may be more than one afferent pathway.

Vanhoutte. During stimulation of laryngeal nerves there are changes in ventilation that might affect the airways.

Widdicombe. We controlled for this by repeating the experiments in paralyzed and artificially ventilated dogs and showed the same bronchoconstrictor response.

Nadel. Does vagal output from the CNS travel via separate fibers to airway muscle and glands?

Widdicombe. Irritation of the larynx causes bronchoconstriction and tracheal mucus secretion, whereas irritation of the nasopharynx causes bronchodilation and tracheal mucus secretion. This suggests separate neural pathways.

Kaliner. How can you explain the difference between increased nasal airway resistance (NAR) after histamine bronchial challenge, and the decrease in NAR after cold air hyperventilation challenge or exercise challenge?

Widdicombe. Exercise, hypoxia, and hypercapnia cause an increase in nasal patency presumably by nasal vasoconstriction. These are quite different inputs from those seen when bronchial afferent reflexes are stimulated.

References

Barnes, P. J. (1984). The third nervous system in the lung: physiology and clinical perspectives. *Thorax* **39**:561-567.

Bartlett, D. Jr. (1986). Upper airway motor systems. In *Handbook of Physiology,* Section 3, The Respiratory System, vol. II. Edited by N. S. Cherniack and J. G. Widdicombe. Washington, D.C., American Physiological Society, pp. 223-246.

Boggs, D. F., and Bartlett, D. (1982). Chemical specificity of a laryngeal apneic reflex in puppies. *J. Appl. Physiol.* **53**:455-462.

Bryan, A. C., Bowes, G., and Maloney, J. E. (1986). Control of breathing in the fetus and the newborn. In *Handbook of Physiology,* Section 3, *The Respiratory System,* vol. II. Edited by N. S. Cherniack and J. G. Widdicombe. Washington, D.C., American Physiological Society, pp. 621-648.

Bundgaard, A., Schmidt, A., Syabbalo, N. C., and Widdicombe, J. G. (1986). Effects of pulmonary inhalation of water and histamine aerosols on nasal airflow resistance in man. *Eur. J. Respir. Dis.* **68**:248-255.

Coleridge, J., and Coleridge, H. (1984). Afferent vagal C-fiber innervation of the lungs and airways and its function significance. *Rev. Physiol. Biochem. Pharmacol.* **99**:1-110.

Coleridge, H., and Coleridge, J. (1986). Reflexes evoked from the tracheobronchial tree and lungs. In *Handbook of Physiology,* Section 3, The Respiratory System, vol II. Edited by N. S. Cherniack and J. G. Widdicombe. Washington, D.C., American Physiological Society, pp. 395-430.

Collett, P. W. T., Barancatisano, T. P., and Engel, L. A. (1983). Changes in the glottic aperture during bronchial asthma. *Am. Rev. Respir. Dis.* **128**:719-723.

Daly, M. de B. (1986), Interactions between respiration and circulation. In

Handbook of Physiology, Section 3, The Respiratory System, vol. II. Edited by N. S. Cherniack and J. G. Widdicombe. Washington, D.C., American Physiological Society, pp. 529-594.

Das, R. M., Jeffery, P. K., and Widdicombe, J. G. (1979). Experimental degeneration of intra-epithelial nerve fibres in cat airways. *J. Anat.* **128**:259-267.

Davies, A., and Roumy, M. (1982). The effect of transient stimulation of lung irritant receptors on the pattern of breathing in rabbits. *J. Physiol.* **324**: 389-401.

Eccles, R. (1982). Neurological and pharmacological considerations. In *The Nose: Upper Airway Physiology and the Atmospheric Environment.* Edited by D. F. Proctor and I. B. Andersen. Amsterdam, Elsevier, pp. 191-214.

Higenbottam, T., and Payne, J. (1982). Glottis narrowing in lung disease. *Am. Rev. Respir. Dis.* **125**:746-750.

Hoyes, A. D., and Barber, P. (1981). Morphology and response to vagus nerve section of the intra-epithelial axons of the rat trachea. A quantitative ultrastructural study. *J. Anat.* **132**:331-339.

Korpas, J., and Tomori, Z. (1979). *Cough and Other Respiratory Reflexes.* Basel, Karger.

Korpas, J., and Widdicombe, J. G. (1983). Defensive respiratory reflexes in ferrets. *Respiration* **44**:128-135.

Krauhs, J. M. (1984). Morphology of presumptive slowly adapting receptors in dog trachea. *Anat. Rec.* **210**:73-85.

Laitinen, L. A., Laitinen, A., and Widdicombe, J. G. (1987). Parasympathetic nervous control of the tracheal vascular resistance in the dog. *J. Physiol.* **385**:135-146.

Lundberg, J. M., and Saria, A. (1983). Capsaicin-induced desensitization of airway mucosa to cigarette smoke, mechanical and chemical irritants. *Nature* **302**:251-253.

Lung, M. A., and Widdicombe, J. G. (1987). Lung reflexes and nasal vascular resistance in the anesthetized dog. *J. Physiol.* **386**:465-474.

Mathew, O. P., Sant'Ambrogio, G., Fisher, J. T., and Sant'Ambrogio, F. B. (1984). Laryngeal pressure receptors. *Respir. Physiol.* **57**:113-122.

Meyrick, B., and Reid, L. (1971). Nerves in rat intra-acinar alveoli: an electron microscopic study. *Respir. Physiol.* **11**:367-377.

Nadel, J. A. (1980). Autonomic regulation of airway smooth muscle. In *Physiology and Pharmacology of the Airways.* Edited by J. A. Nadel. New York, Marcel Dekker, pp. 217-257.

Nadel, J. A., and Barnes, P. J. (1984). Autonomic regulation of the airways. *Annu. Rev. Med.* **35**:451-467.

Negus, V. (1929). *The Mechanism of the Larynx.* London, Heinemann.

Pack, R. J., Al-Ugaily, L. H., and Widdicombe, J. G. (1984). The innervation of the trachea and extrapulmonary bronchi of the mouse. *Cell Tissue Res.* **238**:61-68.

Pack, R. J., and Widdicombe, J. G. (1984). Amine-containing cells of the lung. *Eur. J. Respir. Dis.* **65**:559-578.

Phillipson, E. A., and Bowes, G. (1986). Control of breathing during sleep. In *Handbook of Physiology,* Section 3, The Respiratory System, vol. II. Edited by N. S. Cherniack and J. G. Widdicombe. Washington, D.C., American Physiological Society, pp. 649-690.

Phipps, R. F. (1981). The airway mucociliary system. In *Respiratory Physiology III.* Edited by J. G. Widdicombe. Baltimore, University Park Press, pp. 213-260.

Pressman, J. G., and Kelemen, G. (1955). Physiology of the larynx. *Physiol. Rev.* **35**:506-554.

Proctor, D. F., and Andersen, I. B. (Eds.) (1982). *The Nose: Upper Airway Physiology and the Atmospheric Environment.* Amsterdam, Elsevier.

Richardson, P. S., and Phipps, R. J. (1978). The anatomy, physiology, pharmacology and pathology of tracheobronchial mucus secretion and the use of expectorant drugs in human disease. *Pharmacol. Ther.* **3**:441-479.

Sant'Ambrogio, G. (1982). Information arising from the tracheobronchial tree of mammals. *Physiol. Rev.* **62**:531-569.

Sheppard, D., Rizk, N. W., Boushey, H. A., and Bethel, R. A. (1983). Mechanism of cough and bronchoconstriction induced by distilled water aerosol. *Am. Rev. Respir. Dis.* **127**:691-694.

Stransky, A., Szereda-Przestaszewska, M., and Widdicombe, J. G. (1973). The effect of lung reflexes on laryngeal resistance and motoneuron discharge. *J. Physiol.* **231**:417-438.

Szarek, J. L., Gillespie, M. N., Altiere, R. J., and Diamond, L. (1986). Reflex activation of the nonadrenergic noncholinergic inhibitory system in feline airways.

Szereda-Przestaszewska, M., and Widdicombe, J. G. (1973). Reflex effects of chemical irritation of the upper airways on the laryngeal lumen in cats. *Respir. Physiol.* **18**:107-115.

Syabbalo, N. C., Bundgaard, A., Entholm, P., Schmidt, A., and Widdicombe, J. G. (1986). Measurement and regulation of nasal airflow resistance in man. *Rhinology* **24**:87-101.

Tomori, Z., and Widdicombe, J. G. (1969). Muscular, bronchomotor and cardiovascular reflexes elicited by mechanical stimulation of the respiratory tract. *J. Physiol.* **200**:25-50.

Widdicombe, J. G. (1963). Regulation of tracheobronchial smooth muscle. *Physiol. Rev.* **43**:1-37.

Widdicombe, J. G. (1964). Respiratory reflexes. In *Handbook of Physiology,* Section 3, Respiration, vol. I. Edited by W. O. Fenn and H. Rahn. Washington, D.C., American Physiological Society, pp. 585-630.

Widdicombe, J. G. (1986). Reflexes from the upper respiratory tract. In *Handbook of Physiology,* Section 3, The Respiratory System, vol. II.

Edited by N. S. Cherniack and J. G. Widdicombe. Washington, D.C., American Physiological Society, pp. 363-394.

Widdicombe, J. G. (1987). Nervous control of airway tone. In *Bronchial Hyperresponsiveness.* Edited by J. Nadel, R. Pauwels, and P. Snashall. Oxford, Blackwell Scientific, pp. 46-67.

Widdicombe, J. G., and Wells, U. M. (1982). Airway secretions. In *The Nose: Upper Airway Physiology and the Atmospheric Environment.* Edited by D. F. Proctor and I. B. Andersen. Amsterdam, Elsevier, pp. 215-244.

Widdicombe, J. G., Laitinen, A., and Laitinen, L. A. (1986). Parasympathetic nervous control of tracheal vascular resistance in the dog. *Fed. Proc.* **45**: 558.

Wyke, B. D., and Kirchner, J. A. (1978). Neurology of the larynx. In *Scientific Foundations of Otolaryngology.* Edited by R. Hinchcliffe and D. Harrison. London, Heinemann, pp. 546-574.

9

Modulation of Cholinergic Neurotransmission in the Airways

PAUL M. VANHOUTTE

Mayo Clinic, Mayo Medical School
and Mayo Graduate School of Medicine
Rochester, Minnesota

NICHOLAS A. FLAVAHAN*

Mayo Clinic and Mayo Foundation
Rochester, Minnesota

When discussing the action of bronchodilator agents, it generally is assumed that these drugs act directly on airway smooth muscle. In the vascular system it is now well established that endogenous neurohumoral mediators and a variety of pharmacologic agents can cause either contraction or relaxation of the smooth muscle of the blood vessel wall because they involve other cells such as adrenergic neurons (e.g., Westfall, 1977; Vanhoutte et al., 1981) or endothelial cells (e.g., Furchgott, 1983; Vanhoutte et al., 1986b). This chapter summarizes data from the authors' laboratory, which strongly suggests that the same is true at least in canine bronchi. In particular they suggest that prejunctional actions on cholinergic terminals, or release of relaxing factor(s) from epithelial cells, contribute to the regulation of bronchomotor tone (Vermeire and Vanhoutte, 1979; Flavahan et al., 1985; Flavahan and Vanhoutte, 1985).

I. Prejunctional Actions of Catecholamines

Canine bronchi are innervated by both adrenergic and cholinergic nerves (Knight et al., 1981). Stimulation of these nerves in vivo results in bronchodilation and bronchoconstriction, respectively. Activation of autonomic nerves also can be

**Present affiliation*: University College London, London, United Kingdom

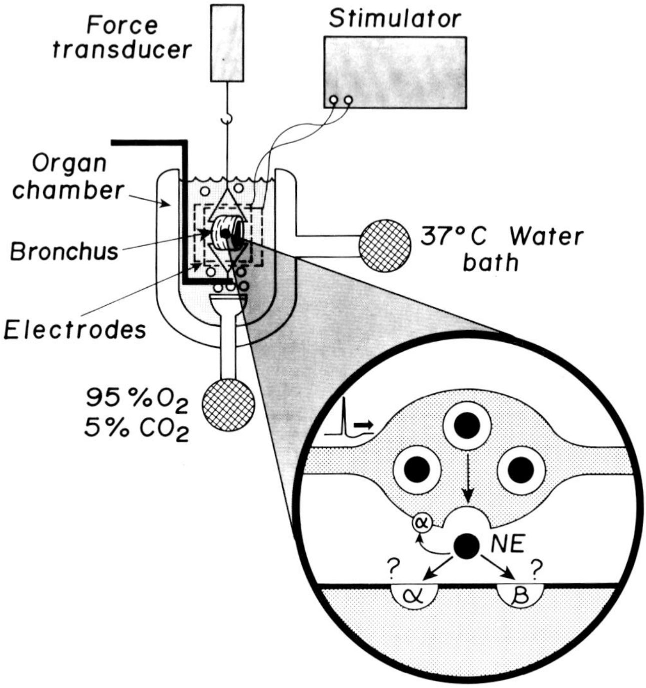

Figure 1 Organ chamber used for the study of isolated rings of canine bronchi. The rings are suspended between two stirrups in an organ chamber filled with Krebs-Ringer bicarbonate solution, maintained at 37°C and continuously oxygenated with a gas mixture containing 95% O_2 and 5% CO_2 (to maintain a constant pH of approximately 7.4). To stimulate the autonomic nerves in the preparation, two platinum electrodes are placed parallel to it. Drugs can also be added to the bath solution, to cause activation or inhibition of either smooth muscle or autonomic nerves.

achieved in vitro by studying rings of canine bronchi in organ chambers and stimulating them electrically (Fig. 1) (Russell, 1978; Vermeire and Vanhoutte, 1979; Russell, 1980). Such stimulation results in contractions of the rings that are not affected by nicotinic blockers (which prevent ganglionic transmission), but are abolished by either tetrodotoxin (which prevents fast Na^+ movements in nerve terminals) or muscarinic antagonists such as atropine (Fig. 2). Thus, it is likely that the electrical impulses cause the release of acetylcholine from cholinergic nerve endings, which in turn stimulates muscarinic receptors on the bronchial smooth muscle; this then initiates the contractile process. Theoretically, by

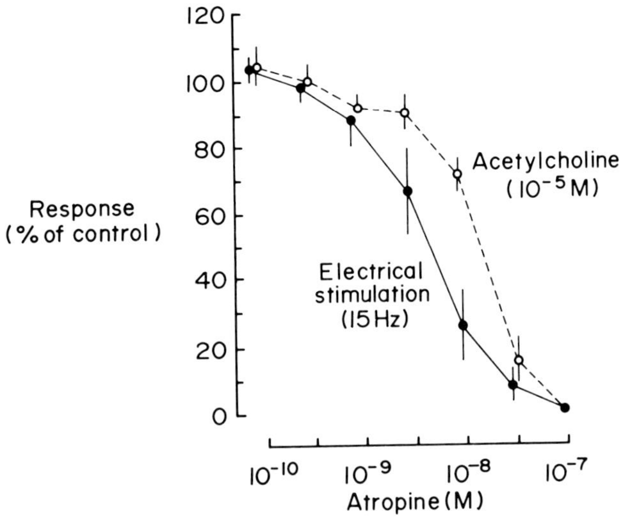

Figure 2 The muscarinic antagonist atropine causes concentration-dependent inhibition of contractions of canine bronchi evoked either by electrical stimulation (15 Hz) or exogenous acetylcholine (10^{-5} M). These experiments illustrate that the transmitter released by the electrical impulses and exogenous acetylcholine act on the same muscarinic receptors on the bronchial smooth muscle (data from Vermeire and Vanhoutte, 1979).

comparing the effect of any drug on the response to such electrical stimulation with that of the same agent on contraction induced by exogenous acetylcholine, one can estimate prejunctional effects (Vanhoutte and Shepherd, 1973; Vanhoutte et al., 1981). Actually, as long as the actual measurement of the overflow of acetylcholine into the extracellular space remains technically impossible in airway smooth muscle, this type of comparison is probably the only reasonable way to examine the prejunctional effects of drugs. Thus, drugs that augment or inhibit the release of acetylcholine without affecting the cholinergic responsiveness of the airway smooth muscle would facilitate or inhibit, respectively, contractions evoked by electrical stimulation without affecting the increases in tension caused by exogenous acetylcholine. Acetylcholine, whether released from cholinergic nerves or added exogenously, contracts canine bronchial smooth muscle by activating the same type of receptor, the M_2-muscarinic receptor (O'Rourke and Vanhoutte, 1986). If the substances involved also have direct effects on the smooth muscle, less clearcut results are obtained. This is the case with beta-adrenergic agonists.

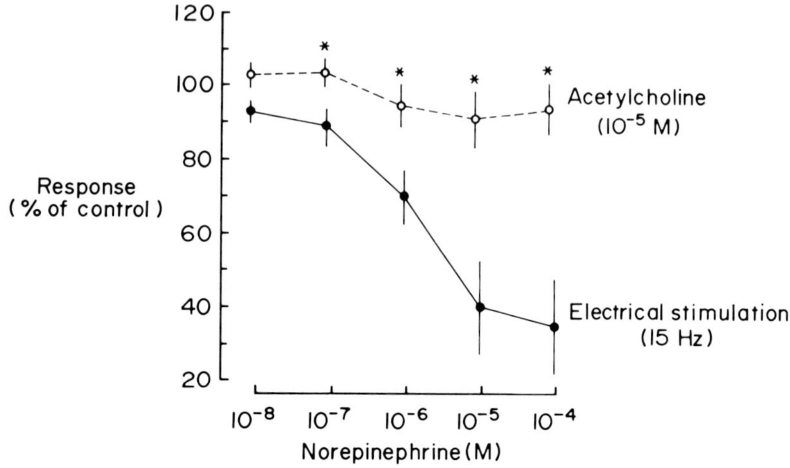

Figure 3 In canine bronchi (without epithelium), the adrenergic neurotransmitter norepinephrine causes significantly larger inhibition of the contractions evoked by electrical field stimulation (15 Hz) than of those caused by exogenous acetylcholine (10^{-5} M) (data from Vermeire and Vanhoutte, 1979).

Indeed, in rings of canine bronchi (in which the epithelium has been removed), both the natural adrenergic neurotransmitter norepinephrine (Fig. 3) and the synthetic beta-adrenergic agonist isoproterenol cause minimal reductions of the contraction to exogenous acetylcholine, but markedly depress that to electrical impulses (Vermeire and Vanhoutte, 1979). These experiments strongly suggest that in the canine bronchi catecholamines cause relaxation of the smooth muscle by virtue of their prejunctional inhibitory effects on cholinergic nerve endings (Vermeire and Vanhoutte, 1979). The effects of both norepinephrine and isoproterenol are suppressed by the beta-adrenergic blocker propranolol, demonstrating that the receptors they activate on both the cholinergic nerve endings and the bronchial smooth muscle are beta-adrenoceptors (Vermeire and Vanhoutte, 1979).

Electrical stimulation causes the release of [^{3}H] norepinephrine in canine bronchi previously incubated with the labeled transmitter (Fig. 4) (Vermeire and Vanhoutte, 1978; Lorenz and Vanhoutte, 1985). When rings of canine bronchi (without epithelium) are stimulated for several minutes, the initial peak-response is not sustained (Fig. 4); the spontaneous decrease in response is prevented by propranolol (Fig. 5). These observations suggest that under certain conditions norepinephrine released from adrenergic nerve endings can act upon prejunctional beta-adrenoceptors of the cholinergic nerve terminals to reduce the release of acetylcho-

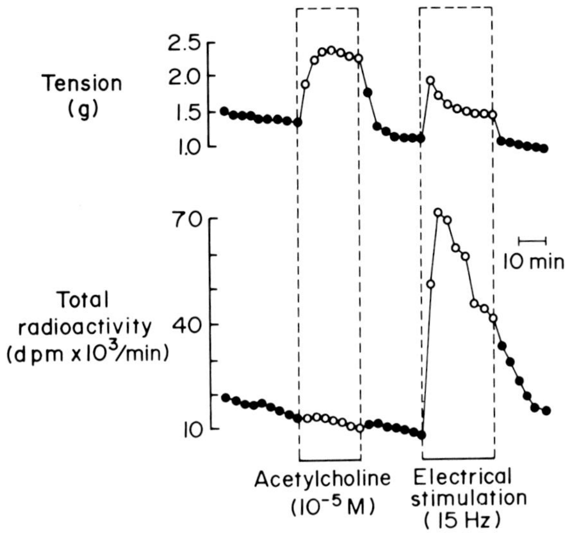

Figure 4 In a canine bronchus previously incubated with [^{3}H] norepinephrine, acetylcholine (10^{-5} M) causes contraction (upper) but no change in the clearance of tritiated compounds (lower). Electrical field stimulation (15 Hz) evokes a rapid increase in tension which is not sustained, and evokes an increased tritium-efflux (data from Vermeire and Vanhoutte, 1979).

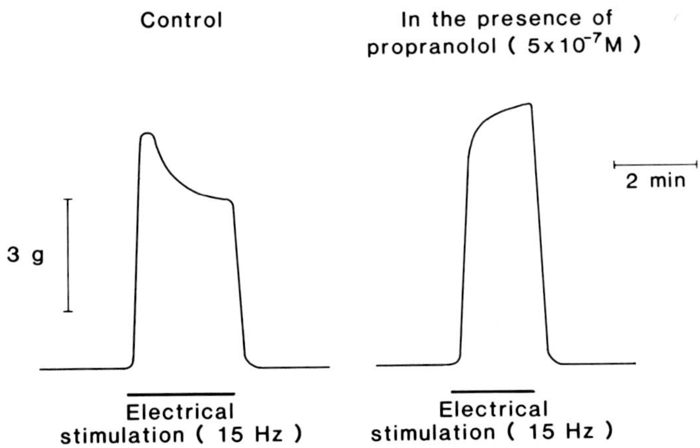

Figure 5 In a ring of canine bronchi, the contraction evoked by electrical stimulation (15 Hz) is not sustained (left); addition of propranolol (5×10^{-7} M) reduces the decay of the response (right) (data from Vermeire and Vanhoutte, 1979).

line. This interpretation has been confirmed by the demonstration that the indirect sympathomimetic amine tyramine (given under conditions where the exocytotic release of norepinephrine is prevented by the postganglionic neuronal blocker bretylium tosylate) markedly reduces the response to electrical field stimulation of the cholinergic nerves. Since the effect of tyramine was prevented by the selective $beta_1$-adrenergic blocker metoprolol, but not by the selective $beta_2$-adrenergic antagonist ICI 118,551, the adrenoceptors on the cholinergic nerve terminals probably belong to the $beta_1$-subtype (Lorenz et al., 1986). Under these conditions, pharmacologic displacement of norepinephrine by tyramine does not effect an equipotent response to acetylcholine, which might suggest that nerve-released norepinephrine acts preferentially to inhibit the release of acetylcholine from cholinergic nerves (Lorenz et al., 1986).

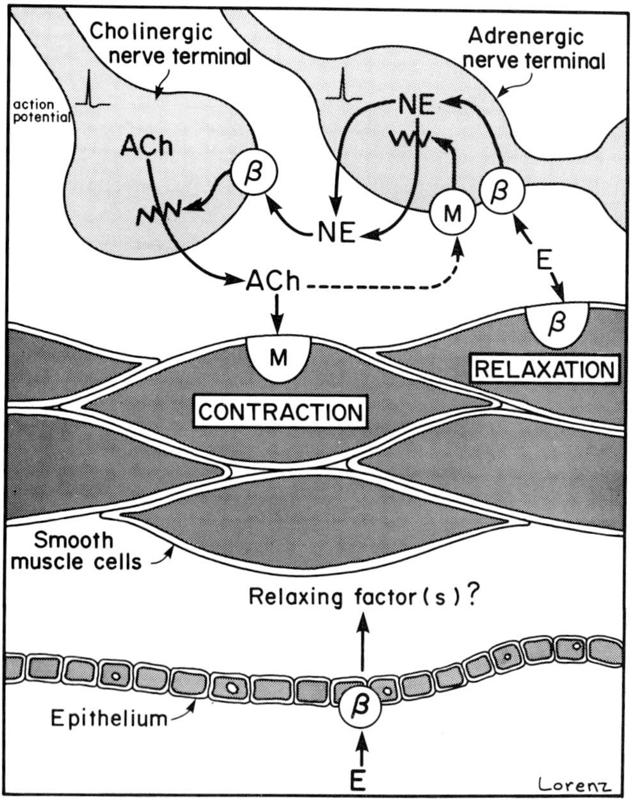

Figure 6 Interactions between adrenergic nerves, bronchial smooth muscle, and epithelial cells in canine bronchi. ACh, acetylcholine; β, beta-adrenergic receptor; E, epinephrine; M, muscarinic receptor; ⩗⩗, interruption.

When extrapolated to the intact organism, the observations in canine bronchi could imply that the inhibitory action of catecholamines on the cholinergic neuroeffector interaction (Fig. 6) explains part of the potent bronchodilator effects of those drugs, and should be considered when exogenous catecholamines reach airway smooth muscle under cholinergic control. Cholinergic and adrenergic nerve terminals are in close apposition in the canine bronchi (Knight et al., 1981). In the intact dog, sympathetic nerve stimulation inhibits the bronchoconstrictor effect of vagal nerve stimulation (Cabezas et al., 1971). Thus, in the case of adrenergic neurogenic bronchodilatation, the norepinephrine released in the vicinity of the cholinergic nerve endings may well interrupt the existing vagal tone (Vermeire and Vanhoutte, 1979; Lorenz et al., 1986). An intense relationship between cholinergic and adrenergic neurotransmitters has been well documented in the cardiovascular system, where acetylcholine causes a profound inhibition of adrenergic neurotransmission (Vanhoutte et al., 1979, 1981; Vanhoutte and Levy, 1982). If the major effect of adrenergic nerves were to inhibit cholinergic neurotransmission, the concept of a neurogenic sympathetic inhibitory control of bronchomotor tone would be compatible with a relative paucity of adrenergic nerve endings in the vicinity of bronchial smooth muscle (see chapter by Laitinen in this volume).

II. Modulatory Role of the Epithelium

The vascular endothelium can profoundly modulate the responsiveness of isolated blood vessels to a variety of vasoactive agents (Furchgott, 1983; Vanhoutte et al., 1986b). Thus endothelial cells may contribute to vascular hyperreactivity and vasospasm (Vanhoutte and Cohen, 1983; Vanhoutte and Houston, 1983). Similarly, damage to or dysfunction of respiratory epithelial cells may contribute to bronchial hyperreactivity in asthma and airway infection (Nadel, 1983; Hogg and Eggleston, 1984). Indeed, the absence of epithelial cells markedly affects the reactivity of the underlying bronchial smooth muscle.

This conclusion was reached from experiments in which only the epithelial layer of canine bronchi was removed by gentle mechanical rubbing (Fig. 7) (Flavahan et al., 1985). The mechanical removal of the epithelium renders the bronchial rings hyperresponsive to histamine, 5-hydroxytryptamine, and acetylcholine (Fig. 8). The potentiation cannot be explained by the disappearance of a major diffusion barrier, or by removal of a major site of enzymatic destruction of the bronchoactive substances (see Fig. 8). The most likely explanation for the potentiation of bronchoconstrictor responses is that the bronchial epithelium releases a factor (or factors) that causes inhibition of bronchial smooth muscle tone. Preliminary bioassay experiments demonstrate that this is the case (Fig. 9) (Flavahan and Vanhoutte, 1985). Bioassay of potential epithelial relaxant factors produces variable results and it is possible that the release of the factor(s) is polarized to-

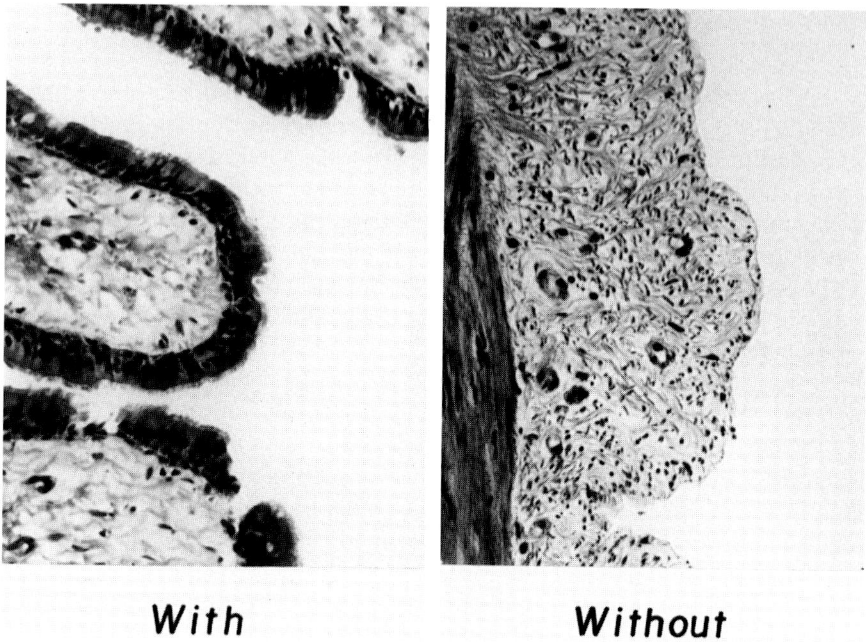

Figure 7 Histologic section demonstrating that gentle rubbing (right) of the luminal surface of canine bronchi denudes the preparation from epithelial cells (from Flavahan, et al., *Journal of Applied Physiology,* 1985, by permission).

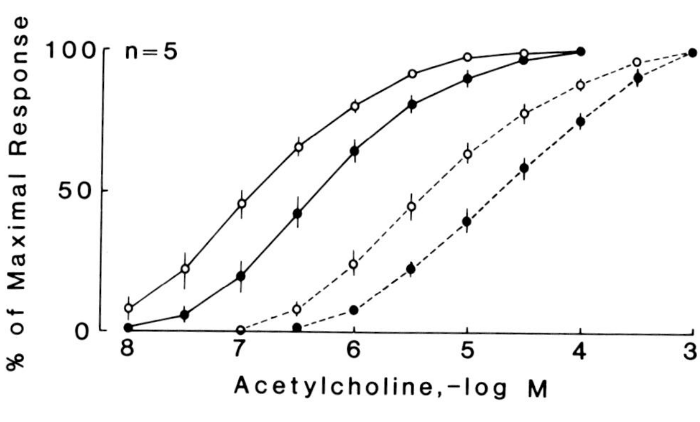

Figure 8 Effect of removal of the epithelium on concentration-response curves to acetylcholine in canine bronchi. The rings with epithelium are shown as solid symbols, and those without as open symbols. The dotted lines show the responses under control conditions, the solid lines those after inhibition of acetylcholinesterase (the major enzyme responsible for the breakdown of the cholinergic transmitter). Note in both cases a marked shift to the left of the concentration-response curve after removal of the epithelium (from Flavahan et al., *Journal of Applied Physiology,* 1985, by permission).

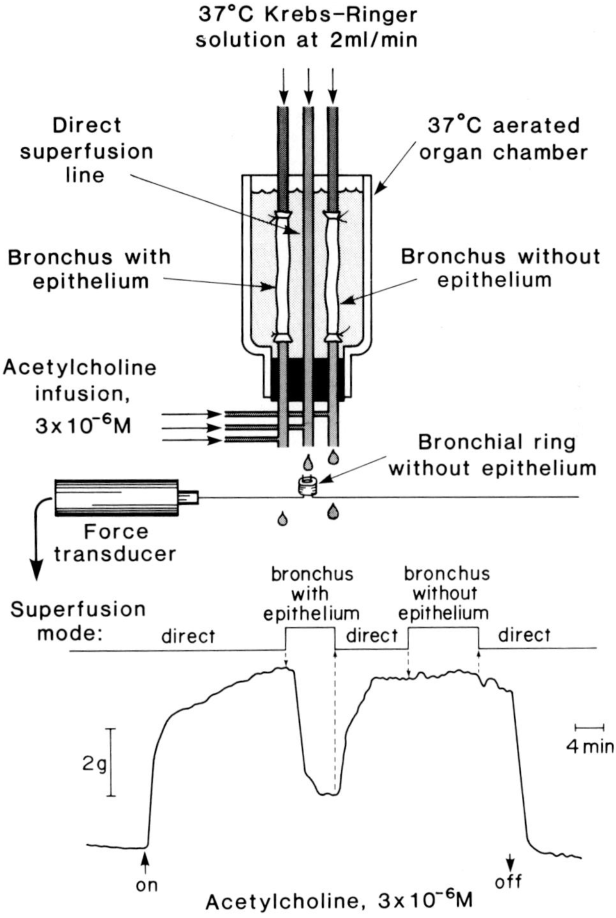

Figure 9 Bioassay experiment in which a ring of canine bronchus without epithelium (and contracted with acetylcholine) is superfused with Krebs-Ringer biocarbonate solution flowing through either a bronchus with epithelium (first arrow; note the marked relaxation), a stainless steel tube (direct; note the reversal of the relaxation), or a bronchus without epithelium (note the absence of relaxation). This demonstrates that the bronchial epithelium can release a potent inhibitory factor (Flavahan and Vanhoutte, unpublished observations).

ward the smooth muscle. The inhibitory effect of the endothelium may be mediated in part by a product of cyclooxygenase, since inhibitors of the enzyme reduce (but do not abolish) the potentiating effect of the removal of the endothelium (Flavahan et al., 1985).

The inhibitory effect of the epithelium is present not only during contractions of the bronchial smooth muscle evoked by exogenous acetylcholine but also during stimulation of the cholinergic nerve endings (Flavahan et al., 1985). In rings with epithelium, the spontaneous decay after the initial peak response to sustained electrical field stimulation is prominent. Removal of the epithelium causes an augmented peak response to lower frequencies of stimulation, and markedly reduces the spontaneous decay of the response (Fig. 10). These results suggest strongly that the epithelial factor interferes also with activation of the bronchial smooth muscle caused by endogenous acetylcholine.

We do not know yet whether the bronchoconstrictor agonists used cause the release of the relaxing factor(s) when they reach the epithelium or whether this release is continuous. The similar parallel shift to the right of the concentration-response curves to acetylcholine, serotonin, and histamine (Flavahan et al., 1985) would favor the latter interpretation and so would the preliminary bioassay studies (Fig. 9). By contrast, the fact that, at least at higher stimulation frequencies, the peak response to cholinergic activation is not reduced (Fig. 10) may suggest that nerve-released acetylcholine has to reach the epithelial cells first, before they release the inhibitory factor(s). Alternatively, the inhibitory factor(s) may dissociate between two distinct components in the neurogenic response (e.g., the release of a second neurotransmitter; see chapter by Burnstock in this volume).

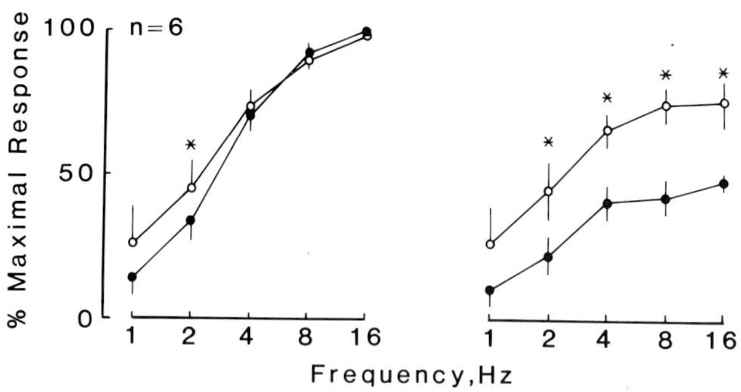

Figure 10 Effect of the removal of the epithelium on the peak (left) and the decayed response (right) to electrical stimulation (at increasing frequencies) of canine bronchi. Solid symbols denote rings with, and open symbols those without epithelium (from Flavahan et al., *Journal of Applied Physiology*, 1985).

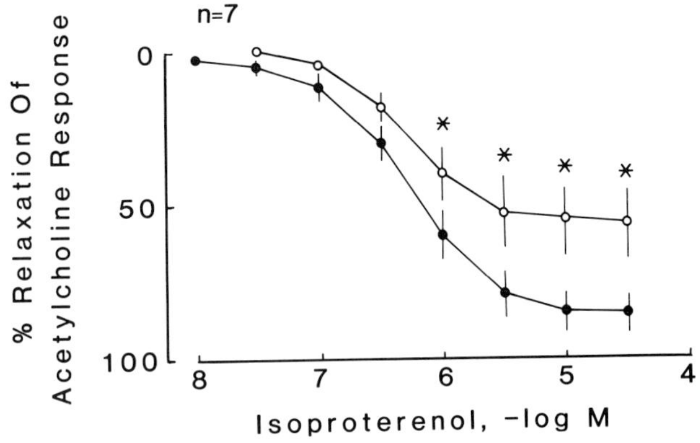

Figure 11 Reduction in rings without epithelium (open symbols) compared to intact rings (solid symbols) of canine bronchi of the relaxation induced by increasing concentrations of isoproterenol (from Flavahan et al., *Journal of Applied Physiology,* 1985).

The removal of the epithelium not only augments the contraction evoked by a variety of bronchoconstrictor agonists, but also reduces the relaxations evoked by isoproterenol (Fig. 11) (Flavahan et al., 1985). This increased responsiveness to isoproterenol in intact compared with epithelium-denuded preparations could be due in part to activation of epithelial beta-adrenoceptors. The respiratory epithelium has a high density of beta-adrenoceptors compared with bronchial smooth muscle (Xue et al., 1983; Carstairs et al., 1984, 1985). A facilitatory role of the epithelial cells on beta-adrenergic inhibition of bronchial smooth muscle, whether or not it involves activated release of epithelium-derived relaxing factor(s), would be of particular relevance for the aerosol administration of beta-adrenergic agonists.

Hyperreactivity of the bronchial wall to a number of constrictor agents, as well as an impaired responsiveness to beta-adrenergic agonists, are common findings in patients with asthma and infection of the airways (Hogg and Eggleston, 1984; Barnes, 1983; Nadel, 1983). Epithelial dysfunction is associated with the pathogenesis of these conditions, suggesting that damage to the airway epithelium may play a predominant role in causing the hyperreactivity, because of a decreased ability of the respiratory epithelium to release epithelium-derived relaxing factor(s). This interpretation is strongly supported by the preliminary findings that the major basic protein of eosinophils, which is believed to play a major role in certain types of inflammation and hyperreactivity of the airways (Gleich and Loegering, (1984), augments the responsiveness of isolated airways only if the epithelial cells are present (Vanhoutte et al., 1986a).

Acknowledgments

The authors thank Mrs. Janet Beckman for secretarial assistance and Mr. Robert Lorenz and Mrs. Helen Hendrickson for preparing the illustrations.

Discussion

Laitinen. What is known of the pharmacology of epithelium-derived relaxant factors?

Vanhoutte. We have not yet optimized conditions for its bioassay.

Barnes. The effect of airway epithelial removal is relatively less than vascular endothelial removal but could have a large effect on airway resistance. Have any experiments been performed on airway function in vivo?

Vanhoutte. In canine airways the effect of epithelial removal is not small.

Barnes. The putative epithelial derived relaxant factor is clearly different from endothelial-derived relaxant factor since the latter is inhibited by nordihydroguaiaretic acid and mepacrine, but (in bovine airways) neither of these compounds (nor indomethacin) influences the effect of epithelial removal (Barnes et al., *Br. J. Pharmacol.* **86**:685-692, 1985.

Vanhoutte. We have reached the same conclusion.

Barnes. You demonstrated that the presynaptic beta-receptor on airway cholinergic nerves is of the beta$_1$ receptor subtype in dogs. In humans, clinical studies suggest that beta$_2$, rather than beta$_1$ antagonists cause bronchoconstriction in asthmatics.

Vanhoutte. Human bronchial smooth muscle may contain more beta$_2$ receptors than that in the dog.

Widdicombe. It would be interesting to know if norepinephrine had a presynaptic inhibitory effect on cholinergic nerves to submucosal glands, where both beta-agonists and methacholine are excitatory.

Nadel. Murlas et al. (*J. Auton. Nerv. Syst.* **2**:23-37, 1980) showed that near airway glands adrenergic vesicles were often in close approximation to cholinergic vesicles, but that most vesicles are considerably different from gland cells.

References

Barnes, P. G. (1983). Pathogenesis of asthma: a review. *J. R. Soc. Med.* **76**:580-586.

Cabezas, G. A., Graf, P. D., and Nadel, J. A. (1971). Sympathetic versus parasympathetic nervous regulation of airways in dogs. *J. Appl. Physiol.* **31**: 651-655.

Carstairs, J. R., Nimmon, A. J., and Barnes, P. J. (1984). Autoradiographic localisation of β-adrenoceptors in human lung. *Eur. J. Pharmacol.* **103**: 189-190.

Carstairs, J. R., Nimmo, A. J., and Barnes, P. J. (1985). Autoradiographic visualization of beta-adrenoceptor subtypes in human lung. *Am. Rev. Respir. Dis.* **132**:541-547.

Flavahan, N. A., and Vanhoutte, P. M. (1985). The respiratory epithelium releases a smooth muscle relaxing factor. *Chest* **87** (suppl):189S-190S.

Flavahan, N. A., Aarhus, L. L., Rimele, T. J. A., and Vanhoutte, P. M. (1985). The respiratory epithelium inhibits bronchial smooth muscle tone. *J. Appl. Physiol.* **58**:834-838.

Furchgott, R. F. (1983). Role of the endothelium in responses of vascular smooth muscle. *Circ. Res.* **53**:557-573.

Gleich, G. J., and Loegering, D. A. (1984). Immunobiology of eosinophils. *Annu. Rev. Immunol.* **2**:429-459.

Hogg, J. C., and Eggleston, P. A. (1984). Is asthma an epithelial disease? *Am. Rev. Respir. Dis.* **129**:207-208.

Knight, D. S., Hyman, A. L., and Kadowitz, P. J. (1981). Innervation of intrapulmonary airway smooth muscle of the dog, monkey and baboon. *J. Autonomic Nervous System* **3**:31-43.

Lorenz, R. R., and Vanhoutte, P. M. (1985). Exocytotic release and pharmacological displacement of ^{3}H-norepinephrine in canine bronchi. *Fed. Proc.* **44**:734.

Lorenz, R. R., Danser, A. J., van den Ende, R., Flavahan, N. A., and Vanhoutte, P. M. (1986). Endogenous norepinephrine activates inhibitory prejunctional beta$_1$-adrenoceptors on cholinergic nerves in canine bronchi. XXX Congress of International Union of Physiological Sciences, Vancouver, Canada.

Nadel, J. A. (1983). Bronchial reactivity. *Adv. Intern. Med.* **28**:207-223.

O'Rourke, S. T., and Vanhoutte, P. M. (1986). M_2-muscarinic receptors mediate contraction of canine bronchi by acetylcholine. *Pharmacologist* **28**:157.

Russell, J. A. (1978). Responses of isolated canine airways to electric stimulation and acetylcholine. *J. Appl. Physiol.* **45**:690-698.

Russell, J. A. (1980). Noradrenergic inhibitory innervation of canine airways. *J. Appl. Physiol.* **48**:16-22.

Vanhoutte, P. M., and Cohen, R. A. (1983). The elusory role of serotonin in vascular function and disease. *Biochem. Pharmacol.* **32**:3671-3674.

Vanhoutte, P. M., and Houston, D. S. (1985). Platelets, endothelium and vasospasm. *Circulation* **72**:728-734.

Vanhoutte, P. M., and Levy, M. N. (1982). Prejunctional cholinergic modulation on adrenergic neurotransmission and the cardiovascular system. In *Excitation and Neural Control of the Heart.* Edited by M. N. Levy and M. Vassalle. Bethesda, MD, The American Physiological Society, pp. 243-255.

Vanhoutte, P. M., and Shepherd, J. T. (1973). Venous relaxation caused by acetylcholine acting on sympathetic nerves. *Circ. Res.* **32**:259-267.

Vanhoutte, P. M., Coen, E. P., De Ridder, W. J., and Verbeuren, T. J. (1979). Evoked release of endogenous norepinephrine in the canine saphenous vein. Inhibition by acetylcholine. *Circ. Res.* **45**:608-614.

Vanhoutte, P. M., Verbeuren, T. J., and Webb, R. C. (1981). Local modulation of the adrenergic neuroeffector interaction in the blood vessel wall. *Physiol. Rev.* **61**:151-247.

Vanhoutte, P. M., Flavahan, N., Slifman, N. R., and Gleich, G. J. (1986a). Eosinophil granule major basic protein causes hyperreactivity of respiratory muscle in the presence but not in the absence of epithelial cells. Proceedings, IUPS, p. 488.

Vanhoutte, P. M., Rubanyi, G. M., Miller, V. M., and Houston, D. S. (1986b). Modulation of vascular smooth muscle contraction by the endothelium. *Annu. Rev. Physiol.* **48**:307-320.

Vermeire, P. A., and Vanhoutte, P. M. (1979). Inhibitory effects of catecholamines in isolated canine bronchial smooth muscle. *J. Appl. Physiol.* **46**: 787-791.

Westfall, T. C. (1977). Local regulation of adrenergic neurotransmission. *Physiol. Rev.* **57**:659-728.

Xue, Q.-F., Maurer, R., and Engel, G. (1983). Selective distribution of beta- and alpha$_1$-adrenoceptors in rat lung visualized by autoradiography. *Arch. Int. Pharmacodyn. Ther.* **266**:308-314.

10

Airway Parasympathetic Ganglia

BENGT-ERIC SKOOGH
University of Göteborg
Göteburg, Sweden

I. General Concepts

There are still relatively few published studies on airway ganglia. However, ganglia in other organs have been studied quite extensively, mainly by neurophysiological techniques. Such studies have shown that ganglia are structures in which neural signals can be modulated. Both inhibition and facilitation of ganglionic transmission have been demonstrated, mediated by both endogenous and exogenous substances (for reviews see Haefely, 1980, and Volle, 1980). Information now appearing on airway ganglia indicates that these may also be targets for similar modulatory influences.

Classically, autonomic ganglia are classified into sympathetic, parasympathetic, and enteric ganglia (Langley, 1921). Parasympathetic and enteric ganglia are both situated in close proximity to the end organs and both release acetylcholine from their postganglionic nerve endings. Aside from these similarities, there are sufficient dissimilarities between parasympathetic ganglia and enteric ganglia to justify classification enteric ganglia as a third subdivision of the autonomic nervous system (Wood, 1983). Enteric ganglia serve in an integrated system that seems to be more complicated and more independent of the central nerve system than other cholinergic nerve systems (Wood, 1981). Thus, there are good reasons to assume that many of the findings obtained from enteric ganglia will not hold true for other cholinergic ganglia, such as the parasympathetic ganglia in the airways.

Airway parasympathetic ganglia are located in the airway wall mainly posteriorly in large airways (Larsell, 1922; Gooding Elftman, 1943; Fischer, 1964; Spencer and Leof, 1964). This relative inaccessability may explain why study of these neural elements has been largely neglected before. Little is presently known about their functions. However, in recent years description of a technique for vital staining (Grillo and Nadel, 1980) that does not affect ganglionic transmission (Skoogh et al., 1983) promoted identification of ganglion cells for neurophysiological recordings (Baker et al., 1982; Cameron and Coburn, 1981). These neurophysiological techniques were further developed for recordings from unstained ganglia in vitro (Baker et al., 1983a,b) and in vivo (Mitchell et al., 1983). An in vitro ganglion-tracheal smooth muscle preparation has been developed that will allow study of the interphase between electrical activity in ganglion cells and in smooth muscle cells (Cameron and Coburn, 1984). In vitro tracheal nerve-muscle preparations have been developed that will allow study of the end organ (smooth muscle) response to both pre- and postganglionic nerve activation (Skoogh et al., 1982; Blackman and McCaig, 1983; Skoogh et al., 1986), giving an indirect assessment of ganglionic transmission. Thus, we are at present rapidly gaining more information about the physiology of airway ganglia.

II. Morphology

Preganglionic parasympathetic axons, whose cell bodies are in medulla oblongata, pass down the vagus and synapse on ganglion cells located in the airway wall. The postganglionic axons innervate the smooth muscle, submucosal glands, and blood vessels of the airways (Richardson, 1979). In humans, ganglion cells are scattered along the peribronchial nerve plexus down to the level of smaller bronchi, although they are most abundant in large airways (Larsell, 1922; Larsell and Dow, 1933).

Most studies on the morphology of airway ganglia have been performed on the trachea in rat, guinea pig, monkey, ferret, and human tracheas, ganglia have been observed in chains extended along the length of the trachea near the lateral borders of the posterior membrane (Fischer, 1964; Coburn, 1984a). In a detailed study on ferret trachea, Baker et al. (1986) extended these observations and identified abundant ganglia, containing one to four ganglion cell bodies, located in the superficial muscle and gland nerve plexus. A few ganglia, containing 10-30 cell bodies, were located dorsally along a longitudinal nerve trunk.

The sympathetic ganglion cells sending postganglionic fibers to the lung are located outside the lung in the stellate and middle cervical ganglia (De Burg Daly and Mount, 1951; Richardson, 1979). However, I have observed small, propranolol-sensitive relaxant responses on administration of the ganglion-stimulating drug 1,1-Dimethyl-4-phenylpiperazinum iodide (DMPP) (Chen et al., 1951) to ferret tracheal rings pretreated with atropine and contracted by serotonin (Skoogh, unpublished observations). This indicates that ferret trachea contains at least a few sympathetic ganglion cells and it raises the concept of short adrenergic neurons for the airways as have been described for the genitourinary tract (Owman et al., 1983).

Morphologic evidence for adrenergic innervation of airway cholinergic has been obtained in some species (Mann, 1971; Richardson and Fergusson, 1976, 1979), indicating a possible interaction between the sympathetic and the parasympathetic nervous system in airway ganglia. However, these few observations are not enough for a firm conclusion. More documentation is certainly needed in this area.

Tracheal ganglia are connected to a dense nerve plexus, and individual ganglion cells show extensive arborization (Baker et al., 1986; Coburn, 1984b) indicating an integrative capacity of this system. At least two different cells types (Baker et al., 1986) and at least two different types of nerve terminals (Coburn, 1984b) have been identified within these ganglia. There is also morphologic evidence of transmitter heterogeneity in airway ganglia, vasoactive intestinal peptide has been found in some airway ganglion cells (Uddman et al., 1978). Thus, morphologic data gathered hitherto indicate that airway ganglia may be capable of complex modulation and integration of neural inputs.

III. Electrical Properties

In autonomic ganglia, stimulation of preganglionic nerves may elicit a sequence of postsynaptic responses in the ganglion neurons. Our knowledge about these events mainly derives from studies on sympathetic ganglia (for reviews see Haefely, 1972; Nishi, 1974; Dun, 1980; Skok, 1980). However, the basic transmission phenomena seem to be basically the same in sympathetic and parasympathetic ganglia. Thus, intracellular potential recordings have shown fast excitatory, (f-EPSP), slow inhibitory (s-IPSP), and slow excitatory (s-EPSP) postsynaptic potentials (Fig. 1). A late s-EPSP has also been described. When the amplitude of the f-EPSP reaches a threshold level, a spike occurs that transmits the signal into the postganglionic fibers. The f-EPSP response is mediated by nicotinic-cholinergic receptors in all ganglia. The only known exception is avian ciliary ganglia, in which both electrical and chemical transmission may occur (Martin and Pilar, 1963).

The mechanisms for the s-IPSP and s-EPSP are more complex. These potentials reflect at least two types of electrically overlapping phenomenas (Haefely,

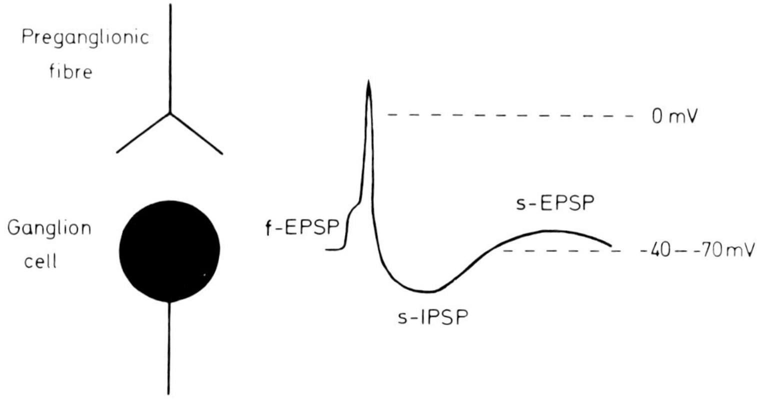

Figure 1 Schematic representation of an intracellular potential recording from a ganglion cell, reflecting the postsynaptic response to a preganglionic stimulus.

1972; Libet, 1979). First, the firing of a spike in the cell is followed by a pure after-potential, which is a direct sequela of the firing and not due to synaptic processes. Second, to this electrogenic after-potential are added receptor-operated slow postsynaptic responses (Eccles and Libet, 1961; Libet, 1979). These latter responses are best observed when the f-EPSP is blocked by a nicotinic blocker, and the ganglion cell then is excited by repetitive preganglionic stimulation (Libet, 1979; Gallagher et al., 1980). The transmitters vary between different ganglia and for several ganglia they are not yet clarified or still controversial. The controversy includes the concept, for some ganglia, of a disynaptic (via an interneuron) mechanism for the s-IPSP (Libet, 1980; Gallagher et al., 1980; Dun, 1980; Wood, 1983). The functional significance of the slow postsynaptic potentials is not yet fully clarified although it seems to be a neuromodulatory action that shifts the level of the ganglion cell excitability (for reviews of slow postsynaptic potentials see Libet, 1979; Skok, 1980, 1983; Dun, 1980; Wood, 1983).

Slow potentials have also been demonstrated in some parasympathetic ganglia in vesical parasympathetic ganglia both s-IPSP and s-EPSP have been recorded after nicotinic receptor blockade and repetitive preganglionic stimulation. These slow potentials were mimicked by iontophoretic application of acetylcholine and blocked by atropine, indicating mediation through muscarinic receptors (Griffith et al., 1981, Gallagher et al., 1982). These studies also demonstrated the significance of slow synaptic potentials for ganglion cell excitability. In spontaneously active cells the frequency of spontaneous spike discharge increased during the s-EPSP and decreased during s-IPSP (Griffith et al., 1981; Gallagher et al., 1982).

Intracellular recordings from airway parasympathetic ganglia in ferrets have shown slow after-potentials suggestive of s-IPSP and s-EPSP (Baker et al., 1982, 1983a,b; Cameron and Coburn, 1981, 1984). However, the synaptic nature of this potential has not yet been firmly established and the transmitter has not been identified. In some ferret airway ganglion cells a calcium- and magnesium-dependent after-hyperpolarization has been observed, which is consistent with this potential being a receptor-mediated s-IPSP (Cameron and Coburn, 1982). Spontaneous discharge has not been demonstrated for airway ganglion cells, as has been observed for enteric ganglia (Wood and Mayer, 1978) and vesical parasympathetic ganglia (De Groat and Booth, 1980; Griffith et al., 1980, 1981; De Groat et al., 1979).

Measurements of electrical constants of the cell membrane in ferret airway ganglia (Baker et al., 1983a,b; Cameron and Coburn, 1984) have provided values of the resting membrane potential, the input resistance, and the time constant similar to earlier published values from mammalian sympathetic ganglia (Nishi, 1974).

IV. Neural Integrative and Modulative Functions of Airway Ganglia

A. The Local Network

There are three types of pathways in autonomic ganglia centrifugal, intrinsic and peripheral reflex. Centrifugal pathways exist in all autonomic ganglia; they are comprised of preganglionic fibers and the neuron that receive preganglionic innervation (Skok, 1983). Intrinsic pathways have not been demonstrated for airway ganglia. Peripheral reflex pathways consist of afferent fibers of peripheral origin and the ganglion cell receiving this afferent innervation. A recent study of neural coordination in ferret trachealis muscle has provided some evidence for the existence of such a pathway in airway nerve plexus (Coburn, 1984b). Electrical stimulation over smooth muscle cells evoked electrical responses of synaptic nature in ganglion cells as far as 20 mm from the stimulation site, indicating a possible afferent pathway for the muscle to the ganglion cell. However, the responses could as well have been evoked by antidromic stimulation of postganglionic nerve fibers also sending collaterals to other ganglion cells. In any case this study showed a wide dissemination within the trachealis nerve plexus of local neural inputs, indicating an integrative capacity of this network. Furthermore, ganglion cell heterogeneity has been demonstrated on the basis of whether or not an action potential could be evoked (Coburn, 1984b), and on the basis of firing pattern: those having inspiratory and those having expiratory rhythms (Mitchell et al., 1983). Thus, neurophysiological studies have demonstrated some conditions for an integrative and modulative function of airway ganglia, although we still know virtually nothing about how this system works.

B. Do Airway Ganglia Act as a Low-Pass Filter?

One of the first neurophysiological observations in the early 1930s was the one-to-one relationship between the preganglionic stimulus and the postganglionic firing, as long as the preganglionic stimulus was supramaximal and at low frequencies. This principle held true both when the recordings were obtained from postganglionic nerves (Bishop and Heinbecker, 1932; Eccles, 1935) and from single or few fibers (Bronk and Pumphrey, 1934; Bronk et al., 1938; Bronk, 1939; Larrabee and Bronk, 1947). Later studies have identified occasional ganglion cells firing multiple spikes after single preganglionic volleys (i.e., Blackman and Purves, 1969). Another early basic observation was that in most ganglia the postganglionic response gradually ceased to follow one-to-one the preganglionic stimulation, when the stimulation frequency was increased above approximately 20 Hz (Bishop and Heinbecker, 1932; Bronk and Pumphrey, 1934; Bronk, 1939). At sustained preganglionic stimulation with stimulation frequencies above 10-20 Hz, the preganglionic transmission also showed a temporal run-down with ganglion cells progressively dropping out of action (Bronk, 1939; Larrabee and Bronk, 1938, 1947; for a review of the older literature and further references see Hillarp, 1959).

Most of the early neurophysiological studies on ganglionic transmission were performed on sympathetic, superior cervical, or stellate ganglia in cat. Extension of these studies to a larger variety of ganglia has provided a more complicated picture than that related above. Still, most ganglion cells start failing to fire when the frequency of preganglionic stimulation is higher than about 15 Hz, and they also show a run-down of the response at sustained preganglionic stimulation (Skok, 1980). However, this pattern varies widely from ganglion to ganglion. Enteric ganglia in guinea pigs may show run-down of the postsynaptic response (f-EPSP) at preganglionic stimulation frequencies as low as 0.1 Hz (Nishi and North, 1973). In frog cardiac ganglion the ganglionic transmission eventually failed when the frequency of preganglionic stimulation was increased to 10-20 Hz (Dennis et al., 1971). In guinea pig thoracic sympathetic ganglia, ganglion cells have been identified responsing to preganglionic stimulation at 30-80 Hz, when many presynaptic fibers were stimulated simultaneously (Blackman and Purves, 1969). In vesical parasympathetic ganglia, transmission fails when the preganglionic activity is below 0.5 Hz and does not fail when the preganglionic stimulation frequency is sustained between 1 and 20 Hz (Booth and DeGroat, 1979). Thus vesical ganglia behave as a high-pass filter that contributes to a switching behavior of the parasympathetic reflex pathway to the urinary bladder (DeGroat and Booth, 1980). Intracellular recordings in vivo from cat airway ganglia have shown that the transmission of preganglionic impulses declines at frequency above 10 Hz in some cells, whereas other cells safely respond to preganglionic impulses above 40-60 Hz (Mitchell, personal communication, 1986).

The filtering in ganglia of high-frequency impulses seems, in most cases to be of little physiological significance since the control of the autonomic effector is exerted at low preganglionic discharge rates, usually not above 10-15 Hz (Bronk et al., 1936; Pitts et al., 1941; Pitts and Bronk, 1942; Folkow, 1952; DeGroat and Ryall, 1969; Manard and Polosa, 1973; DeGroat and Booth, 1980), although impulse frequencies up to 50 Hz has been recorded in preganglionic sympathetic fibers in cat during strong hypothalmic stimulation (Pitts et al., 1941; Pitts and Bronk, 1942), and occasionally in vesical parasympathetic preganglionic neurons during reflex stimulation (DeGroat and Ryall, 1969). However, the low-pass filtering in ganglia is probably of physiological significance in enteric ganglia, which may attenuate preganglionic impulses above 0.1 Hz (Nishi and North, 1973).

The situation might also be different for airway ganglia. Recordings from individual efferent preganglionic fibers in the recurrent laryngeal nerve (possibly also sending fibers to the trachea) and the phrenic nerve have shown two peaks of nerve activity at 87 and 55 Hz. The activity in both the laryngeal and phrenic nerves showed respiratory rhythms (Richardson and Mitchell, 1982). Similar recordings have also been made from pulmonary branches of the vagus, demonstrating respiratory rhythms of the firing also in these fibers (Mitchell et al., 1985). The frequency of the nerve impulses was not reported in this study. It is not known which structures in the lung those fibers supply. If fibers transmitting high-frequency oscillation supply airway ganglia, the ganglionic low-pass filtering effect discussed may be of utmost importance.

In an in vitro nerve-muscle preparation of ferret trachea described elsewhere (Skoogh et al., 1982; Skoogh and Svedmyr, 1986) we have studied the contractile response to pre- and postganglionic stimulation at various frequencies and durations. In this preparation muscle contractions can be induced by preganglionic activation with electrical nerve stimulation or by activation of postganglionic fibers with electrical field stimulation. For nerve stimulation we use the right vagus nerve or simultaneous stimulation of the right vagus and the right superior laryngeal nerve. Induced isometric muscle contractions are recorded by force transducers and are assessed as the developed active tension (peak tension minus resting tension) averaged from three segments of the trachea. Ganglionic blockade by hexamethonium inhibits the response to nerve stimulation, but not the response to field stimulation, whereas blockade at the neuromuscular junction by atropine reduces the response to nerve and field stimulation to the same extent (Skoogh, 1986). Thus, modulation of ganglionic transmission can be assessed by comparing muscle contractions induced by preganglionic activation to muscle contractions induced by postganglionic activation.

In a series of experiments we studied the contractile responses to supramaximal, short-lasting (20 sec every 2 min) stimulations at various frequencies. Up to a stimulation frequency of 24 Hz, the contractile response increased with increasing stimulation frequency both for pre- and postganglionic activation. At higher frequencies the response to postganglionic activation increased further. In contrast, the response to nerve stimulation decreased above 24 Hz, reflecting a filtering in airway ganglia at these impulse frequencies (Fig. 2). Shorter stimulation periods (10 sec) gave smaller contractions, but the shape of the frequency-response curve was the same as in Figure 2. The parallel shift of the two curves in Figure 2 probably reflects that field stimulation activates all postganglionic fibers, whereas nerve stimulation only activates the neurons supplied by the right vagus and superior laryngeal nerves.

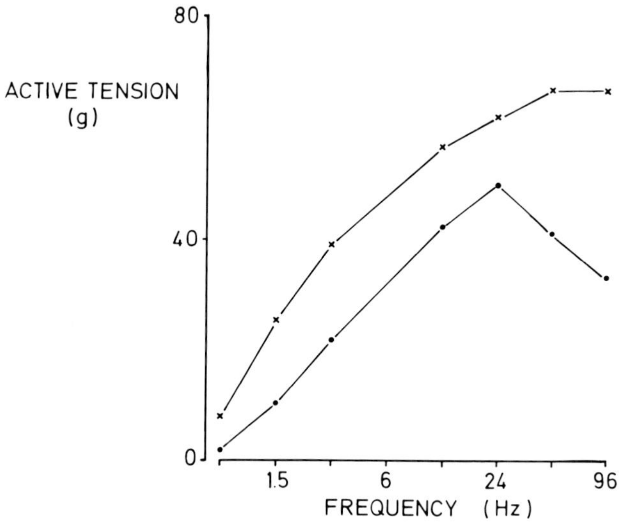

Figure 2 The in vitro contractile response in ferret trachea to preganglionic activation by nerve stimulation (●) and postganglionic activation by field stimulation (X) at various frequencies. Supramaximal currents were used. The duration of each stimulation was 20 sec at the frequencies indicated in figure. The right vagus nerve and the right superior laryngeal nerve were stimulated simultaneously. Neural release of norepinephrine was blocked by 3 μM guanethidine. Data from one experiment shown.

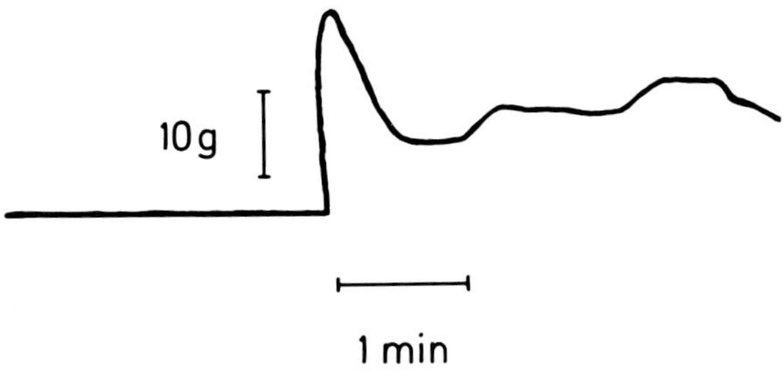

Figure 3 Isometric tracheal smooth muscle contraction introduced by sustained preganglionic activation with nerve stimulation at 48 Hz. The initial rising phase is followed by a run-down of the response with irregular contractions. Recording from one of three 10 mm long segments in an in vitro nerve-muscle preparation of ferret trachea.

Sustained preganglionic activation by nerve stimulation for 3 min gave a stable sustained muscle contraction as long as the stimulation frequency was 6 Hz or below. At 12 and 24 Hz the induced muscle contraction first reached a peak value within 1-2 min and then gradually declined. This run-down was fairly reproducible from time to time. Sustained nerve stimulation at 48 and 96 Hz gave contractions where only the initial (20-30 sec) rising phase was reproducible. The run-down seen after the initial rising phase varied largely both within the same stimulation period (Fig. 3) and when the stimulations were repeated. In contrast, the response to sustained postganglionic activation by field stimulation showed only a slight (about 10%) and reproducible tendency to fatigue at 48 Hz and 96 Hz.

Thus, airway ganglia seem to filter nerve impulses of high frequency. The filtering is more pronounced during sustained stimulation, although more variable, than during the initial 20-30 sec of a stimulation period. Further, this filtering capacity can be modulated by beta-2 agonists (see next section). However, to assess the possible functional and therapeutic significance of this we need more information about the physiological frequency range of the nerve impulses traveling in the efferent preganglionic fibers to the airways and which structures the various pathways supply.

Finally, it should be pointed out that the comparison of the contractile response to pre- and postganglionic stimulation gives an indirect assessment of the overall transmission through airway ganglia. The attenuation, at high stimulation frequencies, of the response to preganglionic activation has most likely a complex basis. Thus, the data in Figure 2 reflect a summation of transmission through frequency-dependent and non-frequency-dependent pathways. Further, the transmission through airway ganglia may be influenced by variations in ganglion cell excitability mediated via slow postsynaptic potentials. The magnitude of these potentials are dependent on the frequency of the preganglionic stimulation (Libet, 1979; Gallagher et al., 1980). Finally, the amount of acetylcholine released per nerve impulse is also frequency-dependent (Nishi et al., 1967; Dennis et al., 1971; Skok, 1980).

V. Effect of General Anesthetics on Ganglionic Transmission

Most general anesthetics depress transmission in sympathetic ganglia (Larrabee and Posternak, 1952; Nistri and Qulliam, 1980). This also holds true for barbiturates, which have been shown to depress synaptic transmission in sympathetic ganglia at 10-fold lower concentrations than those needed to block axonal conduction (Larrabee and Posternak, 1952). The effect of barbiturates is caused by depression of the postsynaptic membrane in the ganglion neuron (Brown and Quilliam, 1964; Exley, 1954), and inhibition of presynaptic acetylcholine release is seen first at considerable higher concentrations (Exley, 1954). In addition, detailed studies of the depressive mechanism of barbiturates in sympathetic ganglia have shown that the effect is strikingly specific for nicotinic receptors in the postsynaptic ganglion membrane (Nicoll, 1978a) and is probably exerted by an action on the sodium-conductance mechanism or the step connecting this mechanism to the nicotinic receptor (Nicoll, 1978b).

Barbiturates have also been shown to depress transmission through parasympathetic ganglia in the airways by an action on the postsynaptic membrane (Skoogh et al., 1982). This has wide implications for all experimental studies that include use of general anesthetics. In studies on anesthetized animals, airway reflexes may be depressed by the anesthetic acting both centrally in the brain and peripherally in airway ganglia (Holtzman et al., 1982).

VI. Effect of Exogenous Catecholamines on Ganglionic Transmission

It has long been known that catecholamines may modulate ganglionic transmission (Marrazzi, 1939). Both depression and, less consistently, facilitation have been reported; these effects appear to be mediated by alpha- and beta-adrenoceptors, respectively (for reviews see DeGroat and Volle, 1966; Haefely, 1969; Volle, 1980; Brown and Caulfield, 1981).

The alpha-mediated depression of transmission is more frequently and consistently observed and has been demonstrated for sympathetic ganglia (Marrazzi, 1939; Matthews, 1956; McIsaac, 1966; DeGroat and Volle, 1966; Medgett, 1983), vesical parasympathetic ganglia (DeGroat and Saum, 1972; DeGroat, 1975; DeGroat and Booth, 1980) and enteric ganglia (Nishi and North, 1973; Wood and Mayer, 1979). At least in sympathetic ganglia, two different alpha-mediated effects have been reported: postsynaptic hyperpolarization (DeGroat and Volle, 1966; Haefely, 1969; Cole and Shinnick-Gallagher, 1981) and inhibition of transmittor release (Christ and Nishi, 1969, 1971a,b; Nishi, 1970; Capuzzo et al., 1983). However, the weighted evidence clearly indicates that depression of ganglionic transmission is mediated through the presynaptic alpha-receptors (Haefely, 1969; Volle, 1980; Brown and Caulfield, 1981). The effect has a rapid onset (Haefely, 1969; Medgett, 1983) and is most pronounced at low stimulation frequencies (Matthews, 1956; McIsaac, 1966). The ionic mechanism appears to be inhibition of inward calcium currents both for the pre- and postsynaptic effect (for references see Brown and Caulfield, 1981).

The studies on the effect of beta-adrenoceptor stimulation on ganglionic transmission have shown conflicting results. Both inhibition (Suzuki and Volle, 1978; Quenzer et al., 1979) and facilitation (Matthews, 1956; DeGroat and Folle, 1966; Haefely, 1969; Madgett, 1983) have been observed on administration of isoproterenol, although facilitation seems to be the most readily observed effect. The discrepancies may be explained by differences in both techniques and species. In rat superior cervical ganglia beta-adreneroceptor stimulation depresses ganglionic transmission in normal Krebs solution, whereas facilitation is observed in a low Ca/high Mg solution (Brown and Dunn, 1983) or when the transmission is depressed by a concomitant alpha inhibition (Madgett, 1983). In cat, superior cervical ganglion facilitation was only seen of submaximal preganglionic stimulation (Matthews, 1956). The facilitation is most pronounced at high stimulation frequencies (Matthews, 1956; Haefly, 1969), and has a slower onset and a longer duration than the alpha-mediated inhibition (Matthews, 1956; Haefely, 1969; Medgett, 1983). The beta-adrenoceptor mediating this effect has been classified into the beta-2 subtype (Haefley, 1969; Brown and Dunn, 1983). The facilitation has been attributed to a postsynaptic depolarization (DeGroat and Volle, 1966; Haefely, 1969) or augmented transmitter release (Brown and Dunn, 1983). Brown and Dunn (1983) found that beta-adrenoceptor stimulation caused a depolarization both pre- and postsynaptically, but concluded that neither of these effects explained the facilitation.

A. Beta-2 Adrenoceptor Stimulation Inhibits Ganglionic Transmission in Airway Parasympathetic Ganglia

We have used the nerve-muscle preparation described above to study the effect of exogenous catecholamines on ganglionic transmission in airway ganglia. In a series of experiments, only one stimulation frequency was used. Thus, every 2 min short-lasting isometric muscle contractions were induced alternating by

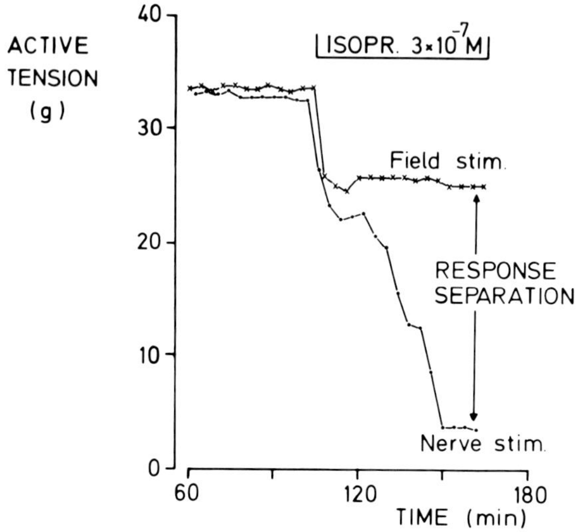

Figure 4 Effect of 0.3 μM isoproterenol on the responses to nerve stimulation (12 Hz for 20 sec) (●) and the response to field stimulation (12 Hz for 20 sec) (X). The response separation seen after 20–30 min exposure indicates inhibition of ganglionic transmission. Data are from one experiment.

activation of preganglionic nerve fibers with electrical stimulation of the vagus nerve (12 Hz for 20 sec) or activation of postganglionic fibers with field stimulation (12 Hz for 20 sec). During the control period before drug application, the two contractions were matched by reducing the current for field stimulation.

A beta-adrenoceptor agonist (isoproterenol) applied to the nerve muscle preparation initially (within 4-6 min) reduced the responses to pre- and postganglionic activation to the same extent, indicating an effect on postganglionic structures (i.e., smooth muscle). After 20-30 min exposure the response to preganglionic activation was further reduced, indicating an additional effect on ganglionic transmission (Fig. 4). This additional inhibition of preganglionic activation by isoproterenol showed a concentration/response relationship in the range 0.1-1 μM (Skoogh and Svedmyr, 1986). In further experiments preincubation with a beta-2 adrenoceptor antagonist (ICI 118.551 0.1 μM) shifted this concentration/response curve about 10 times to the right.

Preincubation with a beta-1 adrenoceptor antagonist (Practolol 10 μM) had only a slight effect on the concentration/response curve (Skoogh and Svedmyr, 1986). In two experiments preincubation with an alpha-adrenoceptor antagonist (phenoxybenzamine 0.1 μM for 20 min) did not inhibit the effect of isproterenol on ganglionic transmission (unpublished observations).

Electrical stimulation of the vagus nerve activates ganglia by presynaptic transmitter release, while the ganglion-stimulating drug DMPP (Chen et al., 1951) activates the postsynaptic cell membrane directly. Using a separate in vitro tracheal ring preparation we studied the effect of isoproterenol on the response to stimulation of the ganglion cell by DMPP and the response to activation of the postganglionic fibers by field stimulation. Sixty min exposure to isoproterenol reduced the response to DMPP to the same extent as the response to field stimulation, which means that they both reflect the smooth muscle effect of isoproterenol (Skoogh et al., 1986). Isoproterenol did not have a further effect on the ganglion cell membrane. This means that the earlier demonstrated inhibition of ganglion transmission must be an effect on the presynaptic level in ganglia with inhibition of transmitter release.

The beta-adrenoceptor-mediated inhibition of ganglionic transmission in ferret airway ganglia observed differs from the earlier inhibition by isoproterenol in rat sympathetic ganglia (Suzuki and Volle, 1978; Quenzer et al., 1979) in at least two aspects. The effect in airway ganglia was exerted at lower isoproterenol concentrations, 0.1-1 μM compared to 10-100 μM. The effect in airway ganglia is clearly presynaptic compared to probably postsynaptic in rat sympathetic ganglia. Further, the effect of isoproterenol in airway ganglia is clearly attributed to beta-2 adrenoceptors, whereas the adrenoceptor classification in rat sympathetic ganglia is ambiguous (Quenzer et al., 1979).

The delayed onset (20-30 min) of the beta-2-mediated inhibition in airway ganglia is another feature that differs from earlier observed ganglionic beta-adrenoceptor effects. However, a delayed onset of catecholamine effects is not unique. In bullfrog sympathetic ganglion cells, epinephrine has been observed to facilitate potassium-induced hyperpolarization of the cell membrane. This effect was not visible until after 5 min and was then gradually intensified, when the application was sustained for up to 60 min. Evidence was given for the effect being an alpha-mediated acceleration of the electrogenic sodium-pump. It was independent of calcium (Akasu and Koketsu, 1978a,b).

Beta-2-adrenoceptor stimulation has been shown to induce a membrane hyperpolarization in rat soleus muscle both in vitro and in vivo via stimulation of the sodium pump (Clausen and Flatman, 1977, 1980; Clausen, 1983). In vivo this effect seems to develop slowly during 30 min (Clausen and Flatman, 1980). Beta-adrenoceptor stimulation by terbutaline is guinea pig soleus muscle has a biphasic effect with an initial rapid depression of induced twitches, followed by a subsequent increase above control levels of the twitches after 20 min exposure. This slower effect was attributed to changes in the intracellular ionic balance due to a beta-2-mediated stimulation of the electrogenic sodium pump (Holmberg and Waldeck, 1980).

We have no data on the possible ionic mechanism for the beta-adrenoceptor-mediated inhibition of ganglionic transmission in ferret airway ganglia. The time course of the effect might indicate a mechanism separate from other ganglionic effects by catecholamines, which probably are exerted via inhibition of inward calcium currents (Brown and Caulfield, 1981).

B. Frequency Dependence of Beta-2-Mediated Ganglionic Inhibition

The earlier studies on the effect of beta-adrenoceptor stimulation on ganglionic transmission were all done using a fixed-stimulation frequency (12 Hz). In another series of experiments we studied the contractile response to field and nerve stimulation at various frequencies, before and after exposure to a beta-2 agonist (Skoogh et al., 1986). Figure 5 (right panel) demonstrates the effect of a low concentration of beta-2 agonist (terbutaline 1 μM) at various stimulation frequencies. At 12 Hz and below, the response to nerve and field stimulation is reduced to about the same extent, indicating an effect only on the smooth muscle. However, at higher stimulation frequencies terbutaline markedly increased the response separation between field and nerve stimulation compared to the left panel

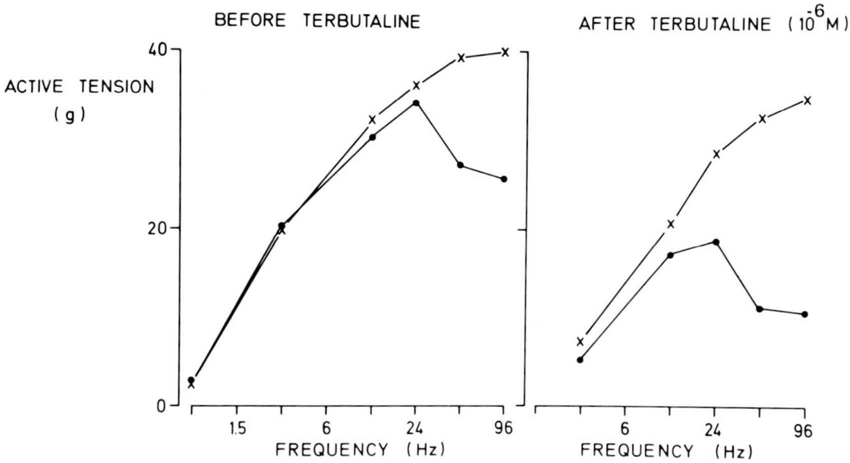

Figure 5 Effect of 1 μM terbutaline on the responses to nerve stimulation (●) and field stimulation (X) at various frequencies. Terbutaline markedly increased (right panel) the response separation (i.e., inhibition of ganglionic transmission) normally seen (left panel) at stimulation frequencies above 24 Hz. The duration of each stimulation was 20 sec with frequencies as indicated in the figure. Before these recordings were obtained, contractions induced by nerve stimulation and by field stimulation were matched for frequencies below 24 Hz by reducing the current for field stimulation.

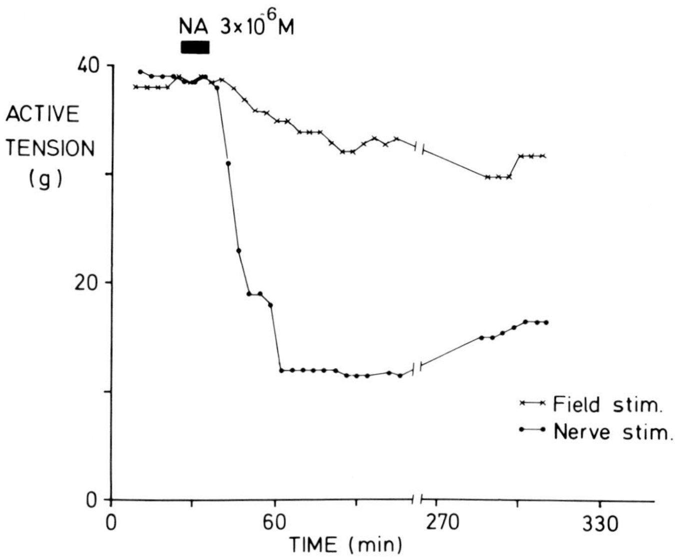

Figure 6 Effect of 3 μM norepinephrine for 10 min on the responses to nerve stimulation (●) and field stimulation (X). Within a few minutes the response to nerve stimulation decreased markedly, whereas the response to field stimulation changed little. This response separation indicates inhibition of ganglionic transmission.

in Figure 5. Thus, beta-2 adrenoceptor stimulation seems to inhibit ganglionic transmission mainly at high frequencies.

C. Alpha-Adrenoceptor Stimulation Inhibits Ganglionic Transmission

Alpha-adrenoceptor stimulation has, by neurophysiological techniques, been shown also to inhibit ganglionic transmission in airway parasympathetic ganglia (Baker et al., 1983a,b). We have reported preliminary data confirming this finding One such experiment is exemplified in Figure 6 (Skoogh, 1986). Further experimentation has shown this effect to be inconsistent. In about half of the experiments 0.3 μM norepinephrine induced a profound inhibition of ganglionic transmission, with a rapid onset of the effect. In the rest of the experiments no such effect could be seen. Propranolol (0.3 μM) does not block the effect, and the effect has not been observed after pretreatment with 0.1 μM phenoxybenzamine for 10 min. However, the inconsistency of the effect does not allow any conclusion to be made from this latter observation. We have not yet found any definite explanation for the variability of inhibition of ganglionic transmission by norepinephrine in this in vitro preparation.

VII. Effect of Neurally Released Catecholamines on Ganglionic Transmission

There is only meager evidence of a physiological role for adrenergic nerves in ganglionic transmission. Some morphologic evidence for such an interaction in airway ganglia has been obtained. At present there are no experimental data on airway ganglia to support this.

In vesical parasympathetic ganglia electrical stimulation of sympathetic fibers in the hypogastric nerve produced both inhibition and facilitation of transmission (DeGroat and Saum, 1971, 1972; DeGroat, 1975). Also reflex-elicited firing in the hypogastric nerves has been shown to induce inhibition of ganglionic transmission in vesical ganglia (DeGroat and Lalley, 1972). It was not possible to demonstrate this effect by stimulation of the hypergastric nerve in vitro (DeGroat et al., 1979).

We have recently improved our nerve-muscle preparation of ferret trachea to include an intact stellate ganglion. This makes it possible to study in vitro the interaction between a possible sympathetic and parasympathetic innervation of the trachea. We have not yet been able to demonstrate such an interaction. However, we have only tested the effect of sympathetic stimulation on the response to supramaximal cholinergic preganglionic stimulation at 3 Hz. Further experimentation must include submaximal cholinergic nerve stimulation at lower frequencies (DeGroat and Saum, 1972).

Acknowledgments

I thank Lena Bernsten for excellent technical assistance. This work has been supported by the Swedish National Association against Heart and Chest Diseases.

Discussion

Barnes. Why does the inhibitory effect of beta-agonists on ganglionic neurotransmission have such a slow onset when the action on airway smooth muscle is rapid?

Skoogh. This may indicate a mechanism other than the normally rapid effect seen with ganglionic inhibition, which is due to inhibition of inward calcium currents. Possibly beta-2 receptors stimulate an electrogenic sodium pump leading to hyperpolarization of the presynaptic terminal, which may have a slow onset.

Coburn. Is it possible that field stimulation and preganglionic stimulation activate different populations of smooth muscle muscarinic receptors as an explanation for the different sensitivities of the two types of response to beta-agonists?

Skoogh. This would not fit with the time course of the effect.

Widdicombe. We need to know patterns of natural discharge in pre- and postganglionic neurons, and to apply these experimental models rather than using artificially selected patterns.

Nadel. Is it possible to measure acetylcholine release?

Burnstock. The difficulty in measuring release of acetylcholine depends on the sensitivity of the assay system as well as the suitability of the tissue stimulated. We have recently used a sensitive chemiluminescent method to measure release of acetylcholine (of the order of 5 pmol) from blood vessel strips and gut following electrical stimulation, but the assay has not been used with airways.

Maklouf. It is possible that isolated muscle cells can be used for bioassay of acetylcholine since they are extremely sensitive with threshold concentrations in the range of 0.1-1 fM.

References

Akasu, T., and Koketsu, K. (1976a). Adrenaline and the electrogenic sodium pump in rana catesbeiana sympathetic ganglion cells. *Experientia (Basel)* **32**:57-59.

Akasu, T., and Koketsu, K. (1976b). The effect of adrenaline on the K^+-activated hyperpolarization of the sympathetic ganglion cell membrane in bullfrogs. *Jpn. J. Physiol.* **26**:289-301.

Baker, D. G., Herbert, D. A., and Mitchell, R. A. (1982). Cholinergic neurotransmission in airway ganglia inhibition by norepinephrine. *Physiologist* **25**: 225.

Baker, D. G., Basbaum, C. B., Herbert, D. A., and Mitchell, R. A. (1983a). Transmission in airway ganglia of ferrets: Inhibition by norepinephrine. *Neurosci. Letts.* **41**:139-143.

Baker, D. G., Mitchell, R. A., and Herbert, D. A. (1983b). Control of airway smooth muscle: Role of the sympathetic nervous system. In *Modelling and Control of Breathing.* Edited by B. J. Whipp and D. M. Wiberg. New York, Elsevier Science Pub. Co., p. 150.

Baker, D. G., McDonald, D. M., and Mitchell, R. A. (1986). The nervous system of the ferret trachea: Its architecture as revealed by acetylcholinesterase histochemistry. *J. Comp. Neur.* **246**:513-526.

Bishop, G. H., and Heinbecker, P. (1932). A functional analysis of the cervical sympathetic nerve supply to the eye. *Am. J. Physiol.* **100**:519-532.

Blackman, J. G., and McCaig, D. J. (1983). Studies on an isolated innervated preparation of guinea-pig trachea. *Br. J. Pharmacol.* **80**:703-710.

Blackman, J. G., and Purves, J. G. (1969). Intracellular recordings from ganglia of the thoracic sympathetic chain of the guinea pig. *J. Physiol.* (*London*) **203**:173-198.

Booth, A. M., and DeGroat, W. C. (1979). A study of facilitation in vesical parasympathetic ganglia of the cat using intracellular recording techniques. *Brain Res.* **169**:388-392.

Bronk, D. W. (1939). Synaptic mechanisms in sympathetic ganglia. *J. Neurophysiol.* **2**:380-401.

Bronk, D. W., and Pumphrey, R. J. (1934). Response of a sympathetic ganglion to high frequency stimulation. *Proc. Soc. Exp. Biol. Med.* **32**:1661-1663.

Bronk, D. W., Ferguson, L. K., Margaria, R., and Solandt, D. Y. (1936). The activity of the cardiac sympathetic centers. *Am. J. Physiol.* **117**:237-249.

Bronk, D. W., Tower, S. S., Solandt, D. Y., and Larrabee, M. G. (1938). The transmission of trains of impulses through a sympathetic ganglion and in its postganglionic nerves. *Am. J. Physiol.* **122**:1-15.

Brown, D. A., and Caulfield, M. P. (1981). Adrenoceptors in ganglia. In *Adrenoceptors and Catecholamine Action.* Part A. Edited by G. Kunos. New York, John Wiley and Sons Ltd., pp. 99-115.

Brown, D. A., and Dunn, P. M. (1983). Depolarization of rat isolated superior cervical ganglia mediated by β_2-adrenoceptors. *Br. J. Pharmacol.* **79**:429-439.

Brown, D. A., and Quilliam, J. P. (1964). Observations on the mode of action of some central depressant drugs on transmission through the cat superior cervical ganglion. *Br. J. Pharmacol.* **23**:257-272.

Cameron, A. R., and Coburn, R. F. (1981). Electrical properties of the cells of the ferret paratracheal ganglion. *Physiologist* **24**:84.

Cameron, A. R., and Coburn, R. F. (1982). Calcium dependence of the after-hyperpolarization of type-A cells of the ferret paratracheal ganglion. *Fed. Proc.* **41**:1356.

Cameron, A. R., and Coburn, R. F. (1984). Electrical and anatomic characteristics of cells of ferret paratracheal ganglion. *Am. J. Physiol.* **246**:C450-C458.

Capuzzo, A., Borasio, P. G., Fabbri, E., Ferretti, M. E., and Trevisani, A. (1983). Alpha-adrenoceptor-mediated inhibition of acetylcholine release in guinea-pig superior cervical ganglion. *Neurosci. Letts.* **43**:215-219.

Chen, G., Portman, R., and Wickel, A. (1951). Pharmacology of 1,1-dimethyl-4-phenylpiperazinium iodide, a ganglion stimulation agent. *J. Pharmacol. Exp. Ther.* **103**:330-336.

Christ, D. D., and Nishi, S. (1969). Presynaptic action of epinephrine on sympathetic ganglia. *Life Sci.* **8**:1235-1238.

Christ, D. D., and Nishi, S. (1971a). Site of adrenaline blockade in the superior cervical ganglion of the rabbit. *J. Physiol.* **213**:107-117.

Christ, D. D., and Nishi, S. (1971b). Effects of adrenaline on nerve terminals in the superior cervical ganglion of the rabbit. *Br. J. Pharmacol.* **41**:331-338.

Clausen, T. (1983). Adrenergic control of Na^{+}-K^{+}-homeostasis. *Acta Med. Scand. Suppl.* **672**:111-115.

Clausen, T., and Flatman, J. A. (1977). The effect of catecholamines on Na-K transport and membrane potential in rat soleus muscle. *J. Physiol.* **270**: 383-414.

Clausen, T., and Flatman, J. A. (1980). β_2-adrenoceptors mediate the stimulating effect of adrenaline on active electrogenic Na-K-transport in rat soleus muscle. *Br. J. Pharmacol.* **68**:749-755.

Coburn, R. F. (1984a). The anatomy of the ferret paratracheal parasympathetic nerve-ganglion plexus. *Exp. Lung Res.* **7**:1-9.

Coburn, R. F. (1984b). Neural coordination of excitation of ferret trachealis muscle. *Am. J. Physiol.* **246**:C459-C466.

Cole, A. E., and Shinnick-Gallagher, P. (1981). Comparison of the receptors mediating the catecholamine hyperpolarization and slow inhibitory postsynaptic potential in sympathetic ganglia. *J. Pharmacol. Exp. Ther.* **217**:440-444.

De Burgh Daly, M., and Mount, L. E. (1951). The origin and nature of bronchomotor fibres in the cervical sympathetic nerves of the cat. *J. Physiol.* **113**: 43-69.

De Groat, W. C. (1975). Nervous control of the urinary bladder of the cat. *Brain Res.* **87**:201-211.

De Groat, W. C., and Booth, A. M. (1980). Inhibition and facilitation in parasympathetic ganglia of the urinary bladder. *Fed. Proc.* **39**:2990-2996.

De Groat, W. C., and Lalley, P. M. (1972). Reflex firing in the lumbar sympathetic outflow to activation of vesical afferent fibres. *J. Physiol. (London)* **226**:289-309.

De Groat, W. C., and Ryall, R. W. (1969). Reflexes to parasympathetic neurons concerned with micturation in the cat. *J. Physiol. (London)* **200**:87-108.

De Groat, W. C., and Saum, W. R. (1971). Adrenergic inhibition in mammals parasympathetic ganglia. *Nature New Biol.* **231**:188-189.

De Groat, W., and Saum, W. R. (1972). Sympathetic inhibition of the urinary bladder of pelvic ganglionic transmission in the cat. *J. Physiol.* **220**:297-314.

De Groat, W. C., and Volle, R. L. (1966). The actions of the catecholamines on transmission in the superior cervical ganglion of the cat. *J. Pharmacol. Exp. Ther.* **154**:1-13.

De Groat, W. C., Booth, A. M., and Krier, J. (1979). Interaction between sacral parasympathetic and lumbar sympathetic impulse to pelvic ganglia. In *Integrative Functions of the Autonomic Nervous System.* Edited by C. McC. Brooks, Koizumi, A. Sato. New York, Elsevier Science Pub. Co., pp. 234-247.

Dennis, M. J., Harris, A. J., and Kuffler, S. W. (1971). Synaptic transmission and its duplication by focally applied acetylcholine in parasympathetic neurons in the heart of the frog. *Proc. R. Soc. Lond. B.* **177**:509-539.

Dun, N. J. (1980). Ganglionic transmission: electrophysiology and pharmacology. *Fed. Proc.* **39**:2982-2989.

Eccles, J. C. (1935). The action potential of the superior cervical ganglion. *J. Physiol.* **85**:179-206.

Eccles, R., and Libet, B. (1961). Origin and blockade of the synaptic responses of curarized sympathetic ganglia. *J. Physiol.* **157**:484-503.

Exley, K. A. (1954). Depression of autonomic ganglia by barbiturates. *Br. J. Pharmacol.* **9**:170.

Fischer, A. W. F. (1964). The intrinsic innervation of the trachea. *J. Anat.* **98**: 117-124.

Folkow, B. (1952). Impulse frequency in sympathetic vasomotor fibres correlated to the release and elimination of the transmitter. *Acta Physiol. Scand.* **25**:49-76.

Gallagher, J. P., Shinnick-Gallagher, P., Cole, A. E., Griffith, W. H. III, and Williams, B. J. (1980). Current hypotheses for the slow inhibitory postsynaptic potential in sympathetic ganglia. *Fed. Proc.* **39**:3009-3015.

Gallagher, J. P., Griffith, W. H., and Shinnick-Gallacher, P. (1982). Cholinergic transmission in cat parasympathetic ganglia. *J. Physiol.* **332**:473-486.

Gooding Elftman, A. (1943). The afferent and parasympathetic innervation of the lungs and trachea of the dog. *Am. J. Anat.* **72**:1-28.

Griffith, W. H. III, Gallagher, J. P., and Shinnick-Gallagher, P. (1980). An intracellular investigation of cat vesical pelvic ganglia. *J. Neurophysiol.* **43**: 343-354.

Griffith, W. H. III, Gallagher, J. P., and Shinnick-Gallagher, P. (1981). Mammalian parasympathetic ganglia fire spontaneous action potentials and transmit slow synaptic potentials. *Adv. Physiol. Sci.* **4**:347-350.

Grillo, M. A., and Nadel, J. A. (1980). Vital staining of tracheal ganglia. *Physiologist* **23**:77.

Haefely, W. E. (1969). Effects of catecholamines in the cat superior cervical ganglion and their postulated role as physiological modulators of ganglionic transmission. In *Progress in Brain Research, Mechanisms of Synaptic Transmission.* Edited by K. Akert and P. G. Waser. Amsterdam, Elsevier, pp. 61-72.

Haefely, W. (1972). Electrophysiology of the adrenergic neuron. In *Handbook of Experimental Pharmacology,* Vol. 33. Edited by H. Blaschko and E. Muscholl. Berlin, Springer Verlag, pp. 661-725.

Haefely, W. E. (1980). Non-nicotinic chemical stimulation of automatic ganglia. In *Pharmacology of Ganglionic Transmission.* Edited by D. A. Kharkevich. New York, Springer-Verlag, pp. 313-357.

Hillarp, N.-Å. (1959). Peripheral autonomic mechanisms. In *Handbook of Physiology,* section 1: Neurophysiology. Vol. II. Edited by J. Field. Bethesda, MD, American Physiological Society, pp. 979-1006.

Holmberg, E., and Waldeck, B. (1980). On the possible role of potassium ions in the action of terbutaline on skeletal muscle contractions. *Acta Pharmacol. Toxicol.* **46**:141-149.

Holtzman, M. J., Hahn, H. L., Sasaki, K., Skoogh, B.-E., Graf, P. D., Fabbri, L. M., and Nadel, J. A. (1982). Selective effect of general anesthetics on reflex bronchoconstrictor responses in dogs. *J. Appl. Physiol.* **53**:126-133.

Langley, J. N. (1921). *The Autonomic Nervous System.* Part I. London, W. Heffer and Sons.

Larrabee, M. G., and Bronk, D. W. (1938). Persistent discharge from sympathetic ganglion cells following preganglionic stimulation. *Proc. Soc. Exp. Biol. Med.* **38**:921-922.

Larrabee, M. G., and Bronk, D. W. (1947). Prolonged facilitation of synaptic excitation in sympathetic ganglia. *J. Neurophysiol.* **10**:139-154.

Larrabee, M., and Pasternak, J. M. (1952). Selective action of anesthetics on synapses and axons in mammalian sympathetic ganglia. *J. Neurophysiol.* **15**:91-114.

Larsell, O. (1922). The ganglia, plexuses, and nerve-terminations of the mammalian lung and pleura pulmonalis. *J. Comp. Neurol.* **35**:97-132.

Larsell, G., and Dow, R. S. (1933). The innervation of the human lung. *Am. J. Anat.* **52**:125-146.

Libet, B. (1979). Slow postsynaptic actions in ganglionic functions. In *Integrative Functions of the Autonomic Nervous System.* Edited by C. McC. Brooks, K. Koizumi, and A. Sato. Amsterdam, Elsevier, pp. 197-222.

Libet. B. (1980). Functional roles of SIF cells in slow synaptic actions. In *Histochemistry and Cell Biology of Autonomic Neurons, SIF Cells, and Paraneurons.* Edited by O. Eränkö et al. New York, Raven Press, pp. 111-118.

Mann, S. P. (1971). The innervation of mammalian bronchial smooth muscle: the localization of catecholamines and cholinesterases. *Histochem. J.* **3**: 319-331.

Mannard, A., and Polosa, C. (1973). Analysis of background firing of single sympathetic preganglionic neurons of cat cervical nerve. *J. Neurophysiol.* **36**:398-408.

Marrazzi, A. S. (1939). Electrical studies on the pharmacology of autonomic synapses. II. The action of a sympathomimetic drug (epinephrine) on sympathetic ganglia. *J. Pharmacol. Exp. Ther.* **65**:395-404.

Martin, A. R., and Pilar, G. (1963). Dual mode of synaptic transmission in the avian ciliary ganglion. *J. Physiol. (London)* **168**:443-463.
Matthews, R. J. Jr. (1956). The effect of epinephrine, levarterenol, and DL-isoproterenol on transmission in the superior cervical ganglion of the cat. *J. Pharmacol.* **116**:433-443.
McIsaac, R. J. (1966). Ganglionic blocking properties of epinephrine and related amines. *Int. J. Neuropharmacol.* **5**:15-26.
Medgett, I. C. (1983). Modulation of transmission in rat sympathetic ganglia by activation of presynaptic alpha- and beta-adrenoceptors. *Br. J. Pharmacol.* **78**:017-027.
Mitchell, R. A., Baker, D. G., Basbaum, C. B., and Herbert, D. A. (1983). In vivo recording from cat, tracheal parasympathetic ganglia. *Physiologist* **17**:37.
Mitchell, R. A., Herbert, D. A., and Baker, D. G. (1985). Inspiratory rhythm in airway smooth muscle tone. *J. Appl. Physiol.* **58**:911-920.
Nicoll, R. A. (1978a). Pentobarbital: differential postsynaptic actions on sympathetic ganglion cells. *Science* **119**:451-452.
Nicoll, R. A. (1978b). Sedative-hypnotics: animal pharmacology. In *Handbook of Psychopharmacology.* Vol. 12. Edited by L. L. Iversen, S. D. Iversen, and S. H. Snyder. New York, Plenum Pub. Corp., pp. 187-233.
Nishi, S. (1970). Cholinergic and adrenergic receptors at sympathetic preganglionic nerve terminals. *Fed. Proc.* **29**:1957-1965.
Nishi, S. (1974). Ganglionic transmission. In *The Peripheral Nervous System.* Edited by J. I. Hubbard. New York, Plenum Press, pp. 225-255.
Nishi, S., and North, R. A. (1973). Intracellular recordings from the myenteric plexus of the guinea pig ileum. *J. Physiol. (London)* **231**:471-491.
Nishi, S. et al. (1967). Release of acetylcholine from sympathetic preganglionic nerve terminals. *J. Neurophysiol.* **30**:114-134.
Nistri, A., and Quilliam, J. P. (1980). Ganglion activity of centrally acting neurotropic agents. In *Pharmacology of Ganglionic Transmission.* Edited by D. A. Kharkevich. New York, Springer-Verlag, pp. 359-384.
Owman, C., Alm, P., and Sjöberg, O. (1983). Pelvic autonomic ganglia structure, transmitters, function and steroid influnece. In *Autonomic Ganglia.* Edited by L.-G. Elfvin. New York, John Wiley and Sons Ltd., pp. 125-143.
Pitts, R. F., and Bronk, D. W. (1942). Excitability cycle of the hypothalamus-sympathetic neurone system. *Am. J. Physiol.* **135**:504-522.
Pitts, R. F., Larrabee, M. G., and Bronk, D. W. (1941). An analysis of hypothalamic cardiovascular control. *Am. J. Physiol.* **134**:359-383.
Quenzer, L., Yahn, D., Alkadhi, K., and Volle, R. L. (1979). Transmission blockade and stimulation of ganglionic adenylate cyclase by catecholamines. *J. Pharmacol. Exp. Ther.* **208**:31-36.

Richardson, J. B. (1979). Nerve supply to the lungs. *Am. Rev. Respir. Dis.* **119**: 785-802.

Richardson, J., and Ferguson, C. C. (1976). The fine structure of the ganglia in human lung. *J. Cell Biol.* **70**:48.

Richardson, J. B., and Ferguson, C. C. (1979). Neuromuscular structure and function in the airways. *Fed. Proc.* **38**:202-208.

Richardson, C. A., and Mitchell, R. A. (1982). Power spectral analysis of inspiratory nerve activity in the decerebrate cat. *Brain Res.* **233**:317-336.

Skok, V. I. (1980). Ganglionic transmission morphology and physiology. In *Pharmacology of Ganglionic Transmission.* Edited by D. A. Kharkevich. New York, Springer-Verlag, pp. 9-39.

Skok, V. I. (1983). Fast synaptic transmission in autonomic ganglia. In *Autonomic Ganglia.* Edited by L.-G. Elfvin. New York, John Wiley and Sons Ltd., pp. 265-279.

Skoogh, B.-E. (1986). Parasympathetic ganglia in the airways. *Bull Eur. Physiopathol. Respir.* **22**(Suppl 7):143-147.

Skoogh, B.-E., and Svedmyr, N. (1986). Beta-2-adrenoceptor stimulation inhibits ganglionic transmission in ferret trachea. Manuscript in preparation.

Skoogh, B.-E., Holtzman, M. J., Sheller, J. R., and Nadel, J. A. (1982). Barbiturates depress vagal motor pathway to ferret trachea at ganglia. *J. Appl. Physiol.* **53**:253-257.

Skoogh, B.-E., Grillo, M. A., and Nadel, J. A. (1983). Neutral red stains ganglia in the vagal motor pathway to ferret trachea without ganglionic transmission. *J. Neurosci. Methods* **8**:33-39.

Skoogh, B.-E., Löfdahl, C.-G., and Svedmyr, N. (1986). Beta-2-adrenoceptor stimulation enhances the attenuation in ferret airway ganglia of the response to high frequency vagus nerve stimulation. Manuscript in preparation.

Spencer, H., and Leof, D. (1964). The innervation of the human lung. *J. Anat. London* **98**:599-609.

Suzuki, T., and Volle, R. L. (1978). Transmission blockade and stimulation of ganglion adenylate cyclase by catecholamines in rat superior cervical ganglia. *Naunyn-Schmiedebergs Arch. Pharmacol.* **304**:15-20.

Uddman, R., Alumets, O., Densert, O. Håkansson, R., and Sundler, F. (1978). Occurrence and distribution of VIP nerves in the nasal mucosa and tracheobronchial wall. *Acta Otolaryngol.* **86**:443-448.

Volle, R. L. (1980). Ganglionic actions of anticholinesterase agents, catecholamines, neuro-muscular blocking agents, and local anaesthetics. In *Pharmacology of Ganglionic Transmission.* Edited by D. A. Kharkevich. New York, Springer-Verlag, pp. 385-410.

Wood, J. D. (1981). Physiology of the enteric nervous system. In *Physiology of the Gastrointestinal Tract.* Edited by L. R. Johnson. New York, Raven Press, pp. 1-37.

Wood, J. D. (1983). Neurophysiology of parasympathetic and enteric ganglia. In *Autonomic Ganglia.* Edited by L.-G. Elfvin. New York, John Wiley and Sons Ltd., pp. 367-398.

Wood, J. D., and Mayer, C. J. (1978). Intracellular study of electrical activity of Auerbach's plexus in guinea pig small intestine. *Pflügers Arch.* **374**:265-275.

Wood, J. D., and Mayer, C. J. (1979). Adrenergic inhibition of serotonin release from neurons in guinea pig Auerbach's plexus. *J. Neurophysiol.* **4**: 594-603.

11

Anticholinergic Drugs in Bronchial Asthma

HANS-L. HAHN

University of Würzburg
Würzburg, West Germany

I. Introduction

Baseline bronchomotor tone is maintained by impulses from the vagus nerves. While the contribution of vagal reflexes to chronic human asthma probably is not as large as had once been thought, reflexes and nonreflex cholinergic pathways are undoubtedly involved in bronchial asthma. Consequently, anticholinergic drugs have been found to be of value in the treatment of asthma. We shall review their effects in clinical asthma as well as in experimental ("laboratory") asthma evoked by a variety of agents.

II. Characteristics of Anticholinergic Drugs Available for Clinical Use

A. Chemical Entity, Kinetics, Differences

Figure 1 shows four anticholinergic drugs in frequent clinical use for the treatment of obstructive airway disease. Atropine is the "oldest" drug of the group and is the only tertiary amine, the remaining drugs (and others not shown) are quaternary ammonium compounds. As a tertiary amine, atropine is well ab-

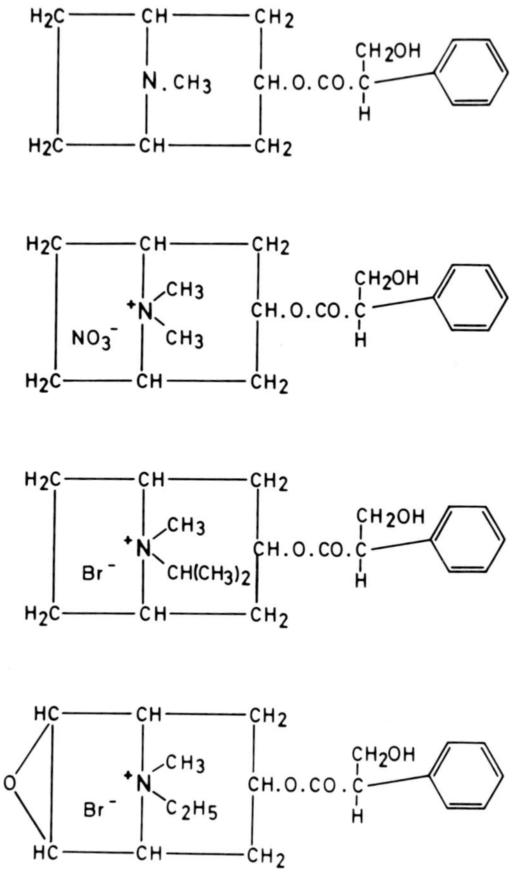

ATROPINE

ATROPINE METHYLNITRATE

IPRATROPIUM BROMIDE

OXITROPIUM BROMIDE

Figure 1 Structural formulae of 4 anticholinergic drugs in common use either for the clinical treatment of airway obstruction or for experimental studies.

sorbed from the gastrointestinal tract and mucosa, is distributed throughout the body, and crosses the blood-brain barrier. In the study by Virtanen et al. (1982), the elimination phase half life of atropine after a single intravenous dose of 0.02 mg/kg was 3-4 hours in most age groups, but was significantly prolonged in subjects over 65 (half life, 10-30 hours) and in children under 2 years (half life, 5-12 hours). Excretion is mainly in the urine. The clinical route used most often is inhalation. Serum levels after inhalation of 0.05 mg/kg atropine sulfate have been measured by Kradjan et al. (1981), who obtained simultaneous measurements of forced expiratory volume (FEV_1) (Fig. 2). Although there was some

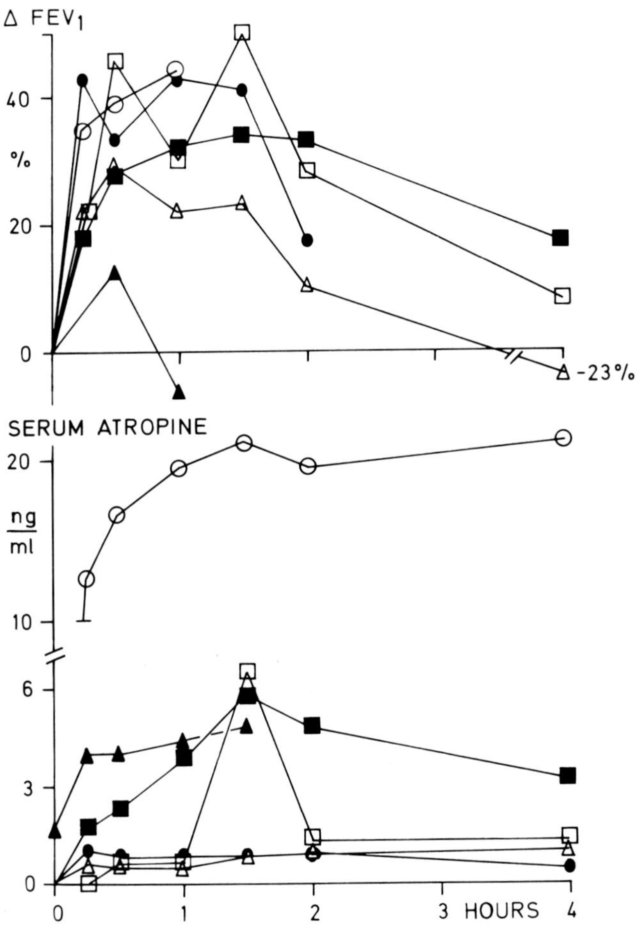

Figure 2 Percent improvement in FEV_1 (top) and serum levels of atropine (bottom) in 6 patients with chronic bronchitis 0.25 to 4 hours after inhalation of 0.05 mg/kg atropine sulfate from a compressor-driven nebulizer; the mass median diameter of the nebulized particles ranged from 2.8 to 4.2 μm (drawn from tabulated data of Kradjan et al., 1981, by permission). Different symbols are used for each patient to permit identification of same patient in top and bottom graph.

relationship between blood level and effect achieved, the relationship was loose. The systemic concentration of the inhaled drug is not a reliable indicator of its local concentration in the lungs, which appears to determine its effects on airway smooth muscle. Blood levels and half life of atropine sulfate are quite similar after inhalation and after intramuscular injection of the same dose, but levels of inhaled atropine are more variable (Harrison et al., 1986).

Ipratropium bromide is very similar to atropine in its effects when given by the intravenous route. Kinetics after intravenous, oral, and inhaled ipratropium have been reported by Rominger (1979). After intravenous administration, the active substance was distributed very rapidly, but excretion started as rapidly. As soon as 10 min after IV application considerable amounts of radioactivity were found in the gut. Following rapid distribution with a steep fall in blood levels, there was a slower elimination phase with a half life of 3.6 hours. By 24 hours, approximately 60% of intravenous ipratropium had been excreted by the kidneys, about 20% in the bile and approximately 5% via the fecal-biliary route. Blood levels after oral administration of 30 mg ipratropium showed a delayed increase with a peak after 3 hours. The peak level represented only 0.2% of the dose. This was not because of poor absorption from the gut. Rather, the drug was absorbed by the gut, but re-excreted immediately by a specific mechanism. The peak was broad and plateau-like, extending from 2 to 7 hours, thereafter blood levels fell slowly to reach baseline levels after 8-12 hours. The calculated half life was 3-4 hours. Essentially the same time course with a somewhat earlier rise in blood levels was seen after inhalation of a high dose (555 μg) of ipratropium bromide, which is not surprising since the major portion of inhaled agents is swallowed and is absorbed from the gastrointestinal tract. The area under the plasma level curve was larger after oral than after inhaled ipratropium. Inhaled radioactive ipratropium appeared in plasma within 2 min and reached a maximum level within 1-3 hours. This level represented only 0.03% of the inhaled dose. The half life was 1½-4 hours. Plasma levels fell below 50% of peak levels after 5 hours and below 17% after 8 hours. While intravenous ipratropium was excreted mainly via the kidneys, 60-70% of oral (and inhaled) ipratropium was excreted in the feces by 24 hr. Total renal excretion after 6 days amounted to 9%, while 89% was excreted in the feces (mean recovery, 96.8%). The recommended single dose is one or two inhalations (20-40 μg).

Both atropine and ipratropium are relatively selective bronchodilators even after intravenous injection. Doses needed to inhibit salivary secretion are 10-fold higher than those required to antagonize acetylcholine-induced bronchoconstriction. Even higher doses are required to induce intestinal relaxation, tachycardia, and smooth muscle relaxation in the bladder. The difference between the concentration causing bronchodilation and the concentration inhibiting salivary secretion increases from 10-fold to 100-fold for atropine and to almost 300-fold for ipratropium bromide when the drugs are inhaled instead of injected (Bauer et al., 1976; Engelhardt, 1979).

B. Dose Response, Route of Administration of Anticholinergic Drugs

In 9 patients with mild asthma (FEV_1, 80-122%) doses of ipratropium bromide increasing from 20 to 60 μg (1-3 puffs from commercial metered dose inhaler) produced increasing improvements in MEF_{40} measured from a partial expiratory flow volume curve (Newcomb et al., 1985). No plateau was seen between the 40 and the 60 μg doses. Other authors using longer intervals between doses have also shown that there is a dose-response effect up to high doses. In those studies in which dose-response curves have been constructed, maximally effective doses for inhaled atropine sulfate and methonitrate ranged from 1000 to 4500 μg, for ipratropium bromide from 80 to 1000 μg, and for glycopyrrolate (1 study) the maximally effective inhaled dose was 1600 μg (Burge et al., 1980; Lulling et al., 1981; Ward et al., 1981; Griffin et al., 1982; Hanley et al., 1986). It appears that the generally recommended dose for ipratropium (20-40 μg) is submaximal for a number of patients. The lowest dose of atropine reaching maximum effect has been found to be lower in mild than in severe disease as one would predict (Lin et al., 1982; Ruffin et al., 1978; Griffin et al., 1982; Ward et al., 1981). Dose also determined duration of effect. The main advantage of increasing dose in the two studies shown in Figure 3 was not the higher peak of the bronchodilator effect, but was maintained bronchodilation at 4 hours (Pak et al., 1982; Allen and Campbell, 1979). This has been confirmed in a more recent study (Friedman et al., 1986).

C. Onset and Time Course of Effects

The effect of ipratropium bromide and of atropine has been found to set in comparatively slowly and to be long lasting. In a number of studies, the onset of the effect of anticholinergic agents ranged from 6 to 60 min and peak effects were seen between 30 and 180 min (Vlagopoulos et al., 1976; Rubbin et al., 1978; Kradjan et al., 1981). The half life of atropine sulfate was 4.1 hr after intramuscular injection and 4-6 hours after inhalation. This would be slightly longer than the half life of ipratropium (1.5-4 hours after inhalation, Rominger, 1979; Harrison et al., 1986).

D. Side Effects

In most studies side effects of anticholinergic drugs have been minimal. On the other hand, few studies were set up to investigate the incidence and duration of side effects in a systematic way, so the recording and reporting of side effects has been largely anecdotal. Of the 26 studies assessed side effects were reported in

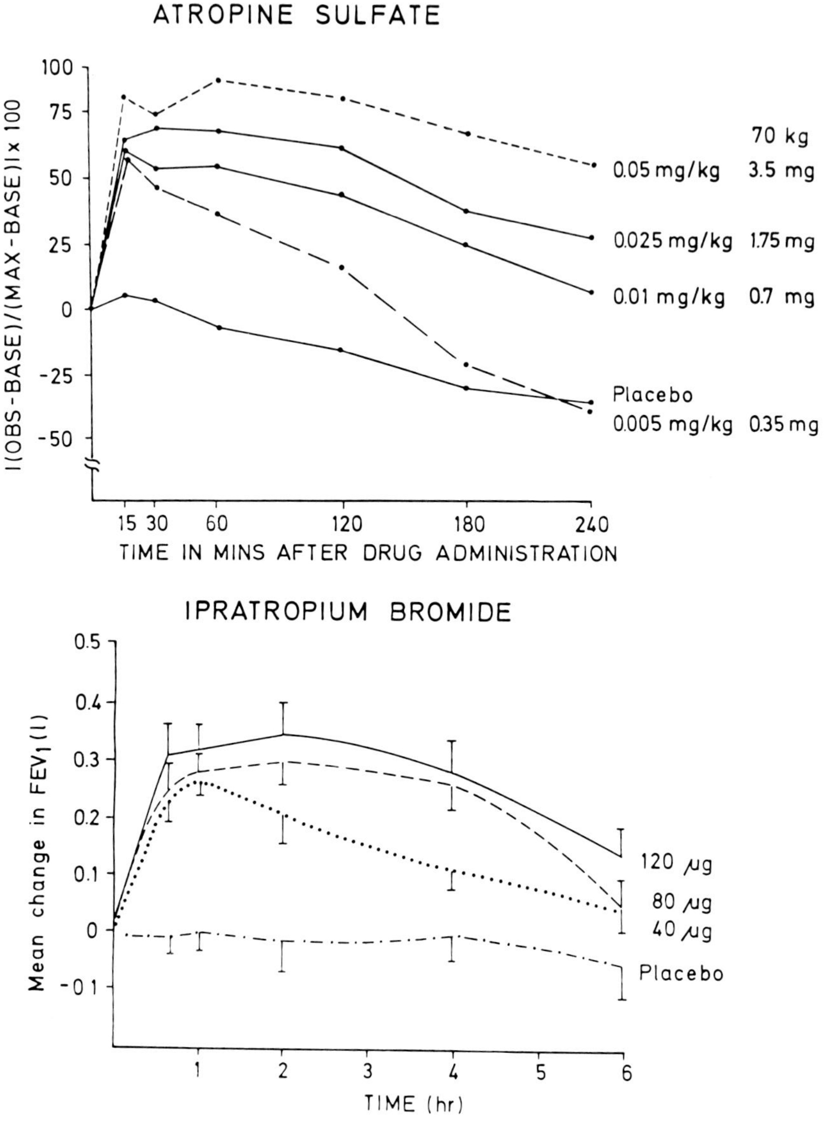

Figure 3 Time and dose-response curves (FEV_1) for atropine (top) and for ipratropium (bottom). Top graph: The bronchodilator response (ordinate) is defined as the percent possible improvement of FEV_1 where "Max" is the best FEV_1 obtained after bronchodilator at any time during the study. Each dose of atropine (indicated) was inhaled on a different day from a compressed air nebulizer (Maximist) using a dosimeter (from Pak et al., 1982, by permission). Bottom graph: Mean increase (± SE) of FEV_1 after different doses of ipratropium (indicated) inhaled by 16 patients with asthma from metered dose inhalers. Each dose was inhaled on a different day (from Allen and Campbell, 1979, by permission). Increasing the dose of inhaled anticholinergic drugs increased not only the peak, but also the duration of the bronchodilator effect. The largest difference in FEV_1 after low and high doses was at 4 hours.

19 (atropine: 10 studies, ipratropium: 9 studies), in the remaining 7 studies side effects were either not mentioned or it was stated that none were observed. Of the side effects reported the most frequent following atropine administration were dry mouth (9 of 10 studies, majority of patients in each study), dizziness, drowsiness, headache or "wobbly feel" (4 of 10), urinary retention (3 of 10 studies, severe problem in 1), tachycardia (2 of 10 studies), blurred vision (2 of 10 studies), excessive thirst (1 of 10 studies). Corresponding figures for ipratropium were as follows: dry mouth 2/9, tachycardia 0/9, dizziness + drowsiness 3/9, urinary retention 0/9, tachycardia (0/9), blurred vision (0/9). Cough was reported in 3 of 9 studies and a decrease in heart rate in a total of five studies on ipratropium (Chapman et al., 1985; Ward et al., 1981; Barber et al., 1977; Sackner et al., 1977; Cockcroft et al., 1982).

High doses of atropine (3.5 mg every 4 hours, total dose 10.5 mg) decreased citric acid-induced salivary flow from 3.6 to 2 g and increased the gastric emptying half time from 65 to 112 min (Botts et al., 1985). A high dose (400 μg) of ipratropium decreased diastolic blood pressure 4-5% in normal subjects, but did not affect systolic blood pressure, heart rate, salivary secretion, and intraocular pressure (Rubbin et al., 1978).

Anisocoria has been observed following inhalation of several anticholinergic preparations (atropine, glycopyrrolate, ipratropium) and has received attention because patients were found to receive needless neurological studies (e.g., Jannum and Nickel, 1986). The symptom has not been observed after intramuscular atropine even in patients in whom it was observed after inhalation of the same dose (Harrison et al., 1986). Aniscoria is therefore believed to be due to a contamination from the inhaled drug. Inhalation of ipratropium bromide through a mask can precipitate angle closure glaucoma (Malani et al., 1982).

As with any drug, there have been occasional incidences of severe and unusual side effects in individual patients. One report by Connolly (1982) lists 3 cases with immediate and prolonged falls in daily peak flow readings reversible only on stopping the drug—manifestation possibly of the paradoxical action of anticholinergic drugs.

E. Mucociliary Clearance Following Anticholinergic Drugs

Animal studies show that mucus secretion can be increased by cholinergic stimuli and that this increase can be blocked by anticholinergic drugs. Most authors have found it difficult, however, to block baseline (unstimulated) secretion by anticholinergic treatment (Gallagher et al., 1975). The effect of cholinergic blockade on airway secretions in humans might therefore depend on the functional status of glands before treatment. If baseline conditions prevail atropine will have no effect. If abnormal (stimulated) secretion is present, atropine will reduce it. In a case report by Wick and Ingram (1976) bronchorrhea with a mucus production of 300-450 ml/day unresponsive to maintenance antibiotic therapy and to sympathomimetic bronchodilators was improved dramatically by 0.4 mg atropine given twice daily. However, in normal subjects and even in patients with asthma or chronic bronchitis effects of atropine on mucus secretion or on mucociliary clearance have been far less dramatic. Atropine and hyoscine have been found in 5 of 6 studies to slow down mucociliary clearance and/or decrease sputum weight or volume by a moderate amount. Complete arrest of particle movement has been reported in only one study (Foster et al., 1976). In contrast, ipratropium as a rule has been found to be devoid of such side effects. In one study clearance rates even improved after inhalation of ipratropium (Ruffin et al., 1978).

III. Effects of Anticholinergic Drugs in Asthma

A. Factors Influencing Response

Dose

Hawkins and Schild (1951) and Russell (1978) showed that a 50% maximal contraction of human and airway smooth muscle was induced with 10^{-6} M acetylcholine, and the maximal contraction was obtained with 10^{-3} M acetylcholine. Since atropine is a competitive antagonist to acetylcholine, 10^{-3} M atropine at maximal cholinergic stimulation would result in only a 50% blockade of the muscarinic receptors of the airways, if the receptor affinity to atropine and acetylcholine were identical. In mammalian brain, the affinity of atropine for binding sites was found to be 20 times that of acetylcholine in one study (Uchida et al., 1978) and 1000 times in another (Burgen et al., 1974). Even if a 1000 times higher affinity of atropine than acetylcholine is considered, the concentration of atropine to block 50% of receptors would be 10^{-6} M, which is 0.67 mg kg^{-1} or 47 mg for a 70 kg man (assuming even distribution of the drug and a specific gravity of 1.0 for the human body). Even this dose for a 50% blockade of the receptors is obviously too high to be used in a human subject. Complete cholinergic muscarinic blockade may be impossible to achieve in vivo. Consequently, in many dose-response studies a maximal dose has not been found (Pak et al., 1982; Gal et al., 1984) even when only effects on baseline bronchomotor tone were studied, effects that are blocked most easily.

Severity of Bronchoconstriction/Importance of Clinical Condition

The effect of bronchodilators—β-adrenergic or anticholinergic—will generally increase with the degree of bronchoconstriction prior to treatment (Astin, 1972; Bandouvakis et al., 1981; Eiser and Guz, 1982). This is true for the mild-to-moderate range of bronchoconstriction while in very severe bronchoconstriction effects of bronchodilating agents tend to fall off again (Hume and Gandevia, 1957; Freedman, 1978). This can affect studies of anticholinergic drugs in two ways: (1) Some comparisons of anticholinergic drugs in asthmatic vs. bronchitic patients are difficult to interpret because of the substantially more severe degree of bronchoconstriction in the latter group (Chick and Jenne, 1977). (2) When cholinergic and adrenergic agents are given sequentially to assess their relative potency, the second drug will appear to offer little additional benefit in patients with only slight bronchoconstriction. Since the first drug achieved all bronchodilation possible a second drug cannot show its worth (Ruffin et al., 1977; Petrie and Palmer, 1975). Crossover and "pattern recognition" designs help in the correct assessment of the relative potency of different drugs as will be discussed later (Ward et al., 1981; Ullah et al., 1981; Karpel et al., 1986).

In acute exacerbations of asthma, cholinergic compounds are less effective than when asthma is in remission. This is a well established finding (Altounyan, 1964; Jolobe and Lane, 1981) although it has recently been reemphasized (McFadden 1986). The mechanism is unclear and may be unrelated to baseline bronchoconstriction.

Baseline vs. Stimulated Cholinergic Effect

This is related to dose. A given dose may be adequate to abolish baseline bronchomotor tone, but may be inadequate to block increases in cholinergic neural drive. In seven nonsmoking volunteers given increasing doses of atropine by inhalation the smallest dose given to each subject (0.13 or 0.26 mg) was sufficient to cause maximal reductions in baseline-specific airway resistance (SRaw). The same dose completely inhibited bronchoconstriction induced by inhalation of 1% methacholine. However, only the highest dose (1.04 mg atropine inhaled) blocked cold air-induced bronchoconstriction in 5 subjects while another two were incompletely blocked even by 2.04 mg (Sheppard et al., 1982). In most studies comparing anticholinergic and beta-sympathomimetic drugs both had the same effect on baseline airway calibre even in studies in which gross differences were found in their effects on induced bronchoconstriction, for example, following allergen administration (Howarth et al., 1985; Hanley et al., 1986). Blockade of induced bronchoconstriction may require doses of anticholinergic drugs well in excess of those required to block baseline bronchomotor tone.

While induced bronchoconstriction is more difficult to block than baseline bronchomotor tone the reverse may be true for mucus secretion from airway submucosal glands. Reduction of baseline secretion by atropine is difficult (Gallagher et al., 1975), inhibition of neurally stimulated secretion by atropine is relatively easy (e.g., Borson et al., 1984).

Dependence of Cholinergic Contribution on Stimulus Strength

Even the same stimulus can have different mechanisms of action at different doses. When histamine was applied to dogs in a divided lung preparation where one side was vagotomized to assess the contribution of vagal mechanisms, low concentrations of histamine applied to both lungs had a significantly greater effect in the control than in the vagotomized lung and the authors estimated about 40% of histamine-induced bronchoconstriction was reflexly mediated. At higher concentrations of histamine there was no difference between the two sides and the contribution from vagal reflexes was estimated to be essentially zero (Shore et al., 1985). Thus, in situations where cholinergic and noncholinergic mechanisms are involved the latter may override the former depending on stimulus strength. Similar phenomena have been reported previously (e.g., Drazen and Austen, 1975).

Route of Administration, Access to Site of Cholinergic Effect

In six asthmatic children the dose of inhaled atropine causing maximal bronchodilation (0.03-0.04 mg kg^{-1}) did not block exercise-induced asthma. Doubling the inhaled dose had no additional effect but when additional atropine (0.35 mg) was injected intramuscularly protection against exercise-induced bronchoconstriction became maximal (Chen et al., 1981). The authors concluded that neither inhaled nor injected atropine reached all cholinergic receptors, but that the maximum effect was achieved by a combination of the two routes, a conclusion also reached by De Troyer et al. (1979) in normal subjects. The route by which cholinergic impulses reach the airways has to be considered also. When the same dose of atropine (0.5 mg) was given by inhalation or intravenously to 6 asthmatic patients the inhaled dose was considerably more effective in blocking bronchoconstriction induced by inhaled methacholine than by hyperventilation with cold air. No such difference could be found for intravenous atropine (Sheppard et al., 1983). A similar difference was found in dogs when inhaled or injected atropine was used to block bronchoconstriction induced by inhaled acetylcholine vs. electrical stimulation of the vagus nerves (Holtzman et al., 1983). The usual test of completeness of cholinergic block following atropine inhalation—inhibition of methacholine-induced bronchoconstriction—can be misleading. Not only may the dose be too low to block an intervention other than methacholine challenge. It may also be the "wrong" route of administration for another stimulus.

Time Course of Effects

Investigators studying effects and/or blood levels of anticholinergic drugs invariably find a slower onset of action and a slower increase in blood levels for anticholinergic drugs than is found for sympathomimetic agents. Tests of pulmonary function performed 10-15 min after application of anticholinergic agents are bound to underestimate their effects (Lulling et al., 1981) although they may still be useful in other respects. If isoproterenol is applied 60 min after atropine the combined effect of the two can be assessed because isoproterenol is applied at the peak of the atropine response. However, if atropine is applied 60 min after isoproterenol (Light and George, 1977) it is almost like studying the effect of atropine alone because of the short action of isoproterenol (Altounyan, 1964).

Anesthesia

This is important in animal studies and in studies on anesthetized patients (e.g., Cheney and Butler, 1970). Anesthetics alter the behavior of sensory receptors in the airways, block reflex pathways, or affect airway smooth muscle contraction. For instance, barbiturates in increasing dosage will inhibit first the afferent, then the efferent arm of pulmonary reflexes (Holtzman et al., 1982) and on the efferent side, inhibit ganglionic transmission at 10-fold lower doses than postganglionic impulses or responses of the effector organ (Skoogh et al., 1982). Relevant effects of other anesthetics have been discussed previously (Hahn and Nadel, 1981).

B. Clinical Asthma

Many patients with chronic bronchitis have airway obstruction that may be improved 20-40% by adrenergic or anticholinergic agonists. Many of those patients could be classified as having asthma. For instance, in the study by Pak et al. (1982), the study population consisted of 10 patients with chronic obstructive pulmonary disease (COPD) who demonstrated at least 15% improvement in FEV_1 following sympathomimetic bronchodilators. According to the authors all patients had "chronic bronchitis as defined by ATS committee on Diagnostic Standards," but the degree of reversibility of their bronchoconstriction and the fact that 3 patients had a history of nonatopic asthma suggests that no clear differentiation was made between asthma and chronic bronchitis. Recent reviews have drawn attention to the high degree of reversibility often found in patients with bronchitis (Gross, 1986). Data on the response of such patients to steroid medication which would greatly aid in the distinction have often not been provided in the papers. For this reason data from patients with chronic bronchitis have been reviewed in the present assessment whenever it was stated or was evident from a publication that a large portion of their airway obstruction was reversible.

Acute Effects of Anticholinergic Agents on Baseline Pulmonary Function

Cholinergic antagonists are effective and long lasting bronchodilators in asthmatic patients, average improvement in FEV_1 after inhaled atropine or ipratropium ranging from 20-30% (e.g., Vlagopoulos et al., 1976; Allen and Campbell, 1979), but reaching 50-60% in more severely affected patient populations (Ward et al., 1981; Burge et al., 1980).

Atopic vs. Nonatopic Asthmatic/Bronchitis Patients

Only one study will be discussed in detail because its results are representative and because it exemplifies some important points of experimental detail. Ullah et al. (1981) studied atopic and nonatopic asthmatic patients. A subgroup of 4 patients from the nonatopic group also had features of chronic bronchitis. Effects of the β-agonist salbutamol and of the anticholinergic drug ipratropium bromide were compared in the two groups. On each of two study days patients received each of the two drugs and only the sequence of application was varied. On a given study day two doses of drug 1 were given before two doses of drug 2 were applied in order to obtain a dose response to each drug and to make certain the plateau of the dose response to drug 1 had been reached before drug 2 was started. The first dose of ipratropium was 80 μg. This was followed 30 min later by a second dose of 40 μg. Corresponding doses for salbutamol were 400 and 200 μg. Average responses for the two groups of patients are shown in Figure 4. Overall, salbutamol was the more effective drug, but the difference between salbutamol and ipratropium was considerably smaller in the nonatopic than in the atopic group and was no longer significant in the subgroup of patients with bronchitis (not shown in Fig. 4). In addition to this statistical assessment, the authors studied individual response patterns allocating individual responses to one of six patterns, two each indicating superiority of ipratropium, of salbutamol or equal effectiveness of either drug (Fig. 5). Despite the statistical superiority of salbutamol analysis of response patterns indicated that 40% of patients had a response to ipratropium equal to or better than that to salbutamol. Although the better response to anticholinergic agents (relative to adrenergic drugs) was more frequent in nonatopic than in atopic patients, analysis of variance revealed that the principal factor determining a favorable response to anticholinergic agents was age, not absence of atopy. In most patients, of course, the two went together, so the distinction may be of little practical value.

This study is particularly valuable for several reasons. (1) A 2 point dose response to each drug was obtained which has several advantages. For instance, it could not be argued that a second dose of the same drug might have achieved the same effect as the other drug. (2) The sequence of drug application was reversed within each patient which is of critical importance: If on day 1 ipratropium has no effect over and above that of salbutamol, ipratropium may appear to be of no value. However, if on day 2 the same occurs with salbutamol which is then given as the second drug the two drugs must be at least equieffective.

Many other studies have limited themselves to one sequence of applications

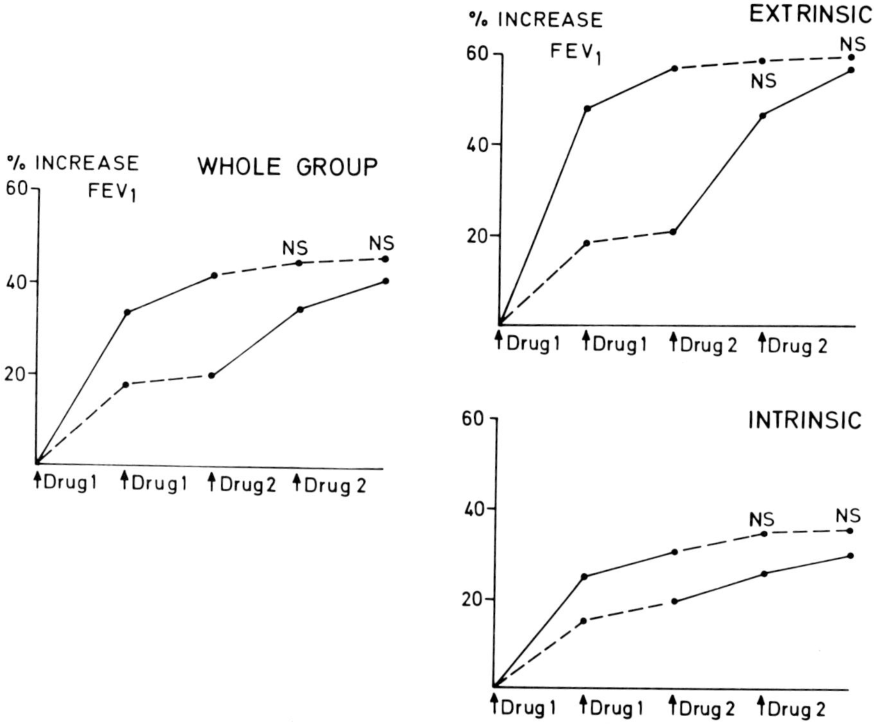

Figure 4 Responses in FEV_1, expressed as % change from baseline for a group of asthmatic patients (left) and for the subgroups with extrinsic and intrinsic asthma (right) following inhalation of salbutamol (solid lines) and of ipratropium bromide (dashed lines). Two doses of each drug were inhaled; doses were 400 μg and 200 μg for salbutamol, 80 μg and 40 μg for ipratropium, NS = difference between FEV_1 after salbutamol and after ipratropium not significant. All other differences were significant (from Ullah et al., 1981, by permission).

obviating valid conclusions as to relative benefit. (3) There was individual in addition to statistical assessment of drug responses (pattern recognition technique), important because a given drug can be consistently better for an individual patient although it may be less effective for the study group as a whole.

Although the study by Ullah et al. (1981) stands out for the reasons stated theirs was not the only and not the first investigation to describe the different responses of atopic and nonatopic asthmatic patients to adrenergic vs. anticholinergic drugs. Most authors addressing this question came to similar conclusions. Anticholinergic drugs are almost as effective as, in some cases more effective than

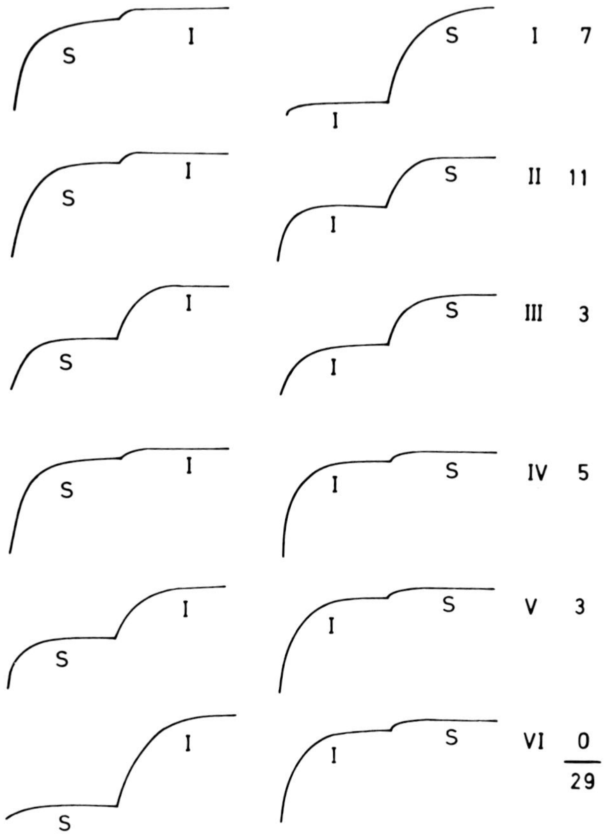

Figure 5 Six possible patterns of response (I-VI) to (a) salbutamol (S) given as the first drug followed by ipratropium (left column) and (b) ipratropium (I) given as the first drug followed by salbutamol (right column). Number of patients exhibiting each response pattern is shown at the right hand margin. Patterns I and II indicate superiority of salbutamol over ipratropium, patterns III and IV indicate equal effectiveness of salbutamol and ipratropium patterns V and VI indicate superiority of ipratropium over salbutamol (from Ullah et al., 1981, by permission).

adrenergic agents in older nonatopic asthmatic or in bronchitic patients while adrenergic and theophylline drugs are more effective in the younger atopic asthmatic patients, especially in exacerbation (Karpel et al., 1986). Reasons for this difference are unclear. It is possible that β-adrenergic drugs have specific antiallergic effects required by atopic, but not by nonatopic or bronchitic patients and lacking in anticholinergic drugs. Some studies would support this concept (Howarth et al., 1985; Woolcock et al., 1986). Another reason may be access of the drugs to their site of action. In practically all studies patients with chronic bronchitis had considerably more severe airway obstruction than patients with atopic asthma. If it is a requirement for effective antiallergic action by β-adrenergic drugs that they reach the periphery of the lung where the highest concentrations of β-adrenoceptors are found (Barnes et al., 1982), then these drugs might be less effective in patients in whom severe baseline bronchoconstriction prevents access to these sites. This mechanism may be valid even if the critical β receptors are located not in smooth muscle but in other target cells, for example, macrophages, neutrophils, or type II cells. A third explanation is related to the fact that the predominant feature of chronic bronchitis is mucus hypersecretion. If a large portion of airway obstruction in chronic bronchitis is due to hypersecretion and to hypertrophy or hyperplasia of secretory cells then anticholinergic drugs which inhibit secretion (at least in higher concentrations) may be more effective in chronic bronchitis than β-agonists which stimulate secretion.

Chronic Studies

The acute response to anticholinergic treatment has been tested before and after chronic treatment. In two studies the acute response to treatment with β-adrengic or theophylline agents was also assessed and these drugs were also part of chronic treatment (Klock et al., 1975; Rebuck et al., 1983). In none of 6 studies was there improvement in the acute response to cholinergic antagonists after chronic treatment and in only one study was baseline pulmonary function improved after chronic treatment with ipratropium bromide (40 μg 4 times daily) for one year (Cockcroft et al., 1982). In another study there was improvement in the acute response to theophylline plus ipratropium following chronic treatment with the same combination for 30 days.

C. Experimental Asthma

Antigen-Induced Asthma

In dogs allergic to *Ascaris suum* antigen allergen-induced bronchoconstriction was abolished in 22 dogs by a rapid infusion of 0.2 mg/kg atropine sulfate starting 20 min after the start of antigen aerosol. Antigen-induced bronchoconstriction was also abolished when atropine (10 mg/ml) was given as an aerosol for 2 min to 10 dogs (Gold et al., 1972). Similar results have not generally been obtained in man. Yu et al. (1972) found inhibition of antigen-induced bronchoconstriction by atropine in 5 of 7 asthmatic patients, but other authors, while finding significant baseline bronchodilation after atropine, did not observe significant protection against allergen-induced bronchospasm if percentage changes were calculated from the new baseline established after atropine. In 8 atopic asthmatic patients inhalation challenge with grass pollen outside the grass pollen season when patients were asymptomatic and required no medication caused reproducible decreases in specific conductance (48.5-49.6%) and FEV_1 (25.5-25.7%) together with increases in plasma histamine and serum neutrophil chemotactic factor. Inhalation of 1 mg ipratropium bromide from a nebulizer and dosimeter caused significant bronchodilation equal to that caused by 200 μg albuterol but, unlike albuterol and cromolyn sodium, did not reduce significantly the allergen-induced % changes in any of the variables measured (Howarth et al., 1985). Even very high doses of atropine inhaled prior to antigen challenge were ineffective against antigen-induced bronchoconstriction in another study although atropine given at the peak of bronchoconstriction reduced bronchospasm as effectively as it did in the study by Yu et al. (Rosenthal et al., 1977). Nobody has been able to resolve this discrepancy which has been noted by other workers as well. Individual variability in the responsiveness to atropine may explain some of the discrepancies observed because there is no doubt that atropine in some patients has a very good protective effect against antigen-induced bronchoconstriction, an effect independent of improvement in baseline lung function (Eiser and Guz, 1982, Fig. 6). Subjects studied by Howarth et al. were only minimally hyperreactive to cholinergic agents which suggests that patient selection may have contributed to the negative results obtained with anticholinergic treatment. However, despite excellent responses to anticholinergic treatment in some individuals (Brown et al., 1984) most studies, in which the effectiveness of atropine against allergen-induced bronchoconstriction was compared with the effectiveness of β-adrenergic drugs the latter were found to be superior.

Exercise-Induced Asthma

Inhalation of 250 μg ipratropium bromide from a nebulizer by 6 patients with asthma caused significant improvement in baseline lung function. Ipratropium did not prevent exercise-induced bronchoconstriction but caused a parallel shift in all dose-response curves (e.g., FEV_1, SGaw, FEF_{50}). In addition, wheezing (recorded by phonopneumography) was significantly less and later in onset (Pasterkamp et al., 1985). Of another 8 studies reviewed in which exercise, no voluntary hyperventilation was used as the bronchoconstrictive stimulus, a moderate to good protective effect of anticholinergic drugs was found in 5 but 3 failed to find any protective effect although baseline lung function was clearly improved. Individual variability in the response to anticholinergic drugs, dose of drug, and route of application may explain different results.

Hyperventilation-Induced Asthma

After a single rapid maximal inspiration, specific conductance decreased in each of 6 patients with airways obstruction (mean decrease, 38%, $p < 0.001$). The re-

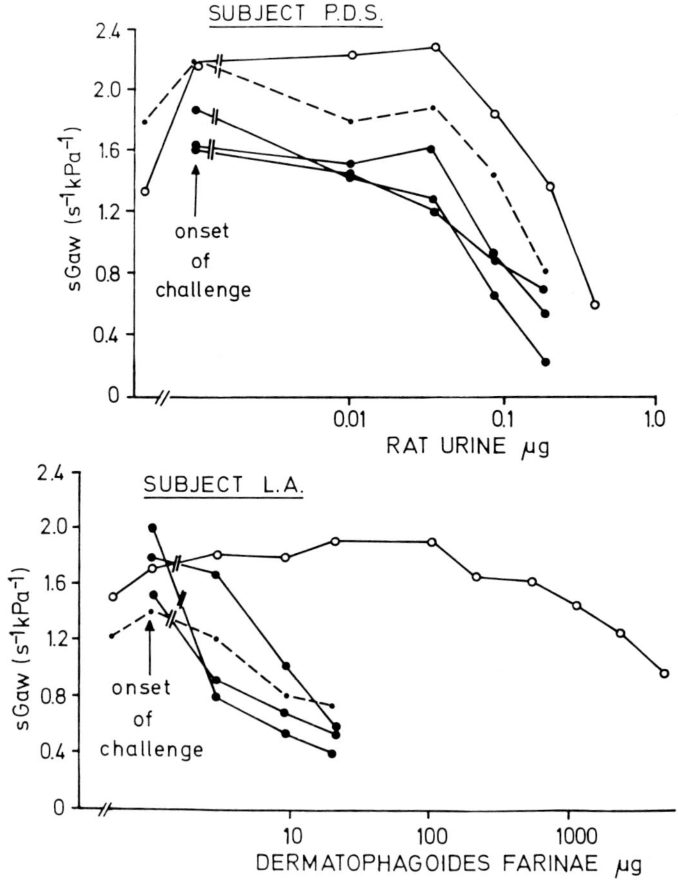

Figure 6 Effects of placebo (dashed lines) and atropine (solid lines, open circles) on antigen dose-response curves of subjects P.D.S. and L.A. Specific conductance (SGaw) is plotted against cumulative dose of antigen in μg. Solid lines and closed circles represent multiple control runs on different days to cover a wide range of baseline values before antigen challenge—including baseline values better than those seen after atropine pretreatment. Results of the study show that (a) atropine is effective against allergen-induced bronchoconstriction in individual patients (b) it is not the effect of atropine on baseline airway calibre that determines its effectiveness (from Eiser and Guz, 1982, by permission).

sponse was abolished by 1-2 mg of IV atropine (mean decrease, 4%, $p < 0.1$). The same was found for the bronchoconstrictive effect of single rapid expirations and for bronchoconstriction induced by breathing cold air for 2 min (Simonsson et al., 1967). Although no dose-response curve was constructed in this early study the protective effect of atropine against hyperventilation-induced bronchoconstriction was clearly demonstrated. Effects of atropine have been quantified better in more recent studies and it is accepted now that atropine protects against hyperventilation-induced bronchoconstriction in many, but not in all patients. The protective effect of atropine was demonstrated even in studies where it was denied by the authors themselves. In a study by Griffin et al. (1982) on 7 patients with mild asthma the same degree of bronchoconstriction could be achieved after atropine as after NaCl if only the dose of the stimulus was made high enough (the authors' main point). However, atropine had a clearcut protective effect at equivalent levels of ventilation. Results were weighted by large atropine effects in 3 of the 7 subjects while effects of atropine were only moderate in 4. This is the pattern that has generally been observed: large effects of atropine in some patients, negligible effects in others.

Bronchoconstriction Induced by Specific Substances in Asthmatic Patients

Cholinergic Agonists: Acetylcholine, Methacholine, Carbachol

Effectiveness of anticholinergic agents against bronchoconstriction induced by cholinergic agonists has unequivocally been found to be excellent as one would expect. Prevention by inhaled atropine of the bronchoconstriction induced by inhaled cholinergic agonists should not lead to the conclusion that complete blockade of all cholinergic muscarinic receptors within the respiratory system has been achieved.

Histamine

In most studies anticholinergic drugs have been found to provide partial, rarely complete, protection against histamine-induced bronchoconstriction. Of 11 studies reviewed only 2 failed to find any effect of atropine-like drugs against histamine-induced bronchoconstriction (Laitinen et al., 1979; Woenne et al., 1978). Both reflex and direct effects of histamine on airway smooth muscle tone have been well established. The contribution of these mechanisms varies with the factors described earlier.

Adenosine

Inhaled adenosine caused no change in specific conductance in 6 normal, nonallergic subjects but in a concentration of 6.7 mg/ml reduced specific conductance in 6 allergic and 7 nonallergic asthmatic patients 76% and 72%, respectively, while inhaled guanosine had no effect in either group (Cushley et al., 1983). Ipratropium bromide, 1 mg, inhaled in 4 ml 0.9% NaCl caused a large increase in the provocative concentration of methacholine needed to decrease specific conductance 35% (PC_{35}) from 0.11 to 21.7 mg/ml, but increased the PC_{35} for adenosine only from 1.97 to 2.51 mg/ml (NS) and the PC_{20} for FEV_1 from 2.2 to 3.33

mg/ml ($p < 0.005$). This was a very small effect compared to the effect of isoproterenol which rapidly reversed bronchoconstriction to both adenosine and histamine. It would appear therefore that only a small portion if any of the effect of adenosine is mediated via cholinergic pathways (Mann et al., 1985).

Prostaglandins

Several prostaglandins, such as prostacyclin (PGI_2), prostaglandin F_{2a}, prostaglandin E_2, prostaglandin D_2, and thromboxane A_2 are released after anaphylactic challenge of human lung (Schulman et al., 1981) and are believed to be mediators of bronchial asthma. Prostaglandin F_{2a} was more potent in causing bronchoconstriction in anesthetized dogs than acetylcholine and histamine (Wasserman, 1975) and a considerable portion of its effect was atropine sensitive. This was true whether PGF_{2a} was given intravenously or by inhalation, thus its action involved cholinergic facilitation or a reflex. Similarly, Drazen and Austen (1975) reported that in guinea pigs atropine prevented the early, but not the late bronchoconstrictor response to prostaglandin F_{2a}. Another effect of PGF_{2a} was profuse salivation and this was blocked completely by atropine. The atropine sensitive effect of prostaglandin F_{2a} on salivary secretion was investigated by other groups (Hahn and Patil, 1972, 1974; Taira and Satoh, 1973) and was shown to be blockable by tetradotoxin, an intervention that did not alter the effect of exogenous acetylcholine. Thus PGF_{2a} acts on cholinergic nerves to increase release of acetylcholine. PGD_2 given as an aerosol was equipotent to F_{2a} and reduction of effects by atropine was also comparable for the two substances (approximately 50%) (Wasserman et al., 1980). Effects of inhaled prostaglandin F_{2a} have also been studied in man and partial protection by atropine has been found in man as in animals (Alanko and Poppius, 1973; Patel, 1975). Dose-response curves have been constructed in normal and asthmatic patients by two different groups with similar results. The dose-response curve does not have the usual sigmoid shape. Initial bronchoconstriction (at 1-100 μg/ml) is followed by partial bronchodilation not quite reaching baseline values (100-1000 μg/ml) until at high doses (1000-5000 μg/ml) severe bronchoconstriction is seen. This pattern has been found in normal subjects (Lewis et al., 1983; see Fig. 7) and in asthmatic patients (Fish et al., 1983) and the most likely explanation appears to be that an initial short-lasting irritant effect of PGF_{2a} on pulmonary sensory receptors is followed later by chemically induced bronchoconstriction. Only the early but not the late reaction was reduced significantly 90 min after inhalation of 780 μg ipratropium bromide in the normal subjects (Fig. 7; Lewis et al., 1983), a result similar to the one obtained previously by Mathé and Hedqvist (1975) in asthmatic patients. The pattern was also observed in at least 3 of the 7 asthmatic patients in the study by Fish et al. In the remaining patients there was either no effect of atropine or only a slight rightward shift of the dose-response curve. Thus anticholinergic drugs can inhibit or block the "early" (low dose), but not the "late" (high dose)

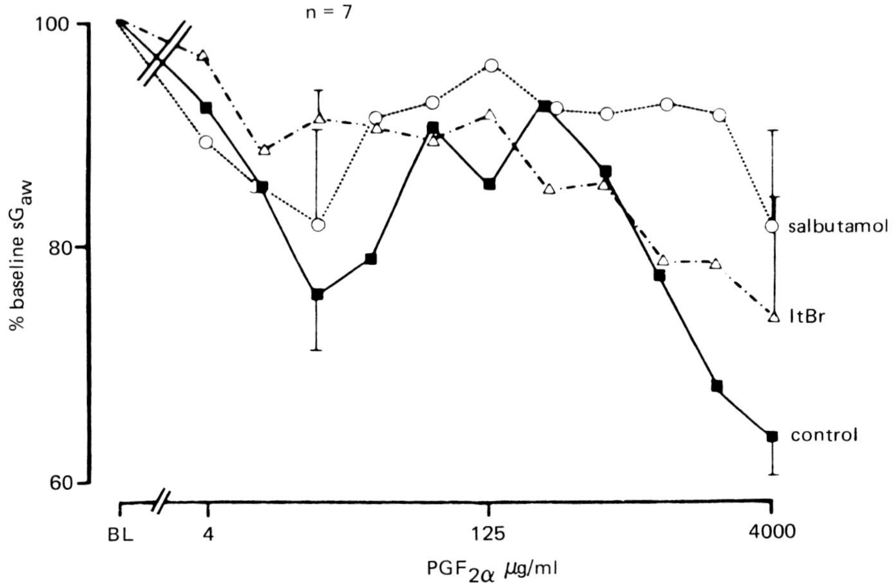

Figure 7 Cumulative dose response to $PGF_{2\alpha}$ inhalation in 7 normal subjects with no premedication (closed squares), 90 min after inhalation of ipratropium bromide (ItBr, mean total dose, 780 μg, open triangles) and 15 min after inhalation of salbutamol (mean total dose, 6100 μg, open circles) (from Lewis et al., 1983, by permission).

response to prostaglandin F_{2a}. The different mechanisms presumably involved in PFG_{2a}-induced bronchoconstriction can explain discrepancies in earlier studies.

Dilator prostaglandins cause diverse effects depending on whether direct or indirect (irritant) effects predominate. Although the direct effect of prostaglandins of the E-series (prostaglandin E_1, E_2) and of the I series (prostaglandin I_2) on airway smooth muscle is relaxation these substances cause cough, irritation of the upper respiratory tract, retrosternal soreness and "paradoxical" bronchoconstriction asthmatic subjects being particularly prone to these effects (Herxheimer and Roetscher, 1971; Kawakami et al., 1973; Mathé and Hedqvist, 1875; Smith and Cuthbert, 1972). In a recent study PGI_2 caused bronchoconstriction in one of seven asthmatic subjects, bronchodilation in two and no change in four (Hardy et al., 1985). Cholinergic blockade blocks such reflex constrictor effects although this has only been studied in the dog thus far (Roberts et al., 1985).

Leukotrienes

The rather short-lived bronchoconstrictor effects of intravenous, but not of inhaled leukotriene D_4 in rats were partially blocked by atropine. However, these effects were also blocked by inhibitors of cyclo-oxygenase and of thromboxane synthetase, so atropine could have acted on systems other than leukotrienes (Hamel et al., 1982). The contractile effect of leukotrienes C_4 and D_4 on isolated human airway smooth muscle could not be blocked by 10^{-6} M atropine (Jones et al., 1982). However, in normal subjects the dose of LTD_4 reducing SGaw 35% increased from 5 to 12.8×10^{-5} M/L after 1.5 mg aerosolized atropine (Smith et al., 1986). It appears that the predominant effect of leukotrienes on isolated airway smooth muscle is direct and is not blockable by atropine. However, leukotrienes have additional effects in vivo both when inhaled and injected and for some of these effects cholinergic pathways are important.

Platelet Activating Factor (PAF)

The degree and time course of PAF-induced bronchoconstriction following intratracheal instillation in baboons was not in any way altered by atropine injected 3 min after PAF application (Denjean et al., 1983). However, the sequence of injections (PAF first, atropine second) would have made it difficult for atropine to have an effect because of its slow onset of action. At this time we do not know if PAF plays an important role as a mediator of human asthma nor if a cholinergic pathway is involved in PAF-induced bronchoconstriction.

Sulfur Dioxide (SO_2)

Results from animal studies have shown a strong effect of high and moderate doses of SO_2 on sensory receptors in lungs and larynx (Roberts et al., 1982; Schultz et al., 1982). Constrictor effects of SO_2 on airway smooth muscle, stimulatory effects on secretion of mucus from tracheal submucosal glands and SO_2-induced rapid shallow breathing have been blocked entirely by atropine or by section of the cervical vagus nerves (Nadel et al., 1965; Hahn et al., 1982; Roberts et al., 1982). Results in man have not been similarly unequivocal. Subcutaneous 1.2-1.8 mg atropine (Nadel et al., 1965) or 7 mg atropine given by inhalation blocked bronchoconstrictor effects of up to 6 ppm SO_2 in normal volunteers and in atopic and asthmatic patients. Ipratropium 80 μg inhibited the bronchoconstriction induced by 10-20 ppm SO_2 only partially (Tan et al., 1982). Up to 4 mg atropine methonitrate inhibited the bronchoconstrictor effects of 8 ppm only in normal subjects, but augmented the bronchoconstrictor effect of 4-8 ppm SO_2 in 3 of 4 asthmatic patients (Snashall and Baldwin, 1982). Thus strong though not complete protection by atropine against SO_2-induced bronchoconstriction has been found in normal individuals while there was less protection in patients with asthma.

Citric Acid

Citric acid induces bronchoconstriction in subjects with airway hyperresponsiveness, but not in those without (Empey et al., 1976; Simonsson et al., 1967; Hirshman et al., 1980, 1984). Changes were prevented completely by IV injection of 1-2 mg atropine (Simonsson et al., 1967). Similar bronchoconstriction was observed and was prevented by atropine inhalation (0.2%, 20 breaths) in normal subjects during viral infections (Empey et al., 1976). Very rapid changes were investigated in these studies in awake subjects in contrast to several studies in anesthetized hyperreactive dogs developing bronchoconstriction in response to prolonged inhalation of citric acid. Atropine was ineffective in these experiments as it was on the bronchoconstriction induced by calcium chelators (Downes and Hirshman, 1983, 1985). Simonsson and Empey studied an effect with the typical features of a reflex: rapid onset and quick adaptation, Hirshman studied a humoral or metabolic event with slow onset and a gradual increase with time. In conclusion, the effects of brief exposures to citric acid can be blocked by atropine, longer exposures act by a different mechanism (tested only in dogs thus far) and are not blocked by atropine.

Distilled Water

Distilled water inhaled from an ultrasonic nebulizer by asthmatic subjects will cause bronchoconstriction (Allegra and Bianco, 1980). This is in contrast to normal subjects who do not respond in this way (e.g., Bianco, 1982; Chadha et al., 1984). Effects on baseline variables were the same for fenoterol and oxytropium bromide in 12 asthmatic patients (Bianco et al., 1983), but oxytropium bromide afforded significantly less protection (29.6%) than fenoterol (62.6%) against the increase in specific airway resistance (SRaw) following inhalation of a distilled water aerosol. The bronchoconstrictor response to distilled water aerosol was unaffected by the IV injection of 1 mg atropine 15 min before challenge or by 1 injection each 30 and 15 min before challenge in patients with asthma or chronic bronchitis (Cheney and Butler, 1968, 1970). In conclusion, bronchoconstriction induced by the inhalation of aerosols of distilled water is little affected by anticholinergic drugs given intravenously or by inhalation.

IV. Longitudinal Distribution of Effect of Anticholinergic Drugs

A. Methodological Factors Influencing Longitudinal Distribution

Some of the differences shown in the literature are due not to inherent differences in airway smooth muscle from different airway generations, but to other influences. They include route of administration, dose of anticholinergic drug, and type of measurement (e.g., bronchograms vs. resistance measurements) as summarized in a previous review (Hahn and Nadel, 1981).

B. Longitudinal Distribution of Cholinergic and Anticholinergic Influences

Experimental Studies

Experimental studies using functional and morphologic methods would appear to give the most precise information on the longitudinal distribution of cholinergic influences. Tantalum bronchography has been most useful for studying the distribution of vagal effects. The bronchoconstrictive effect of vagal stimulation is weakest in the trachea, increases toward the periphery, and is most pronounced in airways 5-1 mm in diameter. Vagally induced bronchoconstriction is weak again or even absent in airways with a diameter less than 1 mm. Several studies agree on this pattern of innervation (Nadel et al., 1971; Hahn et al., 1976; Matsumoto et al., 1985; Inoue et al., 1986). It is likely that the longitudinal distribution of vagal effects does not depend on receptor density but on such nonspecific factors as differences in the amount of smooth muscle in different bronchial generations, mucosal thickness, and creasing of the mucosa in airways (Russell, 1978; Hutt and Wick, 1956; Bouhuys, 1963; Freedman, 1972; James et al., 1986; Inoue et al., 1986). That the distribution of vagal effects may not depend solely on receptor density is also supported by the fact (a) that the same distribution of effects is found whether bronchomotor tone is increased by vagal stimulation (Nadel et al., 1971; Hahn et al., 1976), an infusion of serotonin (Matsumoto et al., 1985), or of leukotriene D_4 (Inoue et al., 1986), (b) that adrenergic and nonadrenergic bronchodilation are most effective in those same airway generations, and (c) that studies of receptor density do not agree at all with the unequivocal functional studies mentioned. Muscarinic receptors are present in high density in smooth muscle of large airways (Cheng and Townley, 1982; Barnes et al., 1983), but decrease toward the periphery so terminal bronchioles are almost devoid of muscarinic receptors (Barnes et al., 1983). Only in bronchi smaller than 1 mm do autoradiographic functional and receptor binding studies agree in that cholinergic muscarinic stimulation is rather ineffective in causing bronchoconstriction (Hahn et al., 1976; Vornanen and Tirri, 1981; Barnes et al., 1983).

Clinical Studies

We do not know how techniques used experimentally correlate with techniques available to the clinician. It is unknown for instance if maximal bronchodilation in the 1-5 mm airways should appear as a peripheral or as a central effect in studies using He-O_2 flow volume curves, the technique employed most frequently in clinical studies. With an even distribution of anticholinergic drug throughout the bronchial tree bronchodilation might appear as predominantly peripheral. An anticholinergic drug given by aerosol and reaching predominantly large airways may appear to dilate central airways, intravenous atropine may add a peripheral effect (De Troyer et al., 1979). Methods for measuring central, peripheral, and overall airway obstruction vary between authors. FEV_1 and conductance measurements, used as indicators of overall bronchial width by some (Hensley et al., 1978; Rubbin et al., 1982; Douglas et al., 1979a), have been used as indicators of central bronchial width by others (Gross, 1975; Chick and Jenne, 1977). An increase in the vital capacity after ipratropium has been interpreted as an effect on smaller airways leading to diminished air trapping. However, a greater FVC increase results in a smaller increase in mean midexpiratory flow rate (MMEF) simply by the nature of the MMEF measurement (Rubbin et al., 1982) and the measurement of MMEF has been invoked by others as a measure of small airways patency. Density dependence of maximal flow, although widely used, has recently been found not to be an accurate predictor of peripheral airway abnormality when density dependence was compared to morphological findings in surgical specimens (Paré et al., 1985). Other clinical techniques for assessing the longitudinal distribution of airway constriction or dilation—useful sometimes in normal subjects—are less reliable in the patient with airways obstruction. Contradictory results have consequently been found in clinical studies.

A preferential effect of inhaled anticholinergic drugs on central airways was found by Ingram et al. (1977) and Hensley et al. (1978) while in three studies from England there was no evidence for a preferential benefit from inhaled ipratropium on central vs. peripheral bronchoconstriction (Partridge and Saunders, 1981; Douglas et al., 1979a,b). Most studies on normal subjects in whom clinical measurements of central vs. peripheral airways obstruction are most reliable suggest there is no preferential effect of atropine on certain airway generations if only the route of administration is such that the drug can reach central and peripheral muscarinic receptors evenly (Vincent et al., 1970; De Troyer et al., 1979; Weiss et al., 1982) and a large number of patient studies support this concept. It is safe to conclude that predictions as to atropine response cannot be made from studies on the longitudinal distribution of airway obstruction.

V. Development of Tolerance to Anticholinergic Drugs

Tolerance to β-sympathomimetic drugs ("tachyphylaxis") has been shown repeatedly to develop in lymphocytes and polymorphonuclear leukocytes upon chronic treatment although no convincing evidence is available to show that the same happens in airway smooth muscle. In fact, it was shown in the same patients that tachyphylaxis to β-agonists develops in polymorphonuclear leukocytes but not in airway smooth muscle (Busse et al., 1985). Does tolerance develop to anticholinergic drugs?

In early studies no tolerance to the effect of the anticholinergic drug ipratropium bromide on baseline lung function was observed and this has recently been confirmed: Methacholine-induced bronchoconstriction was inhibited by inhaled ipratropium just as effectively after 3 weeks of continuous treatment with four inhalations daily as it was before treatment: (Newcomb et al., 1985). Rebuck et al. (1983) tested the acute FEV_1 response to several drug combinations. Chronic combination treatment with fenoterol decreased the acute bronchodilator response, combination treatment with ipratropium did not.

VI. Supersensitivity to Cholinergic Influences Induced by Anticholinergic Drugs

In rat soleus muscle, extrajunctional acetylcholine receptors increase following treatment with alpha-bungarotoxin-induced blockade of cholinergic transmission and following surgical denervation (Drachman et al., 1982). "Up regulation" of muscarinic receptors has likewise been demonstrated in animals after anatomic denervation or after chronic administration of muscarinic antagonists (Emmelin, 1961; Jaffe and Sharpless, 1968; Hata et al., 1980; Taniguchi et al., 1983; Takeyasu et al., 1979; Wise et al., 1980). Short-lasting rebound hyperresponsiveness was observed in 9 patients with mild asthma given 60 μg ipratropium bromide 4 times daily for 3 weeks. As long as 12 hours after ipratropium withdrawal there was still some protection against methacholine-induced bronchoconstriction, but 24 hr after withdrawal there was an increase in methacholine sensitivity which returned to baseline over the next 72 hours (Newcomb et al., 1985). Receptor studies are necessary to prove that the phenomenon is caused by up regulation of cholinergic muscarinic receptors.

VII. Interaction Between Anticholinergic and Other Drugs

A. Corticosteroids

Altounyan (1964) performed serial spirometry measurements on 96 patients with airway obstruction: 60 patients with corticosteroid responsiveness or proven extrinsic asthma ("asthma") and 36 patients with no or a minimal response to corticosteroid treatment ("bronchitis") during varying phases of their disease. In patients with asthma, the response to atropine was as great as, or exceeded, that to isoproterenol when these patients were in relative remission usually achieved by treatment with corticosteroid drugs. The same patients tested when spirometric measurements had deteriorated showed a significant and progressive decline of the atropine response compared with the isoproterenol response (assessed from similar basal conditions). As a rule bronchitic patients responded better to atropine than to isoproterenol which has been confirmed by a number of studies. Similar, but less impressive results were obtained when prednisolone treatment was limited to 3 days (Lightbody et al., 1978). A striking improvement in the response to atropine could also be shown in 8 patients with asthma given a steroid aerosol (beclomethasone dipropionate) for 4-16 weeks (Jolobe and Lane, 1981). The improvement correlated significantly with the features of allergic airways disease: positive skin tests, blood or sputum eosinophilia and nocturnal wheezing and was considered a result of the improvement specifically of the allergic component of reversible airflow obstruction, not a result of the general improvement in lung function observed. The latter interpretation was favored by Altounyan. Although the mechanism of the steroid-induced improvement in the response to atropine remains unclear the phenomenon is established.

B. Theophylline Preparations

In 12 patients with bronchial asthma, 40 μg ipratropium bromide increased the FEV_1 by 0.12 and 0.05 liters, respectively, 30 and 60 min after inhalation when placebo capsules had been given. Ipratropium-induced increases in FEV_1 were 0.27 and 0.33 liters 60 min after oral theophylline in a dose adjusted to cause blood levels in the upper therapeutic range in each subject. Since the effect of ipratropium should have been the same under both circumstances if its effect had only been additive to the effect of theophylline these results suggested synergism between the two drugs (Kreisman et al., 1981). Similar results were obtained by Rebuck et al. (1983). Again this may be due to a general improvement in the patient's condition or to specific improvement in the allergic component of airflow obstruction.

C. Beta-Sympathomimetic Agents

In 16 studies most authors who gave the two drugs alone and in combination found the combination more effective than either drug alone, some did not (Pavia et al., 1979; Rubbin et al., 1977; Petrie and Palmer, 1975; Ingram et al., 1977), and some found that it varies with the individual (Ullah et al., 1981; Brown et al., 1984). The main reasons for the discrepancy may have been severity of disease and clinical status (exacerbation vs. remission), type of disease (asthma vs. bronchitis), and dose of anticholinergic drug. In severe disease, when bronchitis predominated and when high doses of atropine or ipratropium were given, the combination of adrenergic and anticholinergic drugs was usually superior to either drug given alone (Ward et al., 1981; Douglas et al., 1979a). When asthma predominated and the disease was in acute exacerbation, benefit from atropine was limited (Karpel et al., 1986).

Cholinergic agonists may be of additional benefit in patients who have become unresponsive to isoproterenol. Better bronchodilation was reached by 0.05 mg/kg atropine sulfate aerosol given 60 minutes after isoproterenol (average maximum improvement in FEV_1, 19.2%) than by isoproterenol alone in such patients (improvement in FEV_1, 5.9% measured 15 min after inhalation) (Marini and Lakshminarayan, 1980).

VIII. Paradoxical Effects of Anticholinergic Drugs

It has been known for some time that small doses of atropine cause effects opposite to those seen after "normal" therapeutic doses, that is, in low concentrations atropine behaves as a cholinergic agonist, not as an antagonist. These effects have recently been confirmed for atropine (0.1-1.0 μg/kg) by Fryer and Maclagan (1986) who extended their observations to ipratropium bromide which was found to have an even more potent paradoxical effect than atropine. At 1 μg/kg ipratropium doubled the bronchoconstriction induced by vagal stimulation measured as an increase in pulmonary inflation pressure in urethane-anesthetized guinea pigs. The drug appears to have a similar paradoxical effect on fluid secretion from the airways. This effect appears to extend into a concentration range at which the predominant effect on airway smooth muscle is dilation (Bauer et al., 1976; Engelhardt, 1979) which may indicate different dose-response relationships for effects on glands and on smooth muscle or differences in accessibility to the site of action. The effect could very well explain why ipratropium up to the high dose of 200 μg (10 puffs of regular metered dose inhaler) improves radioaerosol clearance in bronchitic subjects and in normal people (Ruffin et al., 1978) or at least does not inhibit clearance (Francis et al., 1977; Sackner et al., 1977) while therapeutic doses of atropine in most studies either decrease (Annis et al., 1976; Sackner et al., 1977) or even arrest mucociliary transport (Foster et al., 1976). Paradoxical effects of anticholinergic drugs might also explain the transient hypersensitivity of patients to cholinergic stimuli following cessation of ipratropium therapy (Newcomb et al., 1985) which is in contrast to the apparent lack of desensitization to chronic anticholinergic therapy reported by the same (and other) authors. If there is up regulation of receptors after cessation of therapy one would normally expect down regulation during therapy. A report on three patients developing immediate and prolonged falls in daily peak flow rates on treatment with ipratropium bromide, reversible only on stopping therapy, may be similarly explained (Connolly, 1982) as may be the initial bronchoconstriction occurring after inhalation of ipratropium bromide and oxitropium bromide before bronchodilation sets in (Lulling et al., 1981). Finally, paradoxical effects of this type may explain the decrease in heart rate following ipratropium which is in contrast to the tachycardia seen after atropine (see under side effects).

Several mechanisms can explain paradoxical effects of anticholinergic drugs. The secretory effect of ipratropium could be explained by unopposed sympathetic drive stimulating gland secretion, but this does not explain why higher doses of the same drug inhibit secretion. An inhibitory effect of atropine on cholinesterases was observed by Lüllmann et al. (1952). The most likely explanation may be the presence of postganglionic muscarinic inhibitory receptors in pulmonary parasympathetic nerves observed in the guinea pig and cat. Blockade of these receptors by gallamine (0.1 to 5 mg/kg) resulted in potentiation of the bronchoconstrictor effects of vagal stimulation and of postganglionic stimulation (transmural stimulation of the tracheal tube or injection of dimethylphenylpiperazinium, DMPP) in vivo (Fryer and Maclagan, 1984; Blaber et al., 1985) and following pre- and postganglionic stimulation of the tracheal tube in vitro (Faulkner et al., 1986) while the bronchoconstrictor effects of acetylcholine were not potentiated. The muscarinic agonist, pilocarpine, in low concentrations (10 ng to 1 μg/kg) had the opposite effect to gallamine and inhibited contractions of the tracheal tube induced by pre- and postganglionic nerve stimulation.

References

Alanko, K., and Poppius, H. (1973). Anticholinergic blocking of prostaglandin-induced bronchoconstriction. *Br. Med. J.* **1**:294.

Allegra, L., and Bianco, S. (1980). Non-specific bronchoreactivity obtained with an ultrasonic aerosol of distilled water. *Eur. J. Respir. Dis.* **106** (Suppl.):41-49.

Allen, C. J., and Campbell, A. H. (1979). Dose response of ipratropium bromide assessed by two methods. *Thorax* **34**:137-139.

Altounyan, R. E. C. (1964). Variation of drug action on airway obstruction in man. *Thorax* **19**:406-415.

Annis, P., Landa, J., and Lichtiger, M. (1976). Effects of atropine on velocity of tracheal mucus in anesthetized patients. *Anesthesiology* **44**:74-77.

Astin, T. W. (1972). Reversibility of airways obstruction in chronic bronchitis. *Clin. Sci.* **42**:725-733.

Bandouvakis, J., Cartier, A., Roberts, R., Ryan, G., and Hargreave, F. E. (1981). The effect of ipratropium and fenoterol on methacholine- and histamine-induced bronchoconstriction. *Br. J. Dis. Chest* **75**:295-305.

Barber, P. V., Chatterjee, S. S., and Scott, R. (1977). A comparison of ipratropium bromide, deptropine citrate and placebo in asthma and chronic bronchitis. *Br. J. Dis. Chest* **71**:101-104.

Barnes, P. J., Basbaum, C. B., Nadel, J. A., and Roberts, J. M. (1982). Localization of β-adrenoreceptors in mammalian lung by light microscopic autoradiography. *Nature* **299**:444-447.

Barnes, P. J., Nadel, J. A., Roberts, J. M., and Basbaum, C. B. (1983). Muscarinic receptors in lung and trachea: autoradiographic localization using [^{3}H]-quinuclidinyl benzilate. *Eur. J. Pharmacol.* **86**:103-106.

Bauer, R., Püschmann, S., and Wick, H. (1976). Wirkung von (8r)-3α-Hydroxy-8-isopropyl-1αH,5αH-tropaniumbromid-($\pm$)-tropat (Ipratropiumbromid) auf

Spasmen des Tracheobronchialbaumes und die Bronchialsekretion, die Speichelsekretion, EKG und Herzfrequenz. *Arzneim.-Forsch.* **26**:981-985.

Bianco, S. (1982). Bronchial hyperreactivity in response to inhalation of ultrasonically nebulised solutions of distilled water and saline. *Br. Med. J.* **284**: 417-418.

Bianco, S., Robuschi, M., Damonte, C., Allegra, L., and Pasargiklian, M. (1983). Prevention of the bronchoconstriction induced by an ultrasonic mist of distilled water by fenoterol and oxitropium bromide. In *Role of Anticholinergic Drugs in Obstructive Airway Disease.* Edited by G. Schultze-Werninghaus and J. G. Widdicombe. München, Gedon u. Reuss Verlag, pp. 92-100.

Blaber, L. C., Fryer, A. D., and Maclagan, J. (1985). Neuronal muscarinic receptors attenuate vagally-induced contraction of feline bronchial smooth muscle. *Br. J. Pharmacol.* **86**:723-728.

Borson, D. B., Charlin, M., Gold, B. D., and Nadel, J. A. (1984). Neural regulation of $^{35}SO_4$-macromolecule secretion from tracheal glands of ferrets. *J. Appl. Physiol.* **57**:457-466.

Botts, L. D., Pingleton, S. K., Schroeder, C. E., Robinson, R. G., and Hurwitz, A. (1985). Prolongation of gastric emptying by aerosolized atropine. *Am. Rev. Respir. Dis.* **131**:725-726.

Bouhuys, A. (1963). Effect of posture in experimental asthma in man. *Am. J. Med.* **34**:470-476.

Brown, I. G., Chan, C. S., Kelly, C. A., Dent, A. G., and Zimmerman, P. V. (1984). Assessment of the clinical usefulness of nebulised ipratropium bromide in patients with chronic airflow limiations. *Thorax* **39**:272-276.

Burge, P. S., Harries, M. G., and I'Anson, E. (1980). Comparison of atropine with ipratropium bromide in patients with reversible airways obstruction unresponsive to salbutamol. *Br. J. Dis. Chest* **74**:259-262.

Burgen, A. S. V., Hiley, C. R., and Young, J. M. (1974). The properties of muscarinic receptors in mammalian cerebral cortex. *Br. J. Pharmacol.* **51**:279-285.

Busse, W. W., Sharpe, G., Smith, A., Arbabian, M., Borgen, L., and Ruoho, A. (1985). The effect of procaterol treatment on beta-adrenergic bronchodilation and polymorphonuclear leukocyte responsiveness. *Am. Rev. Respir. Dis.* **132**:1194-1198.

Chadha, T. S., Birch, S., Allegra, L., and Sackner, M. A. (1984). Effects of ultrasonically nebulized distilled water on respiratory resistance and Breathing pattern in normals and asthmatics. *Bull. Eur. Physiopathol. Respir. Clin. Respir. Physiol.* **20**:257-262.

Chapman, K. R., Smith, D. L., Rebuck, A. S., and Leenen, F. H. H. (1985). Hemodynamic effects of inhaled ipratropium bromide, alone and combined with an inhaled beta$_2$-agonist. *Am. Rev. Respir. Dis.* **132**:845-847.

Chen, W. Y., Brenner, A. M., Weiser, P. C., and Chai, H. (1981). Atropine and exercise-induced bronchoconstriction. *Chest* **79**:651-656.

Cheney, F. W., and Butler, J. (1968). The effects of ultrasonically-produced aerosols on airway resistance in man. *Anesthesiology* **29**:1099-1106.

Cheney, F. W., and Butler, J. (1970). The effects of ultrasonic aerosols on the total respiratory resistance of the intubated patient. *Anesthesiology* **32**: 456-458.

Cheng, J. B., and Townley, R. G. (1982). Comparison of muscarinic and beta adrenergic receptors between bovine peripheral lung and tracheal smooth muscles: a striking difference in the receptor concentration. *Life Sci.* **30**: 2079-2086.

Chick, T. W., and Jenne, J. W. (1977). Comparative bronchodilator responses to atropine and terbutaline in asthma and chronic bronchitis. *Chest* **72**: 719-723.

Cockcroft, D. W., Cotton, D. J., and Berscheid, B. A. (1982). Long-term efficiency and safety of inhaled Sch 1000, an anticholinergic bronchodilator. *Curr. Ther. Res.* **31**:138-147.

Connolly, C. K. (1982). Adverse reaction to ipratropium bromide. *Br. Med. J.* **285**:934-935.

Cushley, M. J., Tattersfield, A. E., and Holgate, S. T., (1983). Inhaled adenosine and guanosine on airway resistance in normal and asthmatic subjects. *Br. J. Clin. Pharmacol.* **15**:161-165.

Denjean, A., Arnoux, B., Masse, R., Lockhart, A., and Benveniste, J. (1983). Acute effects of intratracheal administration of platelet-activating factor in baboons. *J. Appl. Physiol.* **55**:799-804.

De Troyer, A., Yernault, J.-C., and Rodenstein, D. (1979). Effects of vagal blockade on lung mechanics in normal man. *J. Appl. Physiol.* **46**:217-226.

Douglas, N. J., Davidson, I., Sudlow, M. F., and Flenley, D. C. (1979a). Bronchodilatation and the site of airway resistance in severe chronic bronchitis. *Thorax* **34**:51-56.

Douglas, N. J., Sudlow, M. F., and Flenley, D. C. (1979b). Effect of an inhaled atropinelike agent on normal airway function. *J. Appl. Physiol.* **46**: 256-262.

Downes, H., and Hirshman, A. (1983). Importance of calcium in citric acid-induced airway constriction. *J. Appl. Physiol.* **55**:1496-1500.

Downes, H., and Hirshman, C. A. (1985). Calcium chelators increase airway responsiveness. *J. Appl. Physiol.* **59**:92-95.

Drachman, D. B., Stanley, E. F., Pestronk, A., Griffin, J. W., and Price, D. L. (1982). Neurotrophic regulation of two properties of skeletal muscle by impulse-dependent and spontaneous acetylcholine transmission. *J. Neurosci.* **2**:232-243.

Drazen, J. H., and Austen, K. F. (1975). Atropine modification of the pulmonary effects of chemical mediators in the guinea pig. *J. Appl. Physiol.* **38**:834-838.

Eiser, N. M., and Guz, A. (1982). Effect of atropine on experimentally-induced airway obstruction in man. *Bull. Resp., Clin. Respir. Physiol.* **18**:449-460.

Emmelin, N. (1961). Supersensitivity following "pharmacologic denervation." *Pharmacol. Rev.* **13**:16-37.

Empey, D. W., Laitinen, L. A., Jacobs, L., Gold, W. M., and Nadel, J. A. (1976). Mechanisms of bronchial hyperreactivity in normal subjects after upper respiratory tract infection. *Am. Rev. Respir. Dis.* **113**:131-139.

Engelhardt, A. (1979). Pharmacology and toxicology of atrovent. *Scand. J. Respir. Dis.* **103** (Suppl.):110-115.

Faulkner, D., Fryer, A. D., and Maclagan, J. (1986). Postganglionic muscarinic inhibitory receptors in pulmonary parasympathetic nerves in the guinea-pig. *Br. J. Pharmacol.* **88**:181-187.

Fish, J. E., Newball, H. H., Norman, P. S., and Peterman, V. I. (1983). Novel effects of $PGF_{2\alpha}$ on airway function in asthmatic subjects. *J. Appl. Physiol.* **54**:105-112.

Foster, W. M., Bergofsky, E. H., Bohning, D. E., Lippmann, M., and Albert, R. E. (1976). Effect of adrenergic agents and their mode of action on mucociliary clearance in man. *J. Appl. Physiol.* **41**:146-152.

Francis, R. A., Thomson, M. L., Pavia, D., and Douglas, R. B. (1977). Ipratropium bromide: mucociliary clearance rate and airway resistance in normal subjects. *Br. J. Dis. Chest* **71**:173-178.

Freedman, B. J. (1972). The functional geometry of the bronchi. *Bull. Physiopathol. Resp.* **8**:545-551.

Freedman, B. J. (1978). Patterns of response to bronchodilators in asthma. *Br. J. Dis. Chest* **72**:95-107.

Friedman, M., Hornaday, B. L., Fullton, J. M., and Donohue, J. F. (1986). Dose response effects of ipratropium bromide (Atrovent®) in chronic bronchitis (CB). *Am. Rev. Respir. Dis.* **133** (4, part 2):A 63 (abstr).

Fryer, A. D., and Maclagan, J. (1984). Muscarinic inhibitory receptors in pulmonary parasympathetic nerves in the guinea-pig. *Br. J. Pharmacol.* **83**:973-978.

Fryer, A. D., and Maclagan, J. (1986). Ipratropium bromide potentiates bronchoconstriction induced by vagal nerve stimulation. *Am. Rev. Respir. Dis.* **133**(4, part 2):A 13 (abstr).

Gal, T. J., Suratt, P. M., and Lu, J.-Y. (1984). Glycopyrrolate and atropine inhalation: comparative effects on normal airway function. *Am. Rev. Respir. Dis.* **129**:871-873.

Gallagher, J. T., Kent, P. W., Passatore, M., Phipps, R. J., and Richardson, P. S. (1975). The composition of tracheal mucus and the nervous control of its secretion in the cat. *Proc. R. Soc. Lond. B.* **192**:49-76.

Gold, W. M., Kessler, G.-F., and Yu, D. Y. C. (1972). Role of vagus nerves in experimental asthma in allergic dogs. *J. Appl. Physiol.* **33**:719-725.

Griffin, M. P., Fung, K. F., Ingram, R. H., and McFadden, E. R. (1982). Dose-response effects of atropine on thermal stimulus-response relationships in asthma. *J. Appl. Physiol.* **53**:1576-1582.

Gross. N. J. (1975). Sch. 1000: A new anticholinergic bronchodilator. *Am. Rev. Respir. Dis.* **112**:823-828.

Gross, N. J. (1986). COPD: a disease of reversible air-flow obstruction. *Am. Rev. Respir. Dis.* **133**:725-726.

Hahn, H. L., Graf, P. D., and Nadel, J. A. (1976). Effect of vagal tone on airway diameters and on lung volume in anesthetized dogs. *J. Appl. Physiol.* **41**:581-589.

Hahn, H. L., and Nadel, J. A. (1981). Methods of study of airway smooth muscle and its physiology. In *International Encyclopedia of Pharmacology and Therapeutics.* Section 104. *Respiration Pharmacology.* Edited by J. G. Widdicombe, Oxford, New York, Pergamon Press, pp. 501-543.

Hahn, R. A., and Patil, P. N. (1972). Salivation induced by prostaglandin $F_{2\alpha}$ and modification of the response by atropine and physostigmine. *Br. J. Pharmacol.* **44**:527-533.

Hahn, R. A., and Patil, P. N. (1974). Further observations on the interaction of prostaglandin $F_{2\alpha}$ with cholinergic mechanisms in canine salivary glands. *Eur. J. Pharmacol.* **25**:279-286.

Hahn, H. L., Saski, K., and Nadel, J. A. (1982). Effects of sulfur dioxide on ventilation in conscious dogs. *Am. Rev. Respir. Dis.* **125** (4, part 2):220 (abstr).

Hamel, R., Masson, P., Ford-Hutchinson, A. W., Jones, T. R., Brunet, G., and Piechuta, H. (1982). Differing mechanisms for leukotriene D_4-induced bronchoconstriction in guinea pigs following intravenous and aerosol administration. *Prostaglandins* **24**:419-432.

Hanley, S. P., Garrett, H., Britton, J. R., Hadfield, J., and Tattersfield, A. E. (1986). Differential effects of salbutamol and ipratropium bromide on airway calibre and reactivity to histamine in asthma. *Am. Rev. Respir. Dis.* **133** (4, part 2):A 177 (abstr).

Hardy, C., Robinson, C., Lewis, R. A., Tattersfield, A. E., and Holgate, S. T. (1985). Airway and cardiovascular responses to inhaled prostacyclin in normal and asthmatic subjects. *Am. Rev. Respir. Dis.* **131**:18-21.

Harrison, L. I., Smallridge, R. C., Lasseter, K. C., Goldlust, M. B., Shamblen, E. C., Gam, V. W., Chang, S. F., and Kvam, D. C. (1986). Comparative absorption of inhaled and intramuscularly administered atropine. *Am. Rev. Respir. Dis.* **134**:254-257.

Hata, F., Takeyasu, K., Morikawa, Y., Lai, R.-T., Ishida, H., and Yoshida, H. (1980). Specific changes in the cholinergic system in guinea-pig vas deferens after denervation. *J. Pharmacol. Exp. Ther.* **215**:716-722.

Hawkins, D. F., and Schild, H. O. (1951). The action of drugs on isolated human bronchial chains. *Br. J. Pharmacol.* **6**:682-690.

Hensley, M. J., O'Cain, C. F., McFadden, E. R., and Ingram, R. H. (1978). Distribution of bronchodilatation in normal subjects: beta agonist versus atropine. *J. Appl. Physiol.* **45**:778-782.

Herxheimer, H., and Roetscher, I. (1971). Effects of prostaglandin E_1 on lung function in bronchial asthma. *Eur. J. Clin. Pharmacol.* **3**:123-125.

Hirshman, C. A., Downes, H., and Veith, L. (1984). Airway responses in offspring of dogs with and without airway hyperreactivity. *J. Appl. Physiol.* **56**:1272-1277.

Hirshman, C. A., Malley, A., and Downes, H. (1980). Basenji-Greyhound dog model of asthma: reactivity to *Ascaris suum,* citric acid, and methacholine. *J. Appl. Physiol.* **49**:953-957.

Holtzman, M. J., Hahn, H.-L., Sasaki, K., Skoogh, B.-E., Graf, P. D., Fabbri, L. M., and Nadel, J. A. (1982). Selective effect of general anesthetics on reflex bronchoconstrictor responses in dogs. *J. Appl. Physiol.* **53**:126-133.

Holtzman, M. J., McNamara, M. P., Sheppard, D., Fabbri, L. M., Hahn, H. L., Graf, P. D., and Nadel, J. A. (1983). Intravenous versus inhaled atropine for inhibiting bronchoconstrictor responses in dogs. *J. Appl. Physiol.* **54**:134-139.

Howarth, P. H., Durham, S. R., Lee, T. H., Kay, A. B., Church, M. K., and Holgate, S. T. (1985). Influence of albuterol, cromolyn sodium and ipratropium bromide on the airway and circulating mediator responses to allergen bronchial provocation in asthma. *Am. Rev. Respir. Dis.* **132**:986-992.

Hume, K. M., and Gandevia, B. (1957). Forced expiratory volume before and after isoprenaline. *Thorax* **12**:276-278.

Hutt, G., and Wick, H. (1956). Bronchiallumen und Atemwiderstand. *Zeitschr. Aerosol Forsch. Ther.* **5**:131-140.

Ingram, R. H., Wellman, J. J., McFadden, E. R., and Mead, J. (1977). Relative contributions of large and small airways to flow limitation in normal subjects before and after atropine and isoproterenol. *J. Clin. Invest.* **59**:696-703.

Inoue, H., Ichinose, M., Miura, M., Haraoka, I., and Takishima, T. (1986). Sites of LTD_4-induced bronchoconstriction, and an inhibitory effect of KC404 on cat airways. *Am. Rev. Respir. Dis.* **133** (4, part 2):A 114 (abstr).

Jaffe, J. H., and Sharpless, S. K. (1968). Pharmacological denervation supersensitivity in the central nervous system: a theory of physical dependence. *Res. Publ. Assoc. Nerv. Ment. Dis.* **46**:226-240.

James, A. L., Paré, P. D., Moreno, R., and Hogg, J. C. (1986). Smooth muscle shortening and airway narrowing in porcine tracheal rings. *Am. Rev. Respir. Dis.* **133** (4, part 2):A 113 (abstr.).

Jannun, D. R., and Mickel, S. F. (1986). Anisocoria and aerosolized anticholinergics. *Chest* **90**:148-149.

Jolobe, O. M. P., and Lane, D. J. (1981). Atropine responsiveness in asthma in relation to steroid aerosol therapy. *Br. J. Dis. Chest* **75**:413-416.

Jones, T. R., Davis, C., and Daniel, E. E. (1982). Pharmacological study of the contractile activity of leukotriene C_4 and D_4 on isolated human airway smooth muscle. *Can. J. Physiol. Pharmacol.* **60**:638-643.

Karpel, J. P., Appel, D., Breidbart, D., and Fusco, M. J. (1986). A comparison of atropine surfate and metaproterenol sulfate in the emergency treatment of asthma. *Am. Rev. Respir. Dis.* **133**:727-729.

Kawakami, Y., Uchiyama, K., Irie, T., and Murao, M. (1973). Evaluation of aerosols of prostaglandins E_1 and E_2 as bronchodilators. *Eur. J. Clin. Pharmacol.* **6**:127-132.

Klock, L. E., Miller, T. D., Morris, A. H., Watanabe, S., and Dickman, M. (1975). A comparative study of atropine sulfate and isoproterenol hydrochloride in chronic bronchitis. *Am. Rev. Respir. Dis.* **112**:371-376.

Kradjan, W. A., Lakshminarayan, S., Hayden, P. W., Larson, S. W., and Marini, J. J. (1981). Serum atropine concentrations after inhalation of atropine sulfate. *Am. Rev. Respir. Dis.* **123**:471-472.

Kreisman, H., Frank, H., Wolkove, N., and Gent, M. (1981). Synergism between ipratropium and theophylline in asthma. *Thorax* **36**:387-391.

Laitinen, L. A., Viljanen, A. A., and Viljanen, B. C. (1979). The effects of ipratropium bromide on the histamine inhalation challenge in asthmatic and bronchitic patients. *Scand, J. Respir. Dis.* **103** (Suppl.):215-218.

Lewis, R. A., Hardy, C., and Tattersfield, A. E. (1983). A differential response to low and high dose inhaled prostaglandin $F_{2\alpha}$ in normal subjects. In *Role of Anticholinergic Drugs in Obstructive Airway Disease.* Edited by G. Schultze-Werninghaus and J. G. Widdicombe. München, Gedon u. Reuss Verlag, pp. 84-91.

Light, R. W., and George, R. B. (1977). Oral atropine in the treatment of chronic asthma. *Ann. Allergy* **38**:58-61.

Lightbody, I. M., Ingram, C. G., Legge, J. S., and Johnston, R. N. (1978). Ipratropium bromide, salbutamol and prednisolone in bronchial asthma and chronic bronchitis. *Br. J. Dis. Chest* **72**:181-186.

Lin, M. T., Lee-Hong, E., and Collins-Williams, C. (1982). A clinical trial of the bronchodilator effect of Sch 1000 aerosol in asthmatic children. *Ann. Allergy* **40**:326-332.

Lulling, J., Delwiche, J. P., and Prignot, J. (1981). Early bronchodilating effect of oxitropium bromide in comparison with ipratropium bromide. *Respiration* **42**:188-192.

Lüllmann, H., Förster, W., and Westermann, E. (1952). Über eine "paradoxe" Atropinwirkung an isolierten Organen und ihre statistische Erfassung. *Arch. Exp. Path. Pharmak.* **215**:8-18.

McFadden, E. R. (1986). Critical appraisal of the therapy of asthma—an idea whose time has come. *Am. Rev. Respir. Dis.* **133**:723-724.

Malani, J. T., Robinson, G. M., and Seneviratne, E. L. (1982). Ipratropium bromide induced angle closure glaucoma. *N.Z. Med. J.* **95**:749.

Mann, J. S., Cushley, M. J., and Holgate, S. T. (1985). Adenosine-induced bronchoconstriction in asthma. Role of parasympathetic stimulation and adrenergic inhibition. *Am. Rev. Respir. Dis.* **132**:1-6.

Marini, J. J., and Lakshminarayan, S. (1980). The effect of atropine inhalation in "irreversible" chronic bronchitis. *Chest* **77**:591-596.

Mathé, A. A., and Hedqvist, P. (1975). Effect of prostaglandins F_{2a} and E_2 on airway conductance in healthy subjects and asthmatic patients. *Am. Rev. Respir. Dis.* **111**:313-320.

Matsumoto, N., Inoue, H., Ichinose, M., Ishii, M., Inoue, C., Sasaki, H., and Takishima, T. (1985). Effective sites by sympathetic beta-adrenergic and vagal nonadrenergic inhibitory stimulation in constricted airways. *Am. Rev. Respir. Dis.* **132**:1113-1117.

Nadel, J. A., Cabezas, G. A., and Austin, J. H. M. (1971). In vivo roentgenographic examination of parasympathetic innervation of small airways. Use of powdered tantalum and a fine focal spot X-ray tube. *Invest. Radiol.* **6**: 9-17.

Nadel, J. A., Salem, H., Tamplin, B., and Tokiwa, Y. (1965). Mechanism of bronchoconstriction during inhalation of sulfur dioxide. *J. Appl. Physiol.* **20**:164-167.

Newcomb, R., Tashkin, D. P., Hui, K. K., Conolly, M. E., Lee, E., and Dauphinee, B. (1985). Rebound hyperresponsiveness to muscarinic stimulation after chronic therapy with an inhaled muscarinic antagonist. *Am. Rev. Respir. Dis.* **132**:12-15.

Pak, C. C. F., Kradjan, W. A., Lakshminarayan, S., and Marini, J. J. (1982). Inhaled atropine sulfate. Dose-response characteristics in adult patients with chronic airflow obstruction. *Am. Rev. Respir. Dis.* **125**:331-334.

Paré, P. D., Brooks, L. A., Coppin, C. A., Wright, J. L., Kennedy, S., Dahlby, R., Mink, S., and Hogg, J. C. (1985). Density-dependence of maximal expiratory flow and its correlation with small airway disease in smokers. *Am. Rev. Respir. Dis.* **131**:521-526.

Partridge, M. R., and Saunders, K. B. (1981). Site of action of ipratropium bromide and clinical and physiological determinants of response in patients with asthma. *Thorax* **36**:530-533.

Pasterkamp, H., Tal, A., Leahy, F., Fenton, R., and Chernick, V. (1985). The effect of anticholinergic treatment on postexertional wheezing in asthma studied by phonopneumography and spirometry. *Am. Rev. Respir. Dis.* **132**:16-21.

Patel, K. R. (1975). Atropine, sodium cromoglycate, and thymoxamine in $PGF_{2\alpha}$-induced bronchoconstriction in extrinsic asthma. *Br. Med. J.* **2**:360-362.

Pavia, D., Bateman, J. R. M., Sheahan, N. F., and Clarke, S. W. (1979). Effect of ipratropium bromide on mucociliary clearance and pulmonary function in reversible airways obstruction. *Thorax* **34**:501-507.

Petrie, G. R., and Palmer, K. N. V. (1975). Comparison of aerosol ipratropium bromide and salbutamol in chronic bronchitis and asthma. *Br. Med. J.* **1**:430-432.

Rebuck, A. S., Gent, M., and Chapman, K. R. (1983). Anticholinergic and sympathomimetic combination therapy of asthma. *J. Allergy Clin. Immunol.* **71**:317-323.

Roberts, A. M., Hahn, H. L., Schultz, H. D., Nadel, J. A., Coleridge, H. M., and Coleridge, J. C. G. (1982). Afferent vagal C-fibers are responsible for the reflex airway constriction and secretion evoked by pulmonary administration of SO_2 in dogs. *Physiologist* **25**:226 (abstr).

Roberts, A. M., Schultz, H. D., Green, J. F., Armstrong, D. J., Kaufman, M. P., Coleridge, H. M., and Coleridge, J. C. G. (1985). Reflex tracheal contraction evoked in dogs by bronchodilator prostaglandins E_2 and I_2. *J. Appl. Physiol.* **58**:1823-1831.

Rominger, K. L. (1979). Chemistry and pharmacokinetics of ipratropium bromide. *Scand. J. Respir. Dis.* **103** (Suppl.):116-126.

Rosenthal, R. R., Norman, P. S., Summer, W. R., and Permutt, S. (1977). Role of the parasympathetic system in antigen-induced bronchospasm. *J. Appl. Physiol.* **42**:600-606.

Ruffin, R. E., Cockcroft, D. W., and Hargreave, F. E. (1978). A comparison of the protective effect of fenoterol and Sch 1000 on allergen-induced asthma. *J. Allergy Clin. Immunol.* **61**:42-47.

Ruffin, R. E., Fitzgerald, J. D., and Rebuck, A. S. (1977). A comparison of the bronchodilator activity of Sch 1000 and salbutamol. *J. Allergy Clin. Immunol.* **59**:136-141.

Ruffin, R. E., McIntyre, E., Crockett, A. J., Zielonka, K., and Alpers, J. H. (1982). Combination bronchodilator therapy in asthma. *J. Allergy Clin. Immunol.* **69**:60-65.

Ruffin, R. E., Wolff, R. K., Dolovich, M. B., Rossman, C. M., Fitzgerald, J. D., and Newhouse, M. T. (1978). Aerosol therapy with Sch 1000. Short-term mucociliary clearance in normal and bronchitic subjects and toxicology in normal subjects. *Chest* **73**:501-506.

Russell, J. A. (1978). Responses of isolated canine airways to electric stimulation and acetylcholine. *J. Appl. Physiol.* **45**:690-698.

Sackner, M. A., Chapman, G. A., and Dougherty, R. D. (1977a). Effects of nebulized ipratropium bromide and atropine sulfate on tracheal mucous velocity and lung mechanics in anesthetized dogs. *Respiration* **34**:181-185.

Sackner, M. A., Friedman, M., Silva, G., and Fernandez, R. (1977b). The pulmonary hemodynamic effects of aerosols of isoproterenol and ipratropium in normal subjects and patients with reversible airway obstruction. *Am. Rev. Respir. Dis.* **116**:1013-1022.

Schulman, E. S., Newball, H. H., Demers, L. M., Fitzpatrick, F. A., and Adkinson, N. F., Jr. (1981). Anaphylactic release of thromboxane A_2, prostaglandin D_2, and prostacyclin from human lung parenchyma. *Am. Rev. Respir. Dis.* **124**:402-406.

Schultz, H. D., Roberts, A. M., Hahn, H. L., Nadel, J. A., Coleridge, H. M., and Coleridge, J. C. G. (1982). Mechanism of airway constriction and secretion evoked by laryngeal administration of SO_2 in dogs. *Physiologist* **25**: 226 (abstr).

Sheppard, D., Epstein, J., Holtzman, M. J., Nadel, J. A., and Boushey, H. A. (1982). Dose-dependent inhibition of cold air-induced bronchoconstriction by atropine. *J. Appl. Physiol.* **53**:169-174.

Sheppard, D., Epstein, J., Holtzman, M. J., Nadel, J. A., and Boushey, H. A. (1983). Effect of route of atropine delivery on bronchospasm from cold air and methacholine. *J. Appl. Physiol.* **54**:130-133.

Shore, S. A., Bai, T. R., Wang, C. G., and Martin, J. G. (1985). Central and local cholinergic components of histamine-induced bronchoconstriction in dogs. *J. Appl. Physiol.* **58**:443-451.

Simonsson, B. G., Jacobs, F. M., and Nadel, J. A. (1967). Role of autonomic nervous system and the cough reflex in the increased responsiveness of airways of patients with obstructive airway disease. *J. Clin. Invest.* **46**: 1812-1818.

Skoogh, B.-E., Holtzman, M. J., Sheller, J. R., and Nadel, J. A. (1982). Barbiturates depress vagal motor pathway to ferret trachea at ganglia. *J. Appl. Physiol.* **53**:253-257.

Smith, A. P., and Cuthbert, M. F. (1972). Antagonistic action of aerosols of prostaglandins $F_{2\alpha}$ and E_2 on bronchial muscle tone in man. *Br. Med. J.* **3**:212-213.

Smith, L. J., Kern, R., Patterson, R., Krell, R., and Bernstein, P. R. (1986). Leukotriene D_4-induced bronchoconstriction in normal subjects: mechanism of action. *Am. Rev. Respir. Dis.* **133**(4):A 92 (abstr).

Snashall, P. D., and Baldwin, C. (1982). Mechanisms of sulphur dioxide induced bronchoconstriction in normal and asthmatic man. *Thorax* **37**:118-123.

Taira, N., and Satoh, S. (1973). Prostaglandin $F_{2\alpha}$ as a potent excitant of the parasympathetic postganglionic neurons of the dog salivary gland. *Life Sci.* **13**:501-506.

Takeyasu, K., Uchida, S., Noguchi, Y., Fujita, N., Saito, K., Hata, F., and Yoshida, H. (1979). Changes in brain muscarinic acetylcholine receptors and behavioral responses to atropine and apomorphine in chronic atropine-treated rats. *Life Sci.* **25**:585-592.

Tan, W. C., Cripps, E., Douglas, N., and Sudlow, M. F. (1982). Protective effect of drugs on bronchoconstriction induced by sulfur dioxide. *Thorax* **37**:671-676.

Taniguchi, T., Kurahashi, K., and Fujiwara, M. (1983). Alterations in muscarinic cholinergic receptors after preganglionic denervation of the superior cervical ganglion in cats. *J. Pharmacol. Exp. Ther.* **224**:674-678.

Uchida, S., Takeyasu, K., Ichida, S., and Yoshida, H. (1978). Muscarinic cholinergic receptors in mammalian brain: differences between bindings of acetylcholine and atropine. *Jap. J. Pharmacol.* **28**:853-862.

Ullah, M. I., Newman, G. B., and Saunders, K. B. (1981). Influence of age on response to ipratropium and salbutamol in asthma. *Thorax* **36**:523-529.

Vincent, N. J., Knudson, R., Leith, D. E., Macklem, P. T., and Mead, J. (1970). Factors influencing pulmonary resistance. *J. Appl. Physiol.* **29**:236-243.

Virtanen, R., Kanto, J., Iisalo, E., Iisalo, E. U. M., Salo, M., and Sjövall, S. (1982). Pharmacokinetic studies on atropine with special reference to age. *Acta Anaesthesiol. Scand.* **26**:297-300.

Vlagopoulos, T., Townley, R. G., Ghazanshahi, S., Bewtra, A., and Burke, K. (1976). Comparison of the bronchodilating effects of Sch 1000 with isoproterenol in patients with bronchial asthma. *Ann. Allergy* **36**:223-230.

Vornanen, M., and Tirri, R. (1981). Cholinergic responses in different sections of rat airways. *Acta Physiol. Scand.* **113**:177-182.

Ward, M. J., Fentem, P. H., Smith, W. H. R., and Davies, D. (1981). Ipratropium bromide in acute asthma. *Br. Med. J.* **282**:598-600.

Wasserman, M. A. (1975). Bronchopulmonary responses to prostaglandin $F_{2\alpha}$, histamine and acetylcholine in the dog. *Eur. J. Pharmacol.* **32**:146-155.

Wasserman, M. A., Griffin, R. L., Marsalisi, F. B. (1980). Inhibition of bronchoconstriction by aerosols of prostaglandins E_1 and E_2. *J. Pharmacol. Exp. Ther.* **214**:68-73.

Weiss, J. W., McFadden, E. R., and Ingram, R. H. (1982). Parenteral vs. inhaled atropine: density dependence of maximal expiratory flow. *J. Appl. Physiol.* **53**:392-396.

Wick, M. M., and Ingram, R. H. (1976). Bronchorrhea responsive to aerosolized atropine. *J. Am. Med. Assn.* **235**:1356.

Wise, B. C., Shoji, M., and Kuo, J. P. (1980). Decrease or increase in cardiac muscarinic cholinergic receptor number in rats treated with methacholine or atropine. *Biochem. Biophys. Res. Commun.* **92**:1136-1142.

Woenne, R., Kattan, M., Orange, R. P., and Levison, H. (1978). Bronchial hyperreactivity to histamine and methacholine in asthmatic children after inhalation of Sch 1000 and chlorpheniramine maleate. *J. Allergy Clin. Immunol.* **62**:119-124.

Woolcock, A. J., Cheung, W., and Salome, C. (1986). Relationship between bronchial responsiveness to propranolol and histamine. *Am. Rev. Respir. Dis.* **133** (4, part 2):A 177 (abstr).

Yu, D. Y. C., Galant, S. P., and Gold, W. M. (1972). Inhibition of antigen-induced bronchoconstriction by atropine in asthmatic patients. *J. Appl. Physiol.* **32**: 823-828.

12

Neuropeptides of the Gut

GABRIEL M. MAKHLOUF

Medical College of Virginia
Richmond, Virginia

The quest for biologically active peptides started with the discovery of the first hormone, secretin, and has increased during the last 20 years. Progress in the extraction, purification, and characterization of proteins made available a variety of natural and synthetic peptides. Specific antisera were raised that allowed immunochemical measurement of peptides in blood and tissues and immunocytochemical mapping of peptide-containing cells. Peptides were found to occur in homologous families and to be present in various molecular forms, which are indications of their derivation from larger precursor molecules. The discovery of active peptides in nonmammalian species, particularly in the skin of amphibia, led to the discovery of homologous, cross-immunoreactive counterparts in mammalian tissues. Within the same species, peptides were found to be widely distributed. Some were hormonal peptides synthesized by endocrine cells and released into the circulation to act on distant targets. Others, often homologues of endocrine peptide, were present in neurons of the central and peripheral nervous systems. The identification of neural peptides was facilitated by immunochemical measurements in tissues devoid of endocrine cells (e.g., muscle layers and neural plexuses) and by increasingly precise immunostaining of neural pathways. Recent studies have focused on the coexistence of neuropeptides with each other and with nonpeptide transmitters. The most recent discoveries of hitherto unsuspected peptides have come to light as a result of advances in molecular biology. The entire amino acid sequence of precursor proteins can now be characterized with relative ease and the probable loci of proteolytic cleavage determined. This has led to the realization that biologically active peptides are synthesized as one or more copies of the same peptide or a homologous peptide.

I. Enteric Neuropeptides

Peptide-containing neurons are widely distributed in the peripheral nervous system and are present in the extrinsic (sympathetic and parasympathetic) and intrinsic (intramural) subdivisions that supply the viscera (cardiopulmonary, genitourinary, and digestive systems) and the vasculature (Costa and Furness, 1982; Furness and Costa, 1980; Makhlouf, 1983, 1984; Schultzberg et al., 1983). The neurons are abundantly present in the enteric nervous system, where their location and projections are being mapped with increasing precision by immunostaining. Important features that distinguish the enteric nervous system include a virtual independence from central control and a large diversity of neuronal types and transmitters (Furness and Costa, 1980). The diversity is most evident in relation to the number of peptide neurotransmitters or neuromodulators (Costa and Furness, 1982).

Table 1 lists gut peptides and gives an indication of their presence in neurons and endocrine cells or both. Hormonal peptides with known physiological functions include gastrin, secretin, cholecystokinin, motilin, and the insulinotropic peptide gastric inhibitory peptide (GIP) (Table 2; Walsh, 1981). Other peptides produced by endocrine-like cells of the intestine (peptide YY [PYY], neurotensin, and enteric glucagon) have no defined physiological function. Somatostatin is present in endocrine-like cells of the stomach, intestine, and pancreas and in neurons of the myenteric and submucosal plexuses (Keast et al., 1984). It is not known whether somatostatin released into the circulation from endocrine-like cells subserves a hormonal function. Strong evidence favors a paracrine role, that is, close to the site of release, in the pancreas and stomach (Saffouri et al., 1979). The action is distinct from that of somatostatin derived from myenteric or submucosal neurons.

The main neuropeptides of the gut and their general properties are listed in Table 3.

Table 1 Families of Hormonal and Neural Peptides of the Gut

	Hormonal	Neural
Gastrin	+	
CCK	+	+
Secretin, GIP, Glucagon	+	
VIP/PHI		+
PP, PYY	+	
NPY		+
Tachykinins: SP, SK, NK		+
Bombesins: GRP, Neuromedin B		+
Opioids: dynorphin/met-enk		+
Galanin		+
CGRP		+
Somatostatin	+	+
Neurotensin	+	?
Motilin	+	

CCK, cholecystokinin; CGRP, calcitonin gene-related peptide; GIP, gastric inhibitory peptide; GRP, gastrin-releasing peptide; NK, neuromedin K; NPY, neuropeptide Y; Opioids, dynorphin, leumorphin, α-neoendorphin, leu-enkephalin, met-enkephalin, met-enkephalin-arg-gly-leu; PP, pancreatic peptide; PYY, peptide YY; SK, substance K; SP, substance P; VIP/PHI, vasoactive intestinal peptide/peptide histidine isoleucine.

A. Vasoactive Intestinal Peptide and Peptide with N-Terminal Histidine and C-Terminal Isoleucine

Vasoactive intestinal peptide (VIP) is invariably listed with peptide with N-terminal histidine and C-terminal isoleucine (PHI) because the two peptides are cosynthesized within the same precursor and coreleased from the same nerve terminals (Makhlouf, 1983, 1984). The sequence of VIP is well conserved in all mammals with the notable exception of the guinea pig, whereas the sequence of

Table 2 Properties of Hormonal Peptides of the Gut

Gastrin:	Gastric secretion and growth
Secretin:	Pancreatic electrolyte secretion
Cholecystokinin:	Pancreatic enzyme secretion Gallbladder emptying
GIP:	Insulinotropic hormone
Motilin:	Interdigestive motor cycles
PYY, Neurotensin, enteric glucagon:	Unknown function

Table 3 Properties of Neural Peptides of the Gut

VIP/PHI:	Intestinal secretion; muscle relaxation
Opioid peptides:	Intestinal absorption; propulsion
Tachykinins:	Sensory perception; muscle contraction
Bombesins:	Gastrin release; muscle contraction
NPY:	Intestinal absorption; adrenergic cotransmission
Somatostatin:	Gastrin release; descending interneuron
CGRP:	? Sensory perception
Galanin:	? Sensory perception; muscle contraction?

PHI varies with the species. The corresponding peptide in humans derived from human preproVIP is known as PHM because of its C-terminal methionine amide. VIP/PHI are present exclusively in neurons in contrast to their hormonal homologues, secretin, GIP, and glucagon (Costa and Furness, 1983; Walsh, 1981).

VIP/PHI neurons of the myenteric plexus project either caudad to innervate other neurons within the plexus or directly into the underlying circular muscle layer (Costa and Furness, 1983). VIP/PHI neurons of the submucosal plexus innervate submucosal and mucosal blood vessels and cells (Fig. 1). VIP and PHI are unique among neuropeptides in their ability to cause relaxation of vascular and visceral smooth muscle (stomach, intestine, gallbladder, urinary bladder, uterus, trachea, and systematic vasculature) (Grider et al., 1985a,b; Makhlouf, 1982). The polarity of VIP/PHI neurons and the relaxant property of VIP/PHI suggest that these peptides are the transmitters of inhibitory nerves (Furness and Costa, 1980). The main effect of VIP/PHI on mucosal cells is secretory:

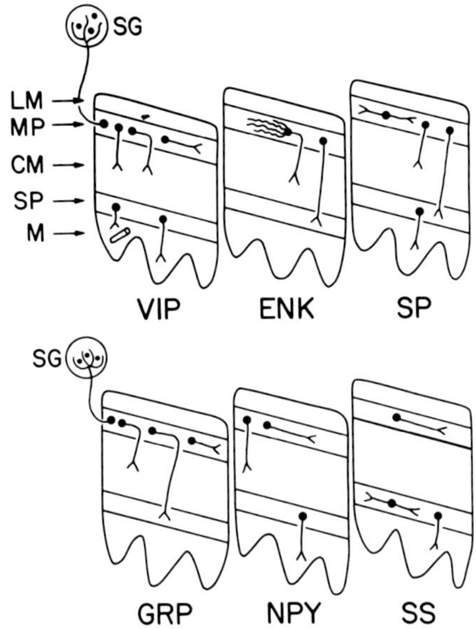

Figure 1 Topography of neurons in the myenteric and submucosal plexuses containing VIP, met-enkephalin (ENK), substance P (SP), mammalian bombesin (GRP), neuropeptide Y (NPY), and somatostatin (SS). Arrows indicate layers in the schematic cross-section of the intestine: longitudinal muscle (LM), myenteric plexus (MP), circular muscle (CM), submucosal plexus (SP), and submucosa/mucosa (M). Left: orad end; Right: caudad end (from Makhlouf, 1986).

mucosal VIP/PHI neurons may constitute the secretory limb of a neural system that regulates electrolyte and water transport in the intestine (Makhlouf, 1984).

B. Opioid Peptides

Derivatives of two opioid precursor proteins, preproenkephalin and preprodynorphin, have been detected in neurons of the gut (Comb et al., 1982; Kakidani et al., 1982). Preproenkephalin yields four copies of Met-enkephalin and one copy each of Met-enkephalin-Arg^6-Phe^7 and Met-enkephalin-Arg^6-Gly^7-Leu^8. Preprodynorphin yields peptides that contain the sequence of Leu-enkephalin such as dynorphin and α-neoendorphin. Met-enkephalin-containing neurons appear to predominate in the myenteric plexus (Furness et al., 1983b). A large number of opioid neurons also contain VIP/PHI, an example of the coexistence of peptides derived from separate precursors (Costa et al., 1985). There is good evidence that dynorphin interacts preferentially with the kappa (κ), Met-enkephalin with the delta (δ), and Leu-enkephalin with the mu (μ) subtype of opiate receptors in smooth muscle cells and cholinergic neurons of the gut (Bitar and Makhlouf, 1982c, 1985).

The main effect of opioid peptides on mucosal function is to enhance intestinal absorption; the effect is mediated predominantly by δ receptors (Kachur et al., 1980). Opioid peptides have three distinct effects on neuromuscular function: Two of these are neurally mediated; the third is a direct contractile effect on smooth muscle cells of the circular muscle layer (smooth muscle cells of the longitudinal muscle layer do not have opiate receptors) (Makhlouf, 1985). The direct effect is clearly demonstrable in isolated gastric and intestinal smooth muscle cells devoid of neural elements (Bitar and Makhlouf, 1982,c, 1985). One neurally mediated effect consists of inhibition of acetylcholine release from cholinergic nerve terminals, as shown by inhibition of electrically induced twitch responses in innervated longitudinal muscle strips. The second neurally mediated effect consists of blockade of inhibitory motor neurons resulting in unmasking of myogenic phasic activity (Grider and Makhlouf, 1983). All three effects contribute to the regulation of intestinal propulsive activity by opioid neurons (Grider and Makhlouf, 1984).

C. Tachykinins

The group of peptides known collectively as tachykinins share the C-terminal pentapeptide sequence Phe-X-Gly-Leu-Met amide (X = variable amino acid residue) and cause rapid (tachy-) contraction of smooth muscle of the intestine and other viscera (Watson, 1984). Until recently, substance P (SP) was thought to be the only mammalian representative of this group of mostly amphibian peptides. It is now known that at least two other tachykinins are present in mammalian tissues, substance K and neuromedin K, also known as neurokinin α and β, respectively (Nawa et al., 1983, Souquet et al., 1985; Watson, 1984). The existence of these homologues in the gut either in association with SP neurons or in separate populations of neurons has not been determined (Costa et al., 1980).

The direct contractile effect of tachykinins on intestinal smooth muscle is brief and is followed by a prolonged effect mediated by release of acetylcholine from cholinergic nerve terminals. At least two subtypes of tachykinin receptors have been identified (Watson, 1984). The existence of one or more receptor subtype on a given target cell (e.g., on a smooth muscle cell) depends on the species. Within the same species, the receptor subtype responsible for direct contraction (i.e., receptor on muscle cell) is different from the receptor subtype responsible for neurally mediated contraction (i.e., receptor on cholinergic neuron). The functional significance of tachykinin neurons has yet to be defined. Recent studies indicate that they may be involved in the ascending contractile component of the peristaltic reflex (Grider and Makhlouf, 1986). Capsaicin-sensitive SP nerve fibers may be involved in sensory perception.

D. Bombesin/Gastrin-Releasing Peptide

Two mammalian homologues of the amphibian bombesin are now known to exist: gastrin-releasing peptide (GRP) and neuromedin B. Bombesin/GRP neurons are found in the myenteric plexus of the intestine where they project caudad into the plexus, as well as into the circular muscle layer (Fig. 1) (Costa et al., 1984; Moghimzadeh et al., 1983). In the stomach, bombesin/GRP neurons, presumably located in the submucosal plexus, project also into the antral (gastrin-secreting) and fundic (acid-secreting) mucosa of the stomach. As the name implies, bombesin/GRP is a potent stimulant of gastrin release. Evidence in support of the functional importance of bombesin neurons in the regulation of gastrin secretion was obtained by showing that neurally mediated gastrin secretion in the isolated vascularly perfused rat stomach is strongly inhibited by addition of bombesin antiserum to the perfusate (Schubert et al., 1985). The other main property of bombesin/GRP is contraction of smooth muscle (Micheletti et al., 1986; Walsh, 1981). However, a neuromuscular function for bombesin GRP in the intestine has yet to be defined.

E. Neuropeptide Y

Neuropeptide Y (NPY) is the neural counterpart of the endocrine peptides, pep-YY (PYY) and pancreatic peptide (PP). NPY neurons are found in the myenteric and submucosal plexuses, especially the latter where they constitute 26% of all neurons (Fig. 1; Furness et al., 1984). NPY is also found in extrinsic adrenergic fibers that innervate gastrointestinal blood vessels. This pattern of coexistence is also found in other viscera and has important implications for the regulation of vascular tone and blood flow (Lundberg et al., 1982). Like its endocrine homologues, NPY is vasoactive, causing vasoconstriction of slow onset and long duration (Lundberg and Tatemoto, 1982). A combination of NPY and norepinephrine mimics the early (norepinephrine-induced) and late (NPY-induced) pattern of vasoconstriction elicited by sympathetic nerve stimulation. The functional role of NPY neurons of the submucosal plexus has not been defined, though recent studies suggest that NPY may be a selective stimulant of intestinal chloride absorption.

F. Somatostatin

Somatostatin neurons are found in the submucosal and myenteric plexuses, where they project caudad within the plexus only (Fig. 1). The topography of myenteric somatostatin neurons suggests that they act as interneurons in descending pathways (see below). The function of submucosal somatostatin neurons that project into the mucosa is not known. The effect of somatostatin on intestinal transport suggests that they may act as a component of the neural system that stimulates absorption. Other possible components of the system include extrinsic adrenergic nerve fibers, as well as intrinsic NPY and opioid nerve fibers supplying the mucosa.

G. Calcitonin Gene-Related Peptide and Galanin

Calcitonin gene-related peptide (CGRP) and galanin are two of the most recently discovered neuropeptides (Makhlouf, 1984; Rokaeus, et al., 1984). Galanin neurons are found in both plexuses but appear to predominate in the submucosal plexus. Galanin neurons are also found in other organs, including the genitourinary and respiratory systems. Galanin and CGRP often coexist in these neurons, where they appear to serve a sensory function. The central distribution of CGRP neurons suggests that they may be involved in the regulation of food intake.

II. Neural Design of the Gut

Several aspects of the neural design of the gut are illustrated in Figure 1 (Costa and Furness, 1982; Furness and Costa, 1980; Makhlouf, 1984). Nerve fibers originating in peptide-containing neurons of the myenteric plexus project into the circular, but not longitudinal, muscle layer, except in specialized segments such as teniae coli. Nerve fibers originating in neurons of the submucosal plexus project into the submucosa, but not into the circular or longitudinal smooth muscle layers. Some nerve fibers originating in neurons of the myenteric or submucosal plexus connect the two plexuses; occasional fibers originating in the myenteric plexus project into the mucosa (Furness et al., 1985). In some instances, fibers originating in intrinsic neurons (e.g., VIP and bombesin/GRP neurons) project outside the gut to paravertebral ganglia. Finally, fibers originating in neurons of sympathetic ganglia project into the gut; some contain norepinephrine while others contain norepinephrine and a peptide, for example, NPY (Costa and Furness, 1982; Makhlouf, 1985; Schultzberg et al., 1983).

Intramural neural pathways are more complex than the discrete pathways illustrated schematically in Figure 1. As noted above, neuropeptides often coexist within the same neurons as a result of synthesis by different precursors. This type of coexistence should be differentiated from that resulting from cosynthesis of two peptides within the same precursor (e.g., cosynthesis of VIP and PHI or substance P and substance K). Examples of peptides that coexist with each other or with other neurotransmitters include the following. Within the gut, VIP/PHI coexists with dynorphin, VIP/PHI with galanin, and NPY, CCK, and somatostatin with acetylcholine (Costa and Furness, 1982; Costa et al., 1985; Furness et al., 1984; Schultzberg et al., 1983). Outside the gut, VIP/PHI coexists with acetylcholine in salivary and sweat glands and NPY, VIP, or somatostatin coexist with norepinephrine in subpopulations of sympathetic neurons (Lundberg et al., 1982; Schultzberg et al., 1983).

The significance of coexistence of peptide and nonpeptide transmitters should be determined separately for each neural pathway. Substances coreleased from the same terminals could act synergistically on postsynaptic receptors. Alternatively, one or both substances could act presynaptically to regulate further release from nerve terminals. Thus, VIP coreleased with acetylcholine from nerve terminals in exocrine glands causes vasodilatation and augments the secretory response to acetylcholine (Lundberg et al., 1980). Additionally, acetylcholine and possibly VIP regulate the release of one or both transmitters from nerve terminals. In the case of NPY and norepinephrine noted above, one transmitter (norepinephrine) is responsible for the initial brief component of the vasoconstrictive response, whereas the other (NPY) is responsible for the sustained component.

III. Criteria for Identification of Peptide Neurotransmitters

Identification of peptides as neurotransmitters requires that several criteria be met. Among these are (1) demonstration of peptide synthesis by a population of neurons; (2) localization of the peptide in these neurons by immunostaining; (3) identification of the target cells innervated by these neurons (neural, smooth muscle, endothelial, mucosal or endocrine cells); (4) characterization of peptide receptors on these cells; and (5) where one or more peptide or nonpeptide neurotransmitters coexist, separation of modulatory from direct action on pre- or postsynaptic targets. These criteria have yet to be met for most enteric neuropeptides. To illustrate the complexity of this process, the example of VIP/PHI and its role in enteric neuromuscular activity is discussed below.

Strong evidence supports the view that VIP/PHI is the mediator of inhibitory descending reflexes in the gut (Furness and Costa, 1980). The reflexes require that a neurotransmitter capable of causing relaxation at neuromuscular junctions be released during peristaltic activity to facilitate the passage of food down the gut. VIP/PHI are the main, perhaps the only, enteric neuropeptides capable of causing relaxation of circular smooth muscle. The relaxant property extends to other viscera and the systemic vasculature (Makhlouf, 1982). As noted in a previous section, immunocytochemical studies have revealed a precise distribution of nerve fibers originating in VIP/PHI neurons of the myenteric plexus. The fibers project caudad within the plexus or into the circular muscle layer (Fig. 1);

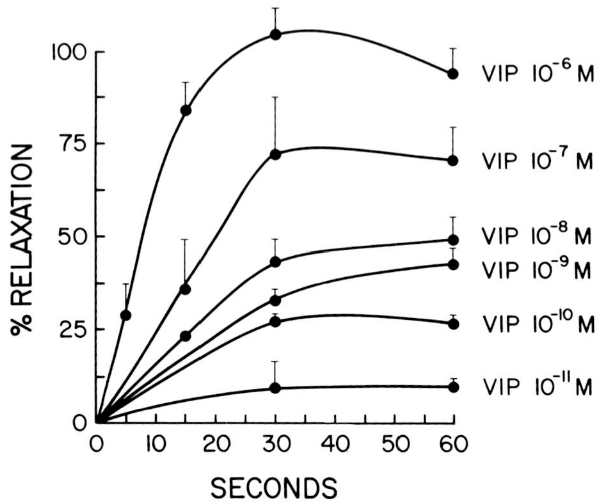

Figure 2 Time course of relaxation induced by different concentrations of VIP in dispersed smooth muscle cells of the guinea pig stomach (from Bitar and Makhlouf, 1982b).

(Costa and Furness, 1983). VIP receptors capable of causing relaxation have been demonstrated in smooth muscle cells isolated from muscle tissues innervated by VIP neurons (Fig. 2; Bitar and Makhlouf, 1982b). The receptors bind [^{125}]VIP specifically; binding is rapid and coincides with the time of optimal relaxation (Bitar and Jensen, 1983). Before the discovery of relaxant neuropeptides with precise, physiologically appropriate polarity, the purine nucleotide ATP was proposed as the neurotransmitter of inhibitory motor neurons in the gut. ATP and related purines also cause relaxation of isolated smooth muscle cells, though specific ATP binding sites have not been demonstrated immunochemically (Bitar and Makhlouf, 1982d; Burnstock, 1979). Field stimulation of smooth muscle strips innervated by VIP/PHI neurons elicits a stimulus-dependent relaxation directly correlated with the amount of VIP released. The neurally induced relaxation is selectively inhibited by VIP antiserum in circular gastric and intestinal muscle, choledochal, lower esophageal, and anal sphincteric muscle, and in teniae coli (Fig. 3; Grider et al., 1985a,b). A photoactivated analogue of ATP, 3′-0-(4-benzoyl) benzoyl ATP, which binds covalently to ATP receptors and inactivates them in the presence of light, blocks ATP-induced relaxation.

The evidence adduced above based on studies of electrically induced relaxation has been corroborated recently by studies in whole organ preparations in which VIP release was induced by radial stretch, a physiologically appropriate peristaltic stimulus. Isolated segments of rat or guinea pig colon subjected to

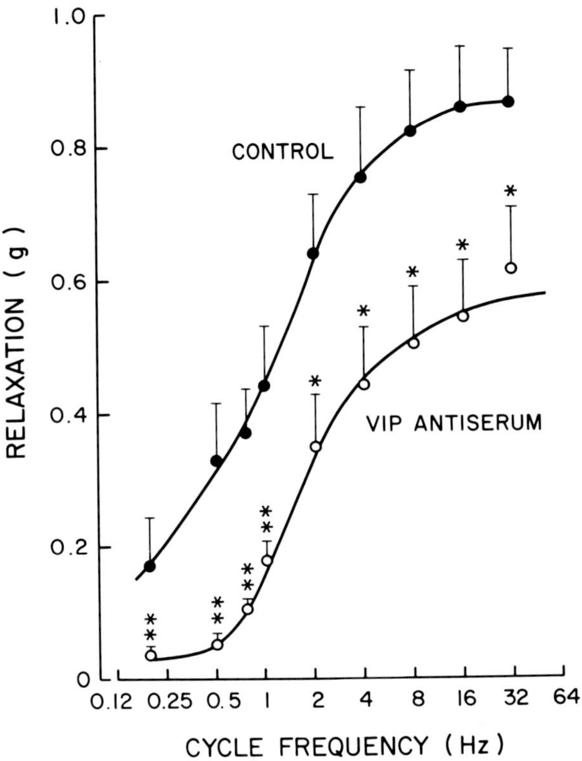

Figure 3 Inhibitory effect of VIP antiserum (final dilution 1:20) on gastric relaxation induced by field stimulation of gastric smooth muscle in the guinea pig. Asterisks denote significant difference from control responses: ** $P < 0.01$; * $P < 0.05$ (from Grider et al., 1985a).

radial stretch at the orad end undergo descending (i.e., caudad) relaxation only, whereas the same segments subjected to radial stretch at the caudad end undergo ascending (i.e., orad) contraction only. In these segments, VIP is released exclusively during descending relaxation and the latter is selectively blocked by VIP antiserum (Fig. 4); Grider and Makhlouf, 1986). The extent of blockade depends on the strength of the stimulus and the concentration of VIP antiserum. Further studies have shown that somatostatin neurons of the myenteric plexus act as facilitatory interneurons that enhance VIP release and descending relaxation (Grider et al., 1986), whereas opioid neurons act to restrict VIP release and descending relaxation (Grider and Makhlouf, 1984). Thus, with precise topography of VIP/PHI neurons as a guide and the ability to assay VIP or immunoneutralize

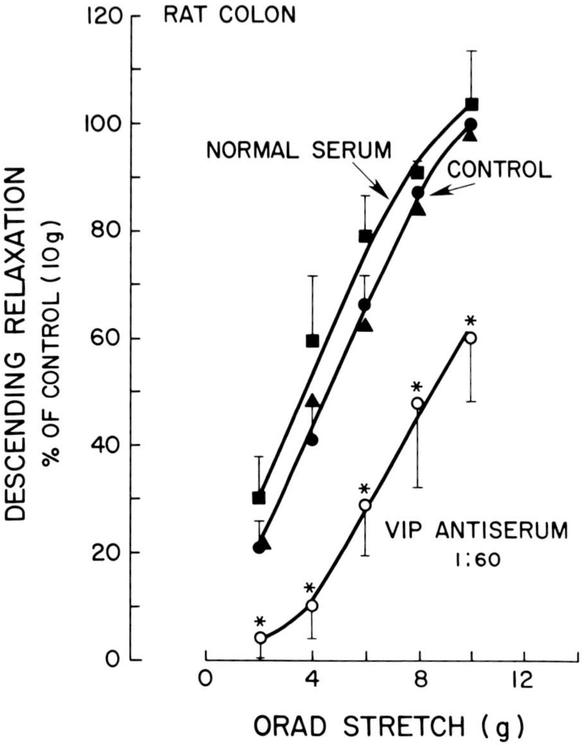

Figure 4 Inhibitory effect of VIP antiserum on descending relaxation in isolated segments of rat colon. Descending (i.e., caudad) relaxation was induced by radial stretch (range, 2-10 g) of the orad end of the segments (from Grider and Makhlouf, 1986).

it as experimental tools, it was possible to demonstrate that VIP/PHI unique in their ability to cause smooth muscle relaxation are the most likely candidates for neurotransmitter(s) of inhibitory motor neurons in the gut.

Acknowledgment

This work was supported by grants AM-15564, AM-28300, and AM-34153 from the National Institutes of Health.

Discussion

Vanhoutte. Would biochemical parameters be more useful to evaluate than length of smooth muscle cells in suspension?

Makhlouf. Cell length is easily measured in cell suspensions and single cells by image-splitting micrometry. The cell responds in a dose-dependent manner, and the effects are reversible and reproducible. Free cytosolic calcium and calcium efflux are precisely related to contraction, and cyclic AMP concentration is correlated with relaxation.

Lundberg. Since PHI is present in the same nerves as VIP, does the antiserum to VIP cross-react with PHI, since these peptides often have the same biologic activity when species-related peptides are used?

Makhlouf. The antiserum used interacts selectively with VIP and the contribution of PHI to relaxation is relatively small (five times less potent than VIP).

Kaliner. Is there any relationship between changes in neuropeptides in GI diseases?

Makhlouf. Abundance of neuropeptides and projections of neurons appear to be abnormal in some diseases. Thus, in achalasia there is a selective absence of VIP-immunoreactive nerves.

Richardson. We have studied the lower esophageal sphincter of normal patients and patients with achalasia. VIP is inactive in both groups, although field stimulation and other agonists are active, suggesting that the neurotransmitter is not VIP in humans.

Makhlouf. The VIP may not have been active for various reasons. A more useful experiment would be to see if VIP antiserum blocks EFS relaxation, as in cat and opossum.

Nadel. What is known of opioid receptors in gut?

Makhlouf. There are opioid receptors on circular but not on longitudinal muscle cells of both guinea pig and human gut, as demonstrated by the ability to cause contraction of isolated muscle cells (Bitar and Makhlouf, 1985). There are also two types of opioid neuroreceptors: one is located on cholinergic nerves and inhibits acetylcholine release, the other is on inhibitory neurons and blocks release of inhibitory neurotransmitter. We have shown that opioid peptides inhibit intestinal VIP release and induce contractile phasic activity.

Burnstock. The question of accessibility of transmitters and agonists to their receptors has been raised many times since "atropine resistance" to responses was claimed in the urinary bladder at the turn of the century. This turned out not to be an accessibility problem, but due to the existence of a noncholinergic excitatory transmitter. In the intestine, nonadrenergic inhibitory responses are fast. This is closely mimicked by exogenous ATP but exogenous VIP causes a slow relaxation, taking several minutes to peak after a latency of 10-20 (Mackenzie and Burnstock, *Eur. J. Pharmacol.* **67**:255-264, 1980). It has been suggested that this lack of mimickry is due to inaccessibility of the peptide to its receptors. However, another peptide, bradykinin, closely mimicks the time course of response. VIP applied to single isolated smooth muscle cells is claimed by Makhlouf to have a comparable time course, but close examination of his figures shows that the time for peak relaxation to exogenous VIP is still considerably longer than relaxation produced by nerve stimulation and ATP. Therefore, inaccessibility does not appear to be the explanation.

Makhlouf. Mimickrey by exogenously applied agent and neurally released agent is not an adequate test. A better approach is the use of selective antisera or antagonists. These clearly show that in stomach, intestine and colon, VIP, not ATP, mediates relaxation (Grider and Makhlouf, 1983, 1984, 1985, 1986).

References

Bitar, K. N., and Jensen, R. T. (1983). Binding of ^{125}I-VIP to isolated gastric smooth muscle cells. *Gastroenterology* **84**:1107A.

Bitar, K. N., and Makhlouf, G. M. (1982a). Receptors on smooth muscle cells: characterization by contraction and specific antagonists. *Am. J. Physiol.* **242**:G400-G407.

Bitar, K. N., Makhlouf, G. M. (1982b). Relaxation of isolated gastric smooth muscle cells by vasoactive intestinal peptide. *Science* **216**:531-533.

Bitar, K. N., and Makhlouf, G. M. (1982c). Specific opiate receptors on isolated mammalian gastric smooth muscle cells. *Nature* **297**:72-74.

Bitar, K. N., and Makhlouf, G. M. (1982d). Purinergic receptors on isolated smooth muscle cells: potentiators of VIP-induced relaxation. *Gastroenterology* **82**:1018A.

Bitar, K. N., and Makhlouf, G. M. (1985). Selective presence of opiate receptors on intestinal circular muscle cells. *Life Sci.* **37**:1545-1550.

Burnstock, G. (1979). Adenosine triphosphate. In *Neurosciences Research, Non-Cholinergic Autonomic Neurotransmission Mechanisms.* Edited by G. Burnstock, M. D. Gershon, T. Hokfelt, L. L. Iverson, H. W. Kosterlitz, and J. H. Szurszewski. Cambridge, MIT Press, pp. 406-414, Bull. 17.

Comb, M., Seeburg, P. H., Adelman, J. et al. (1982). Primary structure of the human Met- and Leu-enkephalin precursor and its mRNA. *Nature* (London) **295**:663.

Costa, M., and Furness, J. B. (1982). Neuronal peptides in the intestine. *Br. Med. Bull.* **38**:247-252.

Costa, M., and Furness, J. B. (1983). The origins, pathways and terminations of neurons with VIP-like immunoreactivity in the guinea-pig small intestine. *Neuroscience* **8**:665-676.

Costa, M., Cuello, C., Furness, J. B., and Franco, R. (1980). Distribution of enteric neurons showing immunoreactivity for substance P in the guinea-pig ileum. *Neuroscience* **5**:323-331.

Costa, M., Furness, J. B., Yanaihara, N., Yanaihara, C., and Moody, T. W. (1984). Distribution and projections of neurons with immunoreactivity for both gastrin-releasing peptide and bombesin in the guinea pig small intestine. *Cell Tissue Res.* **235**:285-293.

Costa, M., Furness, J. B., and Cuello, A. C. (1985). Separate populations of opioid containing neurons in the guinea-pig intestine. *Neuropeptides* **5**: 445-448.

Furness, J. B., and Costa, M. (1980). Types of nerves in the enteric nervous system. *Neuroscience* **5**:1-20.

Furness, J. B., Costa, M., Emson, P. C., Hakanson, R., Moghimzadeh, E., Sundler, F., Taylor, I. L., and Chance, R. E. (1983a). Distribution, pathways and reactions to drug treatment of nerves with neuropeptide Y and pancreatic polypeptide-like immunoreactivity in the guinea pig digestive tract. *Cell. Tissue Res.* **234**:71-92.

Furness, J. B., Costa, M., and Miller, R. J. (1983b). Distribution and projections of nerves with enkephalin-like immunoreactivity in the guinea pig small intestine. *Neuroscience* **8**:653-664.

Furness, J. B., Costa, M., and Keast, J. R. (1984). Choline acetyltransferase and peptide immunoreactivity of submucous neurons in the small intestine of the guinea pig. *Cell Tissue Res.* **237**:329-336.

Furness, J. B., Costa, M., Gibbins, I. L., Llewellyn-Smith, I. J., and Oliver, J. R. (1985). Neurochemically similar myenteric and submucous neurons directly tracted to the mucosa of the small intestine. *Cell Tissue Res.* **241**:155-163.

Grider, J. R., and Makhlouf, G. M. (1983). Tonic and phasic responses of colonic circular muscle to opioid peptides. *Gastroenterology* **84**:1175A.

Grider, J. R., and Makhlouf, G. M. (1984). Regulation of intestinal peristalsis by intramural opioid neurons. *Gastroenterology* **86**:1099A.

Grider, J. R., and Makhlouf, G. M. (1986). Colonic peristalic reflex: identification of VIP as mediator of descending relaxation. *Am. J. Physiol.* **251**: 640-645.

Grider, J. R., Cable, M. B., Said, S. I., and Makhlouf, G. M. (1985a). Vasoactive intestinal peptide (VIP) as neural mediator of gastric relaxation. *Am. J. Physiol.* **248**:73-78.

Grider, J. R., Cable, M. B., Said, S. I., and Makhlouf, G. M. (1985b). Vasoactive intestinal peptide: relaxant neurotransmitter in tenia coli of the guinea pig. *Gastroenterology* **89**:36-42.

Grider, J. R., Arimura, A., and Makhlouf, G. M. (1986). Somatostatin (SS) interneurons of the myenteric plexus facilitate descending relaxation. *Gastroenterology* **90**. In Press.

Kachur, J. F., Miller, R. J., and Field, M. (1980). Control of guinea pig intestinal electrolyte secretion by a δ-opiate receptor. *Proc. Natl. Acad. Sci. USA* **77**:2753.

Kakidani, H., Furutani, Y., Takahashi, H. et al. (1982). Cloning and sequence analysis of cDNA for porcine -neo-endorphin/dynorphin precursor. *Nature* (London) **298**:245.

Keast, J. R., Furness, J. B., and Costa, M. (1984). Somatostatin in human enteric nerves: distribution and characterization. *Cell Tissue Res.* **237**:299-308.

Lundberg, J. M., Tatemoto, K. (1982). Pancreatic polypeptide family (APP, BPP, NPY and PYY) in relation to sympathetic vasoconstriction resistant to α-adrenoceptor blockade. *Acta Physiol. Scand.* **116**:393.

Lundberg, J. M., Anggard, A., Fahrenkrug, J. et al. (1980). Vasoactive intestinal polypeptide in cholinergic neurons of exocrine glands: functional significance of coexisting transmitters for vasodilatation and secretion. *Proc. Natl. Acad. Sci. USA* **77**:1651.

Lundberg, J. M., Terenius, L., Hokfelt, T. et al. (1982). Neuropeptide Y (NPY)-like immunoreactivity in peripheral noradrenergic neurons and effects of NPY on sympathetic function. *Acta Physiol. Scand.* **116**:477.

Makhlouf, G. M. (1982). Role of VIP in the function of the gut. In *Vasoactive Intestinal Peptide.* Edited by S. I. Said. New York, Raven Press, pp. 425-446.

Makhlouf, G. M. (1983). Hormones and neuropeptides of the gut. In *The Gastroenterology Annual 1.* Edited by F. Kern, Jr., and A. L. Blum, Amsterdam-New York-Oxford, Elsevier, 1983, pp. 181-197.

Makhlouf, G. M. (1984). Hormones and neuropeptides of the gut. In *The Gastroenterology Annual 2.* Edited by F. Kern, Jr., and A. L. Blum. Amsterdam-New York-Oxford, Elsevier, 1983, pp. 177-189.

Makhlouf, G. M. (1985). Enteric neuropeptides: role in neuromuscular activity of the gut. *TIPS* **6**:214-218.

Micheletti, R., Bitar, K. N., and Makhlouf, G. M. (1986). Characterization of receptors for bombesin on isolated circular and longitudinal muscle cells of human intestine. *Gastroenterology* **90**:1552.

Moghimzadeh, E., Ekman, R., Hakanson, R., Yanaihara, N., and Sundler, F. (1983). Neuronal gastrin-releasing peptide in the mammalian gut and pancreas. *Neuroscience* **10**:553-563.

Nawa, H., Tadaaki, H., Takashima, H., Inayama, S., and Nakanishi, S. (1983). Nucleotide sequences of clones cDNAs for two types of bovine brain substance P precursor. *Nature* (London) **306**:32-36.

Rokaeus, A., Melander, T., Hokfelt, T., Lundberg, J. M., Tatemoto, K., Carlquist, M., and Mutt, V. (1984). A galanin-like peptide in the central nervous system and intestine of the rat. *Neurosci. Letts.* **47**:161-166.

Saffouri, B., Weir, G. C., Bitar, K. N., and Makhlouf, G. M. (1979). Stimulation of gastrin secretion from the perfused rat stomach by somatostatin antiserum. *Life Sci.* **25**(20):1749-1754.

Schubert, M. L., Saffouri, B., Walsh, J. H., and Makhlouf, G. M. (1985). Inhibition of neurally mediated gastrin section by bombesin antiserum. *Am. J. Physiol.* **248**:G456-G462.

Schultzberg, M., Hokfelt, T., and Lundberg, J. M. (1983). Coexistence of classical transmitters and peptides in the central and peripheral nervous systems. *Br. Med. Bull.* **38**:309-313.

Souquet, J.-C., Grider, J. R., Bitar, K. N., and Makhlouf, G. M. (1985). Receptors for mammalian tachykinins on isolated intestinal smooth muscle cells. *Am. J. Physiol.* **249**:553-538.

Walsh, J. H. (1981). Endocrine cells of the digestive system. In *Physiology of the Gastrointestinal Tract.* Edited by L. R. Johnson, New York, Raven Press, pp. 59-144.

Watson, S. P. (1984). Are the proposed substance P receptors sub-types, substance P receptors? *Life Sci.* **35**:797-808.

13

Distribution, Nature, and Origin of Peptide-Containing Nerves in Mammalian Airways

DAVID R. SPRINGALL, STEPHEN R. BLOOM, and JULIA M. POLAK

Royal Postgraduate Medical School
Hammersmith Hospital
London, United Kingdom

The advent of quantitative radioimmunoassay procedures (Bloom and Long, 1982), and precise antigen localization by immunocytochemistry (Polak and Van Noorden, 1983) has allowed the nature, distribution, and origin of peptides in the airways of humans and other mammals to be investigated (Polak and Bloom, 1982a,b, 1984a). Neuropeptides that have been studied include the neurokinins, vasoactive intestinal polypeptide (VIP), peptide histidine isoleucine (PHI) or the human variant peptide histidine methionine (PHM), neuropeptide tyrosine (NPY), galanin, and calcitonin gene-related peptide (CGRP).

I. Individual Peptides

The following subsections give a brief description of the main characteristics of neuropeptides found in the respiratory tract. For full details readers are referred to chapters by Makhlouf, Said, and Lundberg contained herein.

A. Neurokinins

The neurokinins (tachykinins) are a family of chemically related peptides encoded in a single gene (Nawa et al., 1984). The family includes substance P, neurokinin A, and neurokinin B. The peptides occur in a subpopulation of sensory neurons widely distributed throughout the body and thus originate from primary sensory neurons of dorsal root and other sensory ganglia. Substance P was the first neurokinin to be discovered (von Euler and Gaddum, 1931) and its distribution is known best. Substance P (for details see chapter by Lundberg) has a very broad distribution in neurons of the central and peripheral nervous system (Porter and O'Connor, 1982). The distribution of other neurokinins is becoming more clearly defined.

B. Vasoactive Intestinal Polypeptide/Peptide Histidine Isoleucine or Methionine

These two peptides of 28 (VIP) and 27 (PHI in pig and PHM in humans) amino acids are derived from the same precursor (Itoh et al., 1983; Bloom et al., 1983) and occur in the majority of tissues, including the respiratory tract (Uddman et al., 1978; Christofides et al., 1984), with an identical distribution in most cases. The origin of VIP/PHI(M) nerves is in general similar to that of parasympathetic neurons, with cell bodies located in or around the individual organ. In fact, VIP has been shown to occur in cholinergic neurons (Lundberg et al., 1980a). VIP was discovered prior to PHI and PHM and details of their discoveries and chemical characteristics are given in the Chapter by Said.

C. Neuropeptide Tyrosine

Neuropeptide tyrosine was discovered by Tatemoto et al. (1982) using their classic chemical fragmentation procedures. The 36 amino acid peptide has a tyrosine molecule at each terminus, hence its name. Although originally found in the central nervous system, NPY was later detected in the gut (Ferri et al., 1984) and many other tissues including heart, blood vessels, spleen, genitourinary tract, eye, and respiratory tract (Polak and Bloom, 1984b; Lundberg et al., 1983). NPY is frequently associated with catecholamine-containing tissues including adrenal medulla and pheochromocytomas (Adrian et al., 1983). Indeed, the nucleotide sequence encoding pre-pro-NPY has recently been revealed by recombinant DNA analysis of a pheochromocytoma extract (Minth et al., 1984).

NPY has potent vasoconstrictor properties and has been reported to exist principally in noradrenergic neurons. The amino acid sequence of pre-pro-NPY was predicted from the nucleotide series and this has revealed NPY to be flanked by other peptides (Fig. 1). Antibodies to the C-terminal flanking peptide of NPY (CPON) have recently been raised and used both for radioimmunoassay

20
MetLeuGlyAsnLysArgLeuGlyLeuSerGlyLeuThrLeuAlaLeuSerLeuLeuValCysLeu

40
GlyAlaLeuAlaGluAlaTyrProSerLysProAspAsnProGlyGluAspAlaProAlaGluAsp

60
MetAlaArgTyrTyrSerAlaLeuArgHisTyrIleAsnLeuIleThrArgGlnArgTyrGlyLys

80
ArgSerSerProGluThrLeuIleSerAspLeuLeuMetArgGluSerThrGluAsnValProArg

97
ThrArgLeuGluAspProAlaMetTrp

Figure 1 Amino acid sequence of pre-pro-NPY. The sequence of NPY is underscored in the 97 residue prepromolecule.

(Allen et al., 1985) and immunocytochemistry (Gulbenkian et al., 1986a). As expected, there is a close quantitative relationship between NPY and CPON as shown by radioimmunoassay of extracts of rat adrenal, heart, vasculature, and brain. Furthermore, on immunocytochemical analysis the distribution patterns of both peptides are indistinguishable in rat brain, guinea pig celiac ganglion, and vascular system, and in adrenal medulla of rat (Fig. 2), cat and guinea pig and human pheochromocytomas. Electron microscopic immunocytochemistry has revealed that the peptides are stored in the same neuroendocrine secretory granules.

D. Galanin

The name galanin derives from *g*lycine and *alanin*e present at the N and C terminals, respectively, of this 29 amino acid peptide, which was originally isolated from porcine gastrointestinal tract by Tatemoto et al., (1983). Galanin induces hyperglycemia (McDonald et al., 1985) and enhances muscle tone (Tatemoto et al., 1983). It is not only found in the brain and gut (Rökaeus et al., 1984; Chn'g et al., 1985; Skofitsch and Jacobowitz, 1985) but is also present in other tissues including the adrenal medulla (Terenghi et al., 1986), the genitourinary system (Bauer et al., 1984), and the respiratory tract (Cheung et al., 1985). Galanin occurs in nerves many of which, in certain tissues, show a similar distribution to that of VIP, and their origin is similar to that found for VIP/PHI(M), that is, in cell bodies located in and around the innervated organ.

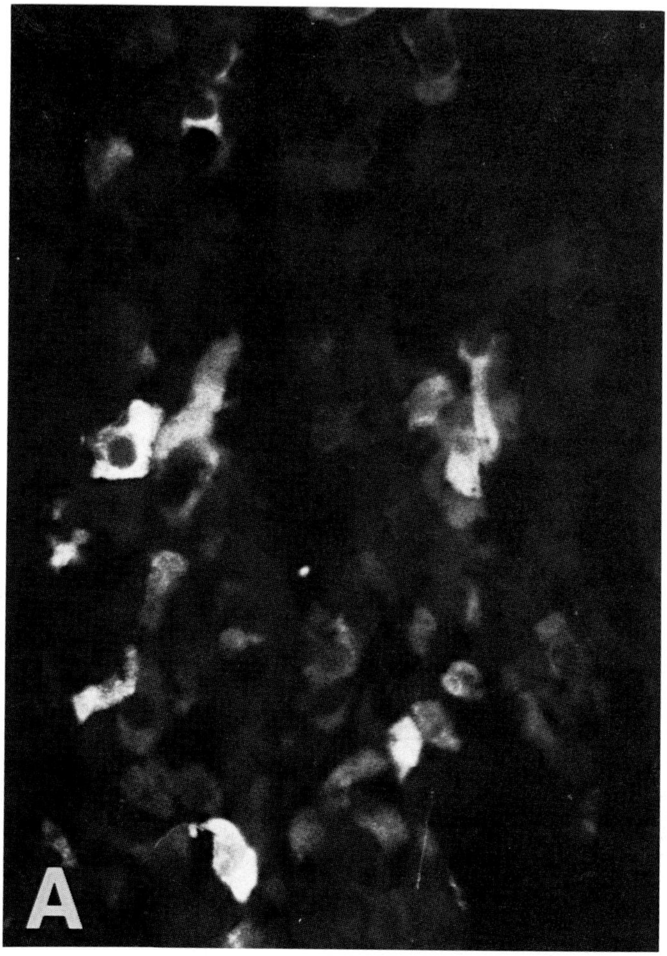

Figure 2 Immunofluorescence micrographs of serial sections of rat adrenal medulla immunostained for (A) C-terminal NPY (CPON) and (B) NPY. Immunoreactivity is seen with both antisera in the same cells (p-Benzoquinone-fixed tissue; ×380).

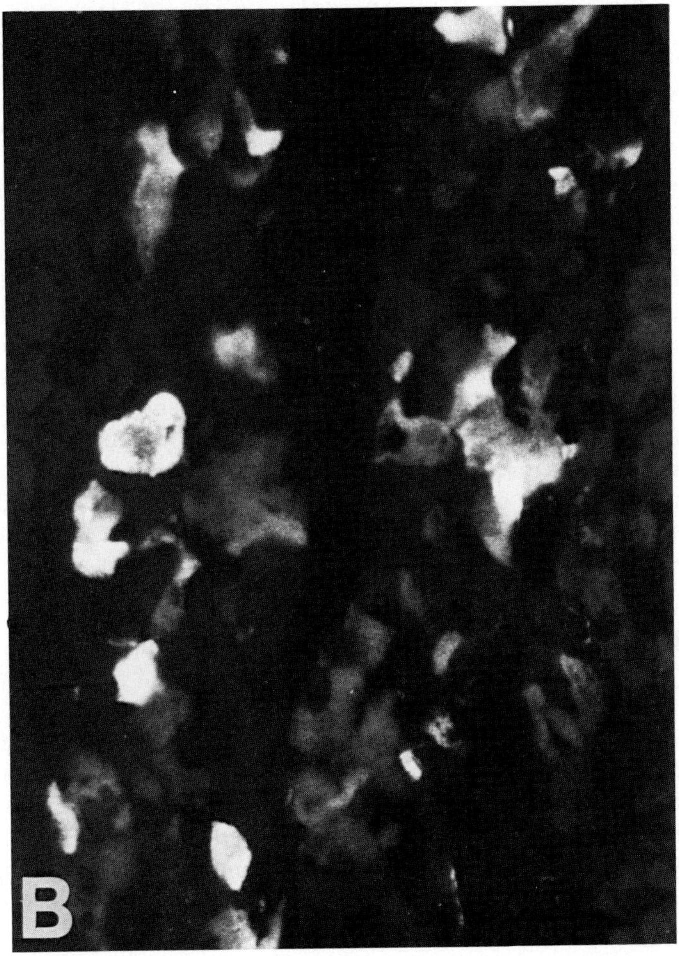

Figure 2 (continued)

E. Calcitonin Gene-Related Peptide

The existence of CGRP was predicted by molecular biologic analysis of the calcitonin gene derived from a rat medullary thyroid carcinoma cell line. The gene was shown to produce a second mRNA transcript that encoded a product of 37 amino acids (Rosenfeld et al., 1983). A variant of CGRP was subsequently isolated from human medullary thyroid carcinoma (Morris et al., 1984), its structure differing from the rat peptide by four amino acid substitutions. Genes encoding separate CGRPs were then discovered for both rat (β-CGRP; Amara et al., 1985) and humans (Edbrooke et al., 1985; Steenbergh et al., 1984), differing from the initially described CGRP sequences by one and three amino acid substitutions, respectively. CGRP immunoreactivity is abundantly and broadly distributed throughout the mammalian body (Clague et al., 1985; Kawai et al., 1985; Rodrigo et al., 1985; Seifert et al., 1985), frequently innervating blood vessel walls (Mulderry et al., 1985), and showing a distribution pattern consistent with sensory neurons (Gibson et al., 1984; Terenghi et al., 1985). In many tissues the coexistence of substance P and α-CGRP in neuronal cell bodies and peripheral axons has been clearly demonstrated (Gibson et al., 1984; Terenghi et al., 1985; Gulbenkian et al., 1986b; Lundberg et al., 1985).

II. Technology for Determination of Neuropeptide Distribution, Nature, and Origin

Previously, basic radioimmunoassay and immunocytochemical techniques were used independently, which permitted the distribution and chemical nature of neuropeptides, including those of the respiratory tract, to be determined. Nowadays, however, chemical and surgical lesioning methods (Heimer and Robards, 1981) may be applied in combination with immunocytochemistry using a broad variety of region-specific antipeptide sera, as well as antibodies to general neuronal markers (such as neurofilament triplet proteins and neuron-specific enolase) to delineate the entire innervation of any organ. The application of these techniques has allowed a more complete understanding, of not only the distribution of neuropeptides within various respiratory tract structures but also their precise origins (e.g., local or extrinsic cell bodies) and nature (e.g., sensory, autonomic). Thus the neurochemical anatomy of each organ is beginning to be determined, thus linking the central nervous system with peripheral tissues such as the respiratory tract. In the following sections we describe established techniques for the determination of the distribution, nature, and origin of neuropeptide-containing nerves within the respiratory tract.

A. Immunocytochemistry of Neuroendocrine Markers

Antibodies to various structural proteins (neurofilaments, chromogranin) or specific enzymes (neuron-specific enolase, choline acetyltransferase, amine-converting enzymes) of the diffuse neuroendocrine system are now available to permit delineation of both neural and endocrine elements of the respiratory tract.

Neuron-Specific Enolase

Neuron-specific enolase (NSE), originally called 14-3-2, was extracted, together with other specific proteins, from brain by Moore (1973). Subsequent characterization by Marangos et al. (1975) revealed that it was present in neurons and had enolase activity; it was therefore called neuron-specific enolase (NSE). Enolase is a large dimeric protein (NSE is approximately 78 kilodaltons) of three possible subunits—α, β, and γ—present in various molecular forms: α-α' (found in muscle), β-β' (present in liver), γ-γ' (NSE), and the hybrid form α-γ. NSE is found broadly distributed throughout the body (Polak and Marangos, 1984), and antibodies to NSE are capable of demonstrating various elements of the diffuse neuroendocrine system.

In the respiratory tract, NSE antibodies stain both neural and endocrine components (Fig. 3) as in other tissues (Sheppard et al., 1983a). It has been used as a marker for determining the developmental pattern of the diffuse neuroendocrine system (Sheppard et al., 1984a), permitting the demonstration of mucosal endocrine cells and nerves even in the early stages of human development. In humans, NSE immunoreactivity was first recorded at 8 weeks of gestation in neuroblasts and mucosal endocrine cells of major airways. This was prior to the appearance of peptide and dopamine-β-hydroxylase immunoreactivity or acetyl cholinesterase activity. Furthermore, NSE immunoreactivity may appear in peripheral neurons at an earlier stage than in neurons of the central nervous system.

Protein Gene Product 9.5

Protein gene product (PGP 9.5) is a recently discovered 27 kilodalton protein (Thompson et al., 1983) originally extracted from the brain and found to be an excellent marker for nerves in many tissues including respiratory tract (Fig. 4). PGP 9.5 antisera also immunostain a variety of endocrine cells, including both single cells and clusters of cells or "neuroepithelial bodies" in the respiratory tract (Fig. 5).

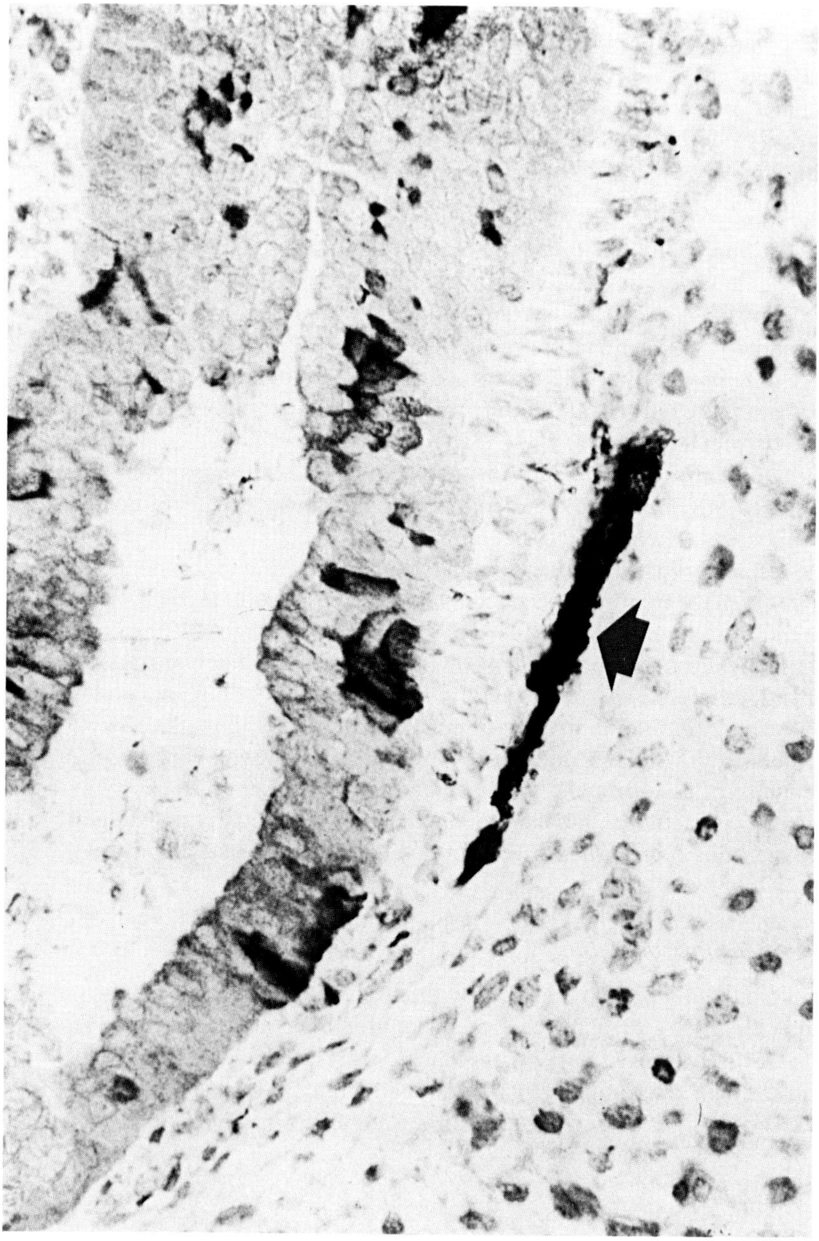

Figure 3 Section of 8-week-old fetal human lung immunostained for neuron-specific enolase by the peroxidase anti-peroxidase technique. Numerous immunoreactive endocrine cells are seen among the epithelial cells of a lobar bronchus, and a fascicle of nerve fibers in the connective tissue is indicated (arrow) (tissue fixed in Bouin's fluid and wax embedded; ×500).

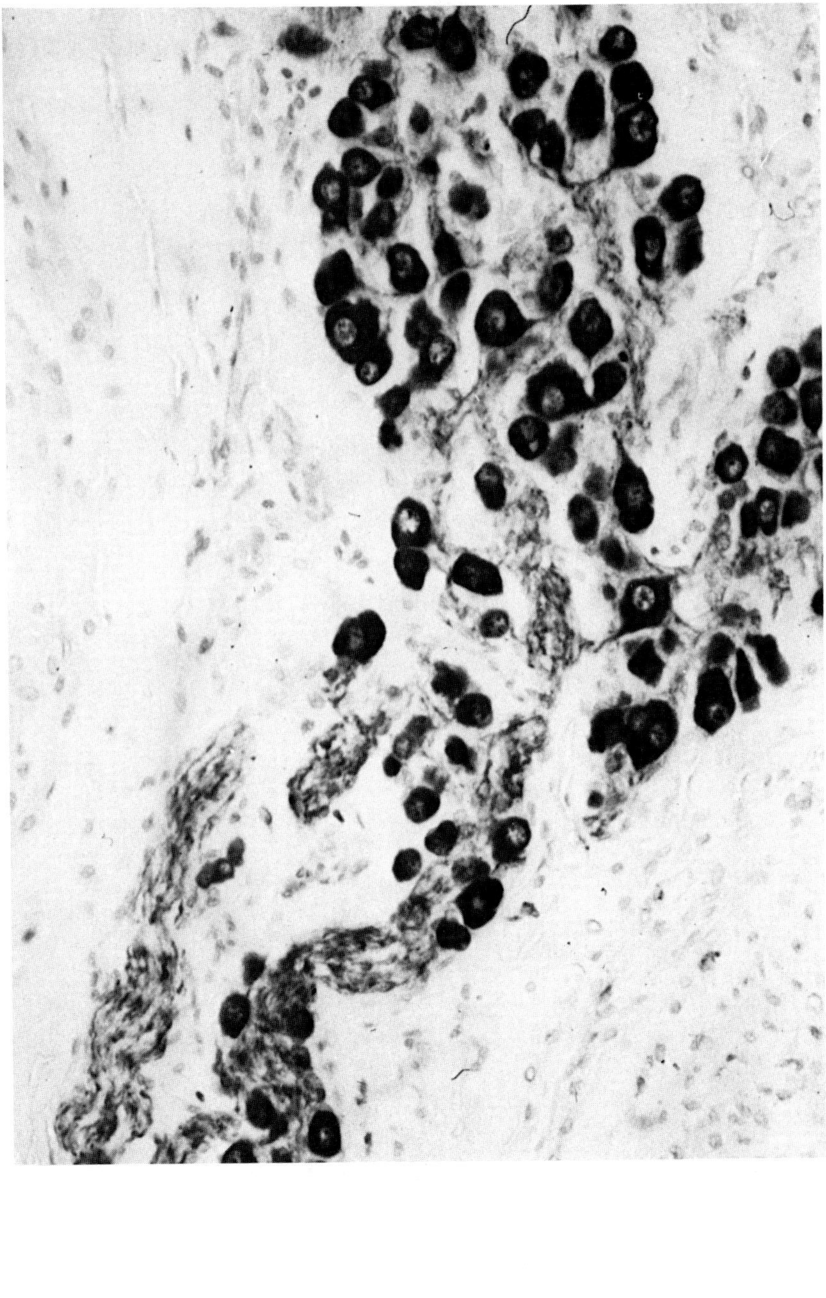

Figure 4 Section of rat lung, immunostained with anti-PGP 9.5 serum by the peroxidase antiperoxidase method, shows immunoreactive nerve fibers and neuronal cell bodies in the anterior pulmonary plexus (tissue fixed in Bouin's fluid and embedded in wax; × 500).

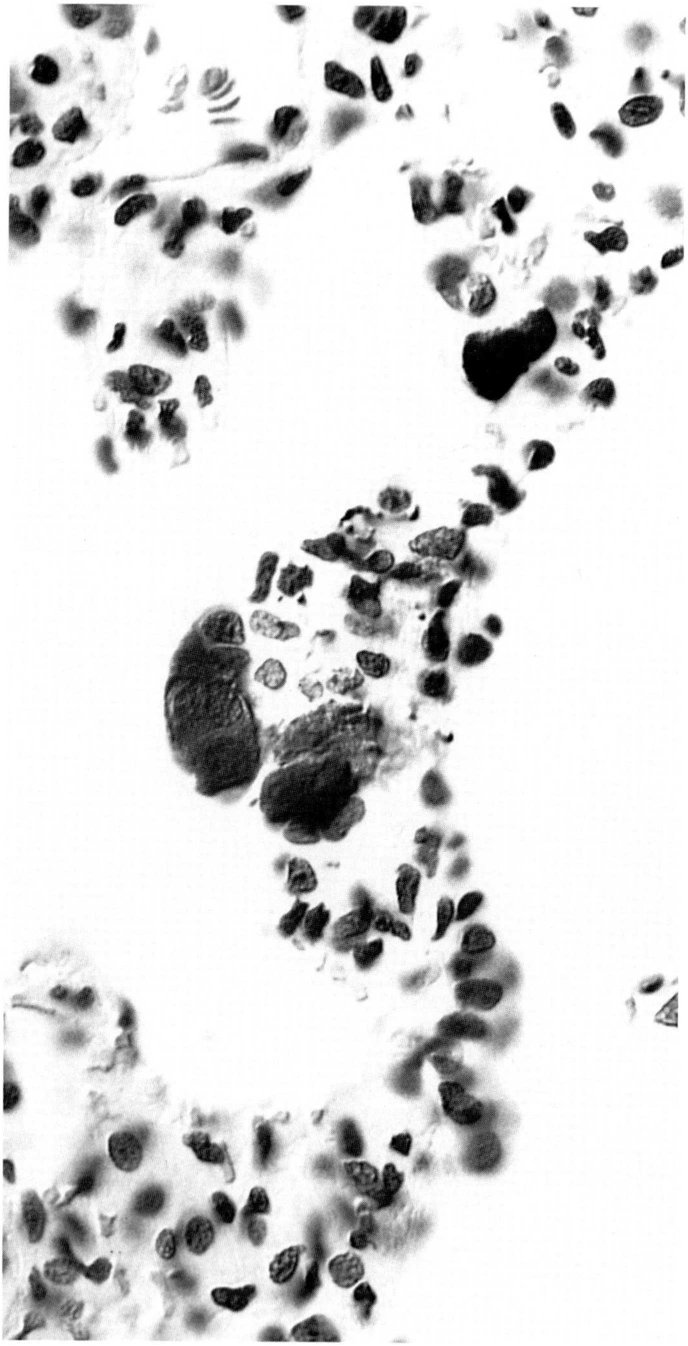

Figure 5 Section of adult rat lung immunostained as in Figure 4. A small group of immunoreactive endocrine cells is seen in an alveolar duct (tissue fixed in Bouin's fluid and wax embedded; ×540).

Neurofilaments

Neurofilaments are component parts of the cytoskeleton of nerves and occur principally in three forms of approximately 68, 150, and 200 kilodaltons (Hoffman and Lasek, 1975). Antibodies to neurofilament triplet proteins, both polyclonal and monoclonal, are excellent for the delineation of the anatomic distribution of nerves within the respiratory tract of man and mammals (Hacker et al., 1985) (Fig. 6). Because of the nature of these cytoskeletal proteins, functional changes within the neuron or nerve fiber are not picked up by these antibodies. They are therefore excellent for straightforward anatomic studies.

Markers for Adrenergic and Cholinergic Innervation

The first two techniques to be used for the delineation of noradrenergic and cholinergic neurons were the Falck et al. (1962) method of formaldehyde-induced fluorescence for the former and cholinesterase histochemistry (Pearse, 1968, 1972). for the latter. Nowadays antibodies to converting enzymes involved in the catecholaminergic and cholinergic pathways (Fig. 7) are widely used. These enzymes include tyrosine hydroxylase (TH), dopamine β-hydroxylase (DBH) (Fig. 8), phenylethanolamine N-methyl transferase (PNMT), and choline acetyl transferase (ChAT).

Specific Peptide Markers

Advances in protein chemistry and molecular biology have made available pure synthetic peptides that have been widely used as antigens. A broad variety of region-specific antibodies that recognize not only the so-called bio-active segment but also the flanking peptides and the whole precursor forms have been raised both for radioimmunoassay and immunocytochemistry. The former, when applied with modern chromatographic procedures, allows for the precise determination of the chemical nature of extractable peptide. Immunocytochemistry, particularly the refinement of techniques at the ultrastructural level, allows determination of the precise tissue distribution for a given peptide (Van Noorden and Polak, 1985), and demonstration of the storage site and secretory granule type (Varndell and Polak, (1984). Electron microscopic immunocytochemistry can also reveal the degree of compartmentalization of peptide molecular forms within single neuroendocrine secretory granules, and thus peptide coexistence can be demonstrated (Gulbenkian et al., 1986b).

There are several methods for the immunocytochemical demonstration of peptide coexistence at the light microscopic level, although the original elution procedures are now less favored. Other techniques are becoming more popular, including reverse face immunostaining (Fig. 9a) the use of antibodies raised in different species (Fig. 9b), the use of serial resin sections less than 1 μm thick,

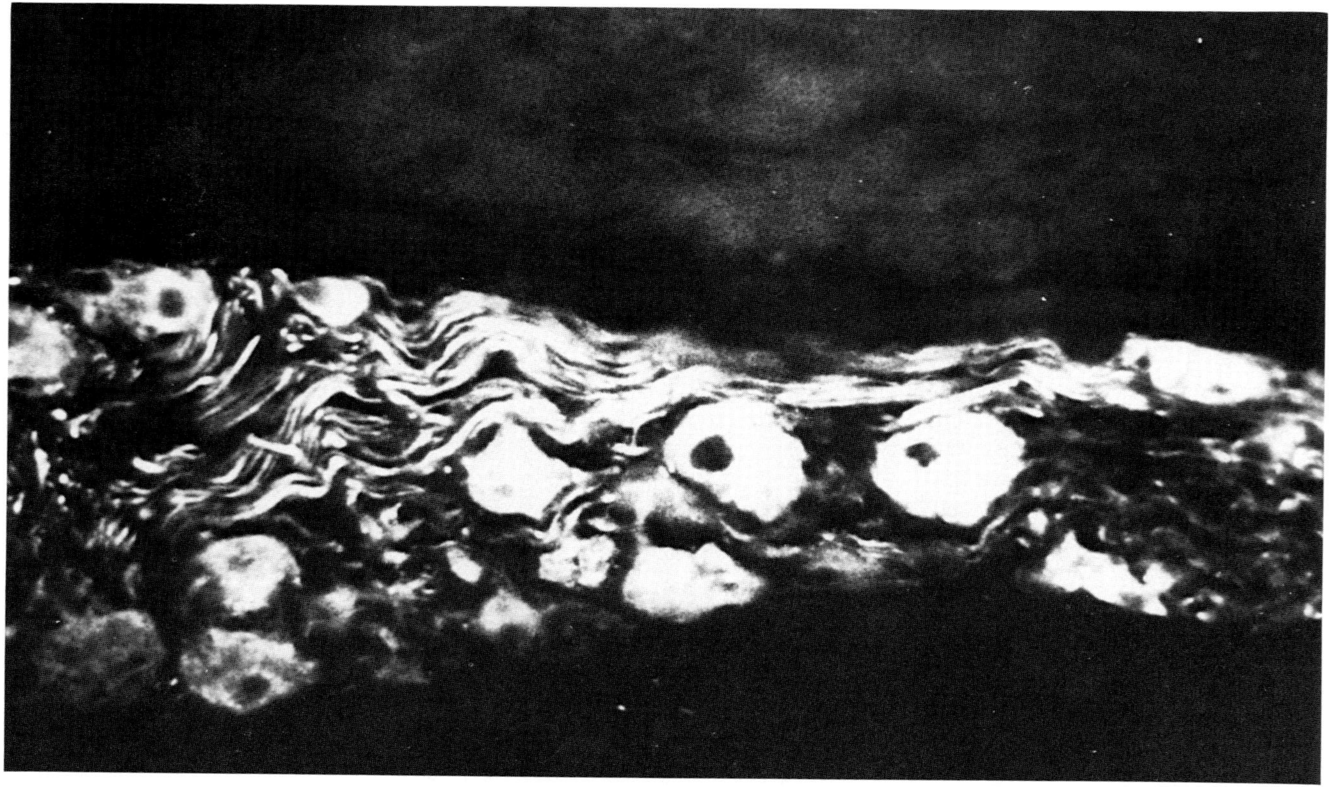

Figure 6 Immunofluorescence micrograph of a section of dog trachea incubated with antineurofilament serum. Nerve fibers and neuronal cell bodies are seen in an extramural ganglion of the upper part of the trachea (p-Benzoquinone-fixed tissue; ×440).

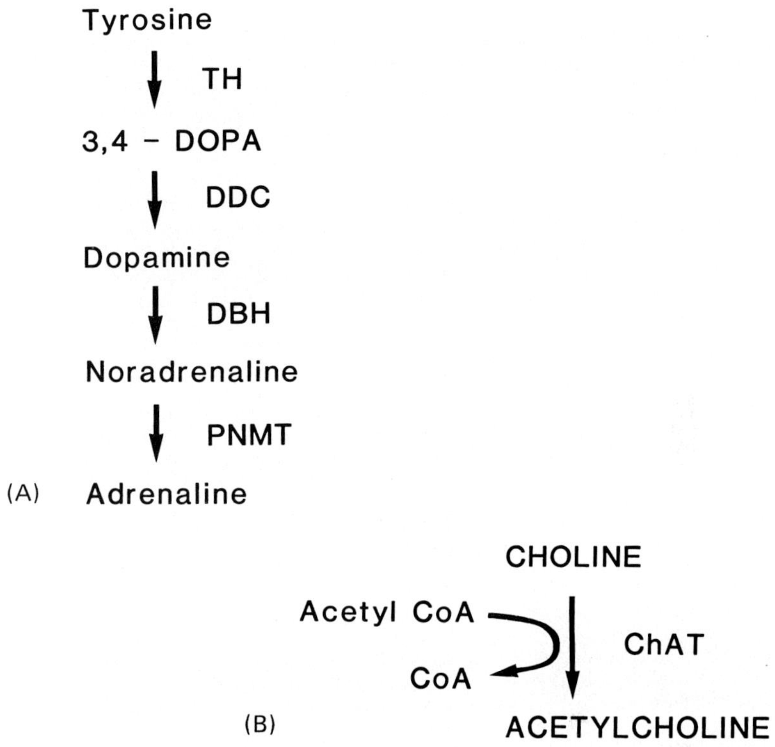

Figure 7 Schematic pathway of catecholamine (A) and acetylcholine (B) biosynthesis. TH, tyrosine hydroxylase; 3,4-DOPA, 3,4-dihydroxy phenylalanine; DDC, dopa decarboxylase; DBH, dopamine-β-hydroxylase; PNMT, phenylethanolamine-N-methyltransferase; ChAT, choline acetyltransferase.

and the recently proposed, but not yet fully validated, technique of Wang and Larsson (1985), involving hot formaldehyde treatment of sections after the first immunostaining (Fig. 9c) to eliminate the possibility of cross-immunostaining.

B. Chemical, Surgical, Neurobiologic, and Tracing Methods Combined with Radioimmunoassay and/or Immunocytochemistry

Pharmacologic manipulations have been used for some time to determine the nature (sensory, autonomic) of a particular peptide immunoreactivity. An extract of the red pepper, capsaicin (8-methyl-N-vanillyl-6-nonenamide) selectively affects sensory (C and fine Aδ) nerve fibers (Fitzgerald, 1983) (Fig. 10). Ap-

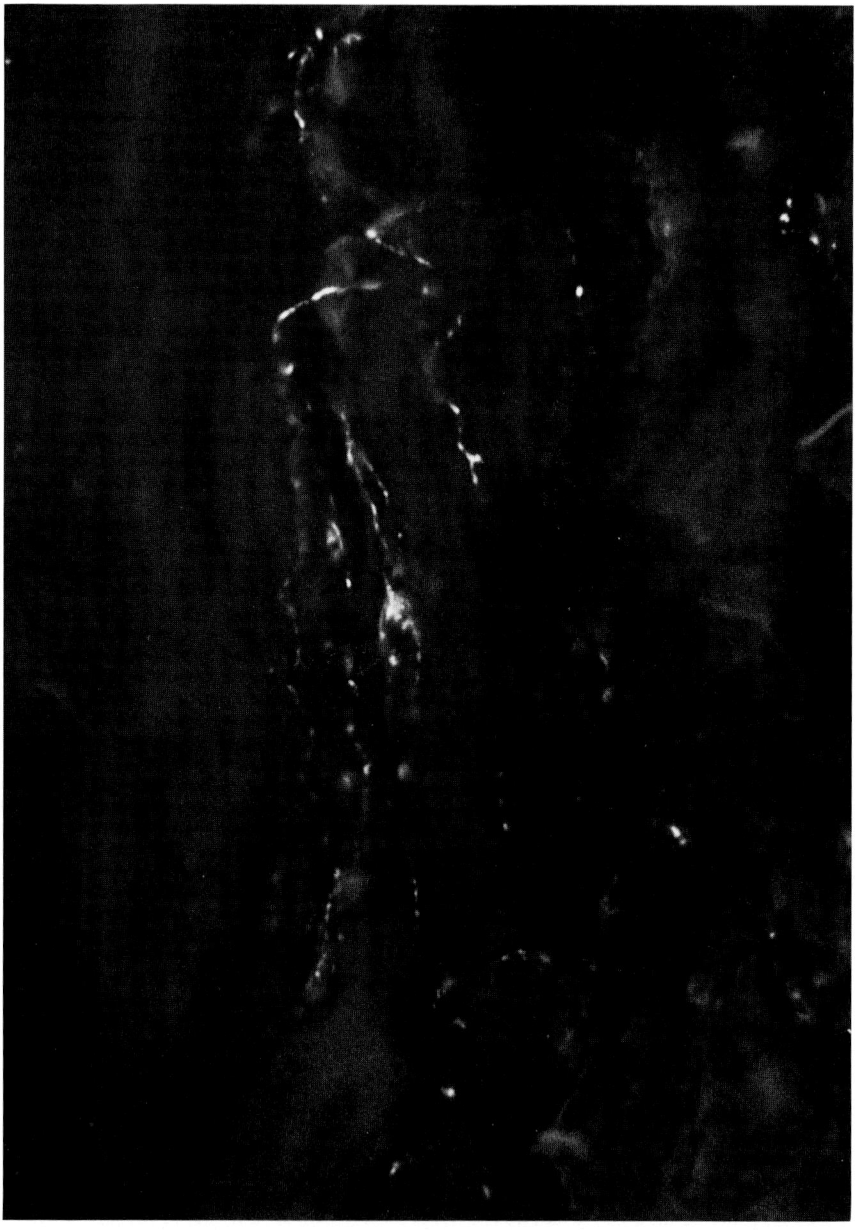

Figure 8 Immunofluorescence micrograph of a section of dog lung immunostained for dopamine-β-hydroxylase shows immunoreactive nerve fibers in the smooth muscle layer of a small bronchus (p-Benzoquinone-fixed tissue; X 460)

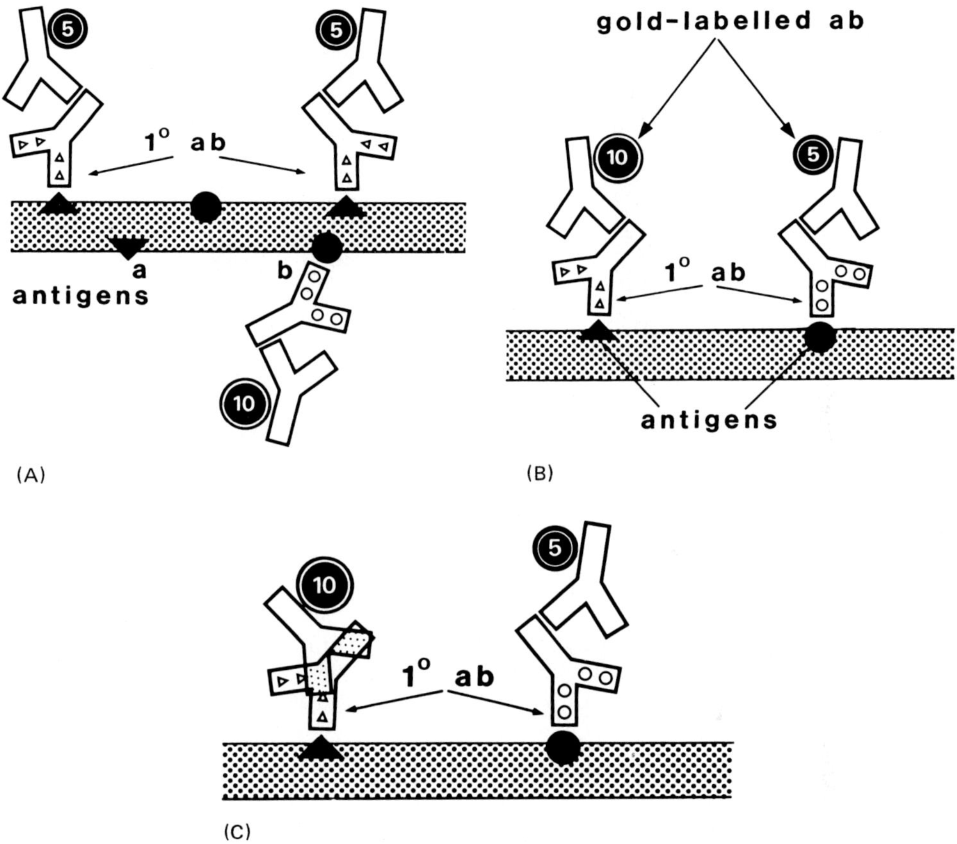

Figure 9 Diagrammatic representations of multiple immunostaining procedures. The illustrations show the methods as used for immunoelectron microscopy, but procedures (B) and (C) can equally well be used at the light microscopic level with different enzyme labels (or chromogens for development) for the two steps. Different sizes of colloidal gold (5 and 10 nm in these diagrams) are used to identify the separate antigens. (A). Modification of the two-surface staining procedure, using immunoglobulin-gold complexes (for review, see Varndell and Polak, 1984). (B) Double immunogold staining method. Primary antisera raised in different species (to avoid cross-reactivity) are differentially localized using antispecies specific Ig sera. (C) Formaldehyde blockade method (Wang and Larsson, 1985). A single immunogold staining is applied and localized with 10 nm gold. The complex is then denatured with formaldehyde vapor (80°C for 1 hr) to render it unreactive to the subsequently applied gold complex (5 nm) gold.

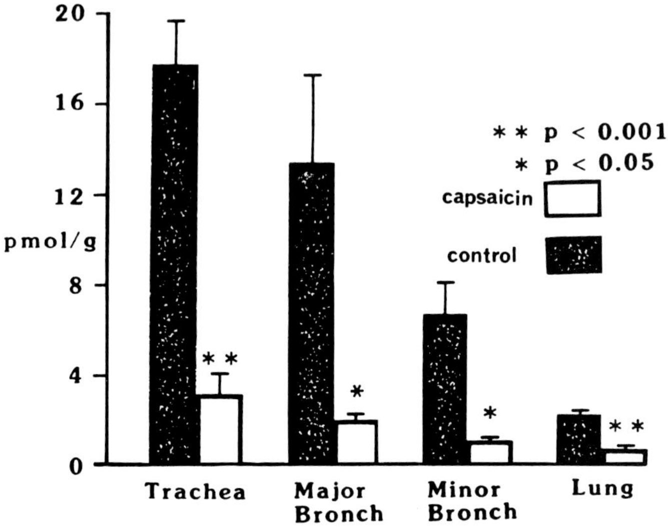

Figure 10 Substance P immunoreactive material in extracts of rat trachea, bronchi, and lungs. Levels in controls are compared with those in animals treated neonatally with systemic capsaicin (50 mg/kg). A significant reduction in substance P levels was found in the capsaicin-treated animals.

plication of capsaicin has been found to deplete both neurokinin and CGRP immunoreactivity (Mulderry et al., 1985; Jessel et al., 1978). Thus the putative sensory nature of substance P and CGRP has been further supported.

For many years 6-hydroxydopamine and reserpine have been known to cause degeneration or degranulation of noradrenergic neurons (Tranzer and Richards, 1971). NPY immunoreactivity is diminished following such treatment and thus the putative coexistence of NPY in noradrenergic neurons is upheld (Morris et al., 1986).

Visualization of nerve cell bodies by basic immunocytochemical means is sometimes difficult because the neurochemicals are mostly stored in electron-dense secretory vesicles that are generally most numerous in nerve terminals. Weak immunostaining of cell bodies may be improved by surgical lesioning (ligation [Fig. 11], denervation) or by systemic or topical treatment of the neuron with colchicine (Dahlström, 1968) or similar compounds that block intracellular transport mechanisms.

Such techniques may also be complemented by nerve tracing (Heimer and Robards, 1981). Tracing methods are based on the ability of a nerve terminal,

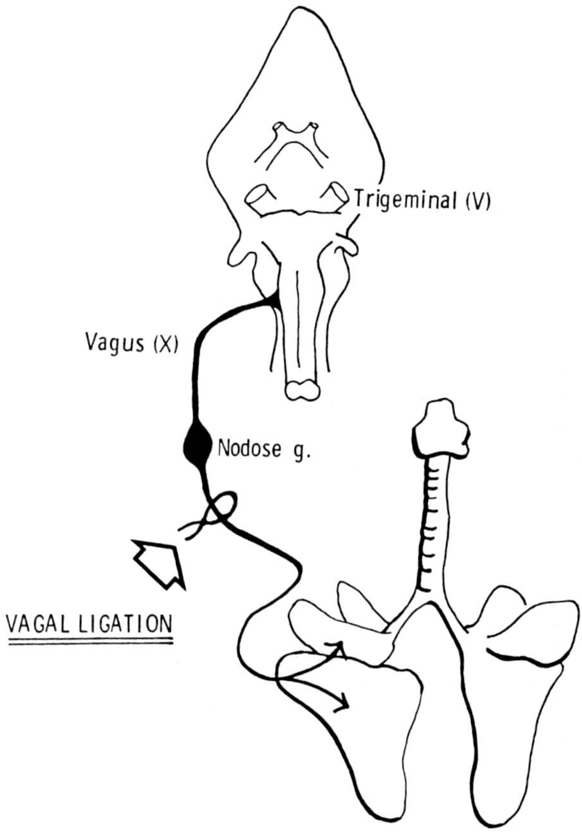

Figure 11 Diagram of vagal innervation of respiratory tract shows ligation point for infranodosal vagal ligation.

sectioned fiber, or micropunctured cell body to take up certain compounds by receptor- or non-receptor-mediated mechanisms. These substances can be transported retrogradely and/or anterogradely in relation to the cell body (Fig. 12). By injecting the tracer into a peripheral tissue and analyzing tissues from the supposed origin of the innervation of the organ, it is possible to reconstruct the neuroanatomic pathway.

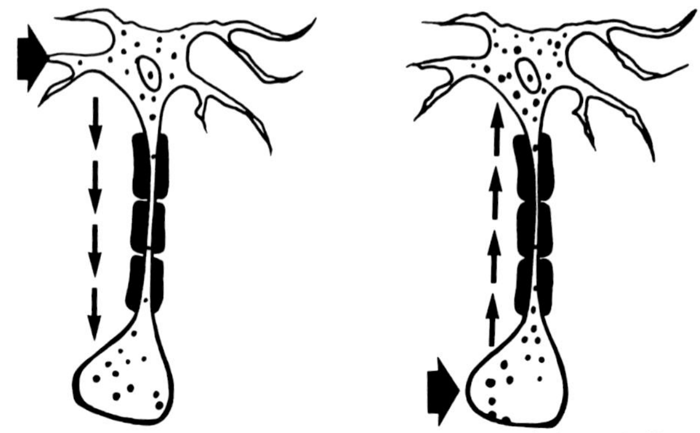

Figure 12 Nerve tracing. Schematic diagram showing retrograde and anterograde transport of tracer in nerves. The tracer substance is taken up by nerve terminals alone or also by fibers of passage, depending on the tracer used.

III. Peptide-Containing Nerves of the Airways

The distribution of individual neuropeptide-containing structures or nerves is described in the following sections. Where possible, reference will be made to species homologies or differences and to the presence or absence in humans.

A. Neurokinins

Substance P was first reported to be present in airway structures of guinea pigs in 1977 (Nilsson et al., 1979), and subsequently in mouse, rat, pig, cat, and humans (Wharton et al., 1979; Ghatei et al., 1982; Hökfelt et al., 1977; Lundberg et al., 1984a) (Fig. 13). Agreement exists between workers that substance P immunoreactivity occurs in a subset of sensory neurons of the respiratory tract, originating mainly from the inferior portion of the nodose ganglion (Katz and Karten, 1980; Lundberg et al., 1980b). That a small proportion of substance P-containing neurons originate from the dorsal root ganglia has not yet been demonstrated by retrograde tracing methods combined with immunocytochemistry, but has been suggested by Lundberg et al. (1984a). However, results obtained from unilateral vagal ligation (Lundberg et al., 1984a; Terenghi et al., 1983) (Fig. 14) just below the nodose ganglion in guinea pigs show that substance-P-like immunoreactive material is still detectable in the ipsilateral lung by radioimmunoassay and immunocytochemistry 3, 7, and 10 days postligation (Fig. 15). This residual material may originate from the contralateral side via the pulmonary plexus and possibly from dorsal root ganglia at the thoracic level.

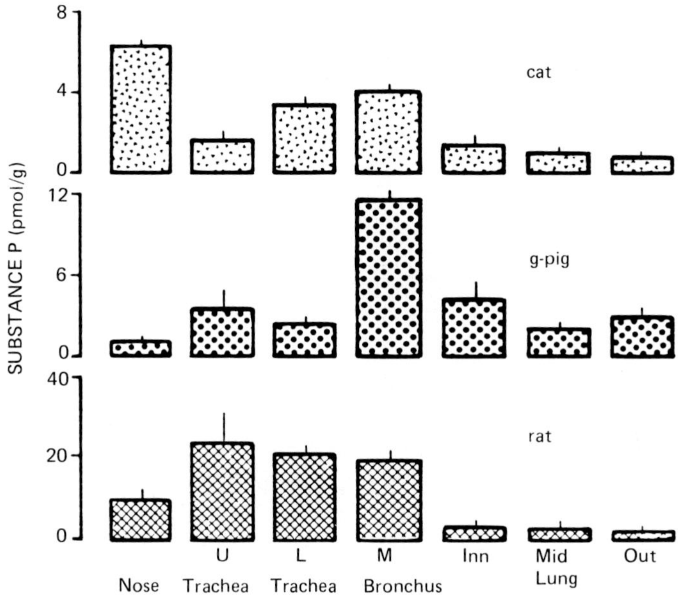

Figure 13 Levels of substance P immunoreactivity in extracts of respiratory tract of cat, guinea pig, and rat.

A similar distribution of substance P immunoreactive nerve fibers has been obtained in all mammalian species so far studied. Immunoreactive nerves are found throughout the respiratory tract down to the level of the bronchiolar wall. Nerve fibers are seen beneath (Fig. 16) and sometimes penetrating the airway epithelium, around vascular and nonvascular smooth muscle and around seromucous glands. However, in the larger mammals such as cat, monkey, and humans, fewer fibers are seen in the airway epithelium and smooth muscle. When extracted and assayed, highest concentrations of substance P were found in the respiratory tract of rat and guinea pig. The chromatographic profile of the extractable material indicates that the majority of substance P immunoreactivity coelutes with synthetic peptide.

Further information on the possible sensory nature of substance-P-immunoreactive nerve fibers comes from experiments after capsaicin treatment of neonatal animals (Sheppard et al., 1983b) (Fig. 17). In rats, a marked depletion of substance P immunoreactivity (up to 86% by radioimmunoassay) was obtained at 3 and 8 months following neonatal systemic administration of capsaicin. This reduction was most marked in the sub- and intraepithelial nerve fibers.

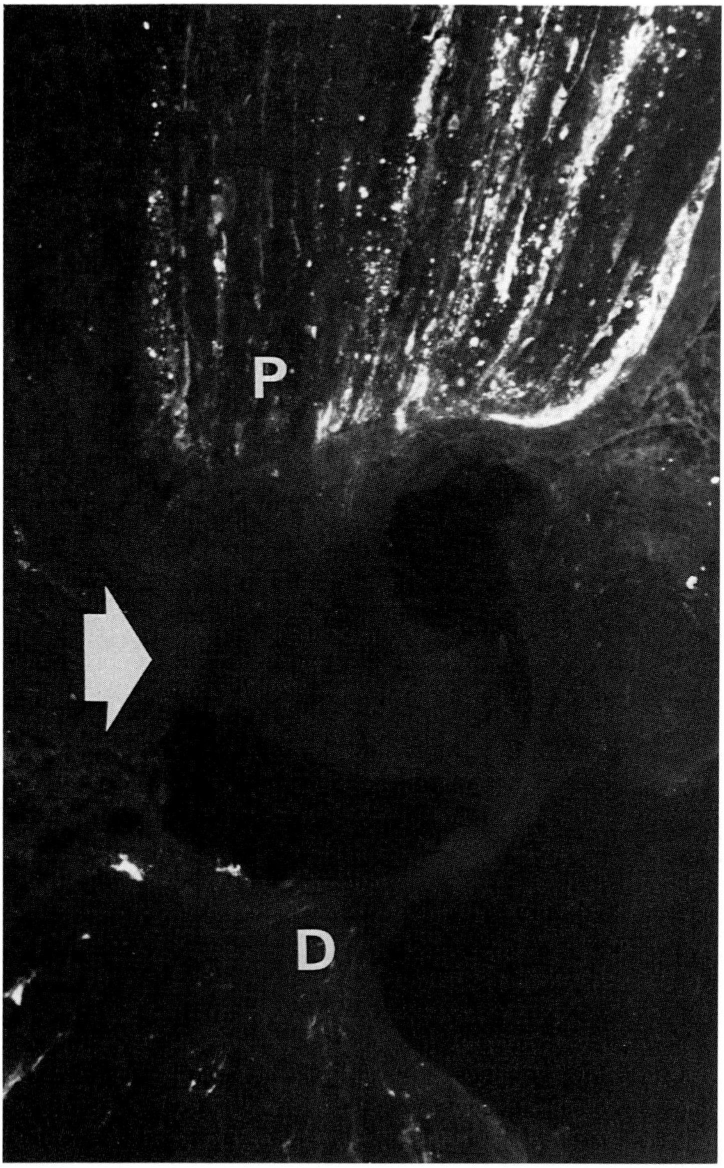

Figure 14 Immunofluorescence micrograph of a longitudinal section of infranodosally ligated rat vagus immunostained for substance P. At 24 hr after ligation, a marked increase of immunoreactive material is seen proximal (P) to the ligation point (arrow). On the distal side (D) a few positive axons were sometimes observed (p-Benzoquinone fixation; ×180).

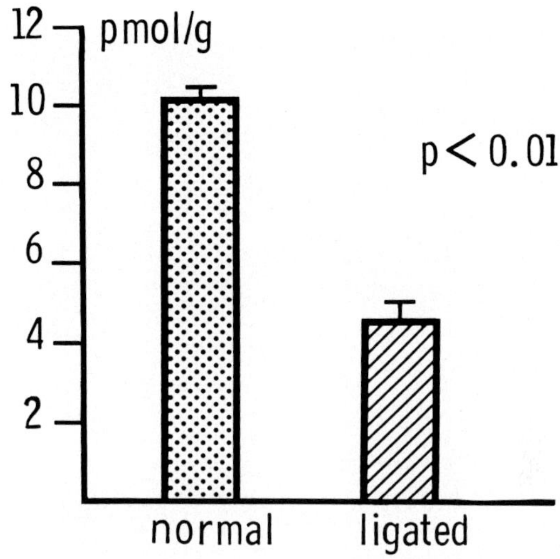

Figure 15 Substance P immunoreactivity in extracts of guinea pig lung. Comparison of tissues from sham-operated controls and animals 10 days after unilateral infranodosal vagal ligation. A significant decrease is seen in the ligated animals.

The presence of substance P in mucosal endocrine cells of guinea pig has also been reported (Sundler et al., 1972) but has yet to be confirmed.

Much less is known about the distribution, nature, and origin of other neurokinins, although reports are now appearing on the existence of an independent neurokinin A and B system in the respiratory tract (Hua et al., 1985). The presence of neurokinin A, neuropeptide K, and an eledoisin-like peptide in capsaicin-sensitive nerves has been demonstrated in guinea pig lung. The immunocytochemical distribution of the nerve fibers containing neurokinin A was identical to those immunoreactive for substance P (Hua et al., 1985).

B. Vasoactive Intestinal Polypeptide/Peptides Histidine [Isoleucine/Methionine]

VIP, PHI, and PHM are discussed together here because of the similar distribution of these peptides, which originate from the same precursor. VIP and PHI(M) are abundant in the upper respiratory tract of cat, dog, pig and ox, and are also found in rat, guinea pig, cattle, and primates including humans (Ghatei et al., 1982; Lundberg et al., 1984b; Dey et al., 1981) (Fig. 18). The chromatographic profile of material extracted from the respiratory tract shows VIP immunore-

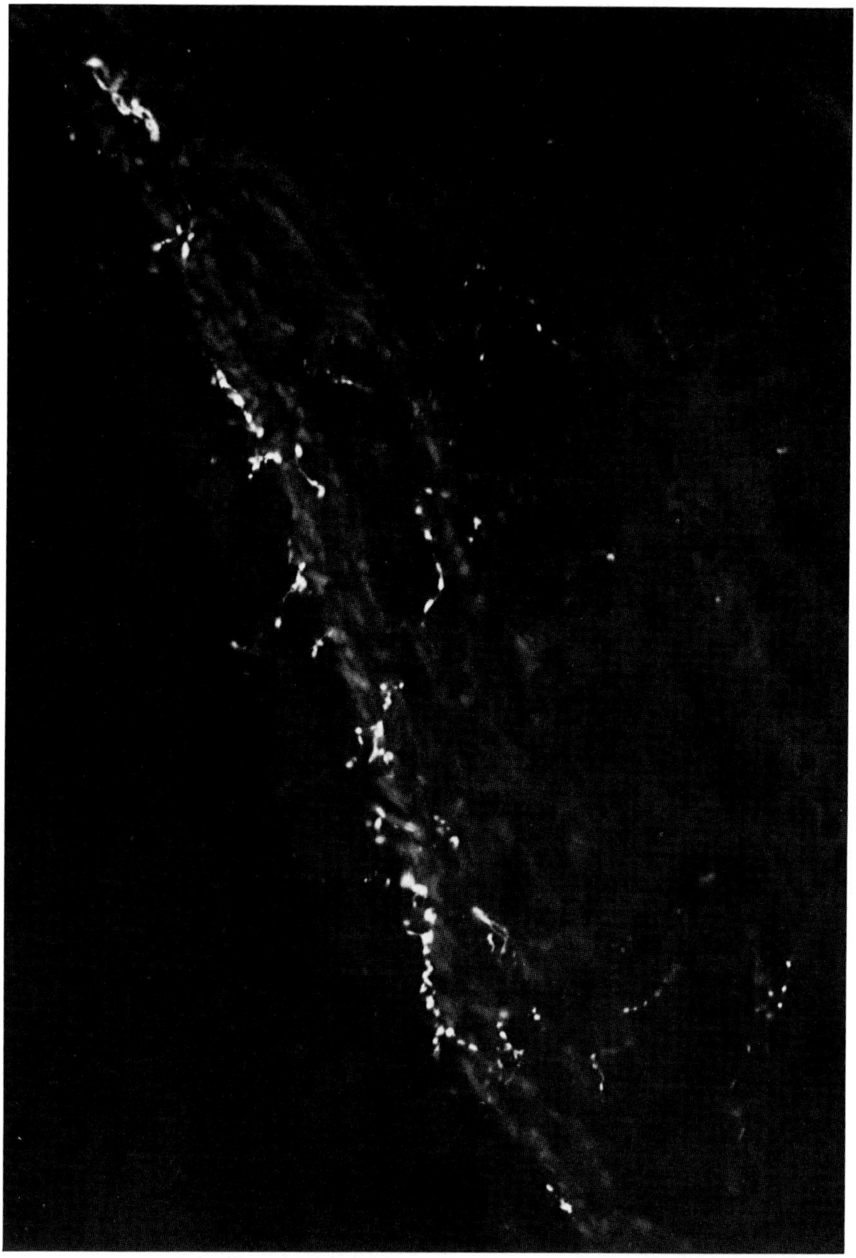

Figure 16 Immunofluorescence micrograph of a section of rat trachea immunostained for substance P. Varicose immunoreactive nerve fibers are seen running beneath and within the epithelium (p-Benzoquinone-fixed tissue; X400).

activity to coelute with the synthetic peptide. However, PHI, especially in extracts of nasal mucosa, shows a different peak of activity due to the presence of an N-terminally extended form (Fig. 19).

VIP/PHI(M) occurs in nerves innervating nasal mucosa, trachea, and main bronchi. Nerve fibers containing these immunoreactivities are most abundant in the cat. In all mammals examined, the immunocytochemical distribution of VIP/PHI(M) is exclusively in nerves found in close association with seromucous glands, smooth muscle, and blood vessels, particularly in upper airways (Fig. 20A). Radioimmunoassay data reveal a range of peptide concentrations between the species, which is largely in accord with the innervation patterns. In the smaller mammals VIP-immunoreactive nerves are found mostly around seromucous glands, predominantly in the trachea, but less frequently in vascular and nonvascular smooth muscle. In the larger species, there is a greater component of VIP innervation in smooth muscle and around blood vessels throughout the respiratory tract.

Local cell bodies containing VIP/PHI(M) are found in the adventitia of the tracheobronchial wall, particularly in the posterior wall of the upper trachea of pig and dog (Figs. 20B and 21). In nasal mucosa, nerve fibers immunoreactive for VIP/PHI(M) originate from cell bodies in the sphenopalatine ganglion that also contain acetylcholine (Lundberg et al., 1980; Ånggard et al., 1979). This is of interest due to the cooperative action of these two substances in enhancing secretion in exocrine glands such as salivary glands and seromucous glands in the respiratory tract, including the nasal mucosa (Lundberg et al., 1981). Differential or simultaneous release of VIP and acetylcholine may be caused, dependent on the frequency of nerve stimulation (Bloom and Edwards, 1980). Furthermore, patients with uncontrollable rhinorrhea due to vasomotor rhinitis have an increased number of nerves immunoreactive to VIP antisera, with an abnormal morphologic pattern in the nasal mucosa (Kurian et al., 1983). The possible function of VIP and PHI(M) as muscle relaxant peptides is further substantiated, and their potential role in the treatment of asthma and cystic fibrosis is supported.

C. Neuropeptide Tyrosine

Neuropeptide tyrosine (NPY)-immunoreactive nerve fibers, although relatively numerous, are found in smaller numbers than other peptidergic nerves of the respiratory tract (Sheppard et al., 1984b). Highest concentrations are found in guinea pig and rat, lower levels in cat, pig, and humans. Within the human respiratory tract the distribution of catecholaminergic neurons, as shown by the use of antibodies to tyrosine hydroxylase and dopamine β-hydroxylase, is indistinguishable from that of NPY, and they show a similar developmental pattern, appearing at gestational week 20. Further proof of the coexistence

Figure 17 Immunofluorescence micrographs of sections of rat lung immunostained with antiserum to substance P. (A) Neonatal systemic capsaicin treatment resulted in a total loss of immunoreactive nerve fibers associated with the smooth muscle of the airways compared with (B) untreated control (p-Benzoquinone-fixed tissue; X 280).

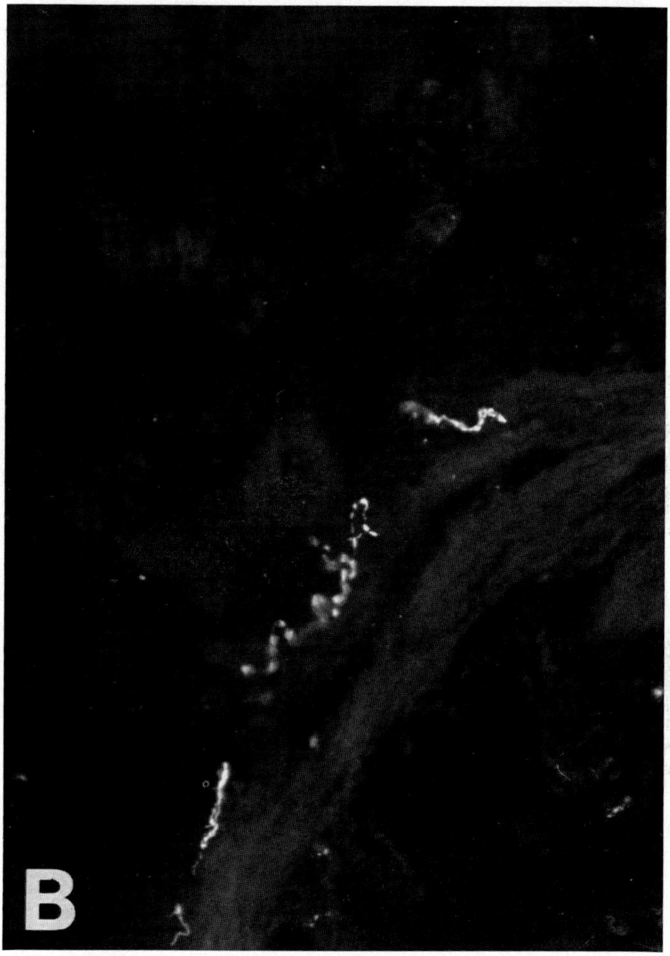

Figure 17 (continued)

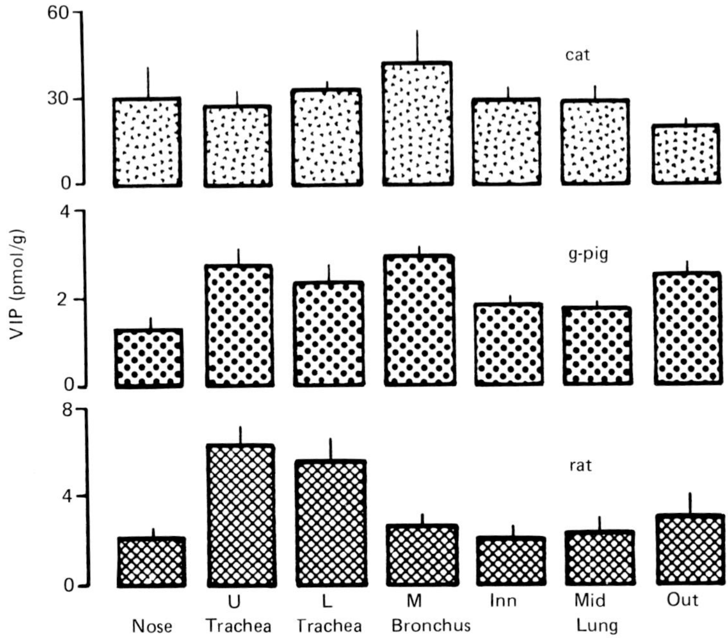

Figure 18 Levels of immunoreactive material detected by radioimmunoassay with anti-VIP serum in extracts of different areas of respiratory tract from cat, guinea pig, and rat.

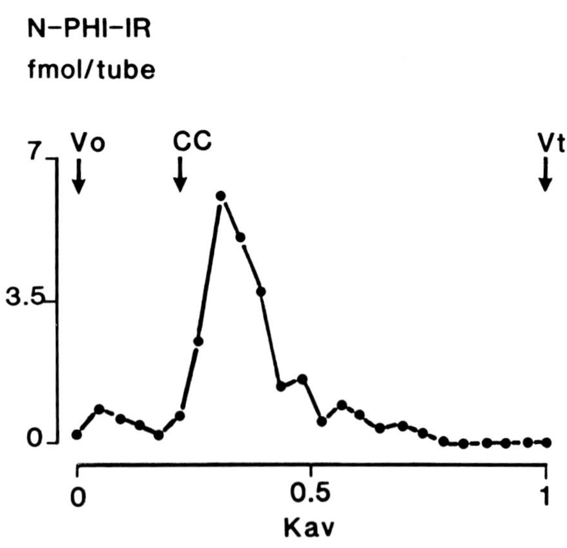

Figure 19 Sephadex G50 profile of an extract of pig nasal mucosa measured with anti-N-terminal PHI serum R8403. Vo, dextran blue; CC, horse heart cytochrome C; Vt, NaI^{125}. Synthetic PHI eluted at $K_{av} = 0.53$.

of norepinephrine and NPY within the same neurons was obtained after treating guinea pigs with 6-hydroxydopamine, which resulted in a depletion of both catecholamines and NPY immunoreactivity. The origin of NPY immunoreactivity has thus been postulated to be neurons in sympathetic ganglia (Lundberg et al., 1983).

D. Galanin

Galanin immunoreactive material was found to have a similar distribution to that of VIP/PHI, particularly in guinea pig, rat, and dog, with lower levels in the pig (Cheung et al., 1985). In all cases, the greatest concentration was in the stem bronchi, and extractable galanin-like immunoreactivity coeluted chromatographically with the synthetic peptide (Cheung et al., 1985). The distribution of galanin in respiratory tract is also similar to that of acetylcholinesterase-positive nerve fibers (i.e., around blood vessels, seromucous glands, and airway smooth muscle (Fig. 22). This suggests that galanin may be present in cholinergic neurons, as does its presence in nerves with a similar distribution to those containing VIP/PHI(M) in nasal mucosa. It has been suggested that galanin coexists with VIP/PHI(M) in cell bodies of neurons in the posterior wall of trachea. Such colocalization has been demonstrated in gut (Bishop et al., 1986).

E. Calcitonin Gene-Related Peptide

This peptide is abundantly distributed throughout the respiratory tract and is the only peptide to be convincingly demonstrated both in mucosal endocrine cells (Fig. 23) and in the innervation of the rat (Cadieux et al., 1986) (Fig. 24). CGRP-immunoreactive material can be extracted from the respiratory tract of many mammalian species including rat, guinea pig, pig, cat, monkey, and humans. Attempts to separate the α and β forms chromatographically in extracted material have been unsuccessful so far, but antisera to rat α-CGRP seem to recognize both forms equally.

In the rat, CGRP-immunoreactive nerves are found around seromucous glands, within the smooth muscle layer of the airways, around blood vessels (both arteries and veins), and beneath as well as within the epithelium of the tracheobronchial tree. CGRP immunoreactivity was also observed in motor end plates of both intrinsic and extrinsic striated muscle of the larynx. Smaller numbers of nerve fibers were seen in similar locations in guinea pig. In humans and monkeys, nerve fibers are restricted to smooth muscle and blood vessels, principally in the trachea and stem bronchi; they are rarely found in lung.

In terms of origin, however, it is possible that substance P and CGRP originate at least partially from different subsets of sensory neurons, CGRP being mostly localized in the jugular ganglion of the rat whereas substance P is reported to derive mostly from the nodose ganglion in guinea pig and rat (Lund-

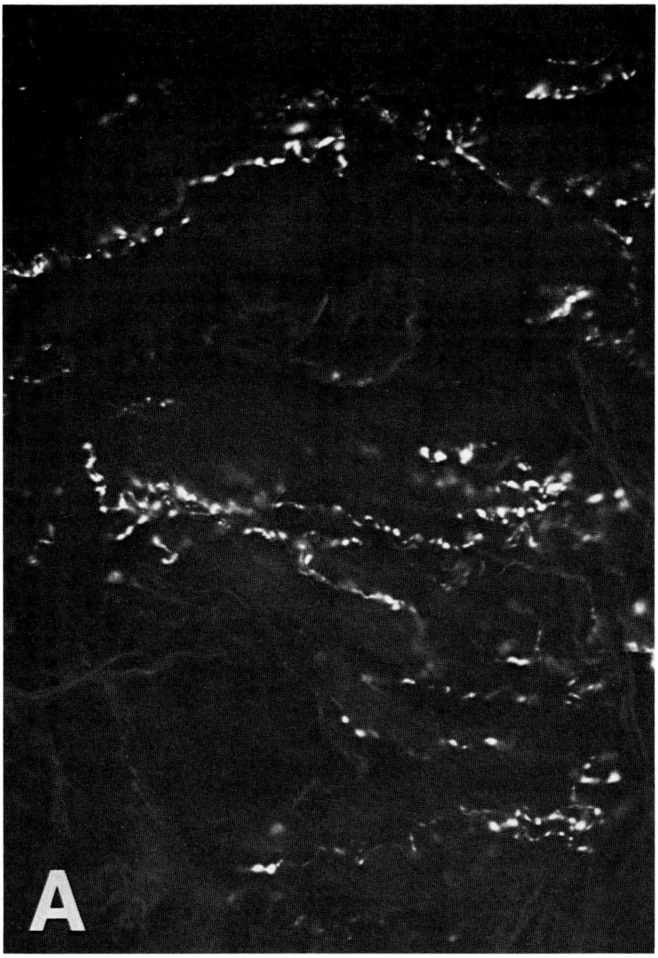

Figure 20 Immunofluorescence micrographs of sections of (A) dog lung and (B) trachea after incubation with anti-VIP serum. Varicose nerve fibers are seen (A) in the smooth muscle of a small intrapulmonary bronchus, and (B) neuronal cell bodies in an extramural ganglion of the trachea (p-benzoquinone-fixed tissue; (A) ×300, (B) ×320).

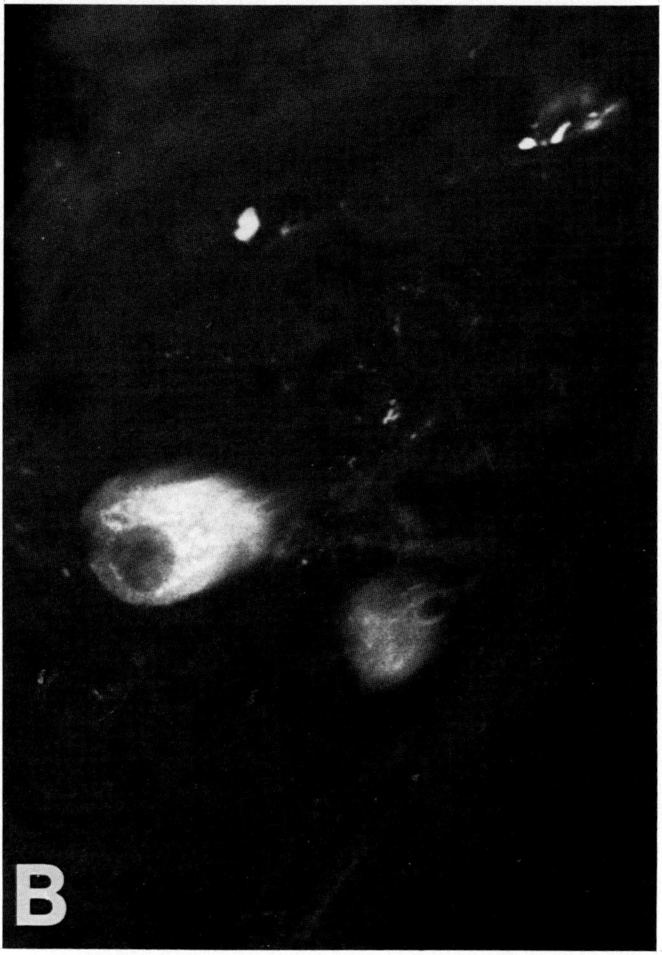

Figure 20 (continued)

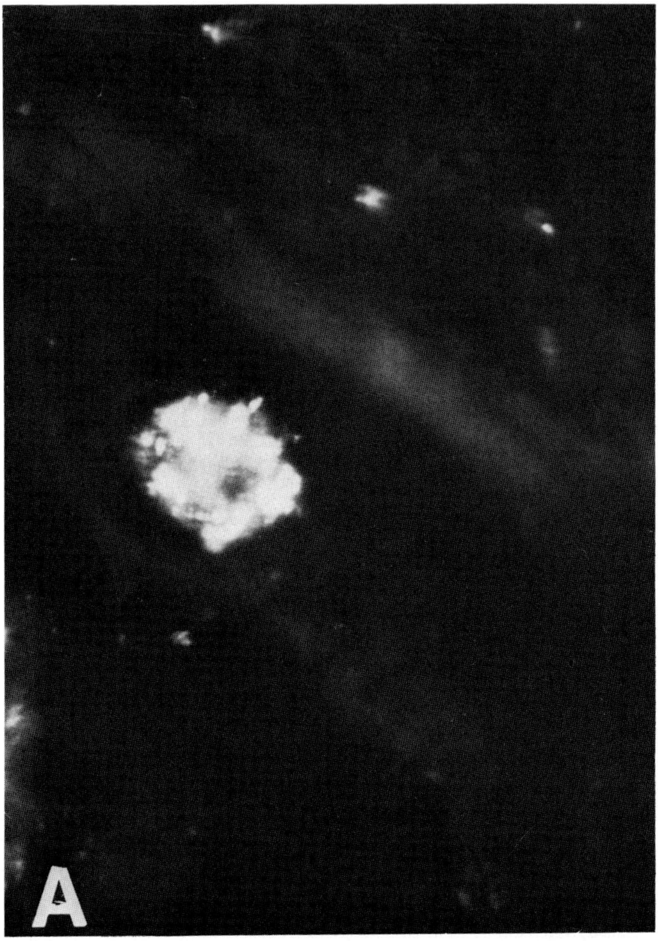

Figure 21 Immunofluorescence micrographs of serial sections of pig trachea immunostained for (A) PHI and (B) VIP. Immunostaining reveals that both peptides are present in the same ganglion cell (p-benzoquinone-fixed tissue; ×320).

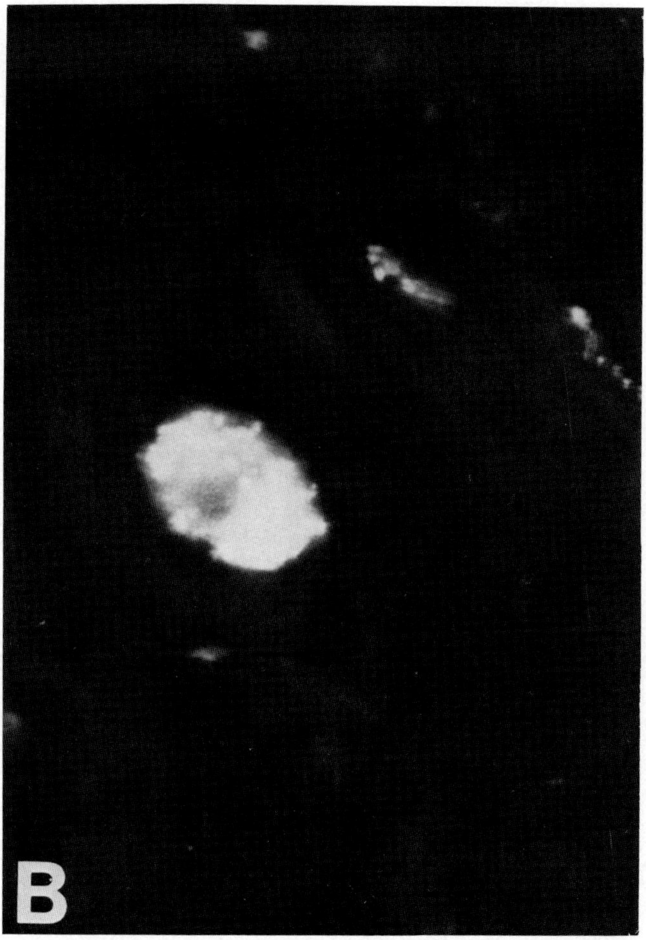

Figure 21 (continued)

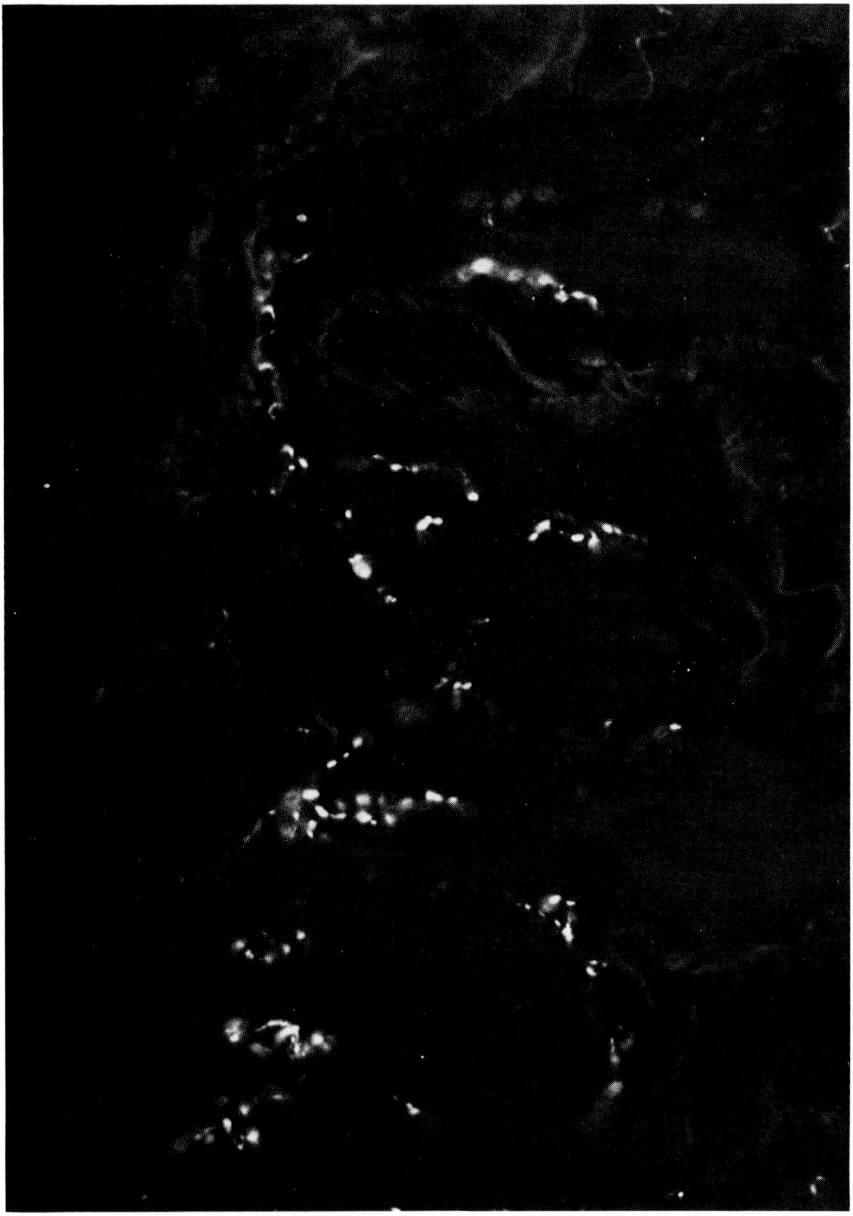

Figure 22 Immunofluorescence micrograph of section of dog lung incubated with antigalanin serum. A network of nerve fibers is seen in the smooth muscle of an intrapulmonary bronchiole (p-benzoquinone-fixed tissue; ×460).

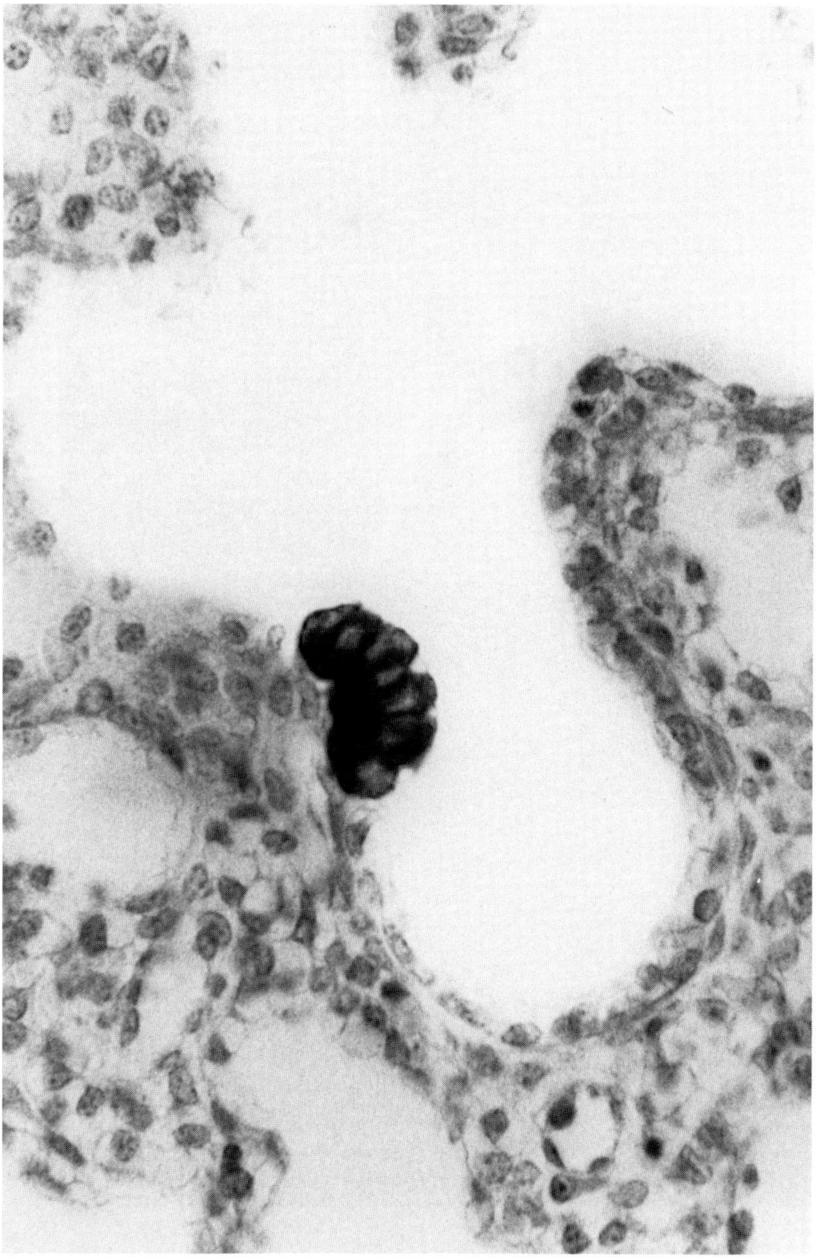

Figure 23 Section of rat lung immunostained with antiserum to CGRP by the peroxidase anti-peroxidase method shows clusters of immunoreactive cells at a bronchioalveolar junction of a 21-day-old fetal rat (tissue fixed in Bouin's fluid and wax embedded; ×600).

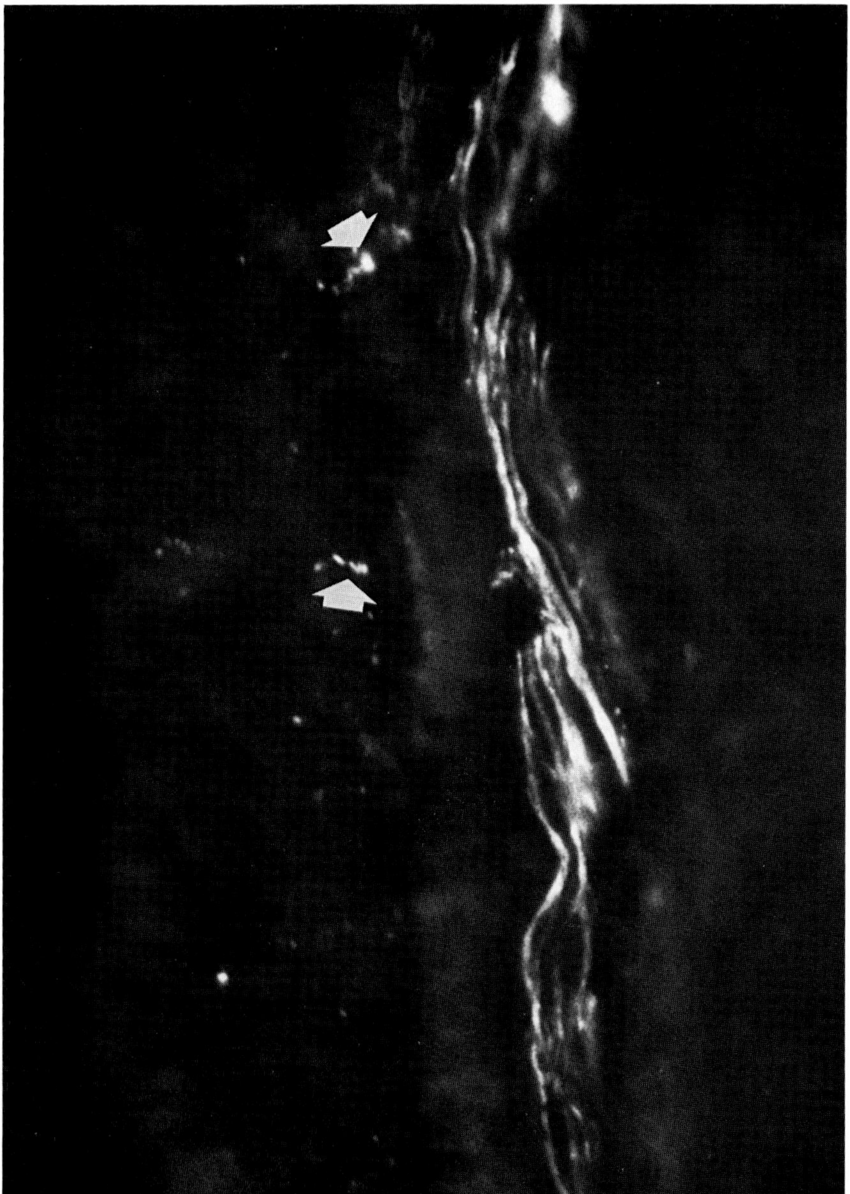

Figure 24 Immunofluorescence micrograph of a section of rat trachea immunostained for CGRP. Immunoreactive nerve fibers are seen among the columnar epithelial cells and in a fascicle in the submucosa (p-benzoquinone-fixed tissue; X 500).

berg et al., 1984a; Terenghi et al., 1983). Colocalization studies in dorsal root and trigeminal and vagal ganglia reveal that although 90% of substance P neurons also contain CGRP, only 50% of all CGRP-immunoreactive neurons in the rat also contain substance P. Therefore, a component of CGRP innervation is not colocalized with substance P. Primary sensory neurons have been found to contain both substance P and CGRP (e.g., rat dorsal root and trigeminal ganglia, urinary system, esophagus, and palate, and the guinea pig cardiovascular system and rat dorsal root ganglia at the electron microscopic level). The sensory nature of these nerves has been demonstrated by neonatal capsaicin administration, which resulted in the almost complete disappearance of CGRP immunoreactivity in the rat respiratory tract. Nerves supplying motor end plates in the larynx were unaffected. Of interest is the fact that a decrease was also obtained in the number of CGRP-immunoreactive endocrine cells in the lung. This supports the hypothesis that they may be under neuronal influence.

Endocrine cells and nerve fibers immunoreactive for CGRP were first detected by days 17 and 18 of gestation, respectively. The former increased in number to a peak at term and then appeared to decrease to a stable population by about postnatal day 21; the latter reached an adult distribution by postnatal day 21.

The majority of CGRP-immunoreactive nerve fibers in the lower respiratory tract of rat have been shown by immunocytochemical analysis, following infranodosal vagal ligation, to originate from the vagal ganglia. The combination of procedures demonstrated a considerable depletion of CGRP immunoreactivity in the respiratory tract, with a concomitant loss of peptide detected by radioimmunoassay. This finding has been further substantiated by preliminary results from retrograde tracing using the fluorescent dye true blue, combined with immunostaining for CGRP, which suggested that the major component of vagal CGRP nerves in the respiratory tract originate from the jugular ganglion. However, the preliminary results also revealed an origin from dorsal root ganglia (levels T_1-T_6) for some nerve fibers in lung tissue, as has been previously demonstrated for substance P.

IV. Conclusions

The presence of nerve terminals containing large (80-100 nm) dense neurosecretory granules in addition to the small electron-lucent agranular vesicles have been recognized in the mammalian respiratory tract for some time. Neurophysiologists suggested that a number of pulmonary responses recorded after nerve stimulation could not be explained by the sole release of the so-called classic neurotransmitters (acetylcholine and norepinephrine). However, it was not until the advent of radioimmunologic and immunocytochemical procedures using specific antipeptide sera that bioactive peptides were convincingly demonstrated and chemically characterized from the respiratory tract. Nowadays the existence of neuropeptides in the respiratory tract is well recognized and it has been hypothesized that the peptides may, in concert with acetylcholine and norepinephrine, serve a modulatory role in lung function. These peptides are present in the innervation and show a broad distribution throughout the respiratory tract. The differences of distribution would suggest that each peptide has a quite distinct and specific set of actions. From the morphologic results on coexistence it must be emphasized that many of the actions seem to be carried out in cooperation with the parallel release of other classic or peptidergic neurochemicals from the same terminal. Alternatively, they may sometimes antagonize or block the release of other putative transmitters.

Advances in neurobiologic procedures, both chemical and surgical, and the combined use of nerve tracing techniques with immunocytochemistry are serving to delineate the sensory nervous system and verify connections of the innervation of the peripheral organs with the central nervous system. The results are also indicating the heterogeneity of the nervous system, in that one neurochemical may have separate actions according to where the nerve terminal is sited and what combination of separate neurochemicals it contains.

Understanding where the peptides are normally localized, where they originate, whether they belong to the autonomic and/or sensory nervous system, as well as an appreciation of species variation, enables appropriate physiological experiments to be designed. Furthermore, data on the neuroanatomic distribution of these numerous active peptides together with their possible functions may help our understanding of their involvement in diseases of the respiratory tract.

Discussion

Burnstock. What percentage of airway ganglion cells are immunoreactive for neuropeptides?

Springall. Only 5-10% of neurones are immunoreactive for galanin (in dog and pig), but a greater number are immunoreactive to VIP/PHI.

Laitinen. What is the time course of depletion of CGRP after ligature of the vagus nerve?

Springall. A decrease is seen after 1 day but is greater after 7 days.

Barnes. Human airways appear to have fewer neuropeptide immunoreactive nerves than several other species. Are there problems with loss of immunoactivity with the delays in fixation caused by surgical resection, with age of patients, or with factors such as cigarette smoking?

Springall. It is certainly possible that loss of immunoreactivity occurs, since blood flow to lung is occluded some time before surgical removal is completed.

Nadel. It is likely that substance P content is not stable in surgical or postmortem human lung over time.

Springall. In animals there is a decrease in substance P in pulmonary tissues after death, but substance P nerve fibers can be immunostained in tissue taken even up to 2 hr after death. It is not known whether this is so in humans.

Vanhoutte. Since CGRP is a potent releaser of endothelium-derived relaxing factor, do CGRP immunoreactive fibers "innervate" endothelial cells?

Springall. CGRP nerve fibers are found in the adventitia of blood vessels.

References

Adrian, T. E., Allen, J. M., Terenghi, G., Bacarese Hamilton, A. J., Brown, M. J., Polak, J. M., and Bloom, S. R. (1983). Neuropeptide Y in phaeochromocytomas and ganglioneuroblastomas. *Lancet* **2**:540-542.

Allen, J. M., Polak, J. M., and Bloom, S. R. (1985). Presence of the predicted C-flanking peptide of neuropeptide Y (CPON) in tissue extracts. *Neuropeptides* **6**:95-100.

Amara, S. G., Arriza, J. L., Leff, S. E., Swanson, L. W., Evans, R. M., and Rosenfeld, M. G. (1985). Expression in brain of a messenger RNA encoding a novel neuropeptide homologous to calcitonin gene-related peptide. *Science* **229**:1094-1097.

Änggård, A., Lundberg, J. M., Hökfelt, T., Nilsson, G., Fahrenkrug, J., and Said, S. (1979). Innervation of cat nasal mucosa with special reference to relations between peptidergic and cholinergic neurons. *Acta Physiol. Scand. Suppl.* **473**:50.

Bauer, F. E., Christofides, N. D., Gu, J., Hacker, G., Tatemoto, K., Polak, J. M., and Bloom, S. R. (1984). Distribution of galanin immunoreactivity in the urogenital tract of man and rat. *Regul. Pept.* **9**:325.

Bishop, A. E., Polak, J. M., Bauer, F. E., Christofides, N. D., Carlei, F., and Bloom, S. R. (1986). The occurrence and distribution of a newly discovered peptide, galanin, in the mammalian enteric nervous systsm. *Gut* **27**:849-857.

Bloom, S. R., and Edwards, A. V. (1980). Vasoactive intestinal polypeptide in relation to atropine resistant vasodilatation in the submaxillary gland of the cat. *J. Physiol.* **300**:41-53.

Bloom, S. R., and Long, R. G. (1982). *Radioimmunoassay of Gut Regulatory Peptides.* London, W. B. Saunders.

Bloom, S. R., Delamarter, J., Kawashima, E., Christofides, N. D., Buell, J., and

Polak, J. M. (1983). Diarrhoea in VIPoma patients associated with co-secretion of a second active peptide (peptide histidine isoleucine) explained by single coding gene. *Lancet* **2**:1163-1165.

Cadieux, A., Springall, D. R., Mulderry, P. K., Rodrigo, J., Ghatei, M. A., Terenghi, G., Bloom, S. R., and Polak, J. M. (1986). Occurrence, distribution and ontogeny of CGRP-immunoreactivity in the rat lower respiratory tract: effect of capsaicin treatment and surgical denervations. *Neuroscience* **19**:605-627.

Cheung, A., Polak, J. M., Bauer, F. E., Cadieux, A., Christofides, N. D., Springall, D. R., and Bloom, S. R. (1985). Distribution of galanin immunoreactivity in the respiratory tract of pig, guinea pig, rat and dog. *Thorax* **40**:889-896.

Chn'g, J. L. C., Christofides, N. D., Anand, P., Gibson, S. J., Allen, Y. S., Su, H. C., Tatemoto, K., Morrison, J. F. B., Polak, J. M., and Bloom, S. R. (1985). Distribution of galanin immunoreactivity in the central nervous system and the responses of galanin-containing neuronal pathways to injury. *Neuroscience* **16**:343-354.

Christofides, N. D., Yiangou, Y., Piper, P. J., Ghatei, M. A., Sheppard, M. N., Tatemoto, K., Polak, J. M., and Bloom, S. R. (1984). Distribution of peptide histidine isoleucine in the mammalian respiratory tract and some aspects of its pharmacology. *Endocrinology* **115**:1958-1963.

Clague, J. R., Sternini, C., and Brecha, N. C. (1985). Localisation of calcitonin gene-related peptide-like immunoreactivity in neurons of the rat gastrointestinal tract. *Neurosci. Letts.* **56**:63-68.

Dahlström, A. (1968). Effects of colchicine on transport of amine storage granules in sympathetic nerves of rats. *Eur. J. Pharmacol.* **5**:111.

Dey, D. A. W., Shannon, W. A., and Said, S. I. (1981). VIP-immunoreactive nerves in airways and pulmonary vessels of dogs, cats and human subjects. *Cell Tissue Res.* **220**:231-238.

Edbrooke, M. R., Parker, D., McVey, J. H., Riley, J. H., Sorensen, G. D., Pettengill, O. S., and Craig, R. K. (1985). Expression of the human calcitonin/CGRP gene in lung and thyroid carcinoma. *EMBO J.* **4**:715-724.

Euler, U. S. von, and Gaddum, J. H. (1931). An unidentified depressor substance in certain tissue extracts. *J. Physiol.* (*Lond.*) **192**:74-87.

Falck, B., Hillarp, N. A., Thieme, G., and Torp, A. (1962). Fluorescence of catecholamines and related compounds condensed with formaldehyde. *J. Histochem. Cytochem.* **10**:348-354.

Ferri, G. L., Ali-Rachedi, A., Tatemoto, K., Bloom, S. R., and Polak, J. M. (1984). Immunocytochemical localisation of neuropeptide Y-like immunoreactivity in extrinsic noradrenergic neurons and intrinsic gut neurons. *Front. Hormone Res.* **12**:81-84.

Fitzgerald, M. (1983). Capsaicin and sensory neurons–a review. *Pain* **15**:109-130.

Ghatei, M. A., Sheppard, M. N., O'Shaughnessy, D. J., Adrian, T. E., McGregor, G. P., Polak, J. M., and Bloom, S. R. (1982). Regulatory peptides in the mammalian respiratory tract. *Endocrinology* **111**:1248-1254.

Gibson, S. J., Polak, J. M., Bloom, S. R., Sabate, I. M., Mulderry, P. K., Ghatei, M. A., McGregor, G. P., Morrison, J. F. B., Kelly, J. S., and Rosenfeld, M. G. (1984). Calcitonin gene-related peptide immunoreactivity in the spinal cord of man and eight other species. *J. Neurosci.* **4**:3103-3111.

Gulbenkian, S., Wharton, J., Hacker, G. W., Varndell, I. M., Bloom, S. R., and Polak, J. M. (1986a). Co-localization of neuropeptide tyrosine and its C-terminal flanking peptide (CPON). *Peptides* **6**:1237-1243.

Gulbenkian, S., Merighi, A., Wharton, J., Varndell, I. M., and Polak, J. M. (1986b). Ultrastructural evidence for the co-existence of calcitonin gene-related peptide (CGRP) and substance P (SP) in secretory vesicles of peripheral nerves in the guinea pig. *J. Neurocytol.* **15**:535-542.

Hacker, G. W., Polak, J. M., Springall, D. R., Ballesta, J., Cadieux, A., Gu, J., Trojanowski, J. Q., Dahl, D., and Marangos, P. J. (1985). Antibodies to neurofilament protein and other brain proteins reveal the innervation of peripheral organs. *Histochemistry* **82**:581-593.

Heimer, L., and RoBards, M. J. (Eds.). 1981). *Neuroanatomical Tract-Tracing Methods.* New York, Plenum Press.

Hoffman, P. N., and Lasek, R. J. (1975). The slow axonal transport. Identification of major structural polypeptides of the axon and their generality among mammalian neurons. *J. Cell Biol.* **66**:351-366.

Hökfelt, T., Johansson, O., Kellerth, J.-O., Ljungdhal, A., Nilsson, G., Nygards, A., and Pernow, B. (1977). Immunohistochemical distribution of substance P. In *Substance P.* Edited by U. S. von Euler and B. Pernow. New York, Raven Press, pp. 117-145.

Hua X.-Y., Theodorsson-Norheim, E., Brodin, E., Lundberg, J. M., and Hökfelt, T. (1985). Multiple tachykinins (neurokinin A, neuropeptide K and substance P) in capsaicin-sensitive sensory neurons in the guinea pig. *Regul. Pept.* **13**:1-19.

Itoh, N., Obata, K., Yanaihara, N., and Okamoto, H. (1983). Human prepro-vasoactive intestinal polypeptide contains a novel PHI-27-like peptide PHM-27. *Nature* **304**:547-549.

Jessel, T. M., Iversen, L. I., and Cuello, A. C. (1978). Capsaicin-induced depletion of substance P from primary sensory neurons. *Brain Res.* **152**:183-188.

Katz, D. M., and Karten, H. J. (1980). Substance P in the vagal sensory ganglia. Localization in cell bodies and pericellular arborizations. *J. Comp. Neurol.* **193**:549-564.

Kawai, Y., Takami, K., Shiosaka, S., Emson, P. C., Hillyard, C. J., Girgis, S., MacIntyre, I., and Tohyama, M. (1985). Topographic localization of calcitonin gene-related peptide in the rat brain: an immunohistochemical analysis. *Neuroscience* **15**:747-763.

Kurian, S. S., Blank, M. A., Sheppard, M. N., Stanley, P. J., Mackay, I. S., Cole, P. J., Bloom, S. R., and Polak, J. M. (1983). Vasoactive intestinal polypeptide (VIP) in vasomotor rhinitis. *IRCS Med. Sci.* **11**:425-426.

Lundberg, J. M., Änggård, A., Fahrenkrug, J., Hokfelt, T., and Mutt, V. (1980a). Vasoactive intestinal polypeptide in cholinergic neurons of exocrine glands: functional significance of co-existing transmitters for vasodilation and secretion. *Proc. Natl. Acad. Sci. USA* **77**:1651-1655.

Lundberg, J. M., Hökfelt, T., Änggård, A., Unväs-Wallensten, K., Brimijoin, S., Brodin, E., and Fahrenkrug, J. (1980b). Peripheral peptide-neuron distribution, axonal transport and some aspects on possible function. *Adv. Biochem. Psychopharmacol.* **22**:25-36.

Lundberg, J. M., Änggård, A., Emson, P., Fahrenkrug, J., and Hökfelt, T. (1981). Vasoactive intestinal polypeptide and cholinergic mechanisms in cat nasal mucosa: studies on choline acetyltransferase and release of vasoactive intestinal polypeptide. *Proc. Natl. Acad. Sci. USA* **78**:5255-5259.

Lundberg, J. M., Terenius, L., Hokfelt, T., and Goldstein, M. (1983). High levels of neuropeptide Y in peripheral noradrenergic neurons in various mammals including man. *Neurosci. Letts.* **42**:167-172.

Lundberg, J. M., Hökfelt, T., Martling, C.-R., Saria, A., and Cuello, C. (1984a). Substance-P immunoreactive sensory nerves in the lower respiratory tract of various mammals including man. *Cell Tissue Res.* **235**:251-261.

Lundberg, J. M., Fahrenkrug, J., Hökfelt, T., Martling, C. R., Larsson, O., Tatemoto, K., and Änggård, A. (1984). Co-existence of peptide HI (PHI) and VIP in nerves regulating blood flow and bronchial smooth muscle tone in various mammals including man. *Peptides* **5**:593-606.

Lundberg, J. M., Franco-Cerceda, A., Hua, X., Hökfelt, T., and Fisher, J. A. (1985). Co-existence of substance P and calcitonin gene-related peptide-like immunoreactivities in sensory nerves in relation to cardiovascular and bronchoconstrictor effects of capsaicin. *Eur. J. Pharmacol.* **108**:315-319.

McDonald, T. J., Dupre, J., Tatemoto, K., Greenberg, G. R., Radzuik, J., and Mutt, V. (1985). Galanin inhibits insulin secretion and induces hyperglycaemia in dogs. *Diabetes* **34**:192-196.

Marangos, P. J., Zomzely-Neurath, C., Luc, D. C. M., and York, C. (1975). Isolation and characterisation of the nervous system specific protein 14-3-2 from rat brain. *J. Biol. Chem.* **250**:1884-1901.

Minth, C. D., Bloom, S. R., Polak, J. M., and Dixon, J. E. (1984). Cloning, characterization, and DNA sequence of a human cDNA encoding neuropeptide tyrosine. *Proc. Natl. Acad. Sci. USA* **81**:4577-4581.

Moore, B. W. (1973). Brain specific proteins. In *Proteins of the Nervous System.* Edited by D. J. Schneider. New York, Raven Press, pp. 1-12.

Morris, H. R., Panico, M., Etienne, T., Tippins, J., Girgis, S. I., and MacIntyre, I. (1984). Isolation and characterization of human calcitonin gene-related peptide. *Nature* **308**:746-748.

Morris, J. L., Murphy, R., Furness, J. B., and Costa, M. (1986). Partial depletion of neuropeptide Y from noradrenergic perivascular and cardiac axons by 6-hydroxydopamine and reserpine. *Regul. Pept.* **13**:147-162.

Mulderry, P. K., Ghatei, M. A., Rodrigo, J., Allen, J. M., Rosenfeld, M. G., Polak, J. M., and Bloom, S. R. (1985). Calcitonin gene-related peptide in cardiovascular tissues of the rat. *Neuroscience* **14**:947-954.

Nawa, H., Kotani, H., and Nakanishi, S. (1984). Tissue-specific generation of two preprotachykinin mRNAs from one gene by alternative RNA splicing. *Nature* **312**:729-734.

Nilsson, G., Dahlberg, K., Brodin, E., Sundler, F., and Strandberg, K. (1977). Distribution and constrictor effects of substance P in guinea pig tracheobronchial tissue. In *Substance P.* Edited by U. S. von Euler and B. Pernow. New York, Raven Press, pp. 75-81.

Pearse, A. G. E. (1968, 1972). *Histochemistry, Theoretical and Applied.* Third edition (2 vols). Edinburgh, Churchill Livingstone.

Polak, J. M., and Bloom, S. R. (1982a). Regulatory peptides and neuron-specific enolase in the respiratory tract of man and other mammals. *Exp. Lung. Res.* **3**:105-116.

Polak, J. M., and Bloom, S. R. (1982b). Distribution of regulatory peptides in the respiratory tract of man and other mammals. In *Systemic Role of Regulatory Peptides.* Edited by S. R. Bloom, J. M. Polak, and E. Lindenlaub. Symposia Medica Hoechst. Stuttgart, F. K. Schattauer Verlag, pp. 211-227.

Polak, J. M., and Bloom, S. R. (1984a). Regulatory peptides of the respiratory tract: a newly discovered control system. In *Frontiers in Neuroendocrinology.* Vol. 8. Edited by L. Martini and W. E. Ganong. New York, Raven Press, pp. 199-221.

Polak, J. M., and Bloom, S. R. (1984b). Regulatory peptides—the distribution of two newly discovered peptides: PHI and NPY. *Peptides* **5**:79-89.

Polak, J. M., and Marangos, P. J. (1984). Neuron-specific enolase, a marker for neuroendocrine cells. In *Evolution and Tumour Pathology of the Neuroendocrine System.* Edited by S. Falkmer, R. Hakanson, and F. Sundler. Amsterdam, Elsevier Science Publishers, pp. 433-480.

Polak, J. M., and Van Noorden, S. (1983). Immunocytochemistry today: techniques and practice. In *Immunocytochemistry: Practical Applications in Pathology and Biology.* Edited by J. M. Polak and S. Van Noorden. Bristol, Wright PSG, pp. 184-211.

Porter, R., and O'Connor, M. (Eds.). (1982). *Substance P in the Nervous System.* Ciba Foundation Symposium 91, London, Pitman Books Ltd.

Rodrigo, J., Polak, J. M., Fernandez, L., Ghatei, M. A., Mulderry, P. K., and Bloom, S. R. (1985). Calcitonin gene-related peptide (CGRP) immunoreactive sensory and motor nerves of the rat, cat and monkey oesophagus. *Gastroenterology* **88**:444-451.

Rökaeus, A., Melander, T., Hökfelt, T., Lundberg, J. M., Tatemoto, K., Carlquist, M., and Mutt, V. (1984). A galanin-like peptide in the central nervous system and intestine of the rat. *Neurosci. Letts.* **47**:161-166.

Rosenfeld, M. G., Mermod, J. J., Amara, S. G., Swanson, L. W., Sawchenko, P. E., Rivier, J., Vale, W. W., and Evans, R. M. (1983). Production of a novel neuropeptide encoded by the calcitonin gene via tissue-specific RNA-processing. *Nature* **304**:129-135.

Seifert, H., Sawchenko, P., Rivier, J., Vale, W., and Pandol, S. (1985). Calcitonin gene-related peptide: immunohistochemical localization, specific binding and biological actions in the pancreas. *Acta Endocrinol.* **108** (suppl. 267):49-50.

Sheppard, M. N., Kurian, S. S., Henzen-Longmans, S. C., Michetti, F., Cocchia, D., Cole, P., Rush, R. A., Marangos, P. J., Bloom, S. R., and Polak, J. M. (1983a). Neurone-specific enolase and S-100: new markers for delineating the entire innervation of the respiratory tract in man and other mammals. *Thorax* **38**:333-340.

Sheppard, M. N., McGregor, G. P., Kurian, S. S., Hughes, A. G., Tyers, M. B., Morrison, J., Bloom, S. R., and Polak, J. M. (1983b). Systemic administration of capsaicin to neonatal rats induces dramatic depletion of substance P-containing nerve fibres from the lung. In *Substance P–Dublin 1983.* Edited by P. Skrabanek and D. Powell. Dublin, Boole Press, pp. 221-222.

Sheppard, M. N., Marangos, P. J., Bloom, S. R., and Polak, J. M. (1984a). Neuron-specific enolase: a marker for the early development of nerves and endocrine cells in the human lung. *Life Sci.* **34**:265-271.

Sheppard, M. N., Polak, J. M., Allen, J. M., and Bloom, S. R. (1984b). Neuropeptide tyrosine (NPY): a newly discovered peptide is present in the mammalian respiratory tract. *Thorax* **39**:326-330.

Skofitsch, G., and Jacobowitz, M. (1985). Immunohistochemical mapping of galanin-like neurons in the rat central nervous system. *Peptides* **6**: 509-546.

Steenbergh, P. H., Höppener, J. W. M., Zandberg, J., Van de Den, W. J. M., Jansz, H. S., and Lips, C. J. M. (1984). Calcitonin gene related peptide coding sequence is conserved in the human genome and is expressed in medullary thyroid carcinoma. *J. Endocrinol. Metabol.* **59**:358-360.

Sundler, F., Alumets, J., Brodin, E., Dahlberg, K., and Nilsson, G. (1977). Perivascular substance P immunoreactive nerves in tracheobronchial tissue. In *Substance P.* Edited by U. S. von Euler and E. Pernow. New York, Raven Press, pp. 271-273.

Tatemoto, K., Carlquist, M., and Mutt, V. (1982). Neuropeptide Y—a novel brain peptide with structural similarities to peptide YY and pancreatic polypeptide. *Nature* **296**:659-662.

Tatemoto, K., Rökaeus, A., Jörnvall, H., McDonald, T. J., and Mutt, V. (1983). Galanin—novel biologically active peptide from porcine intestine. *FEBS. Lett.* **164**:124-128.

Terenghi, G., McGregor, G. P., Bhuttarcharji, J., Wharton, J., Bloom, S. R., and Polak, J. M. (1983). Vagal origin of substance P-containing nerves in the guinea pig lung. *Neurosci. Lett.* **36**:229-236.

Terenghi, G., Polak, J. M., Ghatei, M. A., Mulderry, P. K., Butler, J. M., Unger, W. G., and Bloom, S. R. (1985). Distribution and origin of calcitonin gene-related peptide (CGRP) immunoreactivity in the sensory innervation of the mammalian eye. *J. Comp. Neurol.* **233**:506-516.

Terenghi, G., Hacker, G. W., Varndell, I. M., Bauer, F. E., Bloom, S. R., and Polak, J. M. (1986). Galanin-immunoreactivity in normal adrenals and phaeochromocytomas. *J. Pathol.* **148**:94A.

Thompson, R. J., Doran, J. F., Jackson, P., Dhillon, A. P., and Rode, J. (1983). PGP 9.5—a new marker for vertebrate neurons and neuroendocrine cells. *Brain Res.* **278**:224-228.

Tranzer, J. P., and Richards, J. G. (1971). Fine structural aspects of the effect of 6-hydroxydopamine on peripheral adrenergic neurons. In *6-Hydroxydopamine and Catecholaminergic Neurons.* Edited by T. Malmfors and H. Thoenen. Amsterdam, North-Holland, pp. 15-31.

Uddman, R., Alumets, J., Deusert, O., Håkanson, R., and Sundler, F. (1978). Occurrence and distribution of VIP nerves in the nasal mucosa and tracheobronchial wall. *Acta Otolaryngol.* **86**:443-448.

Van Noorden, S., and Polak, J. M. (1985). Immunocytochemistry of regulatory peptides. In *Techniques in Immunocytochemistry,* Vol. III. Edited by G. R. Bullock and P. Petrusz. London, Academic Press.

Varndell, I. M., and Polak, J. M. (1984). Double immunostaining procedures. In *Immunolabelling for Electron Microscopy.* Edited by J. M. Polak and I. M. Varndell. Amsterdam, Elsevier Science Publishers, pp. 155-178.

Wang, B. L., and Larsson, L. I. (1985). Simultaneous demonstration of multiple antigens by indirect immunofluorescence or immunogold staining. Novel light and electron microscopical double and triple staining method employing primary antibodies from the same species. *Histochemistry* **83**: 47-56.

Wharton, J., Polak, J. M., Bloom, S. R., Will, J. A., Brown, M. R., and Pearse, A. G. E. (1979). Substance P-like immunoreacte nerves in mammalian lung. *Invest. Cell Pathol.* 2:3-10.

14

Airway Nonadrenergic Noncholinergic Inhibitory Nervous System

LOUIS DIAMOND* and RALPH J. ALTIERE*

University of Kentucky College of Pharmacy
Lexington, Kentucky

Evidence accumulated over the past decade and a half strongly suggests that the intrinsic innervation of mammalian airway smooth muscle includes an inhibitory component that is neither adrenergic nor cholinergic. This so-called nonadrenergic noncholinergic (NANC) inhibitory system has been the subject of several succinct reviews and editorials (Richardson, 1981; Diamond and Gillespie, 1982; Diamond and Richardson, 1982; Barnes, 1984). This chapter summarizes information supporting the existence of a NANC inhibitory system in the airways of various species and reviews the current state of knowledge on NANC neurotransmission and neuromodulation. In addition, recently acquired data from our own laboratory are integrated with the work of other investigators to present an analytical view of how NANC inhibitory nerves are distributed within the tracheobronchial tree, how they can be activated reflexly, and how they may possibly function physiologically to control bronchomotor tone.

**Present affiliation*: University of Colorado School of Pharmacy, Boulder, Colorado

I. Electrical Field Stimulation Experiments: General Considerations

In many in vitro studies of the airway NANC inhibitory system, the effects of electrical field stimulation on isometric tension development by trachaelis or bronchial smooth muscle have been determined in the absence and in the presence of various drugs. In tissues with intrinsic tone or with tone induced by a contractile agonist, the response to field stimulation most often observed is biphasic, consisting of an initial rapid contraction followed by relaxation during stimulation and a further decrease in tension below baseline upon termination of the stimulus, with subsequent slow recovery back to baseline. Addition of antimuscarinic drugs such as atropine or scopolamine to the bathing medium abolishes the excitatory component of the response without affecting the inhibitory component. Subsequent treatment of the tissues with drugs that interfere with adrenergic function, either through postsynaptic receptor blockade (propranolol, phentolamine) or adrenergic neuronal blockade (guanethidine, bretylium) may suppress, but never completely eliminates, field-stimulation-induced relaxations. Similarly, pretreatment of animals with 6-hydroxydopamine, syrosingopine, or reserpine, in doses sufficient to efface catecholamine fluorescence in tracheobronchial smooth muscle, does not abolish these relaxations. When tetrodotoxin (TTX) [a substance that blocks fast sodium channels (Kao, 1972; Catterall, 1980) and thereby inhibits axonal conduction without affecting smooth muscle excitability] is present in the bath fluid, the relaxations are abolished entirely, so long as short pulse durations and low frequencies are used (Fig. 1). The resistance of field-stimulation-induced relaxations to all measures used thus far to inhibit adrenergic function, together with their observed sensitivity to TTX, constitute the present in vitro physiological and pharmacologic evidence for the existence of a NANC inhibitory system in mammalian airway smooth muscle.

II. In Vitro Studies

A. Guinea Pig

The first evidence to suggest the existence of NANC inhibitory nerves in mammalian airways came from studies of electrically field-stimulated tracheal smooth muscle isolated from guinea pigs (Coburn and Tomita, 1973; Coleman, 1973; Coleman and Levy, 1974; Richardson and Bouchard, 1975). In transverse strips of guinea pig trachealis smooth muscle with intrinsic tone, Coburn and Tomita (1973) observed a biphasic response to electrical field stimulation that consisted of an initial contraction followed by a relaxation below baseline tension. Contractions were prevented by atropine, whereas relaxations were not affected by muscarinic cholinergic blockade and were only partially reduced by adrenergic inhibi-

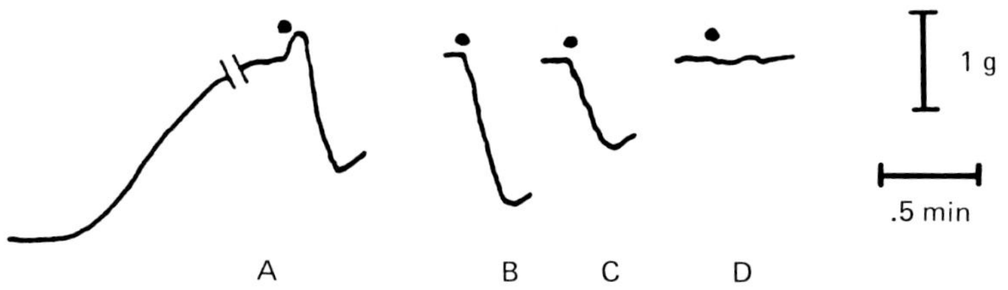

Figure 1 Tracings of representative records showing responses of isolated cat trachea to electrical field stimulation (10 V, 0.3 msec, 4 Hz for 5 sec. Steady-state contraction was induced by 5HT and stimulations lasting 5 sec were applied where indicated by closed circles. A, control biphasic response; B, pretreatment with 10^{-6} M atropine; C, pretreatment with 10^{-6} M atropine, 10^{-6} M propranolol, and 10^{-5} M guanethidine; D, pretreatment with 3×10^{-6} tetrodotoxin. (Reproduced with permission from Altiere et al., 1984b.)

tion with beta receptor antagonists, with bretylium, or by reserpine pretreatment, establishing their nonadrenergic and noncholinergic nature. Tetrodotoxin abolished both phases of the field stimulation-induced response provided pulse durations were short (<0.5 msec). In addition, differences were found in the distribution of adrenergic and NANC inhibitory nerves between the cervical and thoracic ends of the trachea. Propranolol caused a greater reduction in relaxation response in the cervical region compared to the thoracic region. This suggested that the former segment contained both adrenergic and NANC inhibitory nerves while the latter segment contained a preponderance of NANC inhibitory nerves.

The existence of NANC inhibitory nerves in guinea pig trachea also was demonstrated in studies in which changes in luminal pressure were monitored in a tracheal tube preparation stimulated transmurally (Coleman, 1973; Coleman and Levy, 1974). Initial excitatory responses to field stimulation were inhibited by atropine and subsequent inhibitory responses were decreased but not abolished by adrenergic inhibition with propranolol, guanethidine, or by pretreatment of animals with syrosingopine or 6-hydroxydopamine. Different distributions of adrenergic and NANC nerves in the trachea were not observed, perhaps due to the methodology, which consisted of preparing two tracheal tubes from each animal by dividing the trachea in half. TTX abolished NANC inhibitory responses with pulse durations up to 2 msec, documenting their neural origin. Richardson and Bouchard (1975) subsequently verified the existence of a NANC inhibitory nervous system in field-stimulated guinea pig tracheal chain preparations. Further, they were the first to show that activation of the NANC inhibitory system in the presence of atropine, propranolol, and phentolamine reversed contractions induced by histamine or by an antigen to which the guinea pigs had been previously sensitized. Relaxations evoked by field stimulation were abolished by TTX, again evincing their neural origin.

Kalenberg and Satchell (1979) later studied the inhibitory innervation of guinea pig trachea using transverse strip preparations from cervical, middle, and thoracic regions as well as the tracheal tube preparation with intrinsic tone. Field stimulation of tracheal strips before and after adrenergic blockade with guanethidine showed that NANC inhibitory responses formed about 40% of the total maximum relaxation that occurred between 15 and 25 Hz in all segments of the trachea. Similar results were obtained in the tube preparation where NANC relaxations accounted for about 20% of total maximum relaxation. Thus, in contrast to the findings of Coburn and Tomita (1973), the relative contribution of the two inhibitory neural inputs to the total relaxation response appeared to be similar in all regions of the trachea. This study also showed that both adrenergic and NANC inhibitory responses were frequency dependent and that adrenergic nerves were activated at lower frequencies than NANC nerves.

Yip et al. (1981) studied the inhibitory innervation of an in situ cervical tracheal tube preparation in anesthetized, atropinized guinea pigs and obtained results not unlike those of Kalenberg and Satchell (1979) regarding the relative contribution of adrenergic and NANC components to total inhibitory responses. Their preparation was set up to allow stimulation of vagal and sympathetic nerves separately as well as stimulation of the cervical trachea directly via transmural electrodes. These workers confirmed earlier findings of Hammarström and Sjöstrand (1979) that the NANC inhibitory system in guinea pig trachea receives preganglionic innervation from the vagus nerve. In addition, comparisons were made of the relaxation responses to the various modes of stimulation in the absence and presence of beta-adrenergic receptor blockade with propranolol or sotalol. Adrenergic relaxations (via sympathetic nerve stimulation) made up 60-80% of total transmural-stimulation-induced relaxations and NANC relaxations (via vagal nerve stimulation) accounted for the remaining 20-40%. These workers also showed that relaxations produced by simultaneous bilateral sympathetic and vagal stimulation equalled the total relaxation produced by transmural stimulation and that transmural-stimulation-induced relaxation after beta blockade was approximately equal to the NANC relaxation that attended vagal stimulation.

Taylor et al. (1984) recently studied inhibitory nerve responses to field stimulation in guinea pig tracheal chain preparations and, contrary to other investigators, concluded that NANC nerves make up the major inhibitory neural input to this tissue. They also noted, as did Kalenberg and Satchell (1979), that maximum NANC inhibitory responses occurred at higher stimulation frequencies than did total relaxation responses. Despite the minor discrepancies between these various studies, all point to the same conclusion: the guinea pig trachea possesses two inhibitory innervations, one adrenergic, the other nonadrenergic and noncholinergic.

B. Other Nonprimate Species

Studies in guinea pig trachea often make use of the intrinsic tone spontaneously developed by this tissue. Relaxation responses are measured as decreases in tone below baseline level. In contrast, airways from some other species do not develop intrinsic tone and therefore it is necessary to induce a contraction before an inhibitory response can be observed. Reversal of the induced contraction is then taken as a measure of relaxation. Using isolated airway preparations with tone enhanced by a pharmacologic agonist, NANC inhibitory responses have been studied in numerous species (Table 1). Cameron et al. (1983) demonstrated the existence of NANC inhibitory nerves in isolated bovine trachea. Field-stimulation-induced NANC inhibitory responses were observed in tracheal but not in bronchial smooth muscle or in lung parenchymal strips from the rabbit (Satchell, 1982; Doidge and Satchell, 1982). In the same studies, rat tracheal smooth muscle did not exhibit NANC inhibitory responses to field stimulation; rat bronchi were not investigated.

Dog airways appear to lack NANC inhibitory innervation altogether. Suzuki et al. (1976) observed adrenergic but not NANC inhibitory responses in field-stimulated dog tracheal smooth muscle. Russell (1980) showed that beta adrenergic receptor blockade with propranolol caused nearly complete inhibition of field-stimulation-induced relaxations in histamine-contracted dog trachea and bronchi (Fig. 2). Because there were residual TTX-sensitive relaxation responses to high-frequency field stimulation in these tissues, additional studies were conducted in airways isolated from reserpinized animals to determine whether these relaxations were due to increased concentrations of neurally released norepinephrine overcoming receptor blockade or, perhaps, to activation of NANC inhibitory nerves. Field-stimulation-induced relaxations in catecholamine-depleted airways were significantly reduced compared to responses in control tissues and propranolol treatment reduced or abolished the residual relaxations. It was concluded that noradrenergic neurons constitute the primary inhibitory innervation in canine airways and that NANC inhibitory nerves, if present, contribute very little to field-stimulation-induced relaxations. Kannan and Daniel (1980) arrived at the same conclusion based on their electrical field stimulation experiments in isolated dog tracheal smooth muscle. Collectively, these in vitro studies suggest that the principal inhibitory innervation in dog airways is adrenergic and that NANC nerves are either nonexistent or have no significant functional role in regulating airway tone in this species.

The autonomic innervation of sheep airway smooth muscle was investigated by Sheller and Brigham (1982), who examined responses of isolated tracheal segments and lobar bronchial rings to electrical field stimulation. In tissues pretreated with atropine and phentolamine and contracted with 5-hydroxytryptamine (5HT), field stimulation produced frequency-dependent decreases in tone. Both propran-

Table 1 Species Distribution of the Airway NANC Inhibitory System

Species	In vitro studies	In vivo or in situ studies	Reference
Nonprimates			
Guinea pig	+	±[a]	Coburn and Tomita (1973); Coleman and Levy (1973); Chesrown et al (1980); others (see text)
Ferret	+	n.d.	Löfdahl et al. (1986)
Cat	+	+	Altiere et al. (1984b); Diamond and O'Donnell (1980); others (see text)
Sheep	+	n.d.	Sheller and Brigham (1982)
Cow	+	n.d.	Cameron et al. (1983); Palmer et al. (1985b)
Horse	+	n.d.	Richardson (personal communication)
Rabbit	+	n.d.	Satchell (1982)
Chicken	+	n.d.	Bhatla et al. (1980)
Rat	–	n.d.	Satchell (1982)
Dog	–	–	Russell (1980); Hendrix et al. (1983); others (see text)
Pig	–	–	Leff et al. (1985)
Primates			
Monkey	+	+	Satchell (1982); Altiere et al., (1984c)
Baboon	+	n.d.	Middendorf and Russell (1980)
Human	+	n.d.	Richardson and Béland (1976); Davis et al. (1982); others (see text)

n.d., not done.
[a]System demonstrated in situ, not in vivo.

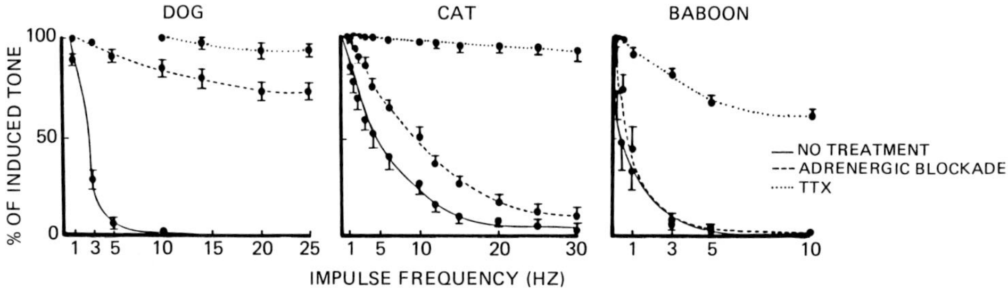

Figure 2 Effects of adrenergic inhibition and tetrodotoxin (TTX) on frequency-dependent relaxation responses to electrical field stimulation in dog, cat, and baboon intrapulmonary airways pretreated with 10^{-6} M atropine (cat) plus 10^{-6} M phentolamine (dog, baboon). Steady-state contractions were induced by histamine (dog, baboon) or 5HT (cat). Stimulus parameters were 15 V, 0.5 msec pulse duration for dog and baboon, and 10 V, 0.3 msec pulse duration for cat airways at variable frequency. Adrenergic inhibition was produced by 10^{-6} M propranolol (dog, baboon) plus 10^{-5} M guanethidine (cat). (Dog and baboon data reproduced with permission from Russell, 1980, and from Middendorf and Russell, 1980; cat data redrawn from Altiere et al., 1984b.)

olol and guanethidine caused significant shifts to the right in relaxation frequency-response curves, suggesting that sheep airways are innervated by both sympathetic and NANC inhibitory nerves. The trachea appeared to have predominantly sympathetic innervation since adrenergic blockade caused a greater than 20-fold increase in the EF_{50} (frequency required to cause a 50% reduction in induced tone) over the control value. The shift in the bronchial relaxation curve was only two- to three-fold, indicating a relatively greater role for NANC inhibitory nerves in this tissue. However, as pointed out by the investigators, relaxation responses observed in the presence of propranolol or guanethidine may have been due to higher-stimulus frequencies releasing sufficient amounts of norepinephrine to overcome beta receptor blockade or adrenergic neuronal blockade. While such actions may occur in the presence of propranolol, they seem unlikely in the presence of guanethidine, since this agent, in the same concentration (10^{-5} M) used by Sheller and Brigham (1982), has been shown to abolish completely field-stimulation-induced, neuronal catecholamine-mediated contractions in cat aorta (Altiere et al., 1984b) and baboon saphenous vein (Middendorf and Russell, 1980). Thus, the shift in frequency-response curves observed in sheep bronchi treated with guanethidine is most likely a manifestation of NANC inhibitory nerve activation.

Experiments in our laboratory have demonstrated the presence of a functional NANC inhibitory system in isolated segments of cat trachea and bronchi contracted with 5HT (Altiere et al., 1984b). In these tissues, field stimulation evoked a biphasic response: a rapid atropine-sensitive contraction followed by a relatively prolonged relaxation. The relaxation phase was characterized by examining the effects of adrenergic inhibition on graded responses over a range of stimulation frequencies. Adrenergic inhibition with propranolol and guanethidine caused small (less than threefold) but significant rightward shifts in relaxation frequency-response curves (Fig. 2). These findings suggested that both adrenergic and NANC nerves contributed to the inhibitory effects of field stimulation.

It should be emphasized that the relative contributions of adrenergic and NANC nerves to total relaxation responses may be difficult to determine from electrical field stimulation studies alone. When the NANC system is incapable of producing maximal relaxation, as in guinea pig trachea (Yip et al., 1981), some estimation can be made of the relative efficacy of each neural inhibitory input (see above). However, when both systems are capable of producing nearly complete reversal of induced tone, as is the case in cat airways, adrenergic blockade may cause little or no change in relaxation frequency-response curves. Small differences may be caused by a variety of factors; for example, different densities of adrenergic and NANC innervation, different sensitivities of each system to activation by field stimulation, unequal responsiveness of smooth muscle tissues to the inhibitory mediators, or additive or synergistic effects. If these factors are not of sufficient magnitude to influence tissue responsiveness to field stimulation significantly, frequency-response curves before and after adrenergic blockade may be the same. As discussed below, these considerations become especially relevant when one is studying primate airways that appear to have only a NANC inhibitory system.

C. Primate Species

The NANC inhibitory system has been demonstrated in the airways of several primate species in which it is believed to provide the principal inhibitory neural control over tracheobronchial smooth muscle. Middendorf and Russell (1980) studied responses to field stimulation in trachea and subsegmental bronchi isolated from baboons. Airways pretreated with atropine and phentolamine to prevent contractile responses exhibited progressive reversal of histamine-induced tone over a narrow range of stimulus frequencies. Adrenergic blockade with propranolol or guanethidine did not significantly alter frequency-response curves (Fig. 2). However, as just noted, a small effect of adrenergic blockade on relaxation frequency-response curves is insufficient evidence to rule out functional adrenergic inhibitory innervation since, if both the adrenergic and NANC systems respond equally over the same range of stimulus frequencies and if both systems are capable of eliciting complete relaxation, adrenergic blockade may have little or no effect on relaxation frequency-response curves. There is, however, additional evidence to suggest that primate airways do not possess significant adrenergic innervation. Middendorf and Russell (1980) showed that tyramine, which acts by releasing norepinephrine from adrenergic nerve terminals, fails to cause relaxation responses in baboon airways. In contrast, tyramine produces a propranolol-sensitive reversal of histamine-induced contractions in dog airways (Russell, 1980). Satchell (1982) also observed field-stimulation-induced relaxation responses in monkey tracheal and bronchial smooth muscle that were unaffected by adrenergic blockade with guanethidine. Fluorescence histochemical studies were unable to reveal the presence of adrenergic fibers in tracheal or bronchial smooth muscle, although adrenergic nerves were observed in vascular smooth muscle of bronchial arteries and in vasa vasorum (Doidge and Satchell, 1982). Together, these findings strongly suggest that the principal inhibitory neural input to nonhuman primate airways is supplied by the NANC system.

The NANC system also is believed to provide the primary inhibitory control over human airways that, like baboon and monkey airways, seem to lack functional adrenergic innervation. The existence of a NANC system in human airways was first reported by Richardson and Béland (1976). Field stimulation of isolated segments of trachea and bronchi evoked cholinergically mediated contractions and in some instances biphasic contraction-relaxation responses. In the presence of atropine and with tone increased by histamine in bronchi, field stimulation caused frequency-dependent relaxation responses that were unaffected by propranolol and partially blocked by TTX. Fluorescence histochemical localization of catecholamines failed to reveal the presence of adrenergic nerves in tracheal or bronchial smooth muscle. Based on the absence of either pharmacologic or histochemical evidence for adrenergic innervation, it was concluded that the NANC system was the principal inhibitory nervous system in human airways smooth muscle. Doidge and Satchell (1982) confirmed these findings in human bronchi. Field-stimulation-evoked TTX-sensitive relaxation responses were unaffected by phentolamine, propranolol or guanethidine.

In most studies of human airway tissue, the effects of adrenergic inhibition on field-stimulation-induced relaxation responses have been determined in the presence of atropine. Hutás et al. (1981) examined the effects of the beta adrenergic receptor antagonist, pindolol, on the biphasic response to field stimulation in human bronchi without atropine. In contrast to the findings of Richardson and Béland (1976), they found that beta blockade partially or completely blocked the relaxation response. Following atropine treatment, pindolol had little effect on the relaxation response to field stimulation, leading these investigators to conclude that the response before atropine was due mainly to activation of adrenergic nerves and that NANC relaxation responses become apparent only after blockade of muscarinic receptors. Daniel et al. (1980) also have presented evidence for adrenergic nerves in human airway smooth muscle. Electron microscopic studies revealed the possible presence of some adrenergic nerves and imipramine treatment was shown to shift the norepinephrine concentration-response curve of bronchi to the left, presumably by inhibiting norepinephrine uptake into adrenergic nerve terminals. Further, the combination of tyramine treatment and electrical field stimulation provoked the release of radiolabeled material from tissues incubated with [^{3}H] 1-norepinephrine. It appeared from these experiments that human airways contained adrenergic nerves capable of taking up and releasing norepinephrine during field stimulation. However, given the extensive evidence from fluorescence histochemical studies indicating the presence of adrenergic nerves in blood vessels in the airways and the absence of such nerves within bronchial smooth muscle, it is most likely that these findings reflect norepinephrine uptake and release from vascular rather than airway smooth muscle adrenergic nerves.

Davis et al. (1982) conducted field stimulation studies in human trachea and bronchi and were unable to demonstrate an adrenergic component to the inhibitory response. Airways with intrinsic tone or with histamine-induced tone responded to field stimulation with biphasic responses that consisted of atropine-sensitive contractions followed by relaxations that were resistant to adrenergic inhibition with phentolamine, propranolol, and/or guanethidine. NANC relaxation responses were abolished by TTX at short pulse durations (<0.5 msec). Scorpion venom, which acts to keep Na^+ channels open, thereby causing nerve depolarization and mediator depletion, also produced biphasic responses and subsequently abolished responses to short-pulse-duration field stimulation. Based on the results obtained with TTX and scorpion venom, it was concluded that NANC relaxation responses were neurally mediated. Studies with the K^+-conductance inhibitors 4-aminopyridine and tetraethylammonium, which potentiate transmitter release by prolonging nerve action potentials, substantiated these conclusions. Both compounds enhanced the excitatory and inhibitory components of the biphasic response to short pulse duration field stimulation. However, TTX- and scorpion-venom-resistant NANC inhibitory responses were evoked by longer-pulse-duration stimulations, suggesting a substantial nonneural component to NANC responses. Taylor et al. (1984) reported essentially the same findings in human bronchi. Atropine-treated preparations with intrinsic tone or with agonist-induced tone responded to field stimulation with frequency-dependent relaxations that were unaffected by propranolol. However, only NANC responses to low-frequency stimulation (<10 Hz) were abolished by TTX; higher-frequency stimulation resulted in TTX-resistant NANC relaxation responses.

III. Tetrodotoxin-Insensitive Relaxations

Determination of whether field-stimulation-induced responses result from activation of neural or muscular elements within a tissue rests on the ability of TTX to inhibit nerve conduction selectively. In most in vitro studies, stimulation parameters are chosen to avoid eliciting TTX-resistant responses so that only nerve-mediated NANC relaxations are observed. However, TTX-insensitive relaxations have been described in many of these studies. Coburn and Tomita (1973) reported TTX-resistant relaxations in guinea pig trachea that were dependent on pulse duration. Stimulations of >0.5 msec evoked relaxations in the presence of TTX and a 5 msec, 20 Hz stimulus produced a TTX-insensitive relaxation that was 23% of total relaxation. We observed NANC relaxations in cat bronchi treated with TTX that were dependent on stimulus voltage and pulse duration (Fig. 3). At high voltages or long pulse durations, TTX-resistant responses accounted for up to 90% of total relaxation. However, by choosing the appropriate stimulation parameters (10 V, 0.3 msec), it is possible to generate complete NANC relaxation frequency-response curves in cat airways that are almost totally abolished by TTX (Fig. 2).

It is intriguing that TTX-resistant relaxations are evoked most readily in primate airways that possess only NANC inhibitory nerves and least readily in canine airways which are devoid of NANC inhibitory nerves. Russell (1980) reported that TTX virtually abolished field-stimulation-induced relaxation in dog airways, whereas TTX-insensitive relaxation in baboon intrapulmonary airways made up nearly 30% of the maximal inhibitory response (Fig. 2) (Middendorf and Russell, 1980). In human airways, TTX-resistant relaxations appear to be the major inhibitory response to field stimulation. Davis et al. (1982) observed frequency-dependent NANC relaxations in human trachea treated with TTX that were equivalent in magnitude to field-stimulation-induced relaxations evoked prior to TTX treatment. Taylor et al. (1984) reported similar findings in human bronchi in which TTX produced only a small rightward shift in NANC relaxation frequency-response curves (Fig. 4). It should be noted that in each of these studies, TTX abolished contractile responses evoked with the same field stimulation parameters that produced TTX-resistant NANC relaxations.

The mechanism underlying TTX-insensitive relaxation is uncertain but several possible explanations have been proposed. Coburn and Tomita (1973) attributed TTX-resistant relaxations to a direct effect of electrical field stimulation on smooth muscle membranes. Based on their findings that TTX was more efficacious in blocking field-stimulation-induced relaxations in human airways denuded of connective tissue, Richardson and Béland (1976) suggested that impaired diffusion of TTX to intrinsic nerves was involved. However, the

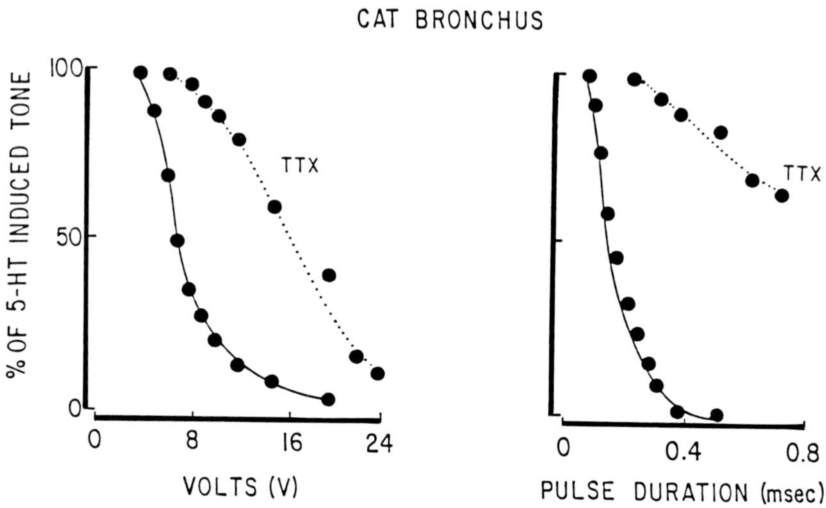

Figure 3 Voltage and pulse duration dependence of NANC relaxations in cat segmental bronchi treated with 10^{-6} M atropine, 10^{-6} M propranolol, and 10^{-5} M guanethidine. After steady-state contraction was induced by 5 HT, electrical impulses were delivered in a cumulative stepwise manner. Stimulus parameters were either 0.3 msec pulse duration, 20 Hz and variable voltage, or 10 V, 20 Hz, and variable pulse duration for a 5 sec period. NANC responses generated in the absence of tetrodotoxin (TTX) are shown by the solid line and in the presence of 3 X 10 M TTX by the broken line. Each point is the mean relaxation response from six experiments. Standard errors (<18%) omitted for sake of clarity. (Data from Altiere et al., 1984b.)

differential sensitivity of cholinergic and NANC responses to the inhibitory effects of TTX make these explanation appear untenable. Perhaps, as suggested by Middendorf and Russell (1980), other nonneural mechanisms are involved, such as release of mediators from secondary cell types insensitive to the effects of TTX. It also is possible that in NANC nerves the process of depolarization is inherently less sensitive to TTX than it is in other autonomic nerves (Fukuda and Kameyama, 1980). Alternatively, field stimulation may directly activate NANC nerve terminals and cause neurotransmitter release by a calcium-dependent mechanism resistant to TTX (Katz and Miledi, 1969). Whatever the mechanism may be, it is clear that TTX-insensitive NANC relaxations are a substantial part of the inhibitory response to field stimulation, particularly in primate airways. In addition to the need to investigate further the mechanisms underlying TTX-resistant relaxations, it is important to determine whether the same or different mediators are involved

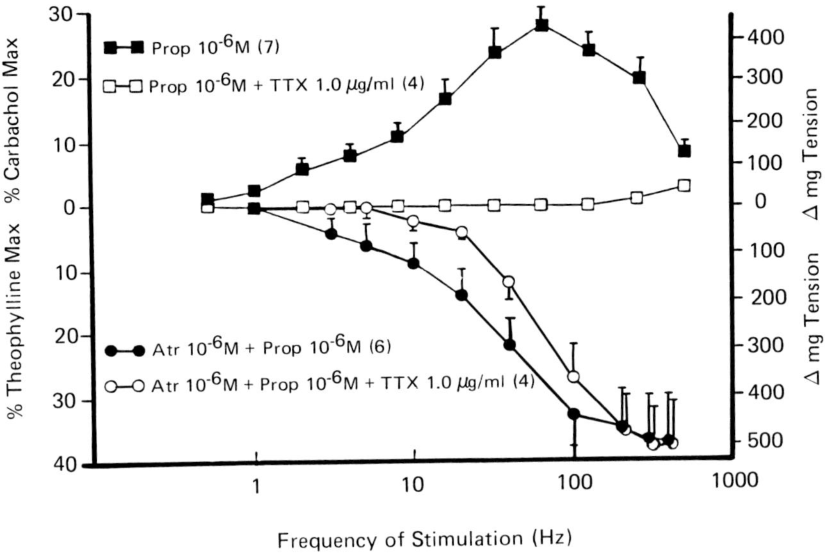

Figure 4 Effect of tetrodotoxin (TTX) on contractile and relaxant response of human bronchial strips with intrinsic tone to electrical field stimulation (70 V, 1 msec pulse duration). Tissues were treated with atropine (Atr) or propranolol (Prop) as indicated. Contractile effects were generated by intermittent field stimulation and relaxant effects by graded continuous stimulation. Contractile responses are expressed in terms of maximal carbachol (10^{-3} M) contractions as determined in paired strips. Relaxations are expressed in terms of maximal relaxation to theophylline (10^{-2} M) as determined in paired strips. Absolute responses as tension in mg are also shown. Each point is the mean ± S.E. of (n) experiments. (From Taylor et al., 1984, with permission.)

in TTX-sensitive and -insensitive responses and whether TTX-resistant NANC relaxations have any physiologically relevant role in the regulation of bronchomotor tone.

IV. Role of Sensory Fibers

Although electrical field stimulation of isolated airways activates all neural elements within the tissue, it usually is presumed that observed responses are mediated through activation of intrinsic postganglionic efferent motor nerves because, in addition to their being sensitive to TTX, they are unaffected by ganglionic blocking agents. However, it is important to recognize that field stimulation also could elicit responses resulting from antidromic firing of afferent fibers and that these responses also would be blocked by TTX and unaffected by ganglionic blockade. Indeed, Trenchard (1983) hypothesized that the airway NANC inhibitory system is an artifact and that responses attributed to stimulation of efferent NANC fibers are actually due to activation of afferent fibers. What is the evidence to support the contention that efferent fibers mediate NANC responses? As will be discussed in the following section, stimulation of the cervical vagus nerve in intact cats produces NANC bronchodilation and this effect is abolished by ganglionic blockade, implying that it is mediated via activation of efferent fibers (Diamond and O'Donnell, 1980). Trenchard (1983) downplayed the significance of this result by pointing out that hexamethonium can block sensory receptor activation. If hexamethonium did act in this way to prevent NANC responses in vivo, one would expect that the agent would act in a similar fashion to prevent NANC responses in vitro. However, this is not the case; hexamethonium has been shown to have no effect on field-stimulation-induced NANC relaxations in guinea pig trachea (Coburn and Tomita, 1973; Coleman and Levy, 1974; Richardson and Bouchard, 1975) or in cat airways (Altiere et al., 1984b).

The ability of ganglionic stimulant drugs to evoke NANC relaxations in isolated airways provides additional evidence that the responses are mediated via activation of postganglionic efferent fibers. Hawkins and Paton (1958) observed nicotine-induced relaxation responses in guinea pig trachea and cat bronchi that were blocked by concentrations of hexamethonium much lower than those required to block the stimulant effects of nicotine on nerve endings. Though these studies were done prior to the advent of beta adrenergic blocking agents, it seems probable that at least some portion of the observed relaxation responses was mediated via NANC inhibitory nerves. Some two decades later, Jones et al. (1980) reexamined the action of nicotine on guinea pig trachea. These investigators observed that nicotine produced a biphasic response consisting of an atropine-sensitive contraction followed by relaxation. The relaxation phase was predominantly adrenergic but also included a residual NANC component. The effects of nicotine were eliminated by TTX, showing that they were neurally mediated, and blocked by hexamethonium, indicating that nicotinic receptors were involved. As pointed out by the investigators, it is improbable that the nicotine-induced adrenergic inhibitory response was mediated through ganglionic excitation, since sympathetic ganglia are anatomically remote from airway smooth muscle tissue. More likely, nicotine acted on receptors located on postganglionic adrenergic nerve terminals to cause TTX-sensitive release of norepinephrine.

The site where nicotine acted to induce NANC relaxations could not be determined but it seems likely that ganglia were involved, for at least two reasons. First, NANC responses in vivo are evoked by stimulating parasympathetic nerves whose ganglia lie within the innervated effector tissue. Therefore, it is reasonable to assume that ganglia of the NANC system also occur within the innervated tissue. Second, as noted above, hexamethonium antagonizes nicotine-induced NANC inhibitory responses in vitro but does not affect NANC relaxations induced by field stimulation. From this it follows that in the experiments of Jones et al. (1980), hexamethonium most likely exerted its inhibitory actions at ganglionic sites rather than at NANC nerve terminals, a view which would be supported by the earlier work of Hawkins and Paton (1958).

Another piece of evidence favoring the notion that NANC inhibitory responses are mediated via activation of efferent rather than afferent fibers was obtained from experiments performed on airway tissues taken from cats subjected to unilateral cervical vagotomy (Altiere and Diamond, 1985a). After allowing 10 days for afferent nerves to degenerate, NANC responses to electrical field stimulation were compared in control and denervated airways. Frequency-response curves generated in vagotomized airways were not different from curves generated in control airways (Fig. 5). Interpretation of these data was constrained by knowledge of the fact that some crossing of vagal fibers occurs within the lungs and some nonvagal sensory fibers remain in vagotomized

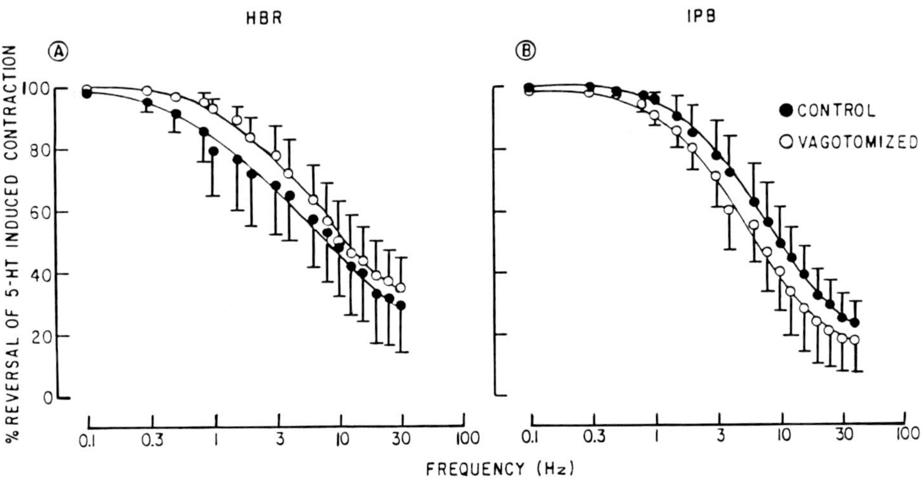

Figure 5 Nerve-mediated NANC relaxation in isolated cat airways 10 days after unilateral left vagotomy. Frequency-dependent relaxation responses were evoked by electrical field stimulation (10 V, 0.3 msec for 5 sec) of cat hilar bronchus (HBR) and intrapulmonary bronchus (IPB) isolated from vagotomized (left) lung and control (right; vagus intact) lung. Tissues were contracted with 5HT and treated with 10^{-6} M atropine, 10^{-6} M propranolol, and 10^{-5} M guanethidine. Data points are means ± S.E. from six experiments.

airway tissues. Nevertheless, when considered in the context of all available evidence, the findings support the contention that airway NANC inhibitory responses are not mediated through stimulation of sensory afferent neurons.

V. In Situ and In Vivo Studies

The in vitro evidence for a functional NANC inhibitory system in the airways of various mammalian species has been verified by in situ and in vivo experiments (Table 1). In all these studies, the principal source of extrinsic control of NANC nerves was localized to preganglionic parasympathetic fibers running in the vagus nerve or branches thereof. Chesrown et al. (1980) and Yip et al. (1981) conducted analogous in situ experiments in anesthetized guinea pigs. They measured pressure changes in an isolated, fluid-filled segment of cervical trachea in response to stimulation of extrinsic autonomic nerves. After atropine treatment, electrical stimulation of the cervical sympathetic or vagal trunks resulted in falls in intraluminal pressure that reflected decreases in trachealis muscle tension. These changes were blocked by hexamethonium, indicating they were due to stimulation of preganglionic fibers. Interruption of the recurrent laryngeal nerves substantially decreased responses to vagal stimulation, while stimulation of the peripheral ends of these nerves caused decreases in intraluminal pressure nearly as large as those seen when the nerves were intact. The effects of sympathetic but not vagal stimulation were reduced markedly in animals that had been chemically sympathectomized with 6-hydroxydopamine or had undergone beta-adrenergic blockade with propranolol or sotalol. The possibility that the relaxations seen during vagal stimulation were due to a decrease in blood flow to the trachealis muscle or that they resulted from the release of a humoral agent from elsewhere in the body was evaluated by clamping the aorta or the superior vena cava or by abruptly stopping the heart with an air bolus or a right ventriculotomy Clamping the aorta caused a small drop in intraluminal pressure, but clamping of the superior vena cava had no effect. Similarly, stopping the circulation did not diminish the decrease in intraluminal pressure evoked by vagal stimulation. It was concluded from these studies that the guinea pig trachealis muscle possesses a dual adrenergic and NANC inhibitory innervation and that the NANC system is supplied by preganglionic cholinergic fibers that reach paratracheal ganglia by traveling primarily in the recurrent laryngeal nerves.

In vivo studies in cats (Diamond and O'Donnell, 1980; Irvin et al., 1980) have documented the existence of airway NANC inhibitory nerves in this species and have shown that they receive preganglionic input from the vagus. These experiments were conducted in anesthetized, paralyzed, and artificially ventilated animals using measurements of lung mechanical function (i.e., lung resistance and dynamic compliance) as indirect indices of changes in airway caliber (Fig.

6). Radiographic evidence also has been obtained for functional NANC inhibitory nerves in cat airways (Fig. 7) (Matsumoto et al., 1985). The protocols followed in each of these studies were basically the same. Because bronchodilator responses cannot be elicited readily in anesthetized animals under basal conditions, the first step was to raise airway smooth muscle tone with an intravenous infusion of a bronchoconstrictive agent. For this purpose, 5HT was used; this agent causes a generalized constriction of the cat tracheobronchial tree. With the tone of the airway musculature increased, the caudal ends of the cut cervical sympathetic and vagal trunks were stimulated electrically. Stimulation on the right and left side produced similar responses. Sympathetic stimulation caused brief bronchodilation (decrease in lung resistance or increase in radiographically measured airway diameter) while vagal stimulation resulted in transient bronchoconstriction followed by relatively prolonged bronchodilation. Atropine abolished vagal bronchoconstriction but did not affect the bronchodilator response to sympathetic or vagal nerve stimulation. Relaxations produced by vagal stimulation were easily differentiated from the more evanescent relaxations caused by sympathetic stimulations. The nonadrenergic nature of vagally mediated relaxations was demonstrated by their persistence following adrenergic inhibition with propranolol and guanethidine. Ganglionic blockade with hexamethonium prevented NANC relaxations, indicating that preganglionic cholinergic fibers were being stimulated and ruling out a possible contributory role for sensory neurons.

The prolonged NANC response to vagal stimulation is not typical of autonomic responses in other tissues, which raised the possibility that it resulted from release of a long-acting humoral agent from the abdominal viscera. However, this theory was dispelled by showing that prolonged NANC bronchodilation continued after the vagal nerves were cut at the point where they transited the diaphragm. Another possible explanation for vagally mediated NANC bronchodilation in the cat is that it results from a specific interaction with 5HT. It is difficult to test this hypothesis in the cat because very few agents are available other than 5HT to produce the requisite level of increased bronchomotor tone. We have used high concentrations of infused histamine (Diamond and O'Donnell, 1980) and prostaglandin $F_{2\alpha}$ (Szarek et al., 1982) to achieve a modest rise in lung resistance and under these conditions we were able to demonstrate small NANC relaxation responses to vagal stimulation. We also have conducted preliminary experiments in anesthetized monkeys (Altiere et al., 1984c) in which we used histamine together with cimetidine (to block the histamine H_2 receptors that mediate bronchodilation) to enhance bronchomotor tone. Here, again, we were able to demonstrate vagally mediated NANC bronchodilator responses, although they were small in comparison to those observed in the cat.

In contrast to the studies described above, in situ and in vivo studies in the dog have provided no evidence for the existence of an airway NANC in-

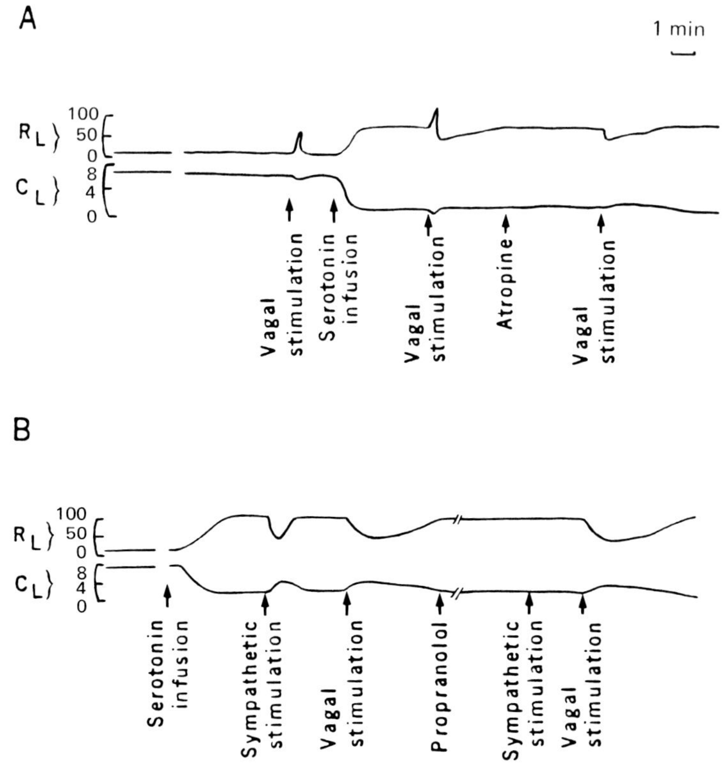

Figure 6 Oscillographic records from two representative experiments in anesthetized, mechanically ventilated cats. (A) Responses to electrical stimulation of the distal end of the cut cervical vagus nerve on three successive occasions (arrows): (i) just prior to beginning an infusion of serotonin, (ii) under steady-state conditions during the infusion, and (iii) after cholinergic blockade with atropine (0.5 mg/kg) during the infusion. (B) Effects of beta-adrenergic blockade with propranolol (0.5 mg/kg) on the responses to electrical stimulation of the caudal end of the cut cervical sympathetic or vagus nerve under steady-state conditions during an infusion of serotonin. The animal was atropinized before the start of the infusion. R_L, lung resistance ($cmH_2O/L/sec$); C_L, dynamic lung compliance (ml/cmH_2O). (From Diamond and O'Donnell, 1980, with permission.)

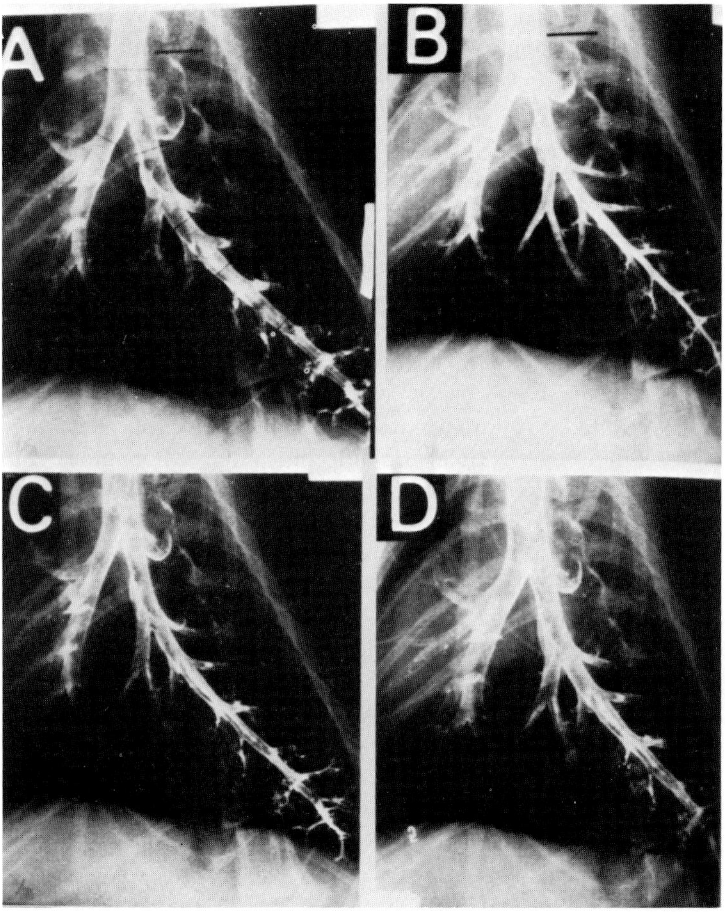

Figure 7 Tantalum bronchograms from one cat. (A) Control bronchogram taken at bilateral sectioning of both cervical vagus and cervical sympathetic nerves after pretreatment intravenously with atropine (3 mg/kg). (B) Bronchogram showing bronchoconstriction induced by serotonin. (C) Bronchogram taken after supramaximal electrical stimulation of bilateral cervical sympathetic nerves, showing β-adrenergic bronchodilation from trachea to small airways. (D) Bronchogram taken after bilateral electrical stimulation of cervical vagus nerves after pretreatment intravenously with propranolol (2 mg/kg), showing bronchodilation similar to that with sympathetic nerve stimulation. (From Matsumoto et al., 1985, with permission.)

hibitory nervous system in these species. Hendrix et al. (1983) examined nerve-mediated inhibitory responses in a canine in situ bronchial smooth muscle preparation by activating postganglionic nerves with intravenous bolus injections of the ganglionic stimulant dimethylphenylpiperazinium (DMPP). Since propranolol nearly abolished the relaxation response to DMPP in dog bronchi, as it previously had been shown to do in dog trachea (Leff et al., 1982), it was concluded that the sympathetic nervous system provided the primary inhibitory innervation to canine airway smooth muscle. Fleetham et al. (1982) sought in vivo evidence for the existence of NANC inhibitory nerves in anesthetized dogs in which airway tone had been enhanced with histamine. Vagal nerve stimulation in the presence of cholinergic or adrenergic blockade did not alter pulmonary resistance or dynamic compliance, indicating an absence of NANC inhibitory innervation.

Porcine airways also appear to be devoid of NANC inhibitory nerves. Leff et al. (1985) simultaneously studied responses of porcine tracheal and bronchial smooth muscle by using a combination of in situ and in vivo methods. Intravenously administered DMPP caused relaxations in the trachea that were completely blocked by propranolol. Likewise, in adrenalectomized animals with airway tone enhanced by histamine, DMPP caused small bronchodilatory responses that were abolished by propranolol. In addition, supramaximal bilateral vagal nerve stimulation failed to elicit airway smooth muscle relaxation following administration of propranolol. These authors concluded that NANC inhibitory nerves are not present in porcine airways.

In summary, the results of the in situ and in vivo studies described herein corroborate and extend previous in vitro studies of the airway NANC inhibitory system. In those species and airways where NANC inhibitory nerves were found in vitro they also were demonstrated in situ or in vivo. Conversely, those species (e.g., dog) and those airways (e.g., guinea pig bronchus) found to lack NANC innervation in vitro also were found to lack NANC innervation when studied in situ or in vivo. A striking feature of the airway NANC-inhibitory system uncovered by these investigations is the prolonged nature of the bronchodilatory response to nerve stimulation. It would appear from this that the common mechanisms for rapidly terminating neurotransmitter action, such as enzymatic degradation and neuronal uptake, are poorly developed or inoperative in the airway NANC inhibitory system. It also is possible that this system operates through a mechanism fundamentally different from the usual forms of synaptic transmission; for example, a neuroparacrine system in which chemical messengers are released from secretory cells and diffuse through the extracellular space to reach their target sites.

VI. Morphologic Studies

Ultrastructural evidence for the existence of NANC innervation in mammalian airways is based on the view that axon profiles of this system are morphologically distinct from other axon profiles. This view was initially expressed by Burnstock (1972), who claimed that NANC nerves in the gastrointestinal tract could be differentiated from adrenergic or cholinergic nerves by the predominant presence in the former of large granular or opaque vesicles 80-200 nm in diameter. Daniel et al. (1977) disputed this claim and argued convincingly that axon varicosities with a predominance of large granular vesicles probably represent chance sections through cholinergic varicosities that contain a heterogeneous distribution of both large granular and small agranular vesicles. The premise that NANC nerves have a distinctive ultrastructural appearance was tested by Gibbins (1982) in 15 different tissues thought from pharmacologic evidence to be innervated by NANC nerves, cholinergic nerves, or both. Gibbins's results substantiated the position of Daniel et al. (1977) in that no consistent ultrastructural differences in terms of proportions or size of vesicles were found between NANC and cholinergic nerves.

The trachea of the guinea pig and cow is known to possess functional NANC innervation, yet varicosities containing a predominance of large granular vesicles rarely are seen in either tissue (Cameron and Kirkpatrick, 1977; Jones et al., 1980). On the other hand, the rat trachea and dog bronchus, which lack functional NANC innervation, have a population of nerve varicosities with a predominance of large granular vesicles (Hoyes and Barber, 1981; Knight et al., 1981). More in keeping with Burnstock's hypothesis, cat, monkey, baboon, and human airways display both functional NANC nerves and some varicosities filled mostly with large granular vesicles (Silva and Ross, 1974; Richardson and Ferguson, 1979; Knight et al., 1981), while dog trachea displays little if any NANC innervation and few if any varicosities with large granular vesicles (Kannan and Daniel, 1980). In light of the generally unclear picture that has emerged from these efforts to correlate morphology and function, it probably is best at this time not to attempt to relate NANC-inhibitory responses of airway smooth muscle tissues with a specific ultrastructural feature of their autonomic innervation.

VII. Electrophysiological Studies

While the presence of the airway NANC-inhibitory system has been well documented in several species and its pharmacologic properties characterized to some extent, relatively little attention has been focused on the system's electrophysiology. Two recent studies examined the electrophysiological effects of NANC nerve stimulation in isolated airways. Ito and Takeda (1982) measured changes in the mechanical and membrane electrical properties of cat tracheal smooth muscle during field stimulation using microelectrode and double sucrose-gap methods. At resting tone, field stimulation of atropinized tissues caused slow membrane hyperpolarization and a reduction in membrane resistance. These changes were prevented by treatment with propranolol. When smooth muscle tone was enhanced with 5HT and the tissues were pretreated with atropine and propranolol, field stimulation caused NANC relaxations but membrane potential and membrane resistance were not affected. Cameron et al. (1983) conducted similar studies in bovine tracheal smooth muscle and found that field stimulation of histamine-contracted tissues caused depolarization and contraction during the period of stimulation. Relaxation responses were recorded when the stimulus was terminated but there was no membrane hyperpolarization (except with prolonged periods of stimulation) and there were no detectable changes in membrane conductance. Propranolol treatment did not affect the field stimulation-induced responses. On the basis of these findings, it would appear that activation of NANC inhibitory nerves by field stimulation is not associated with changes in the electrical properties of airway smooth muscle cell membranes.

VIII. Distribution in the Tracheobronchial Tree

Insights into how NANC inhibitory nerves are distributed along the tracheobronchial tree have been gleaned from three types of experiments: in vivo studies using tests of pulmonary mechanical function, radiographic studies following opacification of the airways, and in vitro studies using electrical field stimulation techniques. These studies have demonstrated differences in both the pattern and degree of functional NANC innervation among various species.

Experiments carried out in our laboratory (Diamond and O'Donnell, 1980) revealed that in the intact, anesthetized, atropine- and propranolol-pretreated cat, vagal stimulation was more effective in reversing the increase in lung resistance induced by an intravenous infusion of 5HT than in reversing the decrease in lung compliance produced by this agent (Fig. 8). On the theoretical assumption that changes in lung resistance reflect primarily changes in the caliber of larger, more central airways while changes in lung compliance are most indicative of dimensional changes in smaller, more peripheral airways (Drazen, 1984), we suggested that NANC inhibitory nerves are more densely concentrated in, or preferentially distributed to, the large airways of cats.

Roentgenograms obtained after insufflation of powdered tantalum have yielded additional information about the distribution of NANC nerves in cat airways. Using a fine focal spot method for magnifying tantalum bronchograms, Matsumoto et al. (1985) were able to measure changes in the diameters of airways as

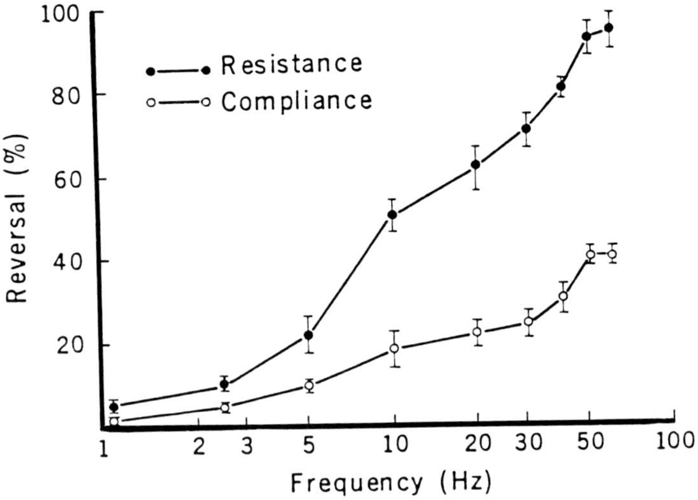

Figure 8 Effects of impulse frequency on vagally mediated reversal of 5HT-induced lung resistance and compliance changes in atropinized cats. Stimulus parameters: 30 V, 2 msec for 5 sec. Each point represents the mean ± S.E. of results from 17 experiments. (From Diamond and O'Donnell, 1980, with permission.)

small as 0.5 mm. They found that stimulation of NANC nerves inhibited 5HT-induced bronchoconstriction from the trachea down to the small bronchioles. The most marked inhibitory effects occurred in midsized airways (2-4 mm in diameter); airways less than 1 mm in diameter were affected least by NANC stimulation.

In vitro studies of the NANC innervation of airways of different sizes have been conducted in tissues obtained from guinea pig, rabbit, cat, cow, monkey, and human. Guinea pig tracheal but not bronchial smooth muscle exhibited NANC relaxation responses to electrical field stimulation (Grundström et al., 1981a). In the latter study, bronchial preparations were used at a resting level of tone. Because it often is necessary to contract airway tissues before relaxation responses can be observed, we conducted similar studies in guinea pig airways contracted with histamine. Field stimulation produced a biphasic response in the trachea but only a contractile response in the primary bronchus (Fig. 9). After adrenergic and muscarinic cholinergic blockade, NANC relaxation responses were observed in trachea but no response was seen in the bronchus, confirming the results of Grundström et al. (1981a). We also conducted several experiments in intact anesthetized guinea pigs with airway tone enhanced by an infusion of histamine, and found that right or left vagal nerve stimulation failed to elicit NANC bronchodilation. This finding is in agreement with the results of an earlier in vivo study that showed no NANC-inhibitory effects of vagal stimula-

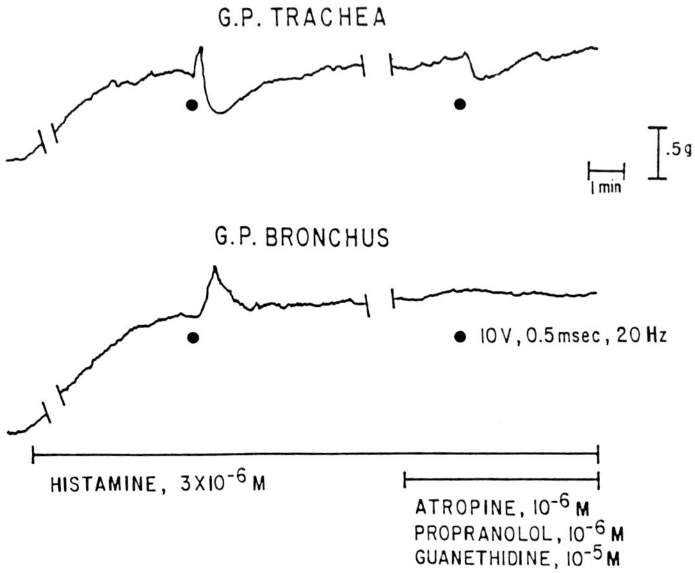

Figure 9 Representative tracings of responses in guinea pig trachea and mainstem bronchus to electrical field stimulation (10 V, 0.5 msec, 20 Hz). Tissues were contracted with histamine and stimulations lasting 10 sec were applied where indicated by closed circles. Field stimulation caused a biphasic response in the trachea and a contractile response in the bronchus. Following muscarinic cholinergic receptor blockade and adrenergic inhibition, field stimulation evoked a NANC relaxation response in the trachea but not in the bronchus.

tion on guinea pig airways below the level of the trachea (Chesrown et al., 1980).

Relaxation responses to electrical field stimulation of intrinsic NANC nerves were studied by us in airway tissues taken from four different levels of the tracheobronchial tree of cats (Altiere et al., 1984b). The frequency of field stimulation that reduced 5HT-induced tone by 50% (EF_{50}) was determined graphically from log frequency-response curves (Table 2). The EF_{50} value for the smallest airway studied (i.e., a segmental bronchus) was significantly greater than that for all other airway segments, indicating a reduced NANC responsiveness with peripheral migration along the airways. Doidge and Satchell (1982) reported that trachea from the rabbit and trachea and extrapulmonary bronchi from the monkey relaxed in response to electrical field stimulation of NANC inhibitory nerves. In the same study, lung parenchymal strips (which are representative in part of fine, peripheral airways) obtained from guinea pig, rabbit, monkey, and human failed to respond to such stimulation. In isolated human

Table 2 Comparison of Electrical-Field-Stimulation-Induced NANC Relaxation Responses in Cat Airways

	TR	HBR	LBR	SBR
log EF_{50}	0.64 ± 0.05	0.60 ± 0.04	0.69 ± 0.04	0.84 ± 0.04*
	(54)	(64)	(66)	(66)

Tissues were treated with 10^{-6} M atropine, 10^{-6} M propranolol, and 10^{-5} M guanethidine. Stimulus parameters: 10 V, 0.3 msec, 0.1-30 Hz for 5 sec. Each value represents the mean ± S.E. of the logarithm of the impulse frequency that reduced 5HT-induced tone by 50% (log EF_{50}). Values in parentheses indicate number of preparations. TR, trachea; HBR, hilar bronchus; LBR, lobar bronchus; SBR, segmental bronchus. (Data taken with permission from Altiere et al., 1984b.)

(Richardson and Béland, 1976; Hutás et al., 1981; Davis et al., 1982) and bovine (Palmer et al., 1985) airways, functional NANC inhibitory nerves were demonstrated from the trachea to the distal bronchi. In bovine airways, NANC inhibitory responses were shown to be greater in large airways than in small airways after correction for weight differences.

Hence, results obtained with a variety of technical approaches and in several different mammalian species all seem to support the general conclusion that NANC-inhibitory nerves exhibit their principal influence upon airways located in the conducting portion of the tracheobronchial tree. Airways in the gas exchange region of the lung appear to be affected minimally by these nerves.

IX. Postulated Neurotransmitters

The most frequently asked question concerning the airway NANC inhibitory system is "What is its neurotransmitter?" Although the answer to this question continues to elude researchers who must work without the availability of a specific pharmacologic antagonist, a number of interesting compounds have come under investigation. Before launching into a discussion of the evidence for or against various candidate mediators, it would be prudent to emphasize that no one, to this date, has demonstrated (e.g., by using superfusion techniques) the release of a pharmacologically active relaxant factor from an airway smooth muscle tissue during stimulation of its NANC-inhibitory innervation. Consequently, the experimental work described below and the conclusions drawn therefrom all are based on the assumption that a transmitter substance is released when NANC nerves are stimulated and that this substance acts at a postsynaptic site to mediate airway smooth muscle relaxation. With this in mind, we can turn our attention to some of the specific chemical compounds that have been studied as possible transmitters of the airway NANC inhibitory system.

As described earlier, there has been speculation that the NANC-inhibitory neurotransmitter may be stored within the large granular vesicles seen on electron microscopy in some axon varicosities associated with airway smooth muscle. Because these vesicles are analogous to those found in other tissues and believed to contain purines or peptides, initial studies have concentrated on these two classes of compounds as potential mediators of NANC responses. Other biologically active endogenous substances such as histamine, dopamine, and cyclooxygenase or lipoxygenase products of arachidonic acid metabolism have been evaluated in our laboratory and rejected as potential mediators, either because they failed to mimic NANC relaxation responses or because agents that antagonized their action did not alter responses to NANC nerve stimulation.

The tracheobronchial tree and the gastrointestinal tract both have endodermic origins and, owing to the widespread interest in the possible role of ATP as an inhibitory neurotransmitter in the gut, early attempts to identify the airway NANC inhibitory transmitter focused on purine nucleotides and nucleosides. Richardson and Bouchard (1975) reported that AMP and ATP caused relaxation of histamine-contracted guinea pig tracheal rings, but further relaxation always was obtained with electrical field stimulation. Coleman and Levy (1974) and Coleman (1976) found that adenosine and ATP produced little or no inhibitory response in an isolated guinea pig tracheal tube preparation until adenosine-uptake-blocking drugs, such as dipyridamole, were added. Then spasmolytic responses to the purines were enhanced and NANC inhibitory nervous responses were potentiated. Satchell (1982) also showed that adenosine, AMP, ADP, and ATP relaxed guinea pig trachea and alluded to unpublished results that confirmed potentiation of NANC inhibitory responses by dipyridamole. Satchell (1984) later reported that adenosine deaminase, the enzyme responsible for terminating the pharmacologic actions of adenosine, antagonized inhibitory responses to both the nucleoside and NANC nerve stimulation in isolated guinea pig tracheal tube preparations treated with dipyridamole. The latter findings constitute the bulk of current evidence supporting adenosine or a related compound as the airway NANC-inhibitory transmitter.

The evidence against a role for purines as transmitters in the airway NANC-inhibitory system is substantial. Subsequent to his earlier report, Coleman (1980) demonstrated that the purine receptor antagonists caffeine and theophylline abolished relaxation responses of the guinea pig tracheal tube preparation to adenosine but did not inhibit NANC relaxation responses. Further doubt has been cast on the notion that adenosine serves as the NANC neurotransmitter in the airways by other investigators who have shown that purine receptor antagonists do not block NANC-inhibitory responses in guinea pig trachea (Grundström et al., 1981a; Karlsson and Persson, 1984), in bovine trachea (Cameron et al., 1983), in the intact cat lung (Irvin et al., 1982), or in isolated human airways (Davis et al., 1982). In addition, several laboratories have been unable to confirm that adenosine uptake inhibitors potentiate NANC relaxations in tissues other than guinea pig trachea (Davis et al., 1982; Ito and Takeda, 1982; Cameron et al., 1983). Still more evidence against purines acting as the NANC-inhibitory transmitter has been provided by the findings that desensitization to purines does not reduce NANC relaxations (Ito and Takeda, 1982); NANC relaxations persist after maximal adenosine relaxations (Karlsson and Persson, 1984); and indomethacin blocks purine but not NANC induced relaxations (Kamikawa and Shimo, 1976; Karlsson and Persson, 1984). Hence, the weight of present evidence, though still not conclusive, points to a mediator other than a purine derivative as the airway NANC-inhibitory neurotransmitter.

Numerous regulatory peptides (e.g., bombesin, calcitonin, cholecystokinin, enkephalin, galanin, neuropeptide Y, peptide histidine isoleucine, somatostatin, substance P, and vasoactive intestinal peptide) have been identified in lung tissue of several species including humans. Some of these peptides have been localized by immunocytochemistry to nerves within the airways. The most widely studied among them is the 28 amino acid peptide, vasoactive intestinal peptide (VIP). This peptide has within its broad spectrum of biological activities the ability to relax airway smooth muscle. The relaxant effect of VIP resembles the relaxation produced by NANC nerve stimulation in that it occurs via a mechanism that is neither adrenergic nor cholinergic and without the involvement of cyclooxygenase products of arachidonic acid metabolism (Diamond et al., 1983). As a consequence, VIP has become a prime candidate for the airway NANC inhibitory transmitter. The myriad actions of VIP in the lung are reviewed elsewhere in this volume; in this section, we summarize the body of evidence that either substantiates or refutes its neurotransmitter function in the airway NANC system.

The evidence implicating VIP as the neurotransmitter of airway NANC nerves is based on the following observations: VIP-immunoreactive nerves and nerve terminals are present in animal and human lungs where they are found, among other locations, in close association with airway smooth muscle (Dey et al., 1981; Polak and Bloom, 1982); VIP mimics the mechanical (Said et al., 1974; Matsuzaki et al., 1980; Said et al., 1982; Wasserman et al., 1982; Cox et al., 1983; Diamond et al., 1983; Altiere and Diamond, 1984; Hand et al., 1984; Karlsson and Persson, 1984; Venugopalan et al., 1984) and electrophysiological (Ito and Takeda, 1982; Cameron et al., 1983) changes produced in airway smooth muscle by NANC nerve stimulation; NANC relaxation responses are diminished in airway tissues that have been desensitized to VIP (Ito and Takeda, 1982; Venugopalan et al., 1984); VIP is released from airway tissues during electrical field stimulation (Matsuzaki et al., 1980; Cameron et al., 1983); and prior incubation of guinea pig trachea with antiserum to VIP reduces field-stimulation-induced NANC relaxations (Matsuzaki et al., 1980). While some of this evidence is direct and irrefutable, a good deal of it has been called into question; moreover, additional data have been advanced that do not support a role for VIP in NANC neurotransmission.

The presence of VIP in airway nerves, though suggestive of a neurotransmitter function, is by no means proof of such a function. This point is perhaps best exemplified by the fact that VIP-immunoreactive nerve fibers have been observed in relation to bronchial smooth muscle in the dog (Dey et al., 1981), a species whose airways have been shown by extensive in vitro and in vivo experiments to have no functional NANC inhibitory innervation (vide supra). The ability of VIP to mimic NANC relaxation of airway smooth muscle has been well documented in a number of species, but even along this front some perplexing issues have emerged.

For instance, when the guinea pig trachea is maximally relaxed by field stimulation of its NANC nerves, exogenous VIP produces additional relaxation; conversely, when the same tissue is exposed to a supramaximal concentration of exogenous VIP, field stimulation of NANC nerves causes further relaxation (Karlsson and Persson, 1984). Davis et al. (1982) also reported an absence of interaction between VIP and NANC relaxations in human airways. Moreover, the proteolytic enzyme, α-chymotrypsin, which abolishes NANC inhibitory responses to electrical field stimulation in dog gastric muscularis mucosa (Angel et al., 1983) and to exogenous VIP in cat airways (Altiere and Diamond, 1985b), does not affect NANC relaxation responses in isolated cat trachea or bronchus (Fig. 10). In the bullfrog lung, where NANC relaxations can be induced readily with a ganglionic stimulant, VIP has nearly no relaxant activity (Downes and Taylor, 1983).

Studies that have assessed the bronchomotor effects of VIP in humans have painted a complex picture. The clinical reports indicate little or no bronchodilator efficacy when VIP is administered by the aerosol route (Bundgaard et al., 1983; Altiere et al., 1984a; Barnes and Dixon, 1984). Whether this lack of efficacy is dose-related, the result of poor bioavailability, or reflective of a relative paucity of VIP receptors in human airways is unclear. In one study in which VIP was given to atopic asthmatic subjects by intravenous infusion, the peptide appeared to effect good bronchodilation (Morice et al., 1983). However, VIP lowers systemic blood pressure and this in turn activates reflex homeostatic mechanisms that could reduce bronchomotor tone coincident with restoration of blood pressure. The effects of VIP also have been studied in isolated human airways with contradictory results. Some authors reported potent relaxant effects (Saga and Said, 1984; Palmer et al., 1986) whereas others

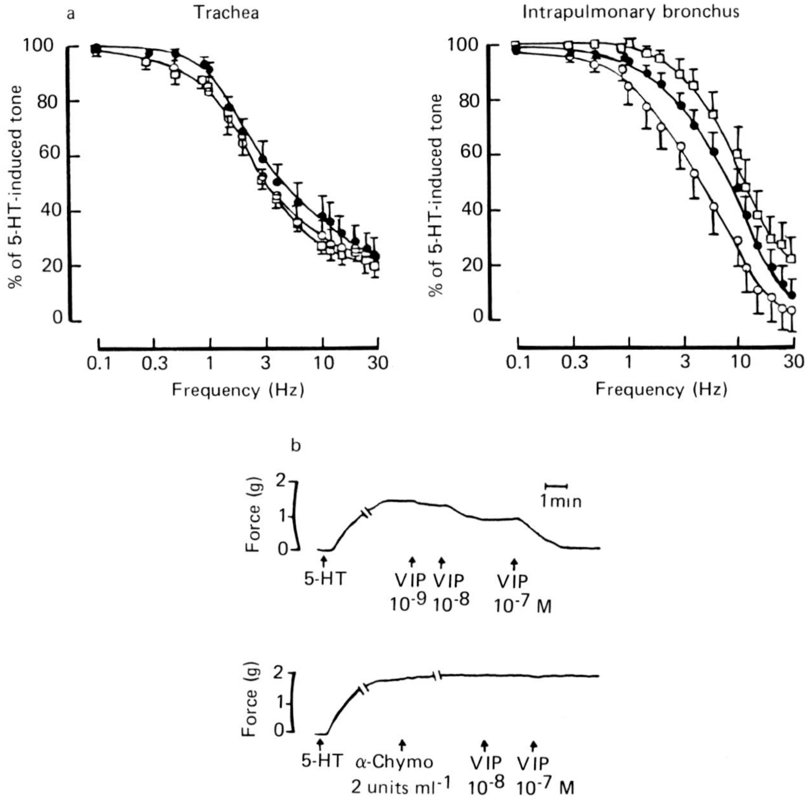

Figure 10 (a) Comparison of frequency-dependent nonadrenergic noncholinergic relaxations (10 V, 0.3 msec, 0.1-30 Hz for 5 sec) in isolated cat trachea and intrapulmonary bronchus pretreated with atropine (10^{-6} M), propranolol (10^{-6} M), and guanethidine (10^{-5} M) before (●) and after exposure to 2 units/ml α-chymotrypsin for 4 min (○) or 20 min (□). Relaxations are expressed as a percentage of 5HT-induced contraction. Each point is the mean ± S.E. of 4 to 11 observations. (b) Relaxation responses to vasoactive intestinal peptide (VIP) in a 5HT-precontracted cat intrapulmonary bronchus incubated with atropine (10^{-6} M), propranolol (10^{-6} M), and guanethidine (10^{-5} M) before and after a 20 min exposure to 2 units/ml α-chymotrypsin. (From Altiere and Diamond, 1985b, with permission.)

found little (Davis et al., 1982) or no (Raffestin et al., 1985) relaxant activity. For the moment, these conflicting accounts of the bronchomotor actions of VIP in human airways resist interpretation and they do little to clarify what role, if any, the peptide plays in NANC neurotransmission.

The experiments carried out to establish a correlation between the electrophysiological effects of VIP and NANC nerve stimulation have yielded interesting but equivocal results. Cameron et al. (1983) recorded no change in conductance and only slight hyperpolarization of the bovine tracheal smooth muscle cell membrane following prolonged NANC nerve stimulation. Similar results were obtained upon exposure of the tissue to high concentrations of VIP. However, Ito and Takeda (1982) working with cat tracheal smooth muscle, noted that the concentrations of VIP required to produce relaxation responses comparable to those evoked to NANC nerve stimulation resulted in significant membrane hyperpolarization that was not observed during field stimulation. Additional studies will be required to resolve these seemingly disparate results.

The data that purport to show a parallel decrease in VIP and NANC nerve-mediated relaxation responses in desensitized airway tissues require careful scrutiny. Ito and Takeda (1982) recorded NANC-induced relaxations of 5HT-contracted cat trachaelis muscle before and after desensitization to VIP (produced by repeated applications of exogenous VIP). These workers found a decrease in the absolute size of the neurally induced NANC relaxation response after desensitization. But close examination of their data reveals that in the process of desensitization a substantial amount of 5HT-induced tone was lost, so that while the magnitude of NANC relaxation decreased after desensitization, the maximum level of relaxation attained did not. It is difficult to conclude from such data that desensitization to VIP reduces the ability of airway smooth muscle to respond to NANC nerve stimulation. The study by Venugopalan et al. (1984) also purported to show loss of responsiveness to NANC nerve stimulation following desensitization (by prolonged incubation with exogenous VIP). However, in these experiments, which were conducted in an intact guinea pig tracheal pouch preparation, there was some question as to the specificity of desensitization since inhibitory responses to sympathetic nerve stimulation also were depressed after VIP incubation.

The demonstrated release of VIP during electrical field stimulation of isolated tracheal smooth muscle (Matsuzaki et al., 1980; Cameron et al., 1983) is an important finding that lends strong support to the contention that the peptide mediates NANC inhibitory responses in the airways. However, enthusiasm for this observation must be tempered by the fact that the source of VIP was not determined in the cited studies, nor was it determined whether the released VIP possessed pharmacological activity. VIP is distributed ubiquitously in the respiratory tract and it is possible that electrical field stimulation promotes its release from extraneous sites in amounts that may or may not be pharmacologically active on airway smooth muscle. Finally, with regard to the experiments reported by Matsuzaki et al. (1980), by showing that NANC-induced relaxations of guinea pig trachea decrease following incubation with VIP antiserum, these investigators have made a potentially signal observation, but their work still requires confirmation by other laboratories and extension into other species, especially humans.

As research into the nature of the airway NANC neurotransmitter continues apace, efforts must be made to avoid adopting a doctrinaire approach. While purines appear to be unlikely NANC neurotransmitter candidates, the case for or against VIP remains unsettled and a host of other peptides await investigation. Because entirely different classes of chemical compounds may eventually come under study, use of the term "peptidergic" should be discouraged, at least for the time being, when reference is made to the airway NANC inhibitory system. Finally and most important, all those engaged in this field of endeavor must be ever mindful and respectful of the fundamental tenets of pharmacology that set forth explicit tests of proof for all putative neurotransmitters (Bowman and Rand, 1980).

X. Neurohumoral Modulation

Interest in neural and humoral modulation of autonomic mechanisms controlling bronchomotor tone has increased in recent years. Modulation of cholinergic and adrenergic neurotransmission in mammalian airways appears to occur via prejunctional inhibitory mechanisms not unlike those that operate in other tissues and organs (Starke, 1981). For instance, in dog trachea prostaglandins inhibit cholinergic transmission (Nakanishi et al., 1976; Ito and Tajima, 1981; Walters et al., 1984) and acetylcholine depresses release of norepinephrine from adrenergic nerve terminals (Russell and Bartlett, 1981). Prostaglandins do not appear to have a role in modulating airway NANC responses because these responses are unaffected by cyclooxygenase inhibition (Coleman and Levy, 1974; Kamikawa and Shimo, 1976; Davis et al., 1982; Altiere et al., 1984b).

We undertook a study to determine whether acetylcholine acted directly or indirectly to modulate or initiate NANC inhibitory responses in cat airways (Altiere et al., 1985). We considered that these were important questions because release of acetylcholine from postganglionic cholinergic nerves was known to occur coincident with activation of the airway NANC-inhibitory system, regardless of whether this was brought about by stimulation of efferent cervical vagus nerves in vivo or by electrical field stimulation of isolated airways in vitro. It was considered that neurally released acetylcholine could act at prejunctional sites in feline airway smooth muscle to regulate release of the NANC transmitter in the same manner that it acts to inhibit NANC neurotransmission in chick rectum (Komori and Ohashi, 1984) or cat submandibular salivary gland (Lundberg, 1981). Alternatively, acetylcholine could elicit NANC relaxation through an atropine-insensitive mechanism by activating postsynaptic nicotinic receptors or by stimulating the release of a relaxant substance from another lung cell type in close proximity to airway smooth muscle. Because the NANC neurotransmitter has not been identified, it was not possible to examine the effects of acetylcholine by measuring stimulation-evoked overflow of transmitter as commonly is done in studies dealing with modulation of adrenergic or cholinergic neurotransmission. Therefore, we examined the effects of acetylcholine on the NANC inhibitory system by observing responses elicited by field stimulation before and during exposure of airways to various pharmacologic agents known to modify its actions.

We found that activation of muscarinic cholinergic receptors by an exogenously applied cholinergic agonist (bethanechol) or by neurally released acetylcholine had no influence on NANC inhibitory responses. From our earlier studies we knew that hexamethonium did not affect field stimulation-induced NANC responses and so we were certain that these responses did not arise from an acetylcholine action on nicotinic receptors on airway smooth muscle cells or on secondary secretory cells. Enhancement of acetylcholine effects by acetylcholinesterase inhibition also did not alter NANC relaxations, further suggesting that the cholinergic neurotransmitter did not serve to regulate NANC neurotransmission. The strongest evidence against a modulatory role for neurally released acetylcholine came from experiments in which hemicholinium was used to deplete nerve terminals of the transmitter. Hemicholinium treatment abolished cholinergically mediated contractile responses to field stimulation but had no effect on frequency-dependent NANC relaxations (Fig. 11). This indicated that the release of acetylcholine per se was not necessary to evoke NANC responses and that acetylcholine had no discernible role in regulating or mediating NANC inhibitory responses. We concluded that NANC relaxation of cat airways is neither dependent upon nor regulated by the neuronal release of acetylcholine.

It remains to be determined whether other neural inputs or endogenous factors can influence NANC neurotransmission in airway smooth muscle. Presynaptic alpha-adrenergic receptors are believed to mediate inhibition of neurotransmitter release in many organs and alpha-2 adrenergic receptor stimulation has been shown to suppress acetylcholine release in guinea pig trachea and human bronchi (Grundström et al., 1981b; Grundström and Andersson, 1985). Likewise, methionine and leucine enkephalins have been reported to inhibit release of acetylcholine from postganglionic parasympathetic neurons in canine tracheal smooth muscle (Russell and Simons, 1985). Whether adrenergic agonists, enkephalins, or a multitude of other substances present in various cell types in

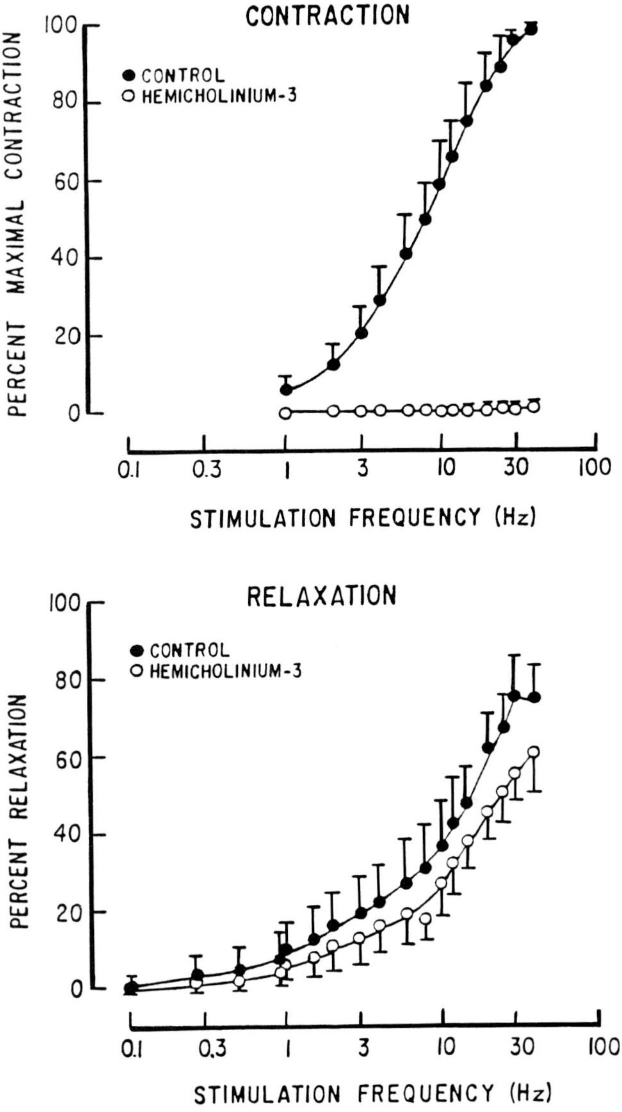

Figure 11 Effects of 5×10^{-4} M hemicholinium on responses of cat intrapulmonary bronchus to electrical field stimulation (10 V, 0.3 msec, 0.1-40 Hz for 5 sec). Tissues were incubated with 10^{-6} M propranolol and 10^{-5} M guanethidine. Top panel, contraction frequency-response curves generated in control and hemicholinium-treated tissues at resting tone. Responses were normalized to first curve maximal contraction. Bottom panel, NANC relaxation frequency-response curves generated in control and hemicholinium-treated tissues contracted with 5HT. Responses were expressed as percent reversal of the induced tone. Each point is the mean ± S.E. of responses from five experiments. (From Altiere et al., 1985, with permission.)

the lung can or do modulate airway NANC inhibitory neurotransmission remains an open question. Perhaps of equal importance is the question of whether the NANC inhibitory system can modulate release in the lung of other neurotransmitters or other pharmacologic mediators.

XI. Reflex Activation

The observation that intrinsic airway NANC inhibitory nerves receive extrinsic input from the vagus raised the question of whether afferent pathways could be identified that either inhibited or activated the motor discharge to this system. To date, no attempts have been made to demonstrate reflex inhibition of the airway NANC inhibitory system. If the system is tonically active this may be possible, but it will require thorough documentation that reflex bronchoconstriction can occur by a mechanism independent of either increased cholinergic or depressed beta adrenergic input to the airway musculature. Once the identity of the neurotransmitter has been established, further experiments may be required to confirm that reflex inhibition of the NANC system is accompanied by diminished transmitter release.

We recently examined the question of whether the airway NANC inhibitory system of the cat could be activated reflexly (Szarek et al., 1986). Two different modes of sensory stimulation were tried: mechanical irritation of the laryngeal mucosa (an area extraordinarily rich in afferent innervation) and bronchoconstriction provoked with bolus intravenous injections of a spasmogen. Total lung resistance or its reciprocal, total lung conductance, was used as the index of airway response. From our first group of experiments we learned that a gentle mechanical stimulus applied to the dorsal surface of the larynx would provoke a biphasic bronchomotor response in cats after their basal lung resistance had been raised by an infusion of 5 HT. Before 5HT, the same stimulus caused only bronchoconstriction. The biphasic response consisted of a transient augmentation of the 5HT-induced bronchoconstriction followed by a prolonged bronchodilation (Fig. 12). After muscarinic cholinergic receptor blockade with atropine, the constriction phase of the response disappeared while the relaxation phase persisted. The relaxation phase was resistant to beta adrenergic receptor blockade with propranolol but was abolished by autonomic ganglionic blockade with hexamethonium and blocked reversibly by cooling the cervical vagi. The bronchomotor response to laryngeal stimulation, as assessed by the first detectable change in transpulmonary pressure following application of the stimulus, began after a short latency that was not different in the absence or presence of atropine; that is, the latency for bronchoconstriction before atropine was the same as for bronchodilation after atropine.

We derived several conclusions from these experiments. First, we con-

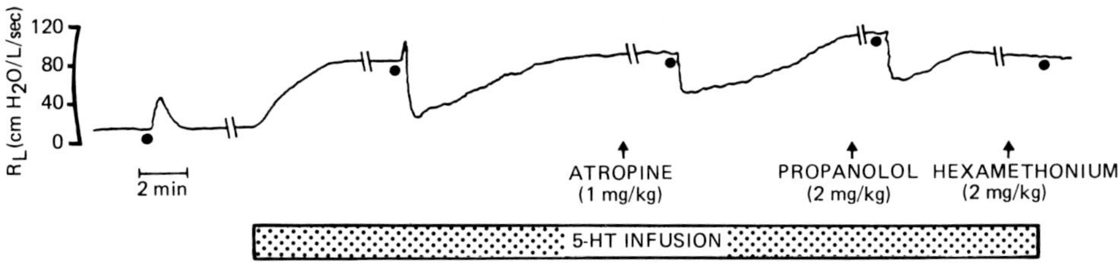

Figure 12 Changes in lung resistance (R_L) caused by mechanical stimulation of the larynx (●) in an anesthetized, artificially ventilated cat. Initially, the larynx was stimulated under basal conditions (far left). Thereafter, baseline airway tone was enhanced by a continuous infusion of 5-hydroxytryptamine (5HT) in order to observe bronchodilatory responses. (From Szarek et al., 1986, with permission.)

cluded that laryngeal stimulation activates not only the well-known vagal cholinergic excitatory pathway to the airways but also the newly described vagal NANC inhibitory pathway. The dilator component of the laryngobronchial reflex is not apparent unless a background of augmented tone is extant at the time of stimulation. Second, because atropine completely prevented the bronchoconstriction phase without affecting the bronchodilation phase of the reflex and because the two responses appeared after the same latency, we concluded that the afferent signal for the NANC component of the reflex must have originated from end organs in the laryngeal epithelium that respond to mechanical stimulation rather than from stretch receptors in the airways that respond to bronchoconstriction (Widdicombe, 1981). As a corollary to this conclusion, the sequelae of bronchoconstriction (e.g., changes in blood gas tensions) also were excluded as possible origins of the initiating stimulus. Finally, because of its susceptibility to vagal cooling and hexamethonium, we concluded that the laryngeal NANC bronchodilator reflex must travel in the vagus and that the efferent limb must traverse a ganglionic synapse enroute to the smooth muscle effector tissue. Recent preliminary reports indicate that a laryngeal NANC bronchodilator reflex analogous to the one found by us in the cat may be operant in human airways. Michoud et al. (1985, 1986) used a bronchoscopy brush to irritate the larynx of subjects who had been pretreated with cholinergic and beta adrenergic blocking agents before inhaling a histamine aerosol. Laryngeal stimulation produced a sharp but short lasting reversal of the increase in lung resistance induced by histamine. These studies used a relatively small number of subjects, but the results are provocative and certainly warrant an expanded investigative effort.

The protocol for our second group of experiments involved challenging

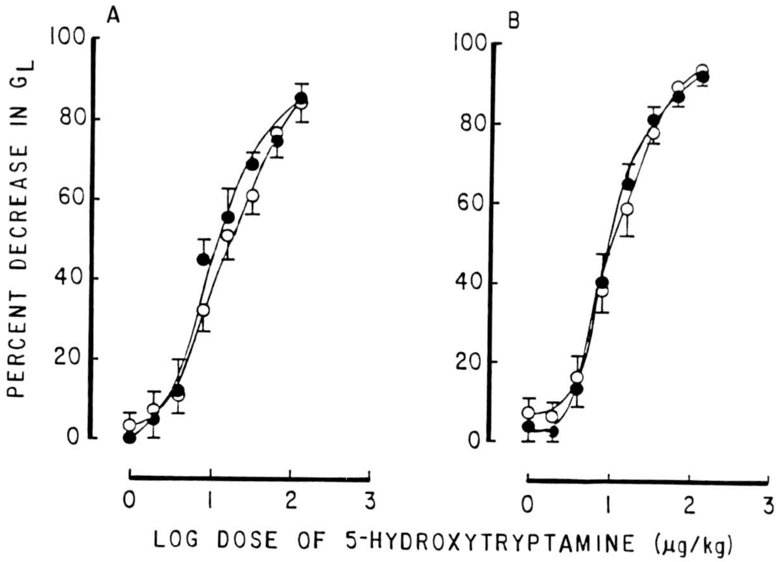

Figure 13 Effects of vagal blockade on changes in lung conductance (G_L) induced by 5-hydroxytryptamine (5HT) in cats pretreated with atropine (1 mg/kg) and propranolol (2 mg/kg). (A) Successive 5HT dose-response curves generated before (●) and after (○) saline administration. (B) Dose-response curves to 5HT before (●) and after (○)vagal blockade produced by administration of hexamethonium (2 mg/kg). Each point represents the mean ± S.E. of results from five experiments. (From Szarek et al., 1986, with permission.)

atropine and propranolol pretreated cats with increasing bolus doses of 5HT and constructing dose-response curves before and after blockade of NANC efferent activity by vagal cooling or with hexamethonium. We reasoned that in animals such as the cat, which have a well-developed NANC inhibitory system, the NANC nerves might be reflexly activated in response to a specific chemical stimulus that evokes bronchoconstriction or by the mechanical process of bronchoconstriction itself. (Here it should be noted that although bronchoconstriction is not a prerequisite for the NANC component of the laryngobronchial reflex, it nonetheless could act as an independent initiating stimulus for another type of NANC reflex originating in the airways.) No differences in the slopes or positions of the 5HT dose-response curves were found before and after blockade of the NANC pathway (Fig. 13) and we thus concluded that neither intravenous 5HT nor the process of airway smooth muscle contraction is capable of initiating reflex activity in the cat NANC inhibitory system. Different results were reported by Aizawa et al. (1982) who carried out nearly identical experiments and reported that very high doses of 5HT evoked more pronounced bronchoconstrictor responses after hexamethonium than before. In plotting their dose-response data, these workers used changes in lung resistance to express airway responses. During intense bronchoconstriction, lung resistance increases sharply toward a theoretically infinite value. As a result, what in fact may be subtle differences in degree of severe obstruction can appear to be very large differences when lung resistance is used as the expression of airway response. We avoided this problem by converting lung resistance to its reciprocal, lung conductance (which can decrease during bronchoconstriction by no more than 100%), before plotting and analyzing our data. Whether or not this accounts for the discrepancy between the two studies remains unclear.

Addressing essentially the same issue as did we and Aizawa et al. (1982), Bai and co-workers (1986) followed the time course of steady-state bronchoconstriction produced by 5HT infusion in atropine- and propranolol-pretreated cats before and after sectioning the cervical parasympathetic nerves. Compared to control animals with intact vagi, parasympathectomized animals exhibited highly variable increases in bronchoconstriction following nerve section. Phentolamine largely eliminated these increases, which led this group of investigators to conclude that they had occurred through an alpha adrenergic mechanism rather than as a consequence of interrupting preganglionic connections to the NANC inhibitory system. In an interesting extension of their study, these workers showed that parasympathectomy increased airway responses to aerosolized 5HT in the presence of atropine, propranolol, and phentolamine, indicating reflex activation of the NANC inhibitory system and demonstrating that the route of administration of a constrictor agent is an important determinant of the type of neural modulation subsequently expressed. We previously speculated that the NANC inhibitory system may function not to counteract ongoing bronchoconstriction but to detect impending bronchoconstriction (by monitoring conditions in the upper airways) and respond as appropriate to moderate its extent or duration (Szarek et al., 1986). If such is the case, it might explain why Bai et al. (1986) were successful in demonstrating NANC-inhibitory modulation of bronchoconstriction induced by aerosolized 5HT but not by infused 5HT.

Widdicombe (1975) has pointed out that the reflex control of airways smooth muscle is integrated in the brainstem and that virtually all inputs to this area can be expected to influence airway caliber. Perhaps it is not surprising then to find sensory pathways from the upper airways that are capable of activating the airway NANC inhibitory system. Be that as it may, it still is important to learn the relative strengths of these reflexes and how they interact with other bronchoactive mechanisms to regulate airway size and responsiveness. Other potentially important sources of afferent input to the NANC inhibitory system also need to be identified and their significance evaluated.

For example, bronchodilator reflexes have been reported to originate in the nasopharynx in response to mechanical stimulation (Tomori and Widdicombe, 1969), in the abdominal viscera in response to chemical irritation (Rybicki et al., 1983), and in the hindlimb muscles in response to static contraction (Kaufman and Rybicki, 1984; Longhurst, 1984). Though it has been presumed that these bronchodilator reflexes depend on withdrawal of cholinergic tone or increased release of catecholamines, it is interesting to speculate that the NANC-inhibitory system may be involved. In addition, the NANC system might play a role in various forms of reflex bronchoconstriction. As just described, mechanical stimulation of the laryngeal mucosa of the cat produces, concurrent with reflex bronchoconstriction, reflex bronchodilation that is mediated via the NANC inhibitory system. Could other bronchomotor reflexes that have been viewed in the past as purely constrictive also possess a NANC dilative component? Studies are needed to determine if NANC inhibitory nerves are activated during reflex bronchoconstriction emanating from such familiar stimuli as hypercapnia; hypoxemia, pulmonary microembolism, edema, or congestion; and inhalation of cold air, pharmacologic agents, dusts, or chemical irritants (Widdicombe, 1975). The potential fecundity of such studies is illustrated by recent preliminary reports (Ichinose et al., 1985, 1986) describing NANC-mediated reflex bronchodilation in cats and humans in response to mechanical stimulation of the dorsal cervical trachea and following intravenous or aerosol administration of the afferent C-fiber stimulant capsaicin.

XII. Functional Significance

From the time of the earliest expository papers on the airway NANC inhibitory system, various authors have offered explanations as to the possible functional role of this system in health and disease. Coburn and Tomita (1973) put forth the suggestion that NANC-inhibitory nerves may be of importance to an effective cough mechanism by controlling the compressibility of the trachea. Richardson and Bouchard (1975) called attention to the fact that the tracheobronchial tree arises from the ventral wall of the foregut and shares certain anatomical and physiological features with the gastrointestinal tract. They emphasized that studies of autonomic nervous regulation of gastrointestinal smooth muscle may bear relevance to airways smooth muscle. For example, in the gut a system of NANC-inhibitory nerves has been identified as the primary neural mechanism responsible for the relaxation phase of peristalsis and for the function of many of the sphincters (Burnstock, 1972). When this system is absent or nonfunctional, as it is in humans with Hirschsprung's disease (Frigo et al., 1973) and achalasia (Smith, 1970), and in experimental animals whose intramural ganglion cells have been destroyed by anoxia (Hukuhara et al., 1961), the smooth muscle develops an uncontrolled myogenic activity that leads to a functional spasm of the tract with obstruction. Thus, to the extent that the pathophysiological consequences of disrupted NANC inhibitory function in the gastrointestinal tract can be extrapolated to the lungs, there is reason to believe that the NANC inhibitory system may play an important physiological role in the regulation of bronchomotor tone.

From a more skeptical perspective, one might ask whether NANC-inhibitory nerves are anything more than evolutionary vestiges, remnants of a primitive inhibitory system that have persisted only because of their innocuousness. A persuasive argument against such a point of view rests upon observations in the baboon (Middendorf and Russell, 1980), monkey (Doidge and Satchell, 1982; Satchell, 1982) and humans (Richardson and Béland, 1976; Doidge and Satchell, 1982; Taylor et al., 1984). In the airways of these primate species, functional adrenergic fibers are absent, leaving the NANC system as the only known source of inhibitory neural control. This has led many investigators to hypothesize that diseases such as bronchial asthma, which are characterized by heightened airway reactivity, may be associated with a defect in the NANC inhibitory system. If such a defect could be demonstrated, it would account for the excessive irritability of the airway musculature in asthma and also would help explain the common but enigmatic clinical observation that beta adrenergic blocking drugs frequently cause bronchospasm in asthmatic subjects but rarely so affect nonasthmatics. Theoretically, this would stem from the fact that nonasthmatic subjects have both a NANC-inhibitory system and circulating catecholamines available to counterbalance episodes of increased bronchomotor tone; lacking this redundancy, asthmatic subjects would be hyperresponsive to bronchoconstrictive stimuli and extraordinarily sensitive to beta adrenergic blockade.

Owing to the inherent difficulty in obtaining asthmatic airway tissue, it has not been possible to test this hypothesis critically. Airway tissues taken from elderly nonasthmatic smokers with bronchogenic carcinoma and a moderate degree of hyperresponsiveness to inhaled methacholine do not show evidence of a defect in NANC inhibitory function (Taylor et al., 1985). How these findings relate, if at all, to the behavior of asthmatic airways is not known. Further, such findings shed no light on the possibility that in asthmatic airways the intrinsic elements of the NANC inhibitory system are present and functional but the capacity to activate them is suppressed; that is, a relative deficiency may exist at the level of sensation or central integration such that asthmatics can not respond appropriately to relevant physiologic stimuli. Richardson (1981) raised the additional intriguing idea that airways hyperresponsiveness may be the result of a pathologic conversion of NANC inhibitory control to NANC-excitatory control. In support of his supposition, he noted that NANC systems in other smooth muscles (e.g., the detrusor muscle of the guinea pig urinary bladder

[Krell et al., 1981]) normally provide excitatory control over the effector tissue.

Most recently, interest in the possible role of the NANC inhibitory system in airways hyperresponsiveness has increased as a result of two new and fundamental observations. First, studies explicitly designed to examine the relationship between in vivo and in vitro responses of human airways smooth muscle to bronchoconstrictive stimuli have revealed that no correlation exists between the two responses (Roberts et al., 1983; Vincenc et al., 1983; Armour et al., 1984a,b; Taylor et al., 1985). Although none of these studies included asthmatic subjects, the general conclusion reached was that airways hyperresponsiveness, as it manifests itself in vivo, is not attributable to an alteration in the intrinsic physiological properties of airway smooth muscle per se (thus strengthening the case for involvement of extrinsic autonomic neural or humoral factors). Second, careful analysis of dose-response curves to inhaled histamine (Woolcock et al., 1984) or methacholine (Sterk et al., 1985a) has shown that unlike asthmatic patients, who respond to increasing cumulative concentrations of an inhaled spasmogen with proportional decreases in pulmonary function, nonasthmatic subjects rapidly reach a plateau on their dose-response curves beyond which further increases in the dose of spasmogen no longer are accompanied by corresponding decreases in pulmonary function. In the case of methacholine challenge, additional experiments have demonstrated that the response plateau is not due to the bronchodilation that follows lung inflation or to the development of tachyphylaxis to cumulative doses of the provocative agent. Because normal bronchial smooth muscle in vitro can shorten to about 20% of its optimal length (Stephens, 1977; Fay, 1983) and because a similar degree of shortening in vivo would result in enormous decreases in pulmonary function, it has been suggested that a powerful inhibiting mechanism (such as the NANC-inhibitory system) normally operates in vivo to prevent excessive bronchoconstriction (Woolcock et al., 1984; Macklem, 1985; Sterk et al., 1985a).

Experiments to test whether specific interdiction by the NANC-inhibitory system is responsible for the limitation of maximal airway narrowing in normal human subjects have been difficult to devise. Sterk et al. (1985b) found little change in methacholine responsiveness in four nonasthmatic subjects following ganglionic blockade with inhaled hexamethonium and arrived at the tentative conclusion that the NANC system was not involved in the limitation of bronchoconstriction. However, blockade of airway ganglia was not confirmed in this study nor was it documented whether the dose of hexamethonium was sufficient to prevent release of adrenal catecholamines. The latter point could be particularly relevant because multiple homeostatic regulatory mechanisms may impinge simultaneously on airway smooth muscle; if so, eliminating only autonomic neural inputs might leave other potent mechanisms (e.g., prostanoids and other locally or systemically released humoral factors) free to exert their modulatory effects. Unfortunately, studies to resolve this issue would require concurrent removal of all known inhibitory controls over airway smooth muscle and could not be performed safely in human subjects. Moreover, studies utilizing available pharmacologic blocking agents cannot rule out the possibility that release of neurotransmitter from NANC inhibitory nerves can, under certain circumstances, occur through a local mechanism totally independent of all extrinsic inputs.

Clearly, experiments to explore possible functional roles of the airway NANC inhibitory system, similar to studies seeking the identity of the NANC neurotransmitter, have been seriously hampered by the lack of a specific pharmacologic antagonist. As a consequence, only circumstantial evidence has been compiled from which definitive conclusions are impossible to draw. In addition to what already has been described here and in the previous section on reflex activation, there are other examples of such circumstantial evidence. These include observations that (1) airway reactivity to 5HT is reduced during continuous stimulation of the cervical vagus nerve in cats pretreated with atropine and propranolol (Aizawa et al., 1982); (2) simultaneous stimulation of sympathetic and NANC inhibitory nerves in atropinized cats produces more pronounced bronchodilation than stimulation of either one individually (Matsumoto et al., 1983); (3) under conditions of acidosis and hypoxia (as might be present in patients with obstructed airways), NANC relaxation responses of isolated guinea pig trachealis muscle are inhibited (Souhrada and Kivity, 1982); and (4) normal human tracheobronchial smooth muscle does not exhibit myogenic activity whereas diseased tissue sometimes shows rhythmic contractions (Richardson, 1981). While these and other observations may be suggestive of a physiological role for the airway NANC inhibitory system, they certainly provide no conclusive proof of such a role. It is unlikely that such proof will be forthcoming until a specific antagonist of the airway NANC inhibitory system is introduced and placed in the hands of eager investigators.

Aside from its role in regulating airway smooth muscle tone, the NANC system may have other physiologically relevant actions in the lung. For example, there is evidence that NANC nerves may influence airway secretions. Peatfield and Richardson (1983) showed that stimulation of vagal nerves increased mucus secretion in cat airways, an action that persisted after administration of cholinergic and adrenergic receptor antagonists. Field stimulation of isolated ferret trachea also causes enhanced secretions and this effect appears to be mediated in part by NANC nerves (Borson et al., 1984). Whether NANC nerves have a corresponding role in regulating mucus secretion in human airways is still unclear (Baker et al., 1985). Finally, NANC nerves have been implicated in pulmonary arterial smooth muscle relaxation (Hamasaki et al., 1983) and in increasing tracheobronchial blood flow (Martling et al., 1985). Sorting out the precise role of NANC nerves in regulating these and perhaps other important aspects of lung function promises to be an arduous task and one that is certain to provide many challenging opportunities for research in the years ahead.

XIII. Conclusion

The presence of a NANC system of inhibitory nerves in mammalian airways is firmly established. Further investigation now is needed to determine the precise functional significance of this system in health and in disease. The central connections of the system require additional study and questions of if and how it is activated or inhibited under normal physiological conditions must be addressed. More information is needed to establish the nature and cellular localization of the neurotransmitter, its biosynthetic-metabolic patterns, the mechanism of its release during nerve stimulation, and the mechanism of its interaction with airway smooth muscle cells. Further research also must be undertaken to determine if the NANC system is of functional importance in regulating other effector tissues in the lung such as blood vessels, glands, or other autonomic neurons.

Acknowledgments

This work was supported by grant no. HL27025 from the National Heart, Lung and Blood Institute.

Dr. Altiere is a Parker B. Francis Foundation Fellow in Pulmonary Research.

Discussion

Makhlouf. Field stimulation releases various transmitters and its effects cannot be equated with the effect of exogenous VIP. A better criterion is to use a selective blocker.

Diamond. A selective inhibitor for either VIP or field stimulation-induced NANC relaxations is not available.

Barnes. Although no VIP antagonist is available, after induction of VIP tachyphylaxis there is reduced NANC relaxation in cat trachea, although sympathetic relaxation and the response to isoproterenol are unchanged, which suggests that VIP may at least account for some of the NANC relaxation (Ito et al., *J. Physiol.* **330**:497-511, 1984).

Persson. In the presence of concentrations of VIP that provided maximal relaxation of guinea-pig trachea, NANC relaxation was not reduced, and addition of VIP to a preparation under sustained NANC inhibition produced a relaxation which equalled the control VIP response (Karlsson, J. A., and Persson, C. G. A., *Acta Physiol. Scand.* **127**:589-598, 1984). This argues against VIP as the transmitter.

Burnstock. Indomethacin blocks the relaxant response to ATP and to VIP in guinea pig trachea, but does not block the NANC relaxation.

Persson. The blocking effect of indomethacin is because resting tone of guinea pig trachea is abolished. If tone is raised by a constrictor mediator the presence of indomethacin will not prevent relaxant effects of VIP, ATP, or NANC.

Widdicombe. The demonstration of reflex activation of the NANC system in airways is important, but if cotransmission is involved it is difficult to see the advantage of simultaneous actions of contractile and relaxant mediators.

Diamond. Simultaneous activation of the NANC system may be important in limiting the extent and duration of vagally mediated bronchoconstriction. In anesthetized cats we have not been able to show reflex activation of the NANC system under basal conditions, which is why tone must be raised with serotonin. It would be intersting to see the effect on increased tone due to other stimuli, such as hypercapnia.

Richardson. Reflex bronchodilatation has been demonstrated in the goose (Callanan et al., *Respir. Physiol.* **22**:157-166, 1974). If, as in other birds such as chicken and duck, the predominant neural mechanism is NANC inhibitory nerves, this could be another example of NANC reflex bronchodilatation.

Laitinen. VIP-immunoreactive nerves are also found around bronchial vessels. Direct injection of VIP into tracheal vessels causes a significant reduction in vascular resistance, so VIP-ergic nerves may regulate bronchial blood flow.

Makhlouf. Field stimulation may not reproduce the effect of nerve activity, and experiments on field stimulation should be supplemented by experiments involving more physiological neural stimuli.

Diamond. The parameters used in electrical field stimulation have not always been carefully selected to avoid tetrodotoxin (TTX)-resistant responses. In isolated cat airways, as field stimulation voltage is increased beyond 10 V or pulse duration increased beyond 0.3 msec, TTX-resistant responses become more and more prominent.

Barnes. Field stimulation of pulmonary vessels gives a large component of relaxation that is TTX-resistant and may be due to the production of free oxygen radicals.

References

Aizawa, H., Matsuzaki, Y., Ishibashi, M., Domae, M., Hirose, T., Shigematsu, N., and Tanaka, K. (1982). A possible role of a nonadrenergic inhibitory nervous system in airway hyperreactivity. *Respir. Physiol.* **50**:187-196.

Altiere, R. J., and Diamond, L. (1984). Comparison of vasoactive intestinal peptide and isoproterenol relaxant effects in isolated cat airways. *J. Appl. Physiol.* **56**:986-992.

Altiere, R. J., and Diamond, L. (1985a). Role of vagal sensory fibers in nonadrenergic noncholinergic inhibitory responses in cat airways. *Am. Rev. Respir. Dis.* **131**:A278.

Altiere, R. J., and Diamond, L. (1985b). Effect of α-chymotrypsin on the nonadrenergic noncholinergic inhibitory system in cat airways. *Eur. J. Pharmacol.* **114**:75-78.

Altiere, R. J., Küng, M., and Diamond, L. (1984a). Comparative effects of inhaled isoproterenol and vasoactive intestinal peptide on histamine induced bronchoconstriction in human subjects. *Chest* **86**:153-154.

Altiere, R. J., Szarek, J. L., and Diamond, L. (1984b). Neural control of relaxation in cat airways smooth muscle. *J. Appl. Physiol.* **57**:1536-1544.

Altiere, R. J., Szarek, J. L., and Diamond, L. (1984c). Neural regulation of bronchomotor tone in the intact monkey. *Physiologist* **27**:244.

Altiere, R. J., Szarek, J. L., and Diamond, L. (1985). Neurally mediated nonadrenergic relaxation in cat airways occurs independent of cholinergic mechanisms. *J. Pharmacol. Exp. Ther.* **234**:590-597.

Angel, F., Go, V. L. W., Schmalz, P. F., and Szurszewski, J. H. (1983). Vasoactive intestinal peptide: a putative transmitter in the canine gastric muscularis mucosa. *J. Physiol. (London)* **341**:641-654.

Armour, C. L., Black, J. L., Berend, N., and Woolcock, A. J. (1984a). The relationship between bronchial hyperresponsiveness to methacholine and airway smooth muscle structure and reactivity. *Respir. Physiol.* **58**:223-233.

Armour, C. L., Lazar, N. M., Schellenberg, R. R., Taylor, S. M., Chan, N., Hogg, J. C., and Paré, P. D. (1984b). A comparison of in vivo and in vitro human airway reactivity to histamine. *Am. Rev. Respir. Dis.* **129**:907-910.

Bai, T. R., Macklem, P. T., and Martin, J. G. (1986). The effects of parasympathetectomy on serotonin-induced bronchoconstriction in the cat. *Am. Rev. Resp. Dis.* **133**:110-115.

Baker, B., Peatfield, A. C., and Richardson, P. S. (1985). Nervous control of mucin secretion into human bronchi. *J. Physiol. (London)* **365**:297-305.

Barnes, P. J. (1984). The third nervous system in the lung: physiology and clinical perspectives. *Thorax* **39**:561-567.

Barnes, P. J., and Dixon, C. M. S. (1984). The effect of inhaled vasoactive intestinal peptide on bronchial reactivity to histamine in humans. *Am. Rev. Respir. Dis.* **130**:162-166.

Bhatla, R., Ferguson, C. C., and Richardson, J. B. (1980). The innervation of smooth muscle in the primary bronchus of the chicken. *Can. J. Physiol. Pharmacol.* **58**:310-315.

Borson, D. B., Charlin, M., Gold, B. D., and Nadel, J. A. (1984). Neural regulation of $^{35}SO_4$-macromolecule secretion from tracheal glands of ferrets. *J. Appl. Physiol.* **57**:457-466.

Bowman, W. C., and Rand, M. J. (1980). *Textbook of Pharmacology.* Oxford, Blackwell Scientific Publications, p. 918.

Bundgaard, A., Enehjelm, S. D., and Aggestrup, S. (1983). Pretreatment of exercise induced asthma with inhaled vasoactive intestinal peptide. *Eur. J. Respir. Dis.* **64**:(Suppl 128) 427-429.

Burnstock, G. (1972). Purinergic nerves. *Pharmacol. Rev.* **24**:509-581.

Cameron, A. R., and Kirkpatrick, C. T. (1977). A study of excitatory neuromuscular transmission in the bovine trachea. *J. Physiol.* (*London*) **270**: 733-745.

Cameron, A. R., Johnston, C. F., Kirkpatrick, C. T., and Kirkpatrick, M. C. A. (1983). The quest for the inhibitory neurotransmitter in bovine tracheal smooth muscle. *Q. J. Exp. Physiol.* **68**:413-426.

Catterall, W. A. (1980). Neurotoxins that act on voltage-sensitive sodium channels in excitable membranes. *Annu. Rev. Pharmacol. Toxicol.* **20**: 15-43.

Chesrown, S. E., Venugopalan, C. S., Gold, W. M., and Drazen, J. M. (1980). In vivo demonstration of nonadrenergic inhibitory innervation of the guinea pig trachea. *J. Clin. Invest.* **65**:314-320.

Coburn, R. F., and Tomita, T. (1973). Evidence for nonadrenergic inhibitory nerves in guinea pig trachealis muscle. *Am. J. Physiol.* **224**:1072-1080.

Coleman, R. A. (1973). Evidence for non-adrenergic inhibitory nervous pathway in guinea-pig trachea. *Br. J. Pharmacol.* **48**:360-361P.

Coleman, R. A. (1976). Effects of some purine derivatives on the guinea pig trachea and their interaction with drugs that block adenosine uptake. *Br. J. Pharmacol.* **57**:51-57.

Coleman, R. A. (1980). Purine antagonists in the identification of adenosine-receptors in guinea-pig trachea and the role of purines in non-adrenergic inhibitory neurotransmission. *Br. J. Pharmacol.* **69**:359-366.

Coleman, R. A., and Levy, G. P. (1974). A non-adrenergic inhibitory pathway in guinea-pig trachea. *Br. J. Pharmacol.* **52**:167-174.

Cox, C. P., Lerner, M. R., Wells, J. H., and Said, S. I. (1983). Inhaled vasoactive intestinal peptide prevents bronchoconstriction induced by inhaled histamine. *Am. Rev. Respir. Dis.* **127**:A249.

Daniel, E. E., Taylor, G. S., Daniel, V. P., and Holman, M. E. (1977). Can non-adrenergic inhibitory varicosities be identified structurally. *Can. J. Physiol. Pharmacol.* **55**:243-250.

Daniel, E. E., Davis, C., Jones, T., and Kannan, M. S. (1980). Control of airway smooth muscle. In *Airway Reactivity: Mechanisms and Clinical Relevance.* Edited by F. E. Hargreave. Ontario, Astra, pp. 80-107.

Davis, C., Kannan, M. S., Jones, T. R., and Daniel, E. E. (1982). Control of human airway smooth muscle: in vitro studies. *J. Appl. Physiol.* **53**:1080-1087.

Dey, R. D., Shannon, W. A., and Said, S. I. (1981). Localization of VIP-immunoreactive nerves in airways and pulmonary vessels of dogs, cats and human subjects. *Cell Tissue Res.* **220**:231-238.

Diamond, L., and Gillespie, M. (1982). The lung nonadrenergic inhibitory nervous system. *Trends Pharmacol. Sci.* **3**:237-239.

Diamond, L., and O'Donnell, M. (1980). A nonadrenergic vagal inhibitory pathway to feline airways. *Science* **208**:185-188.

Diamond, L., and Richardson, J. B. (1982). Inhibitory innervation to airway smooth muscle. *Exp. Lung Res.* **3**:379-385.

Diamond, L., Szarek, J. L., Gillespie, M. N., and Altiere, R. J. (1983). In vivo bronchodilator activity of vasoactive intestinal peptide in the cat. *Am. Rev. Respir. Dis.* **128**:827-832.

Doidge, J. M., and Satchell, D. G. (1982). Adrenergic and non-adrenergic inhibitory nerves in mammalian airways. *J. Autonom. Nerv. Syst.* **5**:83-99.

Downes, H., and Taylor, S. M. (1983). Distinctive pharmacological profile of a nonadrenergic inhibitory system in bullfrog lung. *Br. J. Pharmacol.* **78**:339-351.

Drazen, J. M. (1984). Physiological basis and interpretation of indices of pulmonary mechanics. *Environ. Health Perspect.* **56**:3-9.

Fay, F. (1983). Contractile mechanism of single isolated smooth muscle cells. *Proc. Int. Union Physiol. Sci.* **15**:425.

Fleetham, J., Lazar, N., and Paré, P. (1982). Nonadrenergic noncholinergic airway control in the dog. *Fed. Proc.* **41**:1693.

Frigo, G. M., Del Tacca, M., Lecchini, S., and Crema, A. (1973). Some observations on the intrinsic nervous mechanisms in Hirschsprung's disease. *Gut* **14**:35-40.

Fukuda, J., and Kameyama, M. (1980). Tetrodotoxin-sensitive and tetrodotoxin-resistant sodium channels in tissue cultured spinal ganglia neurons from adult mammals. *Brain Res.* **182**:191-197.

Gibbins, I. L. (1982). Lack of correlation between ultrastructural and pharmacological types of nonadrenergic autonomic nerves. *Cell Tissue Res.* **221**:551-581.

Grundström, N., Andersson, R. G. G., and Wikberg, J. E. S. (1981a). Pharmacological characterization of the autonomous innervation of the guinea pig tracheobronchial smooth muscle. *Acta Pharmacol. Toxicol.* **49**:150-157.

Grundström, N., Andersson, R. G. G., and Wikberg, J. E. S. (1981b). Prejunctional alpha-2-adrenoceptors inhibit contraction of tracheal smooth muscle by inhibiting cholinergic neurotransmission. *Life Sci.* **28**:2981-2986.

Grundström, N., and Andersson, R. G. G. (1985). Inhibition of the cholinergic neurotransmission in human airways via prejunctional alpha-2-adrenoceptors. *Acta Physiol. Scand.* **125**:513-517.

Hamasaki, Y., Saga, T., and Said, S. I. (1983). Autonomic innervation of pulmonary artery: evidence for nonadrenergic, noncholinergic relaxation. *Am. Rev. Respir. Dis.* **127**:300.

Hammarström, M., and Sjöstrand, N. O. (1979). Pathways for excitatory and inhibitory innervation to the guinea-pig tracheal smooth muscle. *Experientia* **35**:64-65.

Hand, J. M., Laravuso, R. B., and Will, J. A. (1984). Relaxation of isolated guinea pig trachea, bronchi and pulmonary arteries by vasoactive intestinal peptide (VIP). *Eur. J. Pharmacol.* **98**:279-284.

Hawkins, D. F., and Paton, W. D. M. (1958). Responses of isolated bronchial muscle to ganglionically active drugs. *J. Physiol.* (*London*) **144**:193-219.

Hendrix, S. G., Munoz, N. M., and Leff, A. R. (1983). Physiological and pharmacological response of canine bronchial smooth muscle in situ. *J. Appl. Physiol.* **54**:215-224.

Hoyes, A. D., and Barber, P. (1981). Morphology and response to vagus nerve section of the intraepithelial axons of the rat trachea. A quantitative ultrastructural study. *J. Anat.* **132**:331-339.

Hukuhara, T., Kotani, S., and Sato, G. (1961). Effects of destruction of intramural ganglion cells on colon motility: possible genesis of congenital megacolon. *Jpn. J. Physiol.* **11**:635-640.

Hutás, I., Hadházy, P., Debreczeni, L., and Vizi, E. S. (1981). Relaxation of human isolated bronchial smooth muscle. *Lung* **159**:153-161.

Ichinose, M., Miura, M., Yafuso, N., Nogami, H., and Inoue, H. (1985). Possible sensory receptor of nonadrenergic inhibitory system. *Am. Rev. Respir. Dis.* **131**:A285.

Ichinose, M., Miura, M., Hataoka, I., Inoue, H., and Takishima, T. (1986). Nonadrenergic bronchodilation in human subjects. *Am. Rev. Respir. Dis.* **133**:A172.

Irvin, C. G., Boileau, R., Tremblay, J., Martin, R. R., and Macklem, P. T. (1980). Bronchodilation: noncholinergic nonadrenergic mediation demonstrated in vivo in the cat. *Science* **207**:791-792.

Irvin, C. G., Martin, R. R., and Macklem, P. T. (1982). Nonpurinergic nature and efficacy of nonadrenergic bronchodilation. *J. Appl. Physiol.* **52**: 562-569.

Ito, Y., and Tajima, K. (1981). Actions of indomethacin and prostaglandins on neuroeffector transmission in the dog trachea. *J. Physiol.* (*London*) **319**:379-392.

Ito, Y., and Takeda, K. (1982). Non-adrenergic inhibitory nerves and putative transmitters in the smooth muscle of cat trachea. *J. Physiol.* (*London*) **330**:497-511.

Jones, T. R., Lefcoe, N. M., and Hamilton, J. T. (1980). Studies of the action of nicotine in guinea-pig tracheal smooth muscle: interaction with β-adrenoceptor antagonists. *Eur. J. Pharmacol.* **67**:53-64.

Kalenberg, S., and Satchell, D. G. (1979). The inhibitory innervation of the guinea-pig trachea: a study of its adrenergic and non-adrenergic components. *Clin. Exp. Pharmacol. Physiol.* **6**:549-559.

Kamikawa, Y., and Shimo, Y. (1976). Pharmacological differences of non-adrenergic inhibitory response and of ATP-induced relaxation in guinea-pig tracheal strip-chains. *J. Pharm. Pharmacol.* **28**:854-855.

Kannan, M. S., and Daniel, E. E. (1980). Structural and functional study of control of canine tracheal smooth muscle. *Am. J. Physiol.* **238**:C27-C33.

Kao, C. Y. (1972). Pharmacology of tetrodotoxin and saxitoxin. *Fed. Proc.* **31**:1117-1123.

Karlsson, J.-A., and Persson, C. G. A. (1984). Neither vasoactive intestinal peptide (VIP) nor purine derivatives may mediate non-adrenergic tracheal inhibition. *Acta Physiol. Scand.* **122**:589-598.

Katz, B., and Miledi, R. (1969). Tetrodotoxin-resistant electrical activity in presynaptic-terminals. *J. Physiol.* (*London*) **203**:459-487.

Kaufman, M. P., and Rybicki, K. J. (1984). Muscular contraction reflexly relaxes tracheal smooth muscle in dogs. *Respir. Physiol.* **56**:61-72.

Knight, D. S., Hyman, A. L., and Kadowitz, P. J. (1981). Innervation of intrapulmonary airway smooth muscle of the dog, monkey and baboon. *J. Autonom. Nerv. Syst.* **3**:31-43.

Komori, S., and Ohashi, H. (1984). Presynaptic, muscarinic inhibition of non-adrenergic, non-cholinergic neuromuscular transmission in the chick rectum. *Br. J. Pharmacol.* **82**:73-84.

Krell, R. D., McCoy, J. L., and Ridley, P. T. (1981). Pharmacological characterization of the excitatory innervation to the guinea pig urinary bladder in vitro: evidence for both cholinergic and nonadrenergic noncholinergic neurotransmission. *Br. J. Pharmacol.* **74**:15-22.

Leff, A. R., Munoz, N. M., and Hendrix, S. (1982). Sympathetic inhibition of histamine-induced contraction of canine trachealis in vivo. *J. Appl. Physiol.* **53**:21-29.

Leff, A. R., Munoz, N. M., Tallet, J., David, A. C., Cavigelli, M. A., and Garrity, E. R. (1985). Autonomic response characteristics of porcine airway smooth muscle in vivo. *J. Appl. Physiol.* **58**:1176-1188.

Löfdahl, C.-G., Lothwall, J., Svedmyr, N., and Skoogh, B.-E. (1986). Frequency-response and current-response characteristics for cholinergic, sympathetic and nonadrenergic noncholinergic stimulation of ferret tracheal smooth muscle. *Am. Rev. Respir. Dis.* **133**:A115.

Longhurst, J. C. (1984). Static contraction of hindlimb muscles in cats reflexly relaxes tracheal smooth muscle. *J. Appl. Physiol.* **57**:380-387.

Lundberg, J. M. (1981). Evidence for coexistence of vasoactive intestinal polypeptide (VIP) and acetylcholine in neurons of cat exocrine glands. Morphological, biochemical and functional studies. *Acta Physiol. Scand.* **112** (Suppl. 496):1-57.

Macklem, P. T. (1985). Bronchial hyporesponsiveness. *Chest* **87**:158S-159S.

Martling, C.-R., Anggard, A., and Lundberg, J. M. (1985). Non-cholinergic vasodilation in the tracheobronchial tree of the cat induced by vagal nerve stimulation. *Acta Physiol. Scand.* **125**:343-346.

Matsumoto, N., Inoue, H., Inoue, C., Ishii, M., Fuyuki, T., Ichinose, M., Sasaki, H., and Takishima, T. (1983). The effective site and mutual cooperation of nonadrenergic inhibitory nervous system in feline airways. *Am. Rev. Respir. Dis.* **127**:A239.

Matsumoto, N., Inoue, H., Ichinose, M., Ishii, M., Inoue, C., Sasaki, H., and Takishima, T. (1985). Effective sites by sympathetic beta-adrenergic and vagal nonadrenergic inhibitory stimulation in constricted airways. *Am. Rev. Respir. Dis.* **132**:1113-1117.

Matsuzaki, Y., Hamasaki, Y., and Said, S. I. (1980). Vasoactive intestinal peptide: a possible transmitter of nonadrenergic relaxation of guinea pig airways. *Science* **210**:1252-1253.

Michoud, M.-C., Amyot, R., and Jeanneret-Grosjean, A. (1985). Bronchodilation induced by laryngeal stimulation in humans. *Am. Rev. Respir. Dis.* **131**:A284.

Michoud, M.-C., Amyot, R., Jeanneret-Grosjean, A., and Couture, J. (1986). Reflex bronchodilatation induced by laryngeal stimulation in humans. *Am. Rev. Respir. Dis.* **133**:A173.

Middendorf, W. F., and Russell, J. A. (1980). Innervation of airway smooth muscle in the baboon: evidence for a nonadrenergic inhibitory system. *J. Appl. Physiol.* **48**:947-956.

Morice, A., Unwin, R. J., and Sever, P. S. (1983). Vasoactive intestinal peptide causes bronchodilatation and protects against histamine induced bronchoconstriction in asthmatic subjects. *Lancet* **2**:1225-1227.

Nakanishi, H., Yoshida, H., and Suzuki, T. (1976). Inhibitory effects of prostaglandin E_1 and E_2 on cholinergic transmission in isolated canine tracheal muscle. *Jpn. J. Pharmacol.* **26**:669-674.

Palmer, J. B., Sampson, A. P., and Barnes, P. J. (1985). Cholinergic and non-adrenergic inhibitory responses in bovine airways: distribution and functional association. *Am. Rev. Respir. Dis.* **131**:A283.

Palmer, J. B., Cuss, F. M., and Barnes, P. J. (1986). VIP and PHM and their role in nonadrenergic inhibitory responses in isolated human airways. *J. Appl. Physiol.* **61**:1322-1328.

Peatfield, A. C., and Richardson, P. S. (1983). Evidence for non-cholinergic non-adrenergic nervous control of mucus secretion into the cat trachea. *J. Physiol. (London)* **342**:335-345.

Polak, J. M., and Bloom, S. R. (1982). Regulatory peptides in the respiratory tract of man and other animals. *Exp. Lung Res.* **3**:313-328.

Raffestin, B., Cerrina, J., Boullet, C., Labat, C., Benvenista, J., and Brink, C. (1985). Response and sensitivity of isolated human pulmonary muscle preparations to pharmacological agents. *J. Pharmacol. Exp. Ther.* **233**: 186-194.

Richardson, J. B. (1981). Nonadrenergic inhibitory innervation of the lung. *Lung* **159**:315-322.

Richardson, J., and Béland, J. (1976). Nonadrenergic inhibitory nervous system in human airways. *J. Appl. Physiol.* **41**:764-771.

Richardson, J. B., and Bouchard, T. (1975). Demonstration of a nonadrenergic inhibitory nervous system in the trachea of the guinea pig. *J. Allergy Clin. Immunol.* **56**:473-480.

Richardson, J. B., and Ferguson, C. C. (1979). Neuromuscular structure and function in the airways. *Fed. Proc.* **38**:202-208.

Roberts, J. A., Raeburn, D., Rodgers, I. W., and Thomson, N. C. (1983). Relationship between in vivo airway responsiveness and in vitro smooth muscle sensitivity to methacholine in man. *Thorax* **38**:705-706.

Russell, J. (1980). Noradrenergic inhibitory innervation of canine airways. *J. Appl. Physiol.* **48**:16-22.

Russell, J. A., and Bartlett, S. (1981). Adrenergic neurotransmissions in airways: inhibition by acetylcholine. *J. Appl. Physiol.* **51**:376-383.

Russell, J. A., and Simons, E. J. (1985). Modulation of cholinergic neurotransmission in airways by enkephalin. *J. Appl. Physiol.* **58**:853-858.

Rybicki, K. J., Longhurst, J. C., and Kaufman, M. P. (1983). Stimulation of splanchnic afferents reflexly relaxes tracheal smooth muscle in dogs. *J. Appl. Physiol.* **55**:427-432.

Saga, T., and Said, S. I. (1984). Vasoactive intestinal peptide relaxes human bronchial and pulmonary arterial smooth muscle. *Clin. Res.* **32**:563A.

Said, S. I., Kitamura, S., Yoshida, T., Preskitt, J., and Holder, L. D. (1974). Humoral control of airways. *Ann. N. Y. Acad. Sci.* **221**:103-114.

Said, S. I., Geumei, A., and Hara, N. (1982). Bronchodilator effect of VIP in vivo: protection against bronchoconstriction induced by histamine or prostaglandin $F_{2\alpha}$. In *Vasoactive Intestinal Peptide.* Edited by S. I. Said. New York, Raven Press.

Satchell, D. (1982). Non-adrenergic non-cholinergic nerves in mammalian airways: their function and the role of purines. *Comp. Biochem. Physiol.* **72C**:189-196.

Satchell, D. G. (1984). Adenosine deaminase antagonizes inhibitory responses to adenosine and non-adrenergic, non-cholinergic inhibitory nerve stimulation in isolated preparations of guinea-pig trachea. *Br. J. Pharmacol.* **83**: 323-325.

Sheller, J. R., and Brigham, K. L. (1982). Bronchomotor responses of isolated sheep airways to electrical field stimulation. *J. Appl. Physiol.* **53**:1088-1093.

Silva, D. G., and Ross, G. (1974). Ultrastructural and fluorescence histochemical studies on the innervation of the tracheo bronchial muscle of normal cats and cats treated with 6-hydroxydopamine. *J. Ultrastruct. Res.* **47**: 310-328.

Smith, B. (1970). The neurological lesion in achalasia of the cardia. *Gut* **11**: 388-391.

Souhrada, J. F., and Kivity, S. (1982). The effect of some factors on the inhibitory nervous systems of airway smooth muscle. *Respir. Physiol.* **48**:297-308.

Starke, K. (1981). Presynaptic receptors. *Annu. Rev. Pharmacol. Toxicol.* **21**: 7-30.

Stephens, N. L. (1977). Airways smooth muscle: biophysics, biochemistry and pharmacology. In *Asthma, Physiology, Immunophysiology and Treatment.* Edited by K. F. Austin and L. M. Lichtenstein. New York, Academic Press.

Sterk, P. J., Daniel, E. E., Zamel, N., and Hargreave, F. E. (1985a). Limited bronchoconstriction to methacholine using partial flow-volume curves in nonasthmatic subjects. *Am. Rev. Respir. Dis.* **132**:272-277.

Sterk, P. J., Daniel, E. E., Zamel, N., and Hargreave, F. E. (1985b). Limited maximal airway narrowing in nonasthmatic subjects: role of neural control and prostaglandin release. *Am. Rev. Respir. Dis.* **132**:865-870.

Suzuki, H., Morita, K., and Kuriyama, H. (1976). Innervation and properties of the smooth muscle of the dog trachea. *Jpn. J. Physiol.* **26**:303-320.

Szarek, J. L., Altiere, R. J., and Diamond, L. (1982). Reversal of prostaglandin $F_{2\alpha}$ induced bronchoconstriction by efferent vagal stimulation. *Pharmacologist* **24**:199.

Szarek, J. L., Gillespie, M. N., Altiere, R. J., and Diamond, L. (1986). Reflex activation of the nonadrenergic noncholinergic inhibitory nervous system in feline airways. *Am. Rev. Respir. Dis.* **133**:1159-1162.

Taylor, S. M., Paré, P. D., and Schellenberg, R. R. (1984). Cholinergic and nonadrenergic mechanisms in human and guinea pig airways. *J. Appl. Physiol.* **56**:958-965.

Taylor, S. M., Paré, P. D., Armour, C. L., Hogg, J. C., and Schellenberg, R. R. (1985). Airway reactivity in chronic obstructive pulmonary disease: failure of in vivo methacholine responsiveness to correlate with cholinergic, adrenergic or nonadrenergic responses in vitro. *Am. Rev. Respir. Dis.* **132**: 30-35.

Tomori, Z., and Widdicombe, J. G. (1969). Muscular, bronchomotor and cardiovascular reflexes elicited by mechanical stimulation of the respiratory tract. *J. Physiol. (London)* **200**:25-49.

Trenchard, D. (1983). The non-adrenergic, vagal efferent system to the lung: does it exist, or is it an artefact. *Med. Hypoth.* **12**:297-301.

Venugopalan, C. S., Said, S. I., and Drazen, J. M. (1984). Effect of vasoactive intestinal peptide on vagally mediated tracheal pouch relaxation. *Respir. Physiol.* **56**:205-216.

Vincenc, K. S., Black, J. L., Yan, K., Armour, C. L., Donnelly, P. D., and Woolcock, A. J. (1983). Comparison of in vivo and in vitro responses to histamine in human airways. *Am. Rev. Respir. Dis.* **128**:875-879.

Walters, E. H., O'Byrne, P. M., Fabbri, L. M., Graf, P. D., Holtzmann, M. J., and Nadel, J. A. (1984). Control of neurotransmission by prostaglandins in canine trachealis muscle. *J. Appl. Physiol.* **57**:129-134.

Wasserman, M. A., Griffin, R. L., and Malo, P. E. (1982). Comparative in vitro tracheal relaxant effects of porcine and hen VIP. In *Vasoactive Intestinal Peptide.* Edited by S. I. Said. New York, Raven Press.

Widdicombe, J. G. (1975). Reflex control of airways smooth muscle. *Postgrad. Med. J.* **51**:(Suppl. 7) 36-45.

Widdicombe, J. G. (1981). Nervous receptors in the respiratory tract and lungs. In *Lung Biology in Health and Disease,* Vol. 17: *Regulation of Breathing.* Edited by T. F. Hornbein. New York, Marcel Dekker, Inc.

Woolcock, A. J., Salome, C. M., and Yan, K. (1984). The shape of the dose-response curve to histamine in asthmatic and normal subjects. *Am. Rev. Respir. Dis.* **130**:71-75.

Yip, P., Palombini, B., and Coburn, R. F. (1981). Inhibitory innervation to the guinea pig trachealis muscle. *J. Appl. Physiol.* **50**:374-382.

15

VIP in the Airways

SAMI I. SAID*

University of Oklahoma Health Sciences Center and VA Medical Center
Oklahoma City, Oklahoma

RICHARD D. DEY

West Virginia University Medical Center
Morgantown, West Virginia

The biological (vasodilator) activity of vasoactive intestinal peptide (VIP) was first discovered in the lung (Said, 1967; Said and Mutt, 1969), but its chemical identity and localization in the lung followed its isolation from intestine (Said and Mutt, 1970, 1972; Mutt and Said, 1974).

VIP levels in the lung as a whole are lower than in brain or gut (Said and Rosenberg, 1976), but VIP in the lung is localized in key sites, has potent activities on all major functions, binds to specific receptors, and appears likely to play an important role in physiology and disease.

I. Localization

The principal localization of VIP-containing neurons in the tracheobronchial tree is in the smooth muscle layer, around submucosal mucous and serous glands, and in the walls of pulmonary and bronchial arteries. Immunoreactive VIP is also present in neuronal cell bodies forming microganglia that provide a source of intrinsic innervation of pulmonary structures.

**Present affiliation*: University of Illinois School of Medicine, Chicago, Illinois

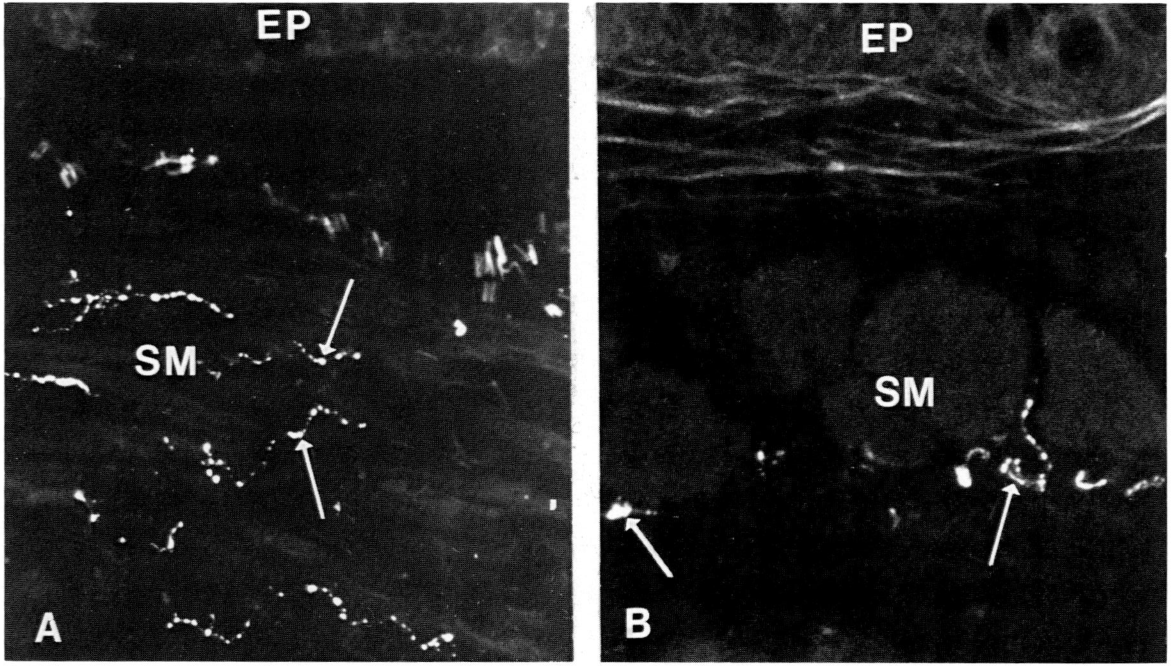

Figure 1 Distribution of VIP-containing nerve fibers in airways from human (A) and canine (B) lung. In human airway, nerve fibers (arrows) penetrate into the smooth muscle layer (SM) and are in close association with small fascicles. In dog airway, nerve fibers (arrows) are located only around the edges of smooth muscle fascicles (SM).

A. Bronchial Smooth Muscle

VIP-containing nerve fibers are found in close association with the smooth muscle layer of airways from the trachea through the small bronchioles. In bronchi from cats and human subjects, VIP-containing nerve fibers come in close contact with and often penetrate into small fascicles of smooth muscle (Fig. 1A). By contrast, VIP innervation in canine bronchial smooth muscle is less extensive, and VIP-containing nerves are distributed predominantly around the periphery of the smooth muscle layer, penetrating only occasionally (Fig. 1B). These species differences may help explain the relatively weak nonadrenergic relaxation observed in canine airways (Russell, 1980).

In a recent ultrastructural immunocytochemical study, VIP-immunoreactivity in the airways was found only in large dense-core vesicles (90-210 nm in diameter) (Laitinen et al., 1985). No VIP-immunoreactivity was observed in terminals containing small agranular vesicles, thought to be cholinergic, or in terminals with small granular vesicles, thought to be adrenergic (Laitinen et al., 1985).

B. Bronchial Glands

The bronchial submucosal glands of cat, dog, and human airways are richly supplied with VIP-containing neurons. In human airways, VIP-containing nerve terminals are closely associated with secretory cells of submucosal gland acini (Fig. 2): the nerves frequently encircle parts of the acinar units and are occasionally observed within the epithelial layer of the gland. No VIP-containing fibers have been observed in the epithelium lining the airways, however.

C. Bronchial Arteries

Like other systemic arteries, bronchial arteries receive a rich supply of VIP-containing nerve fibers, located predominantly at the medial-adventitial junction. The most extensive innervation is seen in the portions of the arteries external to the cartilages, but fibers with VIP-immunoreactivity are also observed along vessels penetrating between cartilaginous plates en route to the bronchial submucosa.

D. Lamina Propria and Epithelium

An extensive network of VIP-containing nerve fibers and nerve terminals is present in the lamina propria (Fig. 3). The close proximity of these fibers and terminals to the epithelial basement membrane explains how VIP released from nerve terminals within the lamina propria could influence epithelial cell function.

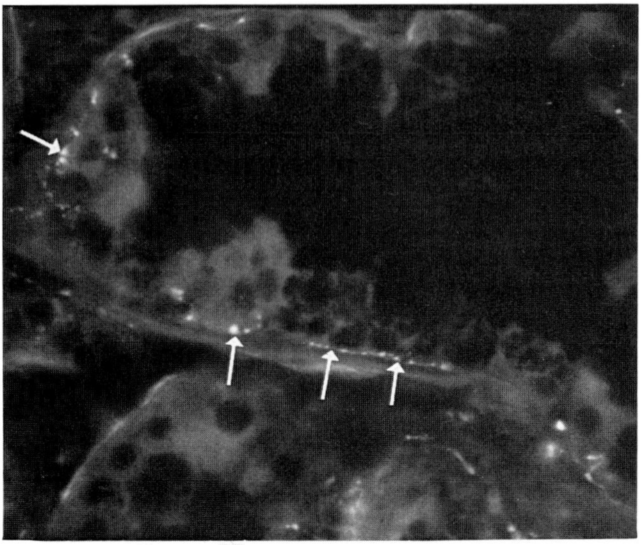

Figure 2 VIP-containing nerve fibers in bronchial submucosal glands from human airway. Nerve fibers (arrows), located in the basal region of the acinar epithelium, are in close association with the secretory cells (X425).

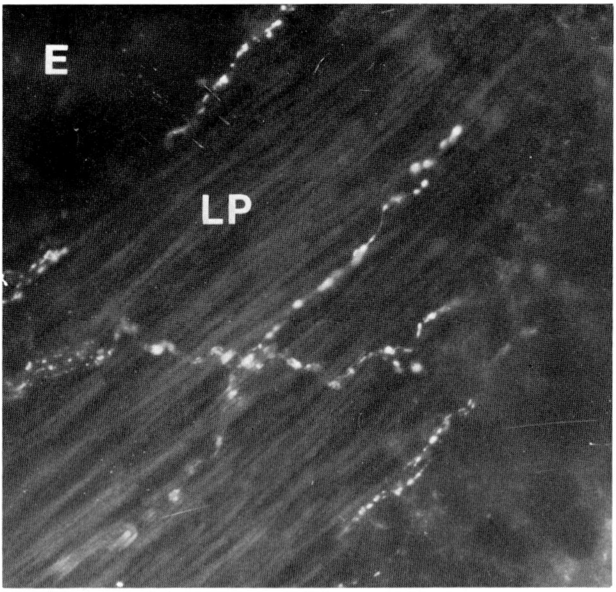

Figure 3 Lamina propria (LP) and bronchial epithelium (E) in an airway from cat lung. An extensive network of VIP-containing fibers is present in the lamina propria but the fibers do not enter the epithelium (X425).

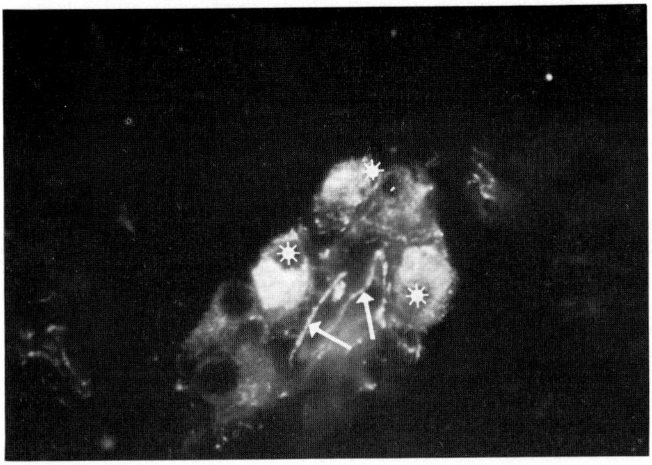

Figure 4 Bronchial ganglion from cat lung. Several of the nerve cell bodies contain intense VIP-like immunoreactivity (*). VIP-containing nerve fibers (arrows) are also present within the ganglion (X 200).

E. Bronchial Ganglia

The airways are innervated from large nerve bundles located external to the cartilages. Collections of nerve cell bodies, forming microganglia, are distributed along these nerve bundles in association with extrapulmonary and larger intrapulmonary bronchi. In lungs of cats, dogs, and humans, many of the nerve cell bodies in the ganglia contain VIP (Fig. 4; Uddman et al., 1978; Uddman and Sundler, 1979; Dey et al., 1981). VIP is also present in verve terminals that contact the nerve cell bodies within the ganglia. Presumably, the nerve fibers supplying the airway smooth muscle, submucosal glands, bronchial arteries, and lamina propria originate from these nerve cell bodies. At least some of these fibers reach the lung through the vagus nerve (Lundberg et al., 1978) and probably originate in the brainstem (Kalia and Mesulam, 1980). The VIP-containing vagal fibers that supply bronchial ganglia could be considered analogous to the preganglionic component of the parasympathetic nervous system, while VIP-containing nerve cell bodies in the bronchial ganglia could be considered postganglionic neurons.

F. Mast Cells

Immunocytochemical and radioimmunologic evidence has been presented for the presence of VIP in murine mast cells and its release with degranulation of these cells (Cutz et al., 1978). The full identity of VIP-like immunoreactivity in mast cells has not been established, however.

II. Colocalization with Other Peptides and Neurotransmitters

The coexistence of peptides and other neurotransmitters in the same neurons is now widely accepted (Lundberg and Hökfelt, 1983). Strong evidence suggests that VIP coexists with acetylcholine in many postganglionic cholinergic neurons supplying exocrine glands and blood vessels. The evidence includes the presence of VIP-immunoreactivity in neurons containing high levels of acetylcholinesterase, and the similarity between the ultrastructural features (especially the diameter of the granular vesicles) of VIP-containing nerve endings and those assumed to be cholinergic (Lundberg et al., 1979, 1980, 1981). As noted by the latter authors, however, acetylcholinesterase may occur in noncholinergic as well as in cholinergic neurons. Confirmation of the cholinergic nature of these neurons, using antisera against choline acetyltransferase, the key enzyme catalyzing acetylcholine synthesis, has been obtained in some sites, including nasal mucosa and submandibular gland (Lundberg et al., 1981; Lundberg and Hökfelt, 1983), but not in others, such as the myenteric or submucosal plexuses in the duodenum (Furness et al., 1984). A recent ultrastructural immunocytochemical study of VIP in the airways (Laitinen et al., 1985) revealed VIP-immunoreactivity in different populations of nerve terminals, some of which were of the "cholinergic type," while others corresponded to the "p-type," containing numerous granular vesicles larger in diameter than those of cholinergic or adrenergic terminals (Baumgarten et al., 1970; Larsson, 1977).

VIP may also be colocalized with other peptides. Using an immunocytochemical technique to colocalize peptides in the same tissue section (Wessendorf and Elde, 1984), we now have evidence that VIP and the undecapeptide substance P (SP) are colocalized in some of the neurons that make up bronchial ganglia (Fig. 5) and also in nerve fibers distributed to bronchial smooth muscle, submucosal glands and the lamina propria (Fig. 6). In general, the number of VIP-containing nerve fibers is greater than SP-containing nerves. While most (possibly all) of the SP-containing fibers also contain VIP, many VIP-containing fibers do not contain SP. Thus, if one assumes that the fibers supplying airway smooth muscle, glands, and lamina propria originate from the intrinsic bronchial ganglia, our findings suggest the presence of two populations of VIP-containing neurons: one containing VIP and the other containing both VIP and SP. Immunocytochemical studies on the ganglia support this conclusion. By contrast, the nerve fibers in airway epithelium contain only SP. These fibers are presumably sensory in nature,

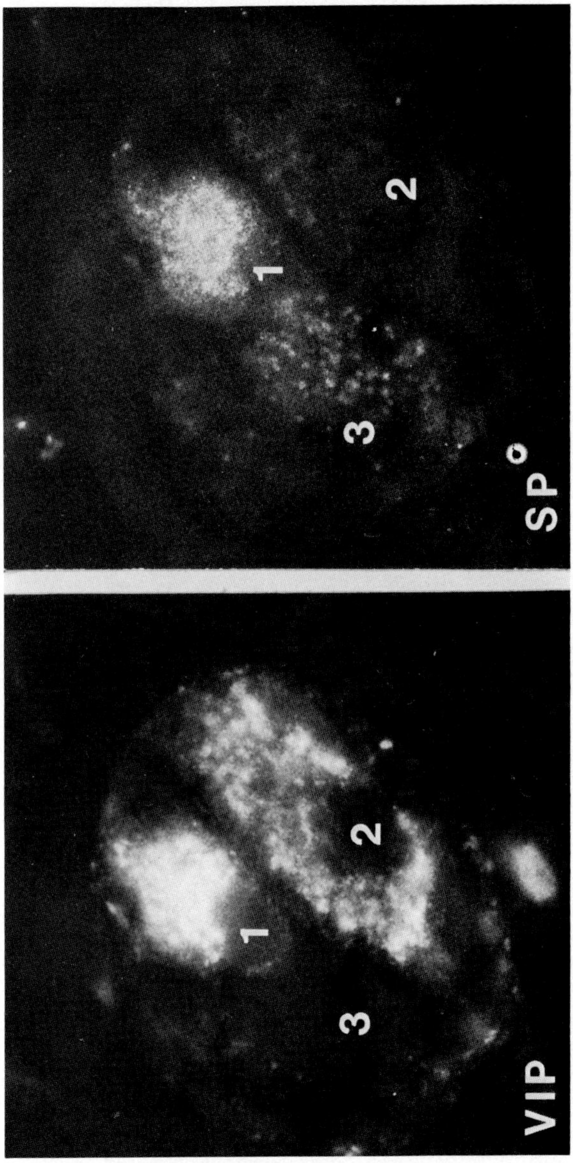

Figure 5 Bronchial ganglion from human lungs showing VIP-like and SP-like immunoreactivity in the same section. One of the nerve cell bodies (1) contains both VIP and SP. A second nerve cell body (2) contains only VIP. A third nerve cell body (3) contains orange autofluorescent pigment, but no VIP- or SP-immunoreactivity (X 1200).

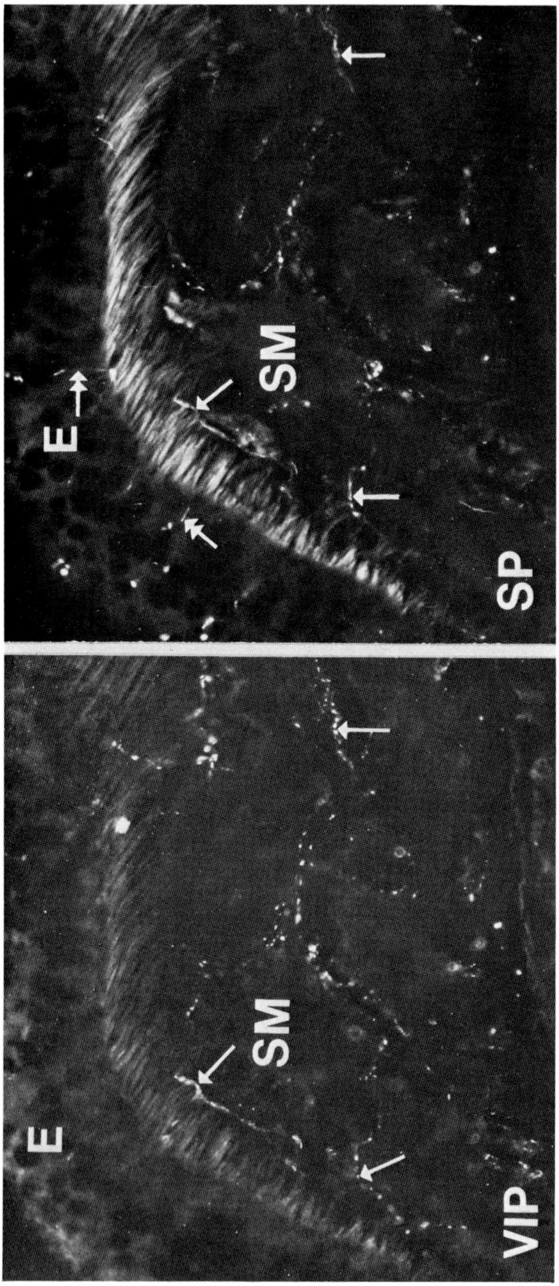

Figure 6 Airway from cat lung showing VIP and SP immunoreactivity in the same section. Several of the nerve fibers (arrows) in the smooth muscle layer (SM) contain both VIP- and SP-like immunoreactivity. On the other hand, only SP-containing nerve fibers (double arrows) are observed in the bronchial epithelium (E) (X 200).

and probably originate from neurons located in the vagal (i.e., nodose) or dorsal root ganglia (Terenghi et al., 1983; Dalsgaard and Lundberg, 1984).

VIP often coexists with a structurally similar peptide, having an N-terminal histidine and a C-terminal isoleucine, called peptide histidine-isoleucine (PHI; Lundberg et al., 1984a; Fahrenkrug et al., 1985). This 27-amino acid residue peptide shows considerable homology (13 identities) to VIP, and both peptides are synthesized from the same precursor molecule (Itoh et al., 1983). The human counterpart of PHI is PHM (peptide histidine methionine), in which the C-terminal residue is methionine instead of isoleucine. In the airways, the distribution of PHI-containing nerve fibers is similar to but less extensive than that of VIP-containing fibers (Lundberg et al., 1984a; Uddman et al., 1985).

III. Actions on Airways

VIP has potent effects on all major structural components of the airways. These actions include those discussed below.

A. Airway Smooth Muscle

In vitro, VIP relaxes isolated tracheal or bronchial segments from guinea pigs, rabbits, dogs, and humans, and prevents or attenuates their contraction by a variety of constrictors, including histamine, $PGF_{2\alpha}$, kallikrein, and leukotriene D_4 (Piper et al., 1970; Said et al., 1974; Wasserman et al., 1982; Ito and Takeda, 1982; Cameron et al., 1983; Hamasaki et al., 1983b). This relaxant action is long-lasting and is unaffected by blockade of adrenergic or cholinergic receptors or of cyclooxygenase activity (Said et al., 1974; Altiere and Diamond, 1984; Hand et al., 1984; Saga and Said, 1984). In vivo, inhaled VIP protects against the bronchoconstriction induced by histamine or prostaglandin $F_{2\alpha}$ in dogs (Said et al., 1982), and by histamine in guinea pigs (Cox et al., 1983). Infused VIP reverses serotonin-induced bronchoconstriction in cats (Diamond et al., 1982). Whether inhaled or infused, VIP has been found to be generally less effective, however, in protecting against asthmatic or histamine-induced bronchoconstriction in human subjects (Morice, 1983; Barnes and Dixon, 1984; Mojarad et al., 1985).

B. Tracheobronchial Secretion

VIP stimulates water and ion transport in canine tracheal epithelium (Nathanson et al., 1983), and stimulates the secretion of sulfated macromolecules by tracheal explants from ferrets (Peatfield et al., 1983) but, paradoxically, inhibits macromolecular secretion in human tracheal explants (Coles et al., 1981).

C. Bronchial and Pulmonary Vessels

VIP dilates the vessels supplying the nose, upper airways (Malm et al., (1980), and trachea and bronchi (Widdicombe, Chap. 8), as well as pulmonary vessels (Hamasaki et al., 1983a; Nandiwada et al., 1985).

D. Immunologic Release of Mediators

VIP has a moderate inhibitory effect on antigen-induced release of histamine from guinea pig lung (Undem et al., 1983).

IV. VIP Receptors in the Airways

Specific receptors for VIP have been identified in membrane preparations of rat, mouse, guinea pig, and human lungs and in human lung tumor cells (Robberecht et al., 1981, Taton et al., 1981).

VIP receptors have been localized immunocytochemically, on the basis of increased cAMP levels, in submucosal serous and mucous glands of the ferret (Lazarus et al., 1983) and in ciliated and basal cells of tracheal epithelium of dog (Lazarus et al., 1983). Use of autoradiographic techniques has confirmed the presence of VIP uptake sites in airways and in alveolar cells (Leroux et al., 1984; Leys et al., 1986). We have found the autoradiographic uptake sites (and, presumably, receptors) of VIP in dog bronchi to be extensively distributed in bronchial epithelium and in bronchial smooth muscle (Table 1).

The binding of VIP to airway sites, as to receptors in other cells and tissues, is coupled to an adenylate cyclase (Amiranoff and Rosselin, 1982). The resultant increase in cyclic AMP levels (Frandsen et al., 1978; Kitamura et al., 1980; Robberecht et al., 1981; Lazarus et al., 1983) probably mediates the biological effects of the peptide.

VIP receptors in the lung have recently been solubilized and partially characterized (Paul and Said, 1986).

V. Release

Immunoreactive VIP is released from isolated guinea pig trachea with transmural (electrical field) stimulation (Matsuzaki et al., 1980). This release is associated with and proportional to tracheal relaxation (Matsuzaki et al., 1980). Both the relaxation and the release are abolished by the neurotoxin tetrodotoxin, but not by adrenergic or cholinergic blockade (Matsuzaki et al., 1980). The airway relaxation is also markedly attenuated by incubation of the tracheal segments with anti-VIP antibodies prior to the transmural stimulation (Matsuzaki et al., (1980).

Table 1 Receptor Binding of ^{125}I-Labeled VIP (25 pmol) to Airway Epithelium and Bronchial Smooth Muscle in Cryostat Sections of Dog Airways

	Binding			
	Total	Specific	Nonspecific	% Specific
Epithelium	554	483	116	79
Smooth muscle	228	143	115	55

Binding, expressed as grains/10 μm^2, was calculated by counting silver grains in autoradiographs.

This VIP release is thus of neural origin and is probably related to the airway relaxation induced by the field stimulation.

VI. Interactions Between VIP and Other Neurotransmitters

Multiple interactions have been demonstrated between VIP and other neurotransmitters. Although most of these interactions have been described in other tissues, many are probably applicable also to the airways. Examples of such interactions include the following.

1. As discussed above, VIP coexists with PHI (or PHM) and, in many neurons, also with acetylcholine (Lundberg et al., 1979, 1981, 1984a,b; Lundberg, 1981; Eckenstein and Baughman, 1984; Pruss et al., 1985). VIP also coexists with substance P in some neurons within the lung.
2. VIP stimulates the release of acetylcholine from myenteric neurons (Yau et al., 1985).
3. VIP release is stimulated by cholinergic agonists (Bitar et et al., 1980; Wang et al., 1986), by pretreatment with atropine (Hedlund et al., 1983), and by dopaminergic agonists (Uvnäs-Moberg et al., 1982), GABA antagonists (Wang et al., 1986), and opiate antagonists (Wang et al., 1986).
4. VIP enhances the affinity of acetylcholine for muscarinic receptors, acetylcholine-induced secretion of saliva (Lundberg et al., 1980), and cholinergic transmission in ganglionic synapses (Kawatani et al., 1965).
5. VIP acts synergistically with norepinephrine to stimulate cAMP production in cerebral cortex (Magistretti and Schorderet, 1984, 1986), and with ATP to relax gastric smooth muscle (Bitar and Makhlouf, 1982).

VII. Physiological Roles in the Lung

The presence of VIP in key locations in the lung and its binding to specific receptors that mediate its potent biological effects strongly suggest physiological regulatory roles for this peptide in the lung. VIP may well be a transmitter of the nonadrenergic, noncholinergic component of the autonomic nervous system (Matsuzaki et al., 1980; Barnes and Palmer, 1986). Activities controlled by this system include major components of relaxation of airways and pulmonary vessels, and of bronchial H_2O, ion, and macromolecular secretion. In addition, VIP may modulate the release (and actions) of mast cell mediators of inflammation (Undem et al., 1983).

The view that VIP is the likely transmitter of nonadrenergic relaxation of airway smooth muscle is supported by the following findings.

1. VIP fulfills many of the criteria of a neurotransmitter.
2. VIP is present in the vagus nerve (Lundberg et al., 1978), whose electrical stimulation after cholinergic and adrenergic blockade leads to bronchodilation.
3. VIP mimics the electrophysiological changes in airway smooth muscle produced by nonadrenergic, noncholinergic nerve stimulation (Ito and Takeda, 1982; Cameron et al., 1983; Karlsson and Persson, 1984).
4. Prolonged incubation of airway smooth muscle with VIP reduces subsequent relaxation by VIP (tachyphylaxis), and also reduces the magnitude of nonadrenergic, noncholinergic relaxation in cats (Ito and Takeda, 1982) and in guinea pigs (Venugopalan et al., 1984).
5. VIP is released on transmural stimulation of guinea pig tracheal segments, in the presence of adrenergic and muscarinic cholinergic receptor blockade, and the release is in direct proportion to the relaxation of these segments (Matsuzaki et al., 1980).
6. This release, along with the associated relaxation, is markedly inhibited by blockade of neurotransmission (Matsuzaki et al., 1980).
7. The relaxation is also greatly reduced by preincubation of the tracheal segments with a specific VIP-antiserum (Matsuzaki et al., 1980).

Certain experimental observations, on the other hand, have been cited against a transmitter role for VIP in nonadrenergic airway relaxation. As noted below, these are not inconsistent with that conclusion, however.

1. Immunoreactive VIP is present in the canine tracheobronchial tree, but the nonadrenergic relaxant system is weak or absent in this species (Russell, 1980). This apparent discrepancy may be explained by the less intimate anatomical relationship between VIP-containing nerves

and airway smooth muscle in dog airways, compared to those of cats or humans (see discussion of localization, above).

2. Guinea pig tracheas that had been fully relaxed by application of VIP could be further relaxed with transmural (electrical field) stimulation (Karlsson and Persson, 1984). This additional relaxation could be due to the release of other relaxant peptides, such as PHI (or PHM), from nerve terminals in the airways. Additionally, electrical field stimulation may, under certain conditions, induce direct (myogenic) relaxation, even after blockade of neurotransmission (Coburn and Tomita, 1973).
3. The proteolytic enzyme α-chymotrypsin, which hydrolyzes VIP in vitro, did not inhibit relaxation induced by electrical field stimulation (Diamond and Altiere, Chap. 14). The negative result with the large-molecular-size enzyme may be explained by its failure to reach the sites of VIP release in sufficient concentrations to degrade the peptide.
4. Human airways exhibit a major component of nonadrenergic relaxation, but human asthmatics, at least in some studies, respond relatively weakly to VIP. The weaker than expected airway relaxation of human asthmatics to inhaled VIP may be attributed to inadequate access of the biologically active peptide to its receptors on airway smooth muscle (due to adsorption on mucus and other secretions, inactivation by airway proteases, or reduced number or affinity of receptors). In support of this explanation, VIP effectively relaxes isolated strips of human bronchi in vitro (Saga and Said, 1984).

VIII. VIP in Relation to Lung Disease

On the basis of experimental and clinical observations, we presented the hypothesis several years ago that a deficiency of VIP (or its biological activity, or receptors) may be present in and contribute to the pathogenesis of two major diseases of the airways and lungs: cystic fibrosis and bronchial asthma (Matsuzaki et al., 1980; Said, 1982).

A. Cystic Fibrosis

The notion that cystic fibrosis may be causally related to a deficiency of VIP is based on the following rationale: (1) VIP-containing nerves richly supply all exocrine organs (Lundberg et al., 1979), the principal organs affected in this disorder; (2) VIP influences all major exocrine function, stimulating water, Cl^-, or HCO_3^- secretion, and macromolecular secretion, and promoting blood flow; (3) VIP binds to specific receptors on exocrine glands, including salivary and sweat glands, bronchial glands, and exocrine pancreas (Amiranoff and Rosselin, 1982). Examined against some of the manifestations of cystic fibrosis, notably the decreased Cl^- permeability in sweat gland ducts (Quinton and Bijman, 1983), the effects of VIP, especially its stimulation of Cl^- secretion, are consistent with the possibility that VIP deficiency may help explain these manifestations.

This hypothesis has recently received support from comparisons of VIP innervation of sweat glands in patients with cystic fibrosis and in normal subjects. Normal sweat glands are well supplied by VIP-immunoreactive nerves, which innervate both the acini and the ducts. In cystic fibrosis patients, however, VIP innervation is significantly decreased around sweat gland acini, and is virtually absent around the ducts (Heinz-Erian et al., 1985).

B. Bronchial Asthma

A similar hypothesis has been proposed, linking the pathogenesis of bronchial asthma to a possible lack of VIP innervation of airway smooth muscle. This proposed link is based on (1) the evidence presented above that VIP may be the transmitter of nonadrenergic relaxation of airways; (2) the dominant, if not exclusive, role of this relaxant system in human airways (Richardson and Beland, 1976); and (3) the speculation that a lack of nonadrenergic relaxation could explain the airway hyperreactivity of bronchial asthma (Richardson, 1979; Matsuzaki et al., 1980).

IX. VIP in the Treatment of Airway Disease

Extensive data from experiments on isolated airway segments in vitro and on anesthetized and unanesthetized animals show that VIP can potently and effectively relax tracheobronchial smooth muscle and prevent or reduce the effect of bronchoconstrictor agents, including histamine, prostaglandin $F_{2\alpha}$ and leukotriene D_4 (Said et al., 1974, 1982; Wasserman et al., 1982; Cox et al., 1983; Hamasaki et al., 1983b). In addition to relaxing airway smooth muscle, VIP also inhibits the immunologic release of mediators from lung slices (Undem et al., 1983).

These properties of VIP, along with its normal presence in the airways as a neuropeptide in close proximity to smooth muscle, bronchial glands, and epithelium, and the presence of specific receptors for it on these sites, make it an excellent candidate as a therapeutic agent in patients with bronchial asthma. Results of several trials to date of VIP in asthma, either as an aerosol or by intravenous infusion, have been only moderately favorable (Morice, 1983; Mojarad et al., 1985) or even less successful (Altiere and Diamond, 1984).

Why has VIP been less effective in human asthmatics than in experimental animals or in vitro? Possible explanations include the inability of aerosolized VIP to reach its airway smooth muscle receptors in sufficient concentrations; degradation or inactivation of the peptide by proteolytic enzymes in bronchial secretions or in bronchial epithelium; and altered responsiveness of asthmatic airways.

Acknowledgments

This work was supported by NIH Research Grants HL-30450, HL-31039, and HL-35656, and by research funds from the Veterans Administration and from the Sarkeys Foundation. The authors thank Brenda Hansel for her expert help with preparation of the manuscript.

Discussion

Barnes. We have not found bronchodilatation after inhalation of VIP in mildly asthmatic subjects (Barnes and Dixon, *Am. Rev. Respir. Dis.* **130**:162-166, 1984), nor when VIP is infused to maximally tolerated doses in normal subjects (who bronchodilate with isoproterenol) (Palmer et al., *Thorax* in press, 1986). This may indicate a problem in access of VIP to receptors in airway smooth muscle because of degradation, diffusion problems, or limitation of dose by cardiovascular effects.

Said. It is possible that an inadequate dose was given by aerosol or that conditions in the asthmatic airway are not as favorable. Using large doses (5-10 μg/kg), we found that at least some asthmatic patients responded to inhaled VIP.

Widdicombe. VIP is a very potent tracheal vasodilator, so it is possible that VIP aerosols may dilate the airway vasculature so that subsequent challenge with bronchoconstrictors, such as histamine, might be less effective because they are more efficiently carried away in the submucosal bloodstream.

Said. Although this is possible, it has been shown in vitro that VIP protects against bronchoconstriction in isolated airway segments devoid of blood supply.

Davis. Does VIP stimulate chloride secretion in sweat ducts?

Said. Sato (personal communication) has found that VIP stimulates sweat secretion in isolated human sweat glands.

Burnstock. Recently we found that VIP release in gut is not calcium-dependent, suggesting that its mechanism of release may be different from that of classic neurotransmitters.

Said. The calcium-dependence of VIP release has been demonstrated in synaptosomes from various parts of the brain (Giachetti et al., *Proc. Natl. Acad. Sci.* **74**: 3424, 1977).

Skoogh. Is VIP present in preganglionic nerve terminals in addition to neuronal bodies in lung?

Said. Probably, because VIP immunoreactivity is found in the vagus nerve.

Barnes. In our in vitro studies VIP is more potent as a relaxant of pulmonary vessels than of airway smooth muscle. Autoradiographic studies show a higher density of VIP-receptors in vascular than in airway smooth muscle (Barnes and Carstairs, *Br. J. Pharmacol.* 87:174, 1986). This may indicate that VIP is more important in regulating bronchial blood flow than airway tone.

Said. In our studies of isolated human bronchi, pulmonary artery, and lung parenchyma, we have found that VIP relaxes bronchial and pulmonary vascular smooth muscle with nearly equal potency, but the *duration* of relaxation was more prolonged in vessels than bronchi. VIP was less potent on lung parenchyma.

References

Altiere, R. J., and Diamond, L. (1984). Comparison of vasoactive intestinal peptide and isoproterenol relaxant effects in isolated cat airways. *J. Appl. Physiol.* **56**:986.

Altiere, R. J., Küng, M., and Diamond, L. (1984). Comparative effects of inhaled isoproterenol and vasoactive intestinal peptide on histamine-induced bronchoconstriction in human subjects. *Chest* **86**:153-154.

Amiranoff, B., and Rosselin, G. (1982). VIP receptors and control of cyclic AMP production. In *Vasoactive Intestinal Peptide.* Edited by S. I. Said. New York, Raven Press, pp. 307-322.

Barnes, P. J., and Dixon, C. M. S. (1984). The effect of inhaled vasoactive intestinal peptide on bronchial reactivity to histamine in humans. *Am. Rev. Respir. Dis.* **130**:162-166.

Barnes, P. J., and Palmer, J. B. D. (1986). Non-adrenergic bronchodilatation. *Clin. Respir. Physiol.* **22**(7):153-161.

Baumgarten, H. G., Holstein, A. F., and Owman, C. (1970). Auerbachs plexus of mammals and man: electron microscopic identification of three different types of neuronal processes in myenteric ganglia of the large intestine from rhesus monkeys, guinea-pigs and man. *J. Zellforsch.* **106**:376-397.

Bitar, K. N., and Makhlouf, G. M. (1982). Relaxation of isolated gastric smooth muscle cells by vasoactive intestinal peptide. *Science* **216**:531-533.

Bitar, K. N., Said, S. I., Weir, G. C., Saffouri, B., and Makhlouf, G. M. (1980). Neural release of vasoactive intestinal peptide from the gut. *Gastroenterology* **79**:1288-1294.

Cameron, A. C., Johnson, C. F., Kirkpatrick, C. T., and Kirkpatrick, M. C. A. (1983). The quest for the inhibitory neurotransmitter in bovine tracheal smooth muscle. *Q. J. Exp. Physiol.* **68**:413-426.

Coburn, R. F., and Tomita, T. (1973). Evidence for nonadrenergic inhibitory nerves in guinea pig trachealis muscle. *Am. J. Physiol.* **224**:1072-1080.

Coles, S. J., Said, S. I., and Reid, L. M. (1981). Inhibition by vasoactive intestinal peptide of glycoconjugate and lysozyme secretion by human airways in vitro. *Am. Rev. Respir. Dis.* **124**:531-536.

Cox, C. P., Lerner, M. R., Wells, J. J., and Said, S. I. (1983). Inhaled vasoactive intestinal peptide (VIP) prevents bronchoconstriction induced by inhaled histamine. *Am. Rev. Respir. Dis.* **127**:249.

Cutz, E., Chan, W., Track, N. S., Goth, A., and Said, S. I. (1978). Release of vasoactive intestinal polypeptide in mast cells by histamine liberators. *Nature* **275**:661-662.

Dalsgaard, S.-J., and Lundberg, J. M. (1984). Evidence for a spinal afferent innervation of the guinea pig respiratory tract as studied by the horseradish peroxidase techniques. *Neurosci. Letts.* **45**:117-122.

Dey, R. D., Shannon, W. A., and Said, S. I. (1981). Localization of VIP-immunoreactive nerves in airways and pulmonary vessels of dogs, cats and human subjects. *Cell Tissue Res.* **220**:231-238.

Diamond, L., Szarek, J. L., Gillespie, M. N., and Altiere, R. J. (1983). In vivo bronchodilator activity of vasoactive intestinal peptide in the cat. *Am. Rev. Respir. Dis.* **128**:827-832.

Eckenstein, F., and Baughman, R. W. (1984). Two types of cholinergic innervation in cortex, one co-localized with vasoactive intestinal polypeptide. *Nature* **309**:153-155.

Fahrenkrug, J., Bek, T., Lundberg, J. M., and Hökfelt, T. (1985). VIP and PHI in cat neurons: co-localization but variable tissue content possible due to differential processing. *Regul. Peptides* **12**:21-34.

Frandsen, E. K., Krishna, G. A., and Said, S. I. (1978). Vasoactive intestinal polypeptide promotes cyclic adenosine 3′, 5′-monophosphate accumulation in guinea pig trachea. *Br. J. Pharmacol.* **62**:367-369.

Furness, J. B., Costa, M., and Keast, J. R. (1984). Choline acetyltransferase- and peptide-immunoreactivity of submucosal neurons in the small intestine of guinea pig. *Cell Tissue Res.* **237**:329-336.

Hamasaki, Y., Mojarad, M., and Said, S. I. (1983a). Relaxant action of VIP on cat pulmonary artery: comparison with acetylcholine, isoproterenol and prostaglandin E_1. *J. Appl. Physiol.* **54**:1607.

Hamasaki, Y., Saga, T., Mojarad, M., and Said, S. I. (1983b). VIP counteracts leukotriene D_4-induced contractions of guinea pig trachea, lung and pulmonary artery. *Trans. Assoc. Am. Physicians* **96**:406-411.

Hand, J. M., Laravuso, R. B., and Will, J. A. (1984). Relaxation of isolated guinea pig trachea, bronchi and pulmonary arteries produced by vasoactive intestinal peptide (VIP). *Eur. J. Pharmacol.* **98**:279-284.

Hedlund, B., Abens, J., and Bartfai, T. (1983). Vasoactive intestinal polypeptide and muscarinic receptors: supersensitivity induced by long-term atropine treatment. *Science* **220**:519-521.

Heinz-Erian, P., Dey, R. D., and Said, S. I. (1985). Deficient vasoactive intestinal peptide innervation in sweat glands of cystic fibrosis patients. *Science* **229**:1407-1408.

Ito, Y., and Takeda, K. (1982). Non-adrenergic inhibitory nerves and putative transmitters in the smooth muscle of cat trachea. *J. Physiol.* **330**:497-511.

Itoh, N., Obata, K., Yanaihara, N., and Okamoto, H. (1983). Human prepro-vasoactive intestinal polypeptide contains a novel PHI-27-like peptide, PHM-27. *Nature* **304**:547-743.

Kalia, M., and Mesulam, M.-M. (1980). Brain stem projections of sensory and motor-components in the vagus complex in the cat: II. Laryngeal, tracheobronchial, pulmonary, cardiac, and gastrointestinal branches. *J. Comp. Neurol.* **193**:467-508.

Karlsson, J.-A., and Persson, C. G. A. (1984). Neither vasoactive intestinal peptide (VIP) nor purine derivatives may mediate nonadrenergic tracheal inhibition. *Acta Physiol. Scand.* **122**:589-598.

Kawatani, M., Rutigliano, M., and De Groat, W. C. (1985). Depolarization and muscarinic excitation induced in a sympathetic ganglion by vasoactive intestinal polypeptide. *Science* **229**:879-881.

Kitamura, S., Ishihara, Y., and Said, S. I. (1980). Effect of VIP, phenoxybenzamine and prednisolone on cyclic nucleotide content of isolated guinea-pig lung and trachea. *Eur. J. Pharmacol.* **67**:219-223.

Laitinen, A., Partanen, M., Hervonen, A., Pelto-Huikko, M., and Laitinen, L. A. (1985). VIP-like immunoreactive nerves in human respiratory tract. *Histochemistry* **82**:313-319.

Larsson, L. I. (1977). Ultrastructural localization of a new neuronal peptide (VIP). *Histochemistry* **54**:173-176.

Lazarus, S. C., Basbaum, C. B., Barnes, P. J., and Gold, W. M. (1983). Mapping of VIP receptors using cAMP immunocytochemistry. *Am. Rev. Respir. Dis.* **127**:274A.

Leroux, P., Vaudry, H., Fournier, A., St.-Pierre, S., and Pelletier, G. (1984). Characterization and localization of vasoactive intestinal peptide receptors in the rat lung. *Endocrinology* **114**:1506-1512.

Leys, K., Morice, A., Hughes, A., Schachter, M., and Sever, P. (1986). Autoradiographic visualisation of VIP receptors in human lung. *Thorax* **41**: 242.

Lundberg, J. M. (1981). Evidence for co-existence of vasoactive intestinal polypeptide (VIP) and acetylcholine in neurons of cat exocrine glands. *Acta Physiol. Scand.* (*Suppl.*) **496**:1-57.

Lundberg, J. M., and Hökfelt, T. (1983). Coexistence of peptides and classical neurotransmitters. *Trends Neurosci.* **6**(8):325-333.

Lundberg, J. M., Hökfelt, T., Nilsson, G., Terenius, L., Rehfeld, J., Elde, R., and Said, S. (1978). Peptide neurons in the vagus, splanchnic, and sciatic nerves. *Acta Physiol. Scand.* **104**:499-501.

Lundberg, J. M., Hökfelt, T., Schultberg, M., Uvnäs-Wallensten, K., Kohler, C., and Said, S. I. (1979). Occurrence of VIP-like immunoreactivity in certain cholinergic neurons of the cat: evidence from combined immunohistochemistry and acetylcholinesterase staining. *Neuroscience* **4**:1539-1559.

Lundberg, J. M., Änggård, A., Fahrenkrug, J., Hökfelt, T., and Mutt, V. (1980). Vasoactive intestinal polypeptide in cholinergic neurons of exocrine glands: functional significance of co-existing transmitters for vasodilation and secretion. *Proc. Natl. Acad. Sci.* **77**:1651-1655.

Lundberg, J. M., Änggård, A., Emson, P., Fahrenkrug, J., and Hökfelt, T. (1981). VIP and cholinergic mechanisms in cat nasal mucosa: studies on choline acetyltransferase and release of vasoactive intestinal peptide. *Proc. Natl. Acad. Sci.* **78**:5255-5259.

Lundberg, J. M., Fahrenkrug, J., Hökfelt, T., Martling, C.-R., Larsson, O., Tatemoto, K., and Änggård, A. (1984a). Coexistence of peptide HI(PHI) and VIP in nerves regulating blood flow and bronchial smooth muscle tone in various mammals including man. *Peptides* **5**:593-606.

Lundberg, J. M., Fahrenkrug, J., Larsson, O., and Änggård, A. (1984b). Co-release of vasoactive intestinal polypeptide and peptide histidine isoleucine in relation to atropine-resistant vasocilation in cat submandibular salivary gland. *Neurosci. Lett.* **52**:37-42.

Magistretti, P. J., and Schorderet, M. (1984). VIP and noradrenaline act synergistically to increase cyclic-AMP in cerebral cortex. *Nature* **308**:208-282.

Magistretti, P. J., and Schorderet, M. (1985). Norepinephrine and histamine potentiate the increases in cyclic adenosine 3′:5′-monophosphate elicited by vasoactive intestinal polypeptide in mouse cerebral cortical slices: mediation by α_1-adrenergic and H_1-histaminergic receptors. *J. Neurosci.* **5**:362-368.

Malm, L., Sundler, F., and Uddman, R. (1980). Effects of vasoactive intestinal polypeptide (VIP) on resistance and capacitance vessels in the nasal mucosa. *Acta Otolaryngol.* (*Stockh.*) **90**:304-308.

Matsuzaki, Y., Hamasaki, Y., and Said, S. I. (1980). Vasoactive intestinal peptide: a possible transmitter of non-adrenergic relaxation of guinea pig airways. *Science* **210**:1252-1253.

Mojarad, M., Grode, T. L., Cox, C. P., Kimmel, G., and Said, S. I. (1985). Differential responses of human asthmatics to inhaled vasoactive intestinal peptide (VIP). *Am. Rev. Respir. Dis.* **131**:281A.

Morice, A. (1983). Vasoactive intestinal peptide causes bronchodilation and protects against bronchoconstriction in asthmatic subjects. *Lancet* **2**:1225-1227.

Mutt, V., and Said, S. I. (1974). Structure of the porcine vasoactive intestinal octacosapeptide: the amino-acid sequence. Use of kallikrein in its determination. *Eur. J. Biochem.* **42**:581-589.

Nandiwada, P. A., Kadowitz, P. J., Said, S. I., Mojarad, M., and Hyman, A. L. (1985). Pulmonary vasodilator responses to vasoactive intestinal peptide in the cat. *J. Appl. Physiol.* **58**(3):1723-1728.

Nathanson, I., Widdicombe, J. H., and Barnes, P. J. (1983). Effect of vasoactive intestinal peptide on ion transport across dog tracheal epithelium. *J. Appl. Physiol.* **55**:1844-1848.

Paul, S., and Said, S. I. (1986). Solubilization of active receptors for VIP from guinea pig lung. *Peptides* **7**(1)(Suppl):147-149.

Peatfield, A. C., Barnes, P. J., Bratcher, C., Nadel, J. A., and Davis, B. (1983). Vasoactive intestinal peptide stimulates tracheal submucosal gland secretion in ferret. *Am. Rev. Respir. Dis.* **128**:89-93.

Piper, P. J., Said, S. I., and Vane, J. R. (1970). Effects on smooth muscle preparations of unidentified vasoactive peptides from intestine and lung. *Nature* **225**:1144-1146.

Pruss, R. M., Moskal, J. R., Eiden, L. E., and Beinfeld, M. C. (1985). Specific regulation of vasoactive intestinal polypeptide biosynthesis by phorbol ester in bovine chromaffin cells. *Endocrinology* **117**:1020-1026.

Quinton, P. M., and Bijman, J. (1983). Higher bioelectrical potentials due to decreased chloride absorption in the sweat glands of patients with cystic fibrosis. *N. Engl. J. Med.* **308**:1185-1189.

Richardson, J. B. (1979). Nerve supply to the lungs. *Am. Rev. Respir. Dis.* **119**:785-802.

Richardson, J., and Beland, J. (1976). Nonadrenergic inhibitory nervous system in human airways. *J. Appl. Physiol.* **41**(5):764-771.

Robberecht, P., Chatelain, P., De Neef, P., Camus, J.-C., Waelbroeck, M., and Christophe, J. (1981). Presence of vasoactive intestinal peptide receptors coupled to adenylate cyclase in rat lung membrane. *Biochem. Biophys. Acta* **678**:76-82.

Russell, J. A. (1980). Nonadrenergic inhibitory innervation canine airways. *J. Appl. Physiol.* **48**:16-22.

Saga, T., and Said, S. I. (1984). Vasoactive intestinal peptide relaxes isolated strips of human bronchus, pulmonary artery, and lung parenchyma. *Trans. Assoc. Am. Physicians* **97**:304-310.

Said, S. I. (1967). Vasoactive substances in the lung. In Proceedings of the Tenth Aspen Emphysema Conference, Aspen, Colorado, June 7-10, 1967, U.S. Public Health Serv. Publication 1787, 223-228.

Said, S. I. (1982). Vasoactive intestinal peptide (VIP) and the lung. In *Systemic Role of Regulatory Peptides.* Edited by S. R. Bloom, J. M. Polak, and E. Lindenlaub. New York, Stuttgart, F. K. Schattauer, pp. 293-300.

Said, S. I., and Mutt, V. (1969). Long acting vasodilator peptide from lung tissue. *Nature* **224**:699-700.

Said, S. I., and Mutt, V. (1970). Polypeptide with broad biological activity: isolation from small intestine. *Science* **169**:1217-1218.

Said, S. I., and Mutt, V. (1972). Isolation from porcine intestinal wall of a vasoactive octacosapeptide related to secretin and to glucagon. *Eur. J. Biochem.* **28**:199-204.

Said, S. I., and Rosenberg, R. N. (1976). Vasoactive intestinal polypeptide: abundant immunoreactivity in neural cell lines and normal nervous tissues. *Science* **192**:907-908.

Said, S. I., Kitamura, S., Yoshida, T., Preskitt, J., and Holden, L. D. (1974). Humoral control of airways. *Ann. NY Acad. Sci.* **221**:103-114.

Said, S. I., Geumei, A., and Hara, N. (1982). Bronchodilator effect of VIP in vivo: protection against bronchoconstriction induced by histamine or prostaglandin $F_{2\alpha}$. In *Vasoactive Intestinal Peptide.* Edited by S. I. Said. New York, Raven Press, pp. 185-191.

Taton, G., Delhaye, M., Camus, J.-C., De Neef, P., Chatelain, P., Robberecht, P., and Christophe, J. (1981). Characterization of the VIP-and secretin-stimulated adenylate cyclase system from human lung. *Pflugers Arch.* **391**:178-182.

Terenghi, G., McGregor, G. P., Bhuttacharji, S., Wharton, J., Bloom, S. R., and Polak, J. M. (1983). Vagal origin of substance P-containing nerves in the guinea pig lung. *Neurosci. Letts.* **36**:229-236.

Uddman, R., and Sundler, F. (1979). VIP nerves in human upper respiratory tract. *Otorhinolaryngology* **41**:221-226.

Uddman, R., Alumets, J., Densert, O., Håkanson, R., and Sundler, F. (1978). Occurrence and distribution of VIP nerves in the nasal mucosa and tracheobronchial wall. *Acta Otolaryngol.* **86**:443-448.

Uddman, R., Luts, A., and Sundler, F. (1985). Nerves fibres containing peptide histidine isoleucine (PHI) in the respiratory tract. *Arch. Otorhinolaryngol.* **242**:189-193.

Undem, B. J., Dick, E. C., and Buckner, C. K. (1983). Inhibition by vasoactive intestinal peptide of antigen-induced histamine release from guinea-pig minced lung. *Eur. J. Pharmacol.* **88**:247-249.

Uvnäs-Moberg, K., Goiny, M., Posloncec, B., and Blomquist, L. (1982). Increased levels of VIP (vasoactive intestinal polypeptide)-like immunoreactivity in peripheral venous blood in dogs following injections of apomorphine and bromocriptine. Do dopaminergic agents induce gastric relaxation and hypotension by a release of endogenous VIP? *Acta Physiol. Scand.* **115**:373-375.

Venugopalan, G. S., Said, S. I., and Drazen, J. M. (1984). Effect of vasoactive intestinal peptide on vagally mediated tracheal pouch relaxation. *Respir. Physiol.* **56**:205-216.

Wang, J., Yaksh, T., Harty, G., and Go, V. (1986). Neurotransmitter modulation of VIP release from cat cerebral cortex. *Am. J. Physiol.* **250**:R104-R111.

Wasserman, M. A., Griffin, R. L., and Malo, P. E. (1982). Comparative in vitro tracheal-relaxant effects of porcine and hen VIP. In *Vasoactive Intestinal Peptide.* Edited by S. I. Said. New York, Raven Press, pp. 177-184.

Wessendorf, M. W., and Elde, R. P. (1985). Characterization of an immunofluorescence technique for the demonstration of coexisting neurotransmitters within nerve fibers and terminals. *J. Histochem. Cytochem.* **33**: 984-994.

Yau, W., Youther, M., and Verdun, P. (1985). A presynaptic site of action of substance P and vasoactive intestinal polypeptide on myenteric neurons. *Brain Res.* **330**:382-385.

16

Bioactive Peptides in Capsaicin-Sensitive C-Fiber Afferents of the Airways

Functional and Pathophysiological Implications

JAN M. LUNDBERG, LARS LUNDBLAD, A. ÄNGGÅRD, C-R. MARTLING, ELVAR THEODORSSON-NORHEIM, PAR STJÄRNE, and TOMAS G. HÖKFELT

Karolinska Institute
Stockholm, Sweden

ALOIS SARIA

University of Graz
Graz, Austria

This chapter summarizes the occurrence and possible functional and pathophysiological roles of multiple neuropeptides, which are present in capsaicin-sensitive C-fiber afferents in the airways. At least four peptides—the tachykinins, substance P, neurokinin A, and neuropeptide K—as well as the calcitonin gene-related peptide (CGRP) have been identified in sensory nerves of the airways. These peptides are likely to be released from peripheral and central branches of sensory nerves upon irritation with certain chemicals, such as capsaicin, vapor-phase components of cigarette smoke, and mediators in the allergic reaction, such as histamine. The peptides induce multiple local effects with individual patterns of bioactivity including vasodilatation, protein extravasation, and bronchoconstriction. These peptide-containing C-fiber afferents are also involved in centrally mediated reflexes including sneezing, cough, exocrine secretion, and hypertension. Pharmacologic blockade of tachykinin-mediated responses can be evoked by substance P analogues with antagonistic activity. This treatment reduces markedly the cigarette-smoke-evoked protein extravasation in the airways. Exposure to high concentrations of capsaicin leads to degeneration of C-fiber afferents and subsequent loss of neuropeptides. In capsaicin-treated animals, protective reflexes as well as local protein extravasation in the mucosa induced by inhalation of certain chemical irritants including cigarette smoke are absent. Furthermore, histamine released from mast cells upon allergen exposure induces flare reaction in the human skin via mediator release from capsaicin-sensitive C-fiber afferents.

I. Biochemical Identification and Characterization of Peptides in Sensory Nerves

Substance P (SP)-like immunoreactivity (LI) has been demonstrated in nerves of the airways in several species, including humans, by immunohistochemistry (Nilsson et al., 1977; Lundberg et al., 1984b) and radioimmunoassay (Lundberg et al., 1983a). Characterization of the SP-LI in the guinea-pig lung by Sephadex G25 chromatography using the SP antiserum K25 indicated an elution pattern similar to synthetic SP. Recent evidence, however, suggests that a whole family of structurally related tachykinins are present in the airways. Thus, Hua et al. (1985b) have demonstrated, using both ion-exchange chromatography and reverse-phase high performance liquid chromatography (HPLC), that SP, neurokinin A (NKA)-, and neuropeptide K (NPK)-like immunoreactivities (LI) as well as a not yet fully identified eledoisin-related peptide are present in capsaicin-sensitive sensory nerves in the lung. Treatment with high doses of capsaicin is known to induce selective degeneration of a population of C-fiber afferents, leaving cholinergic and adrenergic nerves intact (see Janscó et al., 1977, 1981; Szolcsanyi, 1984; Lundblad et al., 1983b). The simultaneous occurrence of SP, NKA, and NPK in sensory nerves can be related to a common precursor form, a so-called preprotachykinin, which contains all these three peptides (Fig. 1).

The calcitonin gene-related peptide (CGRP) is another peptide present in capsaicin-sensitive afferents in the lung (Lundberg et al., 1985a). CGRP has no structural similarity to tachykinins. The possible molecular heterogenicity of the CGRP-LI in airway nerves, however, will yet have to be established using biochemical methods.

II. Tissue Distribution of Tachykinins and CGRP

Using immunohistochemistry, it has been established that both tachykinin-LI (initially using antibodies raised against SP) and CGRP-LI are present in ganglion cells of sensory ganglia and axons known to project to the airways. Thus, many cell bodies of the trigeminal ganglion (Fig. 2a, b) as well as of axons in the trigeminal nerves are tachykinin-immunoreactive (IR). Some of these nerves project to the nasal mucosa (see Lundblad et al., 1983b). Furthermore, cell bodies in the jugular and nodose ganglia as well as axons in the vagal nerves, which innervate the larynx, trachea, and lung, are tachykinin-IR. In addition,

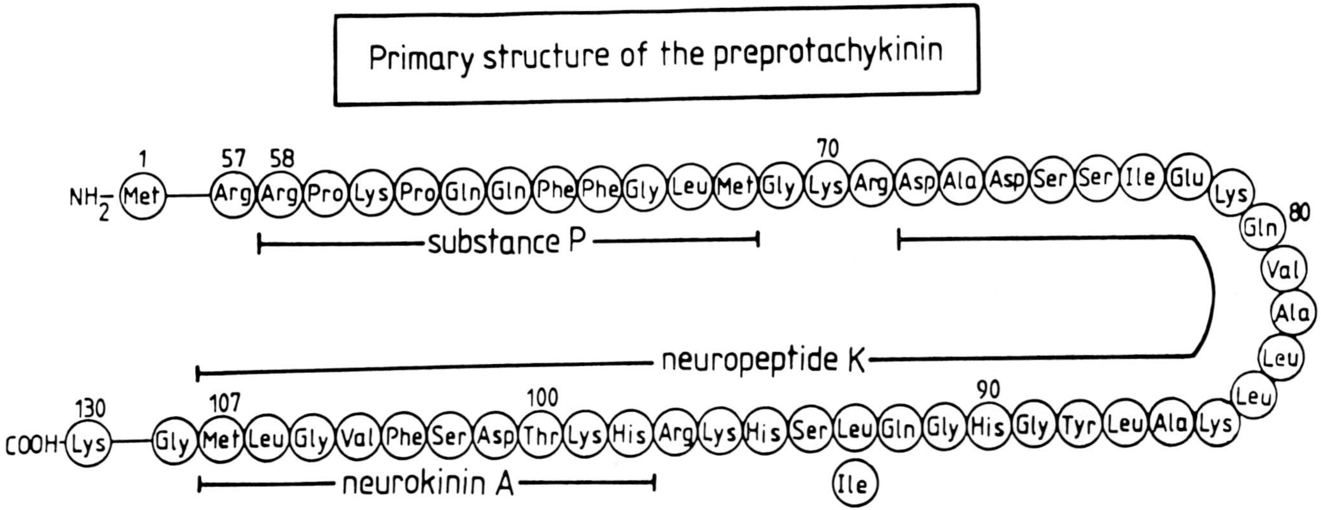

Figure 1 Schematic illustration of the amino acid sequence in position 57-108 of the preprotachykinin precursor in the bovine brain, containing the amino acid sequence of SP, KNA and NPK. (From Hua et al., 1985b.)

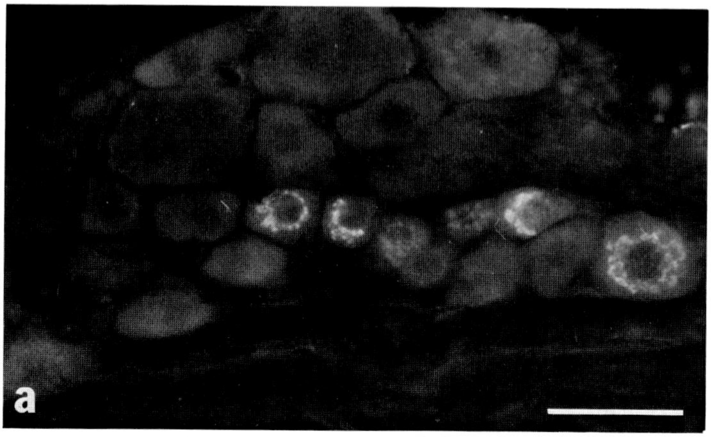

Figure 2 Immunofluorescence micrographs of the trigeminal ganglion (a, b) and nasal mucosa (c, d) of the cat, human nasal mucosa (e, f), and the smooth muscle of a bronchus from the guinea pig lung (g, h) after incubation with antiserum to SP (a, c, g) and CGRP (b, d, e, f, h). Double staining experiments were performed to reveal the simultaneous occurrence of SP-LI and CGRP-LI in the same ganglion cells and nerve fibers in a and b, c, and d as well as g and h, respectively. Thus, the tissue occurrence of antibodies against SP raised in rat was detected by FITC- and antisera against CGRP raised in rabbit by Texas red-labeled second antisera, respectively. Arrowheads in b indicate two CGRP-IR cells, which are only weakly SP-IR (a). Arrow heads in c and d indicate intraepithelial nerve bundles with a varicose fiber, which is branching off towards the lumen. Large arrow heads in e and f indicate CGRP-IR nerves associated with an exocrine duct. Small arrow heads in e indicate perivascular nerves and in f an axon bundle. Asterisk in e indicates lining nasal epithelium. The same nerve fibers in the bronchial smooth muscle of the guinea pig contain both SP- and CGRP-IR (arrow heads in g and h). Bar indicates 50 μm. a and b, c and d, and g and h represent the same magnifications.

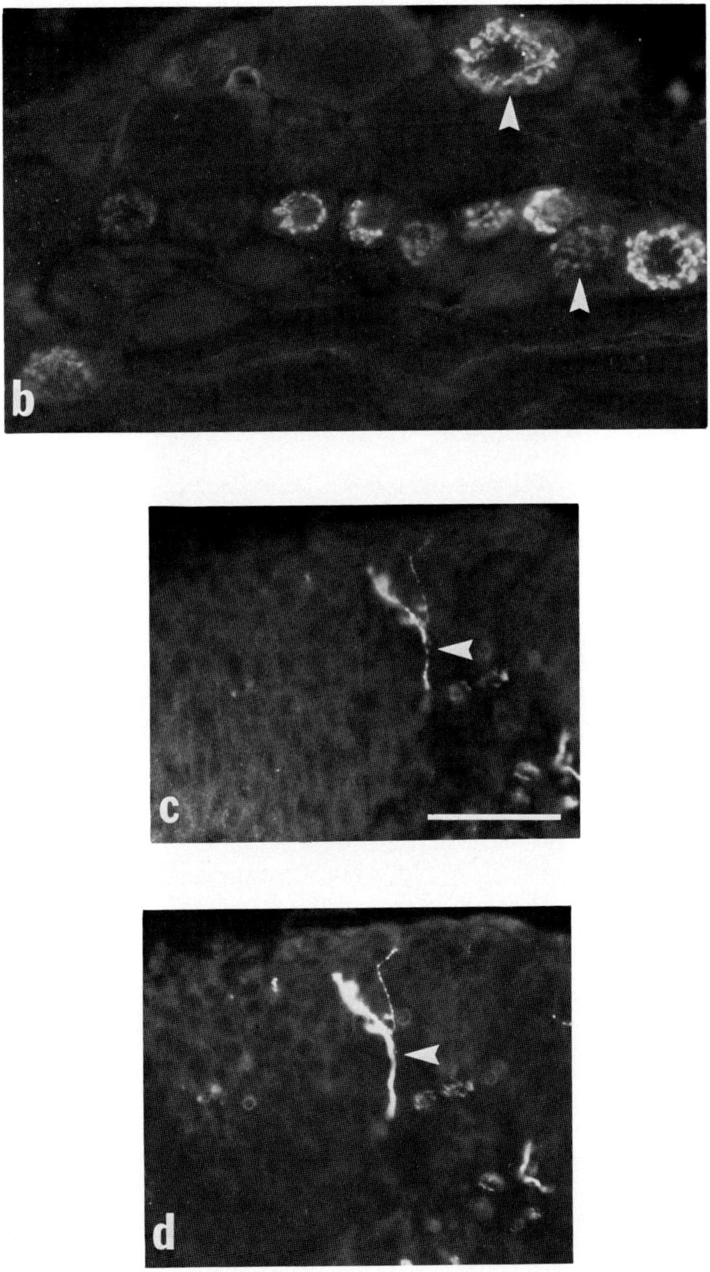

Figure 2 (continued)

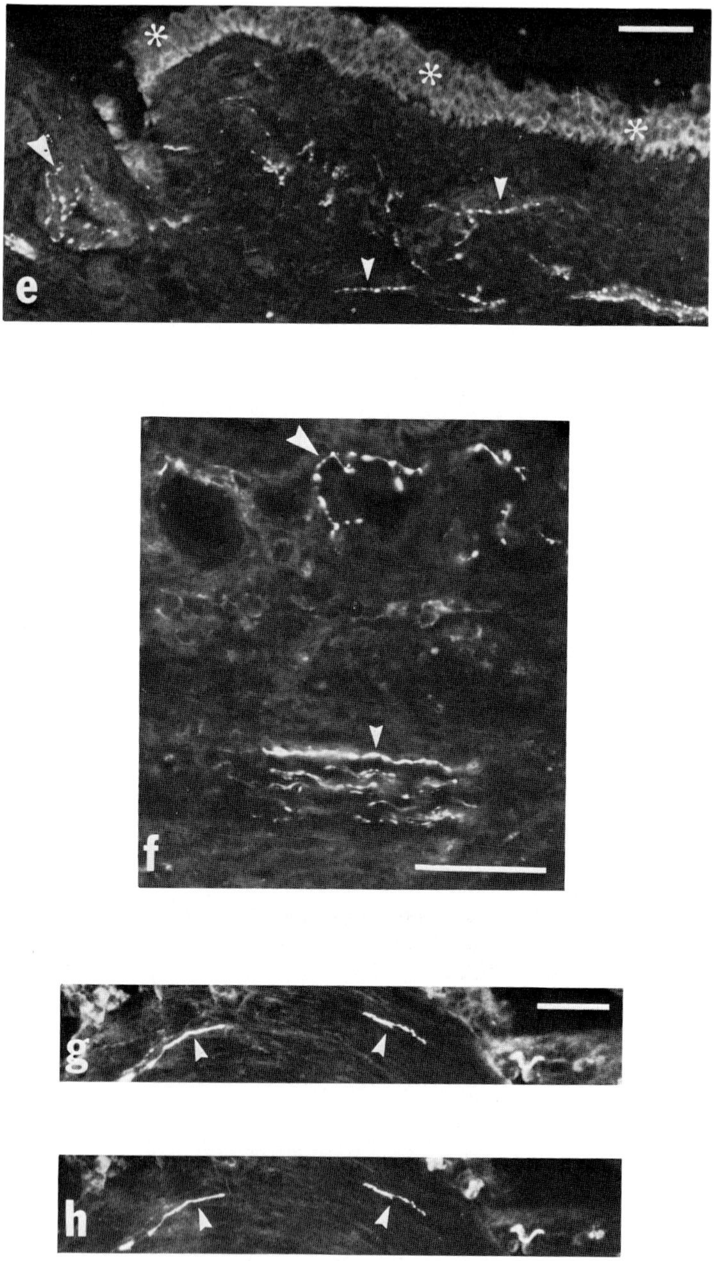

Figure 2 (continued)

functional, histochemical, and biochemical evidence suggests that tachykinin-containing sensory ganglion cells of thoracic spinal ganglia project to the lower airways via sympathetic pathways (Dalsgaard and Lundberg, 1984; Lundberg et al., 1983a; Saria et al., 1985a). Histochemical techniques, using antibodies raised against NKA and SP, have revealed that CGRP coexists with the newly identified tachykinins both in cell bodies in sensory ganglia and terminal areas in the airways (Fig. 2) (see below).

Nerve terminals from tachykinin- and CGRP-containing sensory nerves can be found around local parasympathetic, presumably cholinergic, ganglion cells (the sphenopalatine ganglion innervating blood vessels and exocrine acini of the nasal mucosa and local tracheobronchial ganglia). Furthermore, sensory neuropeptides are present around various types of blood vessels (arteries, arterioles, venous sinusoids, and veins), within the tracheobronchial smooth muscle layers (Fig. 2g, h), close to the exocrine acini and ducts of some species, such as in the rat and human nasal mucosa (Fig. 2e, f) and cat trachea as well as under and within the lining respiratory epithelium (Fig. 2c, d). It has been also possible to demonstrate sensory neuropeptides in fine intraepithelial nerve fibers very close to the surface of the luminal epithelium (see Fig. 2c, d). Thus, irritant chemicals or particles that are inhaled are likely to have easy access to these intraepithelial nerve fibers, which probably represent functional irritant receptor units. Although it has been proposed that axon reflexes within the airways can account for a variety of local reactions (see below), it is difficult to demonstrate that intraepithelial, perivascular, and nerves in the bronchial smooth muscle actually represent branches of the same sensory neuron. It seems likely, however, that the bioactive peptides are present in and can be released from all nerve branches upon activation of irritant receptors.

After capsaicin treatment in adult animals, virtually all nerve fibers containing tachykinin- and CGRP-LI disappear from the airway mucosa. Peptide-containing cell bodies, however, remain in the sensory ganglia, suggesting a damage of axonal branches, but not to the same extent of cell bodies.

In corresponding sensory relay stations of the CNS (i.e., the spinal trigeminal nucleus), the nucleus of the solitary tract and dorsal horn of the spinal cord, very dense networks of tachykinin and CGRP-containing nerve terminals can be seen. Thus, the central branch of the capsaicin-sensitive sensory nerves also seem to contain the same peptides as the peripheral branch. After capsaicin treatment, there is a substantial but not total loss of CGRP-LI in nerve terminals in these central areas in spite of the fact that all CGRP-positive fibers here are probably sensory afferents. This difference from the almost total loss of peptides in peripheral terminal fields after capsaicin treatment indicates that the central branches of the sensory neurons are more resistant to the toxic effects of capsaicin. A less extensive loss of tachykinin fibers than of CGRP-positive nerves is seen in capsaicin-treated animals, most likely due to the occurrence of local, tachykinin-containing neurons in the sensory relay areas, which are not affected by the capsaicin treatment.

The same principles of organization and occurrence of CGRP- and tachykinin-LI hold for the human airways, in the trigeminal and vagal ganglia and terminals in the nasal mucosa (Fig. 2e, f) and lower airways. The number of tachykinin- and CGRP-IR nerves in human trachea and bronchi was, however, less than that in the guinea-pig and rat.

Apart from a nervous localization, CGRP-LI (but not tachykinin-LI) seem to be present in epithelial endocrine cells, so-called neuroepithelial Kultchinsky cells, and in the rat trachea and bronchi.

III. Supply of Peptides to Nerve Endings

In contrast to classic transmitters, peptides are not locally synthetized in nerve endings. Thus, after synthesis in the cell body region, peptides are packed into vesicles and axonally transported at a rate of about 10 mm/hr to nerve terminals. It is likely that some cleavage of the tachykinin precursor occurs along the axon. An interesting feature of the peptide transport is that about 90% of the SP-LI produced in nodose ganglion cells is directed out into the peripheral branches of the vagal sensory neurons (see Brimijoin et al., 1980). This clearly indicates that a major function and turnover for sensory neuropeptides occur in peripheral terminal fields in the airways. Thus, the concept that the only major function of vagal and other sensory neurons is the transduction of afferent signals into the CNS after activation of receptors on peripheral branches may be expanded. As discussed below, release of bioactive peptides from peripheral terminals of sensory nerves upon local irritation suggests that afferent nerves have important local "efferent functions" in the airways.

IV. Release of Peptides from Sensory Nerves

The demonstration of peptide release from sensory nerves is usually difficult due to low peptide levels. Furthermore, radioactive labeling techniques, such as those employed in studies of catecholamine release, cannot be used because peptides are not taken up into nerve terminals after release, but apparently, are mainly locally degraded.

In central primary sensory relay areas, such as the spinal cord where peptides are present in a very dense network of nerve terminals, it has, however, been possible to demonstrate the release of sensory neuropeptides in vitro. Thus, exposure to superfused slices of the thoracic spinal cord to high K^+ or to capsaicin induces a Ca^{2+}-dependent overflow of both tachykinin and CGRP-

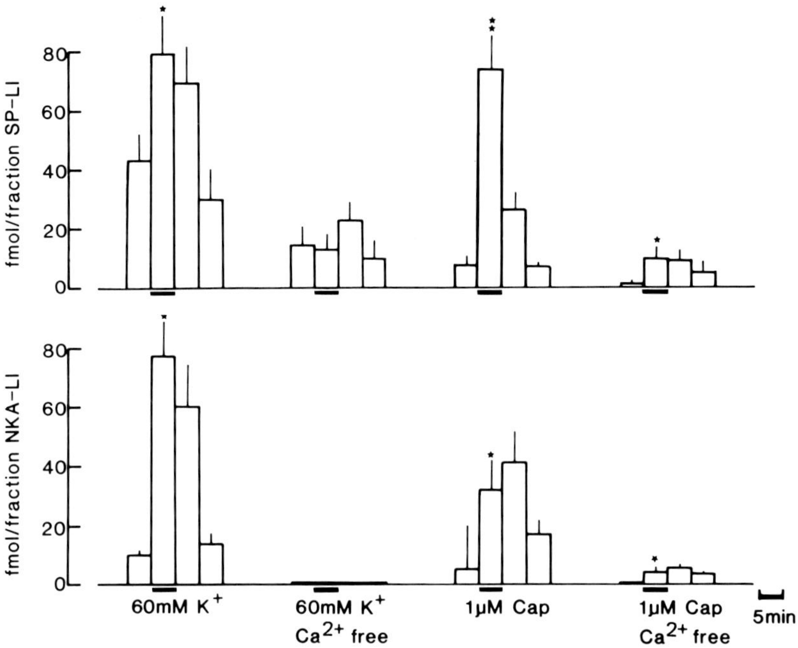

Figure 3 Release of NKA- and SP-LI from the isolated perfused guinea-pig lung in vitro by high K^+ (60 mM) or 1 μM capsaicin. Fractions were collected for 5 min, concentrated on Sep Pak Cartridges, and analyzed by radioimmunoassay. In a Ca^{2+}-free medium, the release of peptides by both K^+ and capsaicin was markedly reduced (from four to six experiments; Saria et al., 1986b). Data are given as means ± S.E.M.

LI into the superfusion medium (Gamse et al., 1979; Hua et al., 1986; Saria et al., 1986a). Chemical characterization of the tachykinin-LI has revealed that both SP (Gamse et al., 1979), NKA, and the eledoisin-LI (Hua et al., 1986) are released by capsaicin. So far, it has not been possible to demonstrate a capsaicin-induced release of NPK-LI. This could indicate that NPK (which contains the NKA sequence at the C-terminal end) represents a precursor peptide, which is not released. Alternatively, NPK may be released only in very low amounts.

The isolated perfused guinea pig lung has recently been used as a model to study the release of peptides from the peripheral branches of sensory neurons. Thus, SP-, NKA- and eledoisin-related material as well as CGRP-LI have been found to be released by high K^+ and capsaicin from the lung (Figs. 3, 4) (Saria et al., 1984, 1986b; Martling et al., 1986b). Furthermore, agents that activate

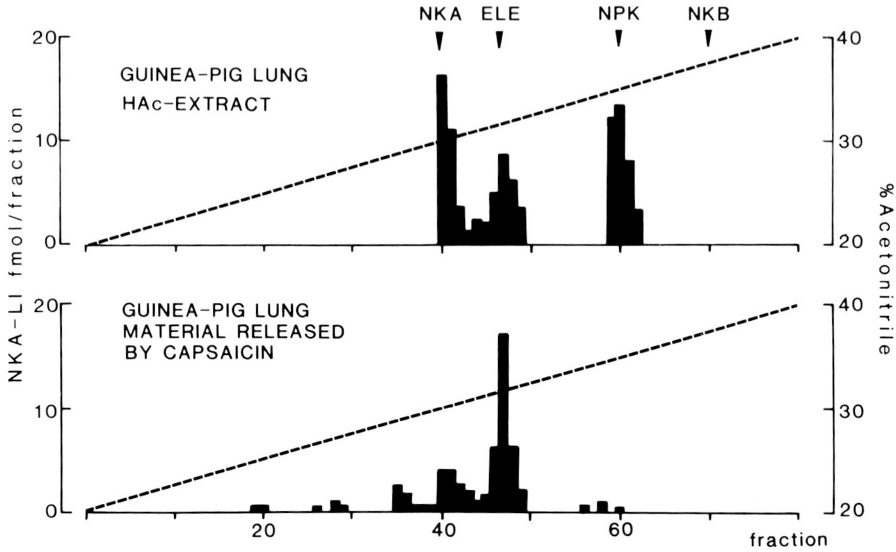

Figure 4 Reversed-phase high performance liquid chromatography of an acetic acid extract of the guinea pig lung (top) or material released by capsaicin from the isolated perfused guinea pig lung. The elution positions for synthetic NKA, eledoisin (ELE), NPK, and neurokinin B (NKB) are indicated by arrow heads. (From Saria et al., 1986b.)

sensory nerves, such as the nicotine analogue dimethylphenyl-piperazine (DMPP), bradykinin, as well as histamine induce the release of tachykinin-LI from the lung (Fig. 5). In addition, electrical stimulation of the vagal nerves causes a release of multiple sensory neuropeptides in the lung (Fig. 6). The data obtained in these experiments represent suggestive evidence that multiple neuropeptides are released upon activation of capsaicin-sensitive nerves in the airways. The capsaicin-induced release of tachykinins in vitro is resistent to tetrodotoxin, suggesting an action independent of nerve impulse propagation and that capsaicin can release mediators directly from sensory nerves at the site of exposure (see Szolcsanyi, 1984; Hua et al., 1986). In the intact animal, however, it seems clear that capsaicin both elicits central reflexes and locally releases sensory neuropeptides, partly via axon reflexes, since, for instance, the protein-extravasation response can be reduced by local anesthetics (Lundberg and Saria, 1983).

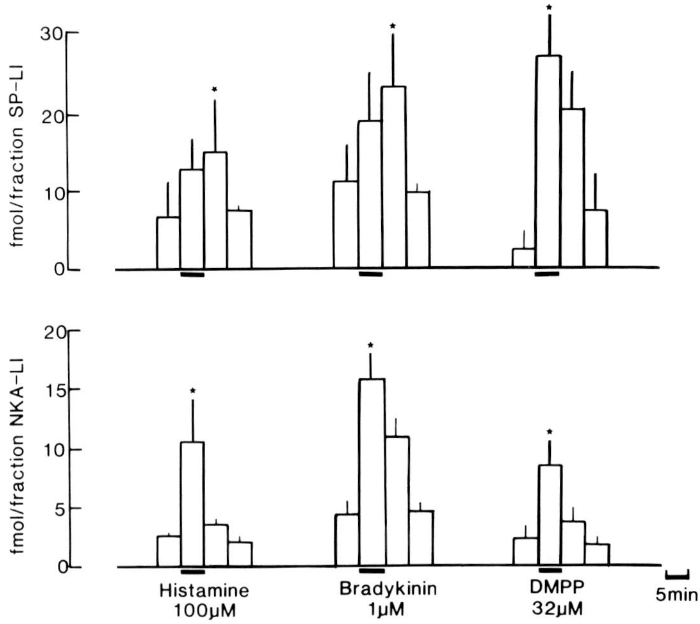

Figure 5 Release of NKA- and SP-LI from the isolated perfused guinea-pig lung by histamine, bradykinin and the stable nicotine analogue DMPP. (From Saria et al., 1986b.)

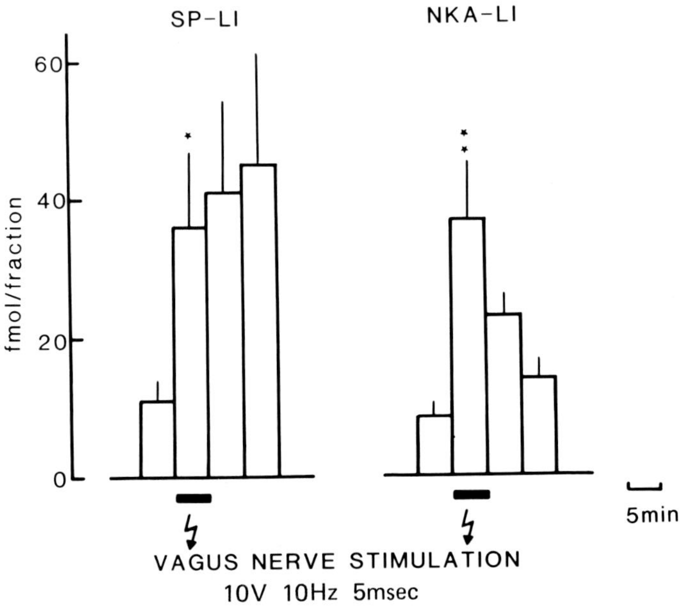

Figure 6 Release of SP- and NKA-LI from the isolated perfused guinea-pig lung by vagal nerve stimulation at 10 Hz for 5 min. (From Saria et al., 1986b.)

V. Comparison of Local Reactions Due to Sensory Nerve Irritation and Effects of Neuropeptides

Several local reactions in the airways can be elicited by irritation of capsaicin-sensitive C-fiber afferents. Thus, capsaicin infused locally into the nasal mucosa (Lundblad et al., 1983a) or applied onto the tracheal epithelium (Martling et al., 1986a) causes increased local blood flow. A vasodilatation response in the nasal mucosa can also be induced by all three tachykinins (SP, NKA, and NPK) as well as by CGRP. SP seems to be the most potent vasodilator agent of these peptides, on a molar basis, in the nasal mucosa of the cat (Lundblad et al., 1986b). There are some peculiarities about the capsaicin-induced vascular response as well as about the mechanism underlying the peptide-mediated vasodilatation. Thus, sometimes capsaicin causes vasoconstriction, which is followed by a long-lasting vasodilatation (see Lundblad et al., 1983a). This biphasic effect does not seem to be mediated via sympathetic or parasympathetic pathways. The mechanisms underlying the peptide-induced relaxation of the vascular smooth muscle have been further studied in vitro. Thus, it is known that the SP-induced relaxation of vascular smooth muscle in vitro is indirect due to release of an endothelium-dependent factor (see Furchott, 1983). When given intraarterially in vivo, SP has an easy access to the endothelium that may underlie at least part of the effects (see Lundblad et al., 1986b). In contrast, the vasodilatory effect of CGRP in vitro does not seem to involve the endothelium to any major extent but may represent a direct action on vascular smooth muscle cells (Edvinsson et al., 1985). Antidromic stimulation of the trigeminal nerve (Lundblad et al., 1983b) results in vasodilatation in the nasal mucosa. Furthermore, vagal nerve stimulation in the presence of a ganglion-blocking agent, to abolish parasympathetic vasodilator mechanisms, also induces vasodilatation in the tracheal mucosa (Martling et al., 1986a). As discussed above, antidromic stimulation of sensory nerves results in release of multiple peptides with vasodilator activity. The relative importance of individual peptides for the nerve-evoked vasodilator response, however, remains to be established, using specific antagonists.

Another important local reaction to antidromic nerve stimulation of sensory nerves or irritation by chemicals is protein extravasation in the mucosa. Tachykinins, especially SP, are very potent in inducing protein extravasation due to leakage in postcapillary venules of the nasal as well as in tracheobronchial mucosa (Lundberg and Saria, 1982a, 1983; Lundblad et al., 1983c; Hua et al., 1984; Lundberg et al., 1984; Persson et al., 1985; Tatemoto et al., 1985). CGRP given in similar amounts as tachykinins does not cause protein extravasation in the airway mucosa (Lundberg et al., 1985a), although it has been reported that CGRP in very high doses can increase the vascular permeability to albumin (Gamse and Saria, 1985). In addition, CGRP can enhance protein extravasation by tachykinins, most likely mainly due to the potent vasodilator activity (Gamse and Saria, 1985; Brain and Williams, 1985). Experiments with SP analogues with antagonistic activity suggest that most of the protein extravasation induced by nerve stimulation (Lundberg et al., 1983d) or cigarette-smoke irritation in the trachea (Lundberg et al., 1983c) is due to tachykinins rather than CGRP. The protein-extravasation reaction seen upon excitation of capsaicin-sensitive sensory nerves is especially pronounced in the airways of the rat and guinea pig. Species differences, however, seem to exist, since observations suggest that vagal nerve stimulation or application of capsaicin into the trachea of cat and dog does not induce protein extravasation in the airway mucosa, as indicated by measurement of Evans blue leakage. This difference can possibly be related to lack of tachykinin receptors on postcapillary venules, since SP does not cause protein extravasation in the trachea of the cat in reasonable intravenous doses. In the human skin, exposure to capsaicin causes severe irritation with a clear-cut, flare reaction (which is assumed to mainly reflect vasodilatation) but no wheal (protein extravasation) (Jancsó et al., 1968; see Lundblad et al., 1986a). This indicates that peptide mediators released from sensory nerves by capsaicin in humans (at least in the skin) do not induce any major protein extravasation by direct actions on postcapillary venules.

Capsaicin and vagal nerve stimulations induce noncholinergic bronchoconstriction in the guinea pig in vivo (Lundberg and Saria, 1982b; Martling et al., 1984). Tachykinins, especially NKA, are very potent bronchoconstrictor agents both in the guinea pig (Hua et al., 1984; Karlsson et al., 1984) and in humans (Lundberg et al., 1985b; Karlsson and Persson, 1985; Martling et al., 1986c). NPK induces a slowly developing, very long lasting bronchoconstrictor effect in vivo (Tatemoto et al., 1985; Hua and Lundberg, 1986). Electrical field stimulation of guinea pig bronchi in vitro has also revealed a long-lasting, atropine-resistant, contractile component, which is sensitive to capsaicin treatment (Lundberg and Saria, 1982b) and blocked by SP analogues with tachykinin-antagonistic activity (Lundberg et al., 1983d; Karlsson et al., 1984). In humans, however, no consistent atropine-resistant contraction has been obtained upon electrical field stimulation of bronchi in vitro (see Lundberg et al., 1983b). This observation does not exclude an important function of sensory neuropeptides in the control of bronchial smooth muscle tone in humans, since powerful opposing bronchodilatory mechanisms may be dominating in atropinized preparations. Bronchodilatory mechanisms seem to be of minor importance in the peripheral airways of the guinea pig, and in this species noncholinergic bronchoconstriction induced by capsaicin-sensitive sensory nerves is easy to demonstrate. Capsaicin-induced bronchoconstriction in vivo is markedly enhanced by propranolol or chlorisondamine treatment in the guinea-pig (Lundberg et al., 1985b; Gamse et al., 1986; Hua and Lundberg, 1986). This suggests that capsaicin induces a sympathetic bronchodilator reflex via beta-adrenergic mechanisms, which partly masks the bronchoconstriction, most likely induced by local release of mediators from sensory nerves.

Species differences also seem to exist with regard to capsaicin- and tachykinin-induced bronchoconstriction. Thus, tachykinins have very poor bronchoconstrictor effects in the rat in vivo and in vitro, although marked protein extravasation is present in the airway mucosa. Furthermore, capsaicin does not seem to contract rat bronchi in vitro. Tachykinins, especially NKA (Lundberg et al., 1983b, 1985b; Karlsson and Persson, 1985; Martling et al., 1986c) are very potent bronchoconstrictor agents on isolated human bronchi. Furthermore, capsaicin seems to cause contraction of human bronchi in vitro (Lundberg et al., 1983b). In vivo, however, capsaicin has been reported to induce cough and retrosternal discomfort but no clear bronchoconstriction (Collier and Fuller et al., 1984) or only a transient, mainly cholinergic, bronchoconstriction (Fuller et al., 1985). However, the existence of capsaicin-activated, sympathetic bronchodilator reflexes has not been elucidated in humans. Furthermore, powerful protective reflexes may impair the spread of inhaled capsaicin to the lower airways in vivo.

Palmer et al. (1985) reported that CGRP was considerably more potent than tachykinins to contract human bronchi in vitro. Conflicting data, however, seem to exist with regard to the bronchial effects of CGRP. Thus, Lundberg et al. (1985a) did not observe any bronchoconstrictor effect of CGRP in the guinea pig. Furthermore, whereas the human form of CGRP is very active to relax human pulmonary arteries in vitro, no effect was obtained by CGRP in either basal or tachykinin-induced increase in smooth muscle tone of isolated human bronchi in vitro (Martling et al., 1986b). Another feature of the CGRP response further questions whether CGRP should induce bronchoconstriction. Thus, both in the vascular smooth muscle (Edvinsson et al., 1985) and heart (Sigrist et al., 1986) CGRP activates adenylate cyclase and raises intracellular cAMP. This change should, if anything, relax the bronchial smooth muscle. However, it has been found that at least in the guinea pig (Lundberg et al., 1985a; Hua and Lundberg, 1986) the bronchial smooth muscle does not respond with any clear-cut relaxation to CGRP in vivo. Thus, whereas CGRP causes a marked inhibition of spontaneous or tachykinin-induced increase in ureteral motility, no change is observed on bronchial smooth muscle tone in the same animals (Hua and Lundberg, 1986). It may be postulated that this difference is related to the occurrence of CGRP receptors mediating smooth muscle relaxation on the ureteral but not bronchial smooth muscle cells. This suggestion is also supported by the finding that capsaicin always induces bronchoconstriction in vivo in the guinea pig, while the ureteral motility is inhibited in low and stimulated in high doses (possibly due to a domination of the CGRP-mediated relaxation at low capsaicin doses) (see Hua and Lundberg, 1986).

Tachykinins (SP and NKA) and capsaicin are known to induce a slow excitatory postsynaptic potential (SEPSP) in sympathetic and parasympathetic, postganglionic neurons (see Saria et al., 1985b). This putative change in membrane potential in, for instance, local cholinergic ganglion cells in the lower airways could, if existing there as well, facilitates cholinergic transmission. The significance for such an effect for the autonomic control of the airways is at present unknown. However, one puzzling observation is worth mentioning in this context. Capsaicin treatment is associated with a reversible impairment of vagal cholinergic bronchoconstriction in the guinea pig (Lundberg et al., 1983a; Martling et al., 1984). Since no signs of loss of markers for cholinergic nerves or changes in muscarinic receptors in the airways were obtained in the capsaicin-treated animals (Martling et al., 1984), it could be of interest to study if this unexplained observation is due to a loss of facilitation of cholinergic, ganglionic transmission by sensory nerves (Fig. 7).

The relationship between tachykinins and inflammatory cells, such as lymphocytes and mast cells has also been interesting. Thus, it is known that specific receptors for SP are present on lymphocytes (see Payan et al., 1984). Furthermore, it is known that SP can release histamine from mast cells in animals (see Sydbom, 1982) as well as in humans (Hägermark et al., 1978; Heavery et al., 1985). The relationship between sensory nerves and mast-cell function, however, is a controversial issue. It was reported by Lembeck and Holzer (1979) that both the vasodilator and protein-extravasation responses to antidromic nerve stimulation and SP in the rat skin were considerably reduced after administration of antihistaminics. However, subsequent studies on the rat trachea have not indicated any involvement of histamine release in the protein-extravasation response to vagal nerve stimulation, SP, or irritation by cigarette smoke (see Lundberg et al., 1983c). Although it seems clear that SP in very high local concentrations in vitro (Sydbom, 1982) or when injected locally into the human skin in vivo (Hägermark et al., 1978) can degranulate mast cells and release histamine, further experimental evidence suggesting that neuropeptides released from sensory nerves can activate mast cells remains to be obtained. Another observation in humans also supports the theory that sensory neuropeptides do not activate mast cells in vivo, since capsaicin applied locally to the skin does not induce any wheal response (which locally injected histamine and antigen-induced mast-cell degranulation clearly promote). As discussed below (and above), the evidence for the reverse relationship, that mast-cell degranulation and histamine activate sensory nerves and release neuropeptides, seems more convincing.

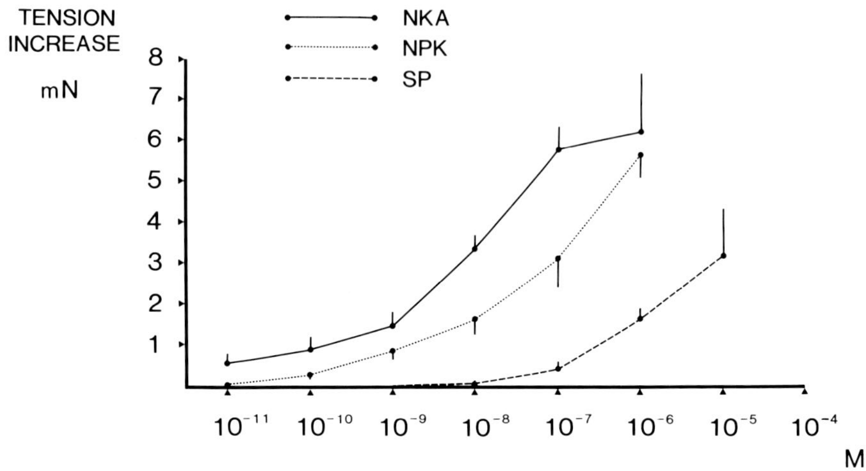

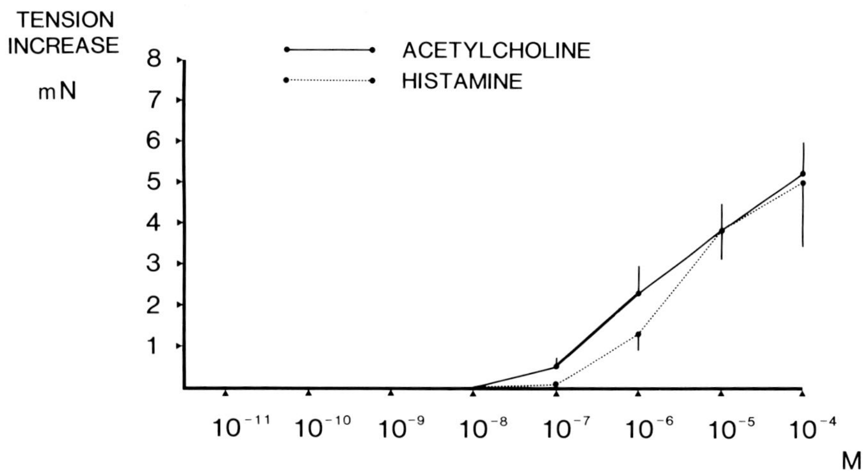

Figure 7 Dose-response curves of contractile effects of tachykinins (NKA, NPK and SP) as well as acetylcholine and histamine on isolated human bronchi (diameter 1-2 mm) in vitro. Tension increase has been given as means ± S.E.M. and represents observations from 6-11 patients. NKA is several orders of magnitude more potent than SP histamine, and acetylcholine in inducing bronchoconstriction. (From Martling et al., 1986c.)

VI. CNS-Mediated Reflexes via Capsaicin-Sensitive Afferents

Irritation of capsaicin-sensitive sensory nerves is followed by rapid protective reflexes, avoidance behavior, and autonomic activation. The importance of capsaicin-sensitive afferents in the response to airway irritation has been extensively studied in the nasal mucosa of capsaicin-treated guinea-pigs, where absence of certain reactions has been taken as evidence for the involvement of capsaicin-sensitive nerves (see Lundblad et al., 1984a, 1985a). Thus, the sneezing response to capsaicin and formalin is absent after capsaicin treatment, while the sneezing induced by nicotine remains to a large extent. Furthermore, the response to mechanical irritation also seems unaffected (Lundblad et al., 1984a). The avoidance behavior (as indicated by nose wipings with the forepaws) to cigarette smoke and ether also seems to be mediated via capsaicin-sensitive nerves (Lundblad et al., 1984a; Lundblad and Lundberg, 1984). The cigarette-smoke-induced avoidance behavior (as well as the protein extravasation, see above) is mediated by vapor-phase chemicals, while the particulate of the smoke containing nicotine seems to have minor importance in this aspect (Lundblad and Lundberg, 1984). Capsaicin is also capable of inducing sneezing upon local application to the nasal mucosa as well as producing cough in humans. Capsaicin induces exocrine secretion in both the nasal and tracheal mucosa (Davies et al., 1982) via cholinergic parasympathetic reflexes. This secretory reaction as well as sensory irritation are also prominent in the human nasal mucosa upon capsaicin exposure (Fig. 8). Sensory neuropeptides, such as SP, can evoke exocrine secretion from salivary, tracheal (Baker et al., 1977), and nasal glands in some species, particularly the rat and dog. However, SP does not induce any nasal (or salivary) secretion in the cat, and the findings in humans remain to be established.

Sympathetic activation with hypertension due to increased peripheral vascular resistance is observed upon irritation of capsaicin-sensitive afferents in the nasal mucosa of the guinea pig (Lundblad et al., 1984b). Furthermore, as mentioned above, evidence suggests that capsaicin activates bronchodilator reflexes via sympathetic pathways (Lundberg et al., 1985b; Gamse et al., 1986; Hua and Lundberg, 1986).

An important question is whether neuropeptides have any important role for the transmission of information from the central sensory terminals to the CNS. It seems clear that tachykinins can excite neurons in, for example, the dorsal horn of the spinal cord (see Yanagisawa et al., 1982). The tachykinin-induced responses are, however, as in the autonomic ganglia, rather slow compared to the rapid signals of sensory afferents. Therefore, it has been postu-

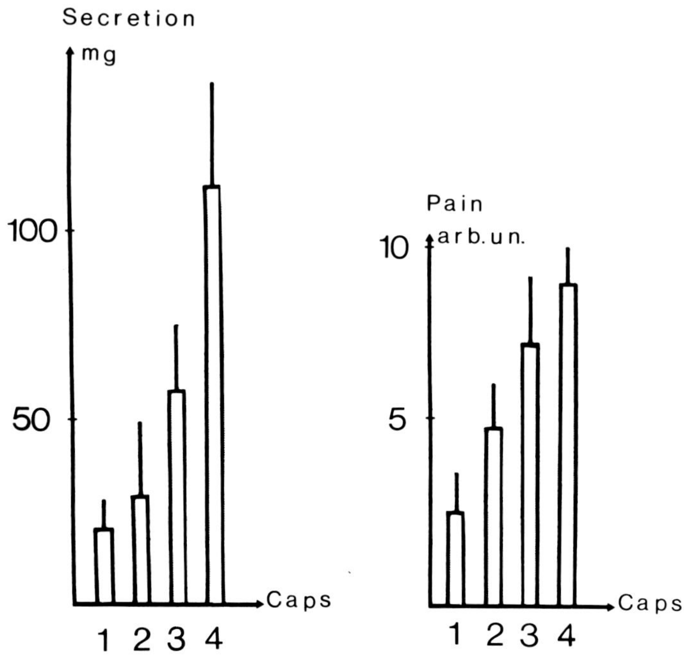

Figure 8 Parallel secretion of mucus from the human nasal mucosa and perceived pain sensation (graded 1-10 in an arbitrary scale) induced by local applications of capsaicin in increasing concentrations. Data are given as means ± S.E.M. (n = 20) and indicate the weight increase of small filter-paper strips inserted into the nasal cavity before capsaicin exposure. The following concentrations were used: 1:3, 2:30, 3:300 and 4:3000 μM, respectively.

lated that the rapid primary transmitter of sensory reflexes is a nonpeptide molecule, possibly an amino acid. When applied close to the central terminals of sensory neurons, capsaicin can initiate the release of neuropeptides, as discussed above. Furthermore, intracisternal administration of capsaicin in vivo elicits exocrine reflex-exocrine secretion (salivation) as well as hypertension (Gamse et al., 1986). Intracisternally applied CGRP has also been found to induce hypertension (Fischer et al., 1983). No clear-cut reflex bronchoconstriction was elicited by intracisternal capsaicin, which suggested that, at least in the guinea pig, vagovagal reflexes are not of any major importance for the capsaicin-induced bronchoconstriction (Gamse et al., 1986; see Lundberg and Saria, 1982b).

VII. Functional and Pathophysiological Significance of Capsaicin-Sensitive Airway Afferents

It seems reasonable to assume that capsaicin-sensitive C-fiber afferents are not very active during basal conditions, while a marked excitation occurs upon local irritation of the airway mucosa by either irritant chemicals or allergic reactions. Several stimuli are known to activate capsaicin-sensitive nerves, as studied by reduction or loss of protein-extravasation responses in capsaicin-treated animals (Table 1). Whereas strong mechanical stimulation by intubation and expansion of the tracheal lumen does not induce a protein-extravasation response, which is dependent on capsaicin-sensitive nerves (Lundberg and Saria, 1983), light mechanical touch causes activation of the C-fibers that are likely to represent polymodal afferents (see Widdicombe, 1981; Coleridge and Coleridge, 1984). Several irritant chemicals excite capsaicin-sensitive nerves. As described above, cigarette smoke is a very powerful activator of these nerves. Furthermore, formalin and ether induce both protein extravasation and bronchoconstriction (ether) via peptide-containing C-fiber afferents (see Lundberg and Saria, 1982a,b). It seems clear that nicotine (and the stable nicotine analogue, DMPP) can activate capsaicin-sensitive C-fibers in the nasal mucosa, eliciting hypertension (Lundblad et al., 1984b), protein extravasation in the trachea (Lundberg et al., 1983e), and tachykinin release from the lung (Saria et al., 1986b). Application of acid solutions also seems to activate capsaicin-sensitive nerves in the tracheobronchial mucosa (unpublished findings), which may have implications for the mucosal reactions upon aspiration of gastric contents (unpublished findings).

Table 1 Chemical Agents Stimulating Capsaicin-Sensitive C-Fiber Afferents in the Airways

Capsaicin
Formalin
Ether
Vapor-phase chemicals of smoke
Nicotine (high-dose)
Bradykinin
Histamine
HCl

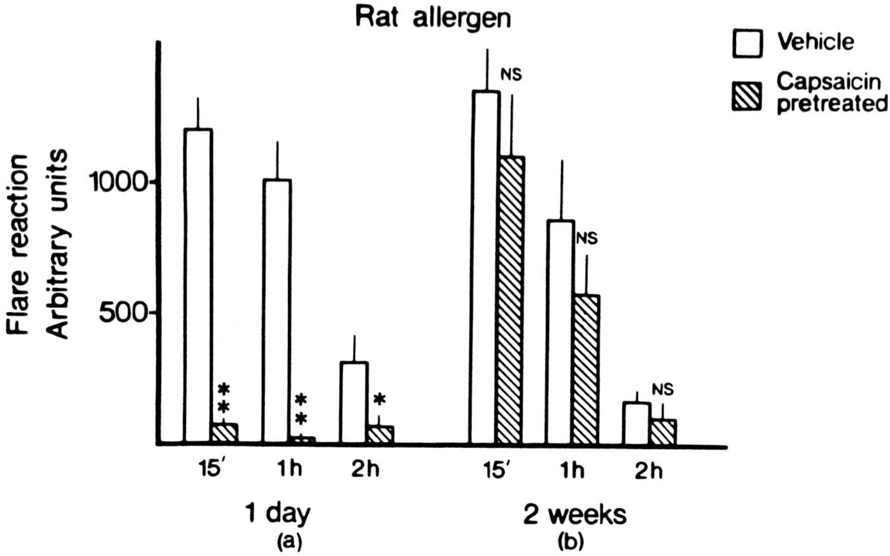

Figure 9 Flare reaction 15 min, 1, and 2 hr after rat-antigen exposure in the human skin in sensitized persons in vehicle (70% alcohol) and capsaicin-treated sides. (a) Two days after completed treatment and (b) 2 weeks after capsaicin treatment. Note the reversible loss of the allergen-induced flare reaction in the human skin after capsaicin treatment. (From Lundblad et al., 1986a.)

As has partly been discussed above, several lines of evidence suggest that capsaicin-sensitive nerves are activated upon mast-cell degranulation in experimental animals (Saria et al., 1983) and in humans (Lundblad et al., 1985b, 1986a). Thus, the protein-extravasation response to histamine in the rat trachea is significantly reduced after capsaicin treatment (Lundberg and Saria, 1983). Furthermore, histamine induces release of tachykinins from the guinea-pig lung (Saria et al., 1986b). The histamine-induced flare reaction in human skin is lost after local capsaicin treatment (Bernstein et al., 1981). In accordance, the flare response in human skin upon antigen challenge in the acute phase of the allergic reaction (which, to a large extent, is also histamine-mediated) is lost after capsaicin treatment (Fig. 9) (Lundblad et al., 1985b, 1986a). The sensory impairment caused by capsaicin treatment of the human skin seems to be reversible, since 2 weeks after completed treatment the flare reaction to allergen exposure had fully recovered (Fig. 9) (Lundblad et al., 1986a). The subjective sensation (itching) accompanying the release of mediators in the allergic reaction was also reduced after capsaicin treatment of the human skin (Lundblad et al., 1986a).

This implies that associated reflexes upon allergic manifestations in the airway mucosa, such as sneezing and exocrine secretion, may also be reduced after capsaicin treatment and damage of the afferent pathways.

Bradykinin is produced by local tissue damage and subsequently activates C-fiber afferents (Kaufman et al., 1980), which at least in the rat seem to be capsaicin-sensitive (Lundberg and Saria, 1983). Furthermore, bradykinin releases the tachykinins from lung afferents (Saria et al., 1986b) and the pupillary contractile response to bradykinin in the eye, can be blocked by SP antagonists (Wahlestedt et al., 1984). It is interesting that bradykinin has potent bronchoconstrictor effects when inhaled by asthmatic subjects but very little effect in normal persons (Simonsson et al., 1973). Furthermore, bradykinin has only minor effects on isolated human bronchi in vitro, suggesting an indirect nervous action in vivo (Fuller et al., 1986).

Leukotrienes are very potent agents for inducing protein extravasation in the airway mucosa (Hua et al., 1985a) and constricting the bronchial smooth muscle (see Dahlén, 1983). However, available evidence does not suggest that the protein extravasation or bronchoconstrictor response to LTC_4 in the guinea pig is reduced after capsaicin treatment.

Is there any evidence that the drugs presently used for treatment of allergic reactions specifically influence sensory neuropeptide mechanisms or the activity of capsaicin-sensitive nerves? It has been reported that disodium chromoglycate (DSCG) inhibits capsaicin-induced activation of C-fiber afferents in the lower airways of the dog (Dixon et al., 1979). A slight reduction of capsaicin-induced sneezings was also seen in the guinea pig after local DSCG application to the nasal mucosa (Lundblad et al., 1984a). In the rat, however, DSCG did not influence the protein-extravasation response to cigarette smoke, which is dependent on capsaicin-sensitive nerves (Lundberg et al., 1983c). Furthermore, the response of lower airways to inhalation of capsaicin in humans is not reduced by pretreatment with DSCG (Fuller et al., 1985). Evidently, capsaicin treatment performed locally can be used at least in human skin to reduce local vascular reactions and possibly also reflex responses to allergens (Lundblad et al., 1985b, 1986a). However, this inhibitory effect of capsaicin treatment was more short-lasting compared to the apparent irreversible effect in the guinea pig (Lundberg et al., 1983a; Lundblad et al., 1985a). With regard to capsaicin treatment of the airway mucosa, whether loss of capsaicin-sensitive mechanisms is beneficial or not is a crucial question. Thus, both local and centrally mediated reflexes are likely to be of importance in protecting against inhalation or reduce the toxic effects of irritants. Under pathophysiological conditions, however, reflex mechanisms may be hypersensitive and exaggerated and have a negative influence when activated in allergic reactions.

In conclusion, capsaicin-sensitive C-fiber afferents in the airways (and other organs) have been characterized both with regard to the release of local bioactive peptides and the importance in local and reflex responses to irritant chemicals and mediators of the allergen reaction. It seems likely that a more complete understanding of the functional importance of these nerves will also help to reveal the pathophysiology of airway disorders.

Acknowledgments

The present studies have been supported by grants from the Swedish Medical Research Council (14X-6554, 17X-5438, 03X-07464, 04X-2887), the American Council for Tobacco Research, the Swedish Tobacco Company, Petrus och Augusta Hedlunds Stiftelse, the Swedish Work Environmental Fund, funds from the Karolinska Institute, and the Austrian Scientific Research Funds (5605). For expert secretarial help, we thank Mrs Hilka Lindberg.

Discussion

Burnstock. In addition to sensory neuropeptides it is likely that ATP is also involved in axon reflexes (Jahr and Jessel, *Nature* **304**:730-733, 1983.

Lundberg. ATP may be coreleased but the marked inhibitory effect of SP antagonists on the protein extravasation response indicates a key role for techykinins.

Makhlouf. In airway smooth muscle the order of potency neurokinin A and SP suggests that the subclass of receptor differs from that in intestinal muscle.

Lundberg. In human bronchi neurokinin A is more potent than SP, suggesting an SP-E receptor, but in pulmonary vessels tachykinins have a similar potency, suggesting SP-P receptors.

Nadel. Could the differences in potency be due to differences or degradation of tachykinins?

Lundberg. Even if the metabolic degradation of neurokinin A and SP is not similar, a 100-fold difference in potency in human bronchi is less likely to depend on differences in metabilism.

Persson. SP antagonists are active in the same concentration range to inhibit bronchoconstriction by nerve stimulation and exogenous neurokinin A, but larger concentrations are necessary to inhibit SP. This suggests, together with the observation that neurokinin A is more potent, that the SP-E receptors is more important.

Makhlouf. In guinea pig intestine the order of potency of tachykinins in eliciting direct contraction is different from that causing acetylcholine release, suggesting different receptor subtypes on nerves and muscles.

Barnes. Are SP-immunoreactive nerves found in distal airways of humans?

Lundberg. SP nerves are found in small bronchioles, although in relatively low numbers in humans.

Nadel. Are there species differences? The increase in airway vascular permeability with electrical stimulation of the vagus occurs within seconds and remains for only a short time. Does this indicate tachyphylaxis?

Lundberg. There are species differences since, while antidromic stimulation produces flare in most species, protein extravasation occurs in guinea pigs and rats, but not cats and dogs. In human skin capsaicin induces flare but not wheal. We have not studied the time course.

Persson. In guinea pig trachea we observe the maximum effect of capsaicin-induced microvascular leakage within 1-3 min, and then recovery. Addition of other mediators is then necessary to keep the leaky gaps open.

Bousquet. Does SP cause bronchoconstriction in humans in vivo?

Barnes. We have looked at the effect of intravenously administered SP in humans, including asthmatic subjects, and no significant bronchoconstriction occurs. However, the profound cardiovascular effects of this peptide limit the dose which can be given. Similarly, by inhalation, we have not seen any effect even with high doses (1 mg), suggesting breakdown or difficulty in diffusing across airway epithelium (Fuller et al., *Thorax* **40**:714, 1985).

References

Baker, A. P., Hillegass, L. M., Holden, D. A., and Smith, W. J. (1977). Effect of kallidin, substance P and other basic polypeptides on the production of respiratory macromolecules. *Am. Rev. Respir. Dis.* **115**:811-817.

Bernstein, J. E., Swift, R. M., Soltani, K., and Lorincz, A. L. (1981). Inhibition of axon reflex vasodilatation by topically applied capsaicin. *J. Invest. Dermatol.* **76**:394-395.

Brain, S. D., and Williams, T. J. (1985). Inflammatory oedema induced by synergism between calcitonin gene-related peptide (CGRP) and mediators of increased vascular permeability. *Br. J. Pharmacol.* **86**:855-860.

Brimijoin, S., Lundberg, J. M., Brodin, E., Hökfelt, T., and Nilsson, G. (1980). Aconal transport of substance P in the vagus and sciatic nerves of the guinea-pig. *Brain Res.* **191**:443-457.

Coleridge, J. C. G., and Coleridge, H. M. (1984). Afferent vagal C-fibre innervation of the lung and airways and its functional significance. *Rev. Physiol. Biochem. Pharmacol.* **99**:1-110.

Collier, J. G., and Fuller, R. W. (1984). Capsaicin inhalation in man and the effects of sodium chromoglycate. *Br. J. Pharmacol.* **81**:113-117.

Dahlén, S.-E. (1983). Pulmonary effects of leucotrienes. *Acta Physiol. Scand.* **118**(Suppl. 512):1-52.

Dalsgaard, C.-J., and Lundberg, J. M. (1984). Vagal and spinal afferent innervation of the guinea-pig lower respiratory tract as studied by the HRP-technique. *Neurosci. Letts.* **45**:117-122.

Davies, B., Roberts, A. M., Coleridge, H. M., and Coleridge, J. C. G. (1982). Reflex tracheal gland secretion evoked by stimulation of bronchial C-fibres in dogs. *J. Appl. Physiol.* **53**:985-991.

Dixon, M., Jackson, D. M., and Richards, I. M. (1979). The effect of sodium chromoglycate on lung irritant receptors and left ventricular receptors in anesthetized dog. *Br. J. Pharmacol.* **67**:569-574.

Edvinsson, L., Fredholm, B. B., Hamel, E., Janson, I., and Verreuhia, C. (1985). Perivascular peptides relax cerebral arteries concomitant with stimulation of cyclic adenosine monophosphate accumulation or release of an endothelium derived relaxing factor in the cat. *Neurosci. Letts.* **58**:213-217.

Fischer, L. A., Kikkawa, D. O., Rivier, J., Amara, S., Evans, R., Rosenfeld, M., Vale, W., and Brown, M. R. (1983). Stimulation of noradrenergic sympathetic outflow by calcitonin gene-related peptide. *Nature (Lond.)* **305**: 534-536.

Fuller, R. W., Dixon, C. M. S., and Barnes, P. J. (1985). The bronchoconstrictor response to inhaled capsaicin in humans. *J. Appl. Physiol.* **85**:1080-1084.

Fuller, R. W., Dixon, C. M. S., Cuss, F., and Barnes, P. J. (1986). In vivo and in vitro assessment of bradykinin induced bronchoconstriction in humans. *Am. Rev. Respir. Dis.* in press.

Furchchott, R. F. (1983). Role of endothelium in responses of vascular smooth muscle. *Circ. Res.* **35**:557-573.

Gamse, R., and Saria, A. (1985). Potentiation of tachykinin-induced plasma Protein extravasation by calcitonin gene-related peptide. *Eur. J. Pharmacol.* **114**:61-66.

Gamse, R., Molnar, A., and Lembeck, F. (1979). Substance P release from spinal cord slices by capsaicin. *Life Sci.* **25**:629-636.

Gamse, R., Martling, C.-R., Saria, A., and Lundberg, J. J. (1986). Bronchial cardiovascular and secretory responses after central administration of capsaicin in the guinea-pig. *Naunyn Schmiedebergs Arch. Pharmacol.* in press.

Hägermark, O., Hökfelt, T., and Pernow, B. (1978). Flare and itch induced by substance P in human skin. *J. Invest. Dermatol.* **71**:233-235.

Heavery, D., Fuller, R. W., Barnes, P. J., and Dollery, C. T. (1985). Histamine, substance P and neurogenic flare in human skin. *Clin. Sci.* **88**:23.

Hua, X.-Y., and Lundberg, J. M. (1986). Dual capsaicin effects on ureteral motility: Low dose inhibition mediated by calcitonin gene-related peptide and high dose stimulation by tachykinins. *Acta Physiol. Scand.* submitted.

Hua, X.-Y., Dahlén, S.-E., Lundberg, J. M., Hammarström, S., and Hedqvist, P. (1985a). Leucotrienes C_4, D_4 and E_4 cause widespread and extensive plasma extravasation in the guinea-pig. *Naunyn Schmiedebergs Arch. Pharmacol.* **330**:136-141.

Hua, X.-Y., Theodorsson-Norheim, E., Brodin, E., Lundberg, J. M., and Hökfelt, T. (1985b). Multiple tachykinins (neurokinin A, neuropeptide K and substance P) in capsaicin-sensitive sensory neurons in the guinea-pig. *Regul. Peptides* **13**:1-19.

Hua, X.-Y., Saria, A., Gamse, R., Theodorsson-Norheim, E., Brodin, E., and Lundberg, J. M. (1986). Capsaicin-induced release of multiple tachykinins (substance P, neurokinin A and eledoisin-like material) from guinea-pig spinal cord and ureter. *Neuroscience* in press.

Jancsó, N., Jancsó-Gabor, A., Szolcsanyi, I. (1968). The role of sensory nerve endings in neurogenic inflammation induced in human skin and in the eye and paw of the rat. *Br. J. Pharmacol. Chemother.* **32**:31-41.

Jancsó, G., Király, E., and Jancsó-Gabor, A. (1977). Pharmacologically induced selective degeneration of chemosensitive primary sensory neurons. *Nature* **270**:741-743.

Jancsó, G., Hökfelt, T., Lundberg, J. M., Kiraly, E., Halasz, N., Nilsson, G., Terenius, L., Rehfeld, J., Steinbusch, H., Verhofstad, H., Elde, R., Said, S., and Brown, M. (1981). Immunohistochemical studies on the effect of capsaicin on spinal and medullary peptide and monoamine neurons using antisera to substance P, gastrin/CCK, somatostatin, VIP, enkephalin, neurotensin and 5-hydroxytryptamine. *J. Neurocytol.* **10**:963-980.

Karlsson, J. A., and Persson, C. G. A. (1985). Effects of different substance P analogues on tachykinin-induced contraction of airway smooth muscle. In *Tachykinin Antagonists.* Edited by R. Håkanson and F. Sundler. New York, Elsevier North-Holland, pp. 181-188.

Karlsson, J. A., Finney, M. B., Persson, C. G. A., and Post, C. (1984). Substance P antagonists and the role of tachykinins in noncholinergic bronchoconstriction. *Life Sci.* **35**:2681-2691.

Kaufman, M. P., Coleridge, H. M., Coleridge, J. C. G., and Baker, D. G. (1980). Bradykinin stimulates afferent vagal C-fibres in intrapulmonary airways of dogs. *J. Appl. Physiol.* **48**:511-517.

Lembeck, F., and Holzer, P. (1979). Substance P as neurogenic mediator of antidromic vasodilatation and neurogenic plasma extravasation. *Naunyn Schmiedebergs Arch. Pharmacol.* **310**:175-183.

Lundberg, J. M., and Saria, A. (1982a). Capsaicin-sensitive vagal neurons involved in control of vascular permeability in rat trachea. *Acta Physiol. Scand.* **115**:521-523.

Lundberg, J. M., and Saria, A. (1982b). Bronchial smooth muscle contraction induced by stimulation of capsaicin-sensitive vagal sensory neurons. *Acta Physiol. Scand.* **116**:473-476.

Lundberg, J. M., and Saria, A. (1983). Capsaicin induced desensitization of the airway mucosa to cigarette smoke, mechanical and chemical irritants. *Nature* **302**:251-253.

Lundberg, J. M., Brodin, E., and Saria, A. (1983a). Effects and distribution of vagal capsaicin-sensitive substance P neurons with special reference to the trachea and lungs. *Acta Physiol. Scand.* **119**:243-252.

Lundberg, J. M., Martling, C.-R., and Saria, A. (1983b). Substance P and capsaicin induced bronchial smooth muscle contraction in human airways. *Acta Physiol. Scand.* **119**:49-53.

Lundberg, J. M., Martling, C.-R., Saria, A., Folkers, K., and Rosell, S. (1983c). Cigarette smoke induced oedema due to activation of capsaicin-sensitive vagal afferents and substance P release. *Neuroscience* **10**:1361-1368.

Lundberg, J. M., Saria, A., Brodin, E., Rosell, S., and Folkers, K. (1983d). A substance P antagonist inhibits vagally induced increase in vascular permeability and bronchial smooth muscle contraction in the guinea-pig. *Proc. Natl. Acad. Sci.* **80**:1120-1124.

Lundberg, J. M., Saria, A., and Martling, C.-R. (1983e). Capsaicin pretreatment abolishes cigarette smoke-induced oedema in rat tracheobronchial mucosa. *Eur. J. Pharmacol.* **86**:317-318.

Lundberg, J. M., Brodin, E., Hua, X.-Y., and Saria, A. (1984a). Vascular permeability changes and smooth muscle contraction in relation to capsaicin-sensitive substance P afferents in the guinea-pig. *Acta Physiol. Scand.* **120**:217-227.

Lundberg, J. M., Hökfelt, T., Martling, C.-R., Saria, A., and Cuello, C. (1984b). Sensory substance P-immunoreactive nerves in the lower respiratory tract of various mammals including man. *Cell Tissue Res.* **235**:251-261.

Lundberg, J. M., Franco-Cereceda, A., Hua, X.-Y., Hökfelt, T., and Fischer, J. A. (1985a). Co-existence of substance P and calcitonin gene-related peptide immunoreactivities in sensory nerves in relation to cardiovascular and bronchoconstrictor effects of capsaicin. *Eur. J. Pharmacol.* **108**:315-319.

Lundberg, J. M., Saria, A., Theodorsson-Norheim, E., Brodin, E., Hua, X.-Y., Martling, C.-R., Gamse, R., and Hökfelt, T. (1985b). Multiple tachykinins in capsaicin-sensitive afferents: occurrence, release and biological effects with special reference to irritation of the airways. In *Tachykinin Antagonists.* Edited by R. Håkanson and F. Sundler, New York, Elsevier North-Holland, pp. 159-169.

Lundblad, L., and Lundberg, J. M. (1984). Cigarette smoke-induced nasal irritation by vapour-phase activation of capsaicin-sensitive neurons. *Toxicology* **33**:1-7.

Lundblad, L., Änggård, A., and Lundberg, J. M. (1983a). Effects of antidromic trigeminal nerve stimulation in relation to sympathetic vasodilation in cat nasal mucosa. *Acta Physiol. Scand.* **119**:7-13.

Lundblad, L., Lundberg, J. M., Brodin, E., and Änggård, A. (1983b). Origin and distribution of capsaicin-sensitive substance P-immunoreactive nerves in the nasal mucosa. *Acta Otolaryngol.* **96**:485-493.

Lundblad, L., Saria, A., Lundberg, J. M., and Änggård, A. (1983c). Increased vascular permeability in rat nasal mucosa induced by substance P and stimulation of capsaicin-sensitive trigeminal neurons. *Acta Orolaryngol.* **96**:479-484.

Lundblad, L., Lundberg, J. M., and Änggård, A. (1984a). Local and systemic capsaicin pretreatment inhibits sneezing and nasal mucosal permeability increase to certain chemical irritants. *Naunyn Schmiedebergs Arch. Pharmacol.* **326**: 254-261.

Lundblad, L., Lundberg, J. M., and Hua, X.-Y. (1984b). Mechanism for reflexive hypertension induced by local application of capsaicin and nicotine to the nasal mucosa. *Acta Physiol. Scand.* **121**:277-282.

Lundblad, L., Brodin, E., Lundberg, J. M., and Änggård, A. (1985a). Effects of nasal capsaicin pretreatment and cryosurgery on sneezing reflexes, neurogenic plasma extravasation, sensory and sympathetic neurons in guinea-pig nasal mucosa. *Acta Otolaryngol.* **100**:117-127.

Lundblad, L., Lundberg, J. M., Änggård, A., and Zetterström, O. (1985b). Capsaicin pretreatment inhibits the flare component of the cutaneous allergic reaction in man. *Eur. J. Pharmacol.* **113**:461-462.

Lundblad, L., Lundberg, J. M., Änggård, A., and Zetterström, O. (1986a). Capsaicin-sensitive nerves and the cutaneous allergy reaction in man: possible involvement of sensory neuropeptides in the flare reaction. *Allergy* submitted.

Lundblad, L., Stjärne, P., Lundberg, J. M., and Änggård, A. (1986b). Vasodilator effects of tachykinins and calcitonin gene-related peptide in cat nasal mucosa. *Acta Otolaryngol.* submitted.

Martling, C.-R., Saria, A., Andersson, P., and Lundberg, J. M. (1984). Capsaicin pretreatment inhibits vagal cholinergic and noncholinergic control of airway mechanic in the guinea-pig. *Naunyn Schmiedebergs Arch. Pharmacol* **325**:343-348.

Martling, C.-R., Gazelius, B., and Lundberg, J. M. (1986a). Vagal nervous control of blood flow in cat tracheal mucosa. *Acta Physiol. Scand.* in press.

Martling, C.-R., Saria, A., Yan, T., Lundberg, J. M., Fischer, J. A., and Hökfelt, T. (1986b). Calcitonin gene-related peptide and the lung: coexistence with substance P, release by capsaicin and biological effects. *Peptides,* submitted.

Martling, C.-R., Theodorsson-Norheim, E., and Lundberg. J. M. (1986c). Occurrence and effects of multiple tachykinins (substance P, neurokinin A and neuropeptide K) on human bronchi. *Life Sciences* submitted.

Nilsson, G., Dahlberg, K., Brodin, E., Sundler, F., and Strandberg, K. (1977). Distribution and constrictor effects of substance P in guinea-pig tracheobronchial tissue. In *Substance P.* Edited by U. S. von Euler and B. Pernow. New York, Raven Press, pp. 57-61.

Palmer, J. B., Cuss, F. M., and Mulderry, P. K. (1985). Calcitonin gene-related peptide is localized to human airway nerves and potently constricts human airway smooth muscle. *Thorax* **40**:713.

Payan, G. P., Levine, J. D., and Goetzl, E. J. (1984). Modulation of immunity and hypersensitivity by sensory neuropeptides. *J. Immunol.* **132**:1601-1604.

Persson, C. G. A., Erjefält, I., and Karlsson, J.-A. (1985). Effects of tachykinins and tachykinin antagonists on the tracheobronchial microcirculation. In *Tachykinin Antagonists.* Edited by R. Håkanson and S. Sundler. New York, Elsevier North-Holland, pp. 171-179.

Saria, A., Lundberg, J. M., Skofitsch, G., and Lembeck, F. (1983). Vascular protein leakage in various tissues induced by substance P, capsaicin, bradykinin, serotonin, histamine and by antigen challenge. *Naunyn Schmiedebergs Arch. Pharmacol.* **324**:212-218.

Saria, A., Theodorsson-Norheim, E., Gamse, R., and Lundberg, J. M. (1984). Release of substance P and substance K-like immunoreactivities from the isolated perfused guinea-pig lung. *Eur. J. Pharmacol.* **106**:207-208.

Saria, A., Martling, C.-R., Dalsgaard, C.-J., and Lundberg, J. M. (1985a). Evidence for substance P-immunoreactive spinal afferents that mediate bronchoconstriction. *Acta Physiol. Scand.* **125**:407-414.

Saria, A., Ma, R. C., and Dun, N. J. (1985b). Neurokinin A depolarizes neurons of the guinea-pig inferior mesenteric ganglia. *Neurosci. Letts.* **60**:145-150.

Saria, A., Gamse, R., Petermann, J., Fischer, J. A., Theodorsson-Norheim, E., and Lundberg, J. M. (1986a). Simultaneous release of several tachykinins and calcitonin gene-related peptide from rat spinal cord slices. *Neurosci. Letts.* **63**:310-314.

Saria, A., Martling, C.-R., Theodorsson-Norheim, E., and Lundberg, J. M. (1986b). Release of multiple tachykinins from sensory nerves in the lung by bradykinin, histamine, nicotine and vagal nerve stimulation. *Am. Rev. Respir. Dis.* submitted.

Sigrist, S., Franco-Cereceda, A., Henke, H., Lundberg, J. M., and Fischer, J. A. (1986). Cardiovascular effects of calcitonin gene-related peptide are mediated by a specific receptor and activation of adenylate cyclase. *Endocrinology* in press.

Simonsson, B. G., Skoogh, B. F., Bergh, N. P., Andersson, R., and Svedmyr, N. (1973). In vivo and in vitro effects of bradykinin on bronchial motor tone in normal subjects and in patients with airway obstruction. *Respiration* **30**:377-388.

Sydbom, A. (1982). Histamine release from isolated rat mast cells by neurotensin and other peptides. *Agents Actions* **12**:91-93.

Szolcsanyi, J. (1984). Capsaicin and neurogenic inflammation: history and early findings. In *Antidromic Vasodilatation and Neurogenic Inflammation.* Edited by L. A. Chahl, J. Szolcsanyi, and F. Lembeck, Hung. Acad. Scipp., pp. 27-55.

Tatemoto, K., Lundberg, J. M., Jörwall, M., and Mutt, V. (1985). Neuropeptide K: isolation, structure and biological activities of a novel brain tachykinin. *Biochim. Biophys. Res. Commun.* **128**:947-953.

Yanagisawa, M., Otsuka, M., Konishi, S., Agaki, H., Folkers, K., and Rosell, S. (1982). A substance P antagonist inhibits a slow reflex response in the spinal cord of the newborn rat. *Acta Physiol. Scand.* **116**:109-111.

Wahlestedt, C., Bynke, G., and Håkanson, R. (1984). Pupillary constriction by bradykinin and capsaicin: mode of action. *Eur. J. Pharmacol.* **106**: 577-583.

Widdicombe, J. (1981). Nervous receptors in the respiratory tract and lungs. In *Lung Biology in Health and Disease,* Vol. 17. Part I. *Regulation of Breathing.* Edited by T. Hornbein, pp. 429-472.

17

Influence of Neurohormones and Neuropeptides on Mast Cells

KASPAR SERTL* and MICHAEL A. KALINER

National Institute of Allergy and Infectious Diseases
Bethesda, Maryland

When allergic asthmatics inhale allergens towards which they have IgE antibodies directed, mast cells are stimulated to release or generate the mediators of anaphylaxis (Table 1). These mediators cause the responses leading to asthma: smooth muscle contraction, mucosal edema, airway inflammation, and mucus secretion as well as contributing to the airway denudation, basement membrane thickening, and goblet cell hyperplasia also characteristic of asthma (Table 2). In this chapter we shall focus on the mast cell and the effect of neurohormones and neuropeptides on the release of the mediators of allergy. Neurohormones of the autonomic nervous system have been studied for more than a decade and much is known of their actions, while the data on neuropeptides are currently evolving. The capacity of these agents to modulate and stimulate mast cell degranulation will be our major focus. Whenever possible, this information will be applied to our knowledge of the relationship between mast cells and asthma.

**Present affiliation*: Max Kade Institute, Vienna, Austria

Table 1 Mast-Cell-Derived Mediators

Preformed, rapidly eluted under physiological conditions
Histamine
Eosinophil chemotactic factors of anaphylaxis (ECF-A)
Neutrophil chemotactic factors (NCF)
Dexoglycosidase[a] (beta-hexosaminidase, beta-D-galactosidase, beta-glucuronidase)
Serotonin[a]
Kininogenase
Arylsulfatase A
Secondary or newly generated mediators
Superoxide anions
Slow-reacting substances of anaphylaxis (SRS-A): LTC, LTD, LTE
Prostaglandins
Monohydroxyeicosatetraenoic acids (HETEs)
Hydroperoxyeicosatetraenoic acids (HPETEs)
Hydroxyheptadecatrienoic acid (HHT)
Thromboxanes
Platelet-activating factor (PAF)
Prostaglandin-generating factor of anaphylaxis (PGF-A)
Preformed granule-associated mediators
Heparin
Chymotrypsin/trypsin
Peroxidase[a]
Superoxidase dismutase
Arylsulfatase B
Inflammatory factors of anaphylaxis (IF-A)[a]

[a]Demonstrated in nonhuman mast cells.

Table 2 Pathologic Changes in Asthma and the Mediators Possibly Responsible

Feature	Proposed Mediator
Bronchospasm	Histamine (H_1 response)
	SRS-A (LTC_4, LTD_4, LTE_4)
	Prostaglandins and thromboxane A_2
	Platelet-activating factor (PAF)
	Acetylcholine
	Bradykinin
Mucosal edema	Histamine (H_1 response)
	SRS-A (LTC_4, LTD_4, LTE_4)
	PGE
	PAF
	Bradykinin
Cellular infiltration (airway hyperreactivity)	Eosinophil chemotactic factors
	Neutrophil chemotactic factors
	Inflammatory factors of anaphylaxis (IF-A)
	HETEs
	LTB_4
Mucus secretion	Histamine (H_2 response)
	Acetylcholine
	Alpha-adrenergic agonists
	Prostaglandins
	HETEs
	SRS-A (LTC_4, LTD_4, LTE_4)
	Macrophage mucus secretagogue (MMS)
	Prostaglandin-generating factor of anaphylaxis (PGF-A)
Desquamation	O_2^-, H_2O_2, OH^-
	Proteolytic enzymes
Basement membrane	O_2^-
Thickening	Proteolytic enzymes

I. Influence of Neurohormones on Mast Cells: Adrenergic Agonists

Mast cells are found in the connective tissue throughout the lung: mast cells constitute about 0.5-1% of the cells in the airway lumen and about 50% of total lung mast cells are found in the submucosa of the airways, while the rest are found in the interalveolar septa. Mast cells are frequently found near nerves, are characteristically one of the cells found in the sheaths of myelinated nerves, and may even be directly innervated (Seyle, 1965; Newson et al., 1983; Skofitsch et al., 1985). However, it is more likely that mast cells may be influenced by neurohormones or neuropeptides reaching the connective tissue from the circulation or from local release from nerve endings or neuroepithelial bodies.

Most of the work to be reviewed has been done on isolated rat peritoneal mast cells or on whole lung preparations of human or rodent tissue. With the recent realization of mast cell heterogeneity (Barrett and Metcalfe, 1987), the existing data on the influence of neurohormones and neuropeptides on mast cells may require reanalysis. For example, all of the studies on human lung mast cell responses in vitro was performed before the recognition of varied mast cell populations. However, recent in vivo studies in humans and dog models of asthma suggest that the earlier in vitro lung studies were accurate.

The classic concept of the autonomic nerve system includes the sympathetic and the parasympathetic nervous systems, with norepinephrine and acetylcholine as the respective neurotransmitters. Under normal conditions, norepinephrine is found only in nerves while epinephrine circulates as a hormone and is not found in nerve fibers. Direct examination of bronchial tissue from a variety of experimental mammals stained specifically for the presence of norepinephrine reveals that the adrenergic supply to bronchial mucosa and musculature is sparse, while that to the nearby vasculature is rich (Mann, 1971), suggesting that the direct action of sympathetic hormones at the level of the bronchial muscle and mucosa is relatively weak. In 1982 some noradrenergic fibers were described for the first time in human bronchial muscles (Partanen et al., 1982). An alternative mechanism for the adrenergic nervous system to modulate bronchial smooth muscle tone might involve inhibitory influences at the level of the parasympathetic ganglion. (McNeill, 1964).

Clinicians have traditionally used adrenergic agonists and cholinergic antagonists for the treatment of asthma. While adrenergic agonists have been generally thought to act as bronchodilators by relaxing smooth muscles, it was observed in 1936 that epinephrine was capable of preventing allergic skin test reactions in humans (Tuft and Brodsky, 1936), while isoproterenol prevented antigen induced histamine release from guinea pig lung in vitro (Schild, 1936). With the knowledge that adrenergic agents were capable of stimulating increases in cyclic AMP in many tissues, the explanation for these earlier observations became obvious. Assem and Schild in 1969 showed that epinephrine prevented the release of histamine during anaphylactic stimulation of isolated human lung. These results were extended by demonstrating a direct relationship between the capacity of beta-agonists to inhibit the immunologic release of histamine and slow-reacting substance from human lung fragments and increase total lung cyclic AMP (Orange et al., 1971a). In the last decade, the relationship between increases in cyclic AMP and the capacity of immunologic stimulation to cause mast cell degranulation has been extended to a variety of models both in vivo and in vitro. This work has recently been extended to preparations of purified human lung mast cells (Peters et al., 1982).

In addition to adrenergic agonists, other agents capable of raising lung cyclic AMP may also influence mast cell reactivity. These agents include cyclic AMP itself, prostaglandin E_1 and E_2 (Tauber et al., 1973), methylxanthines and other inhibitors of phosphodiesterase (Orange et al., 1971b), and cholera toxin (Kaliner et al., 1973). Studies involving cyclic nucleotide changes in purified mast cells have used rat peritoneal mast cells and have analyzed the effect of cyclic AMP active agents on both immunologically and nonimmunologically induced degranulation. Beta-adrenergic stimulation either fails to increase isolated rat peritoneal mast cell cyclic AMP (Kaliner and Austen, 1974) or increases cyclic AMP without inhibition of histamine release (Sullivan and Parker, 1976; Marquardt and Wassermann, 1982). Moreover, mast cells have been demonstrated to have high-affinity beta$_2$-adrenergic receptors on their cell surface and on perigranular membranes (Donlon et al., 1982; Marquardt and Wassermann, 1982; Hughes et al., 1983; Undem and Buckner, 1984). These observations taken together suggest that mast cells, once purified, uncouple their beta-adrenerigic/adenylate cyclase systems or that subcellular pools of cyclic AMP are stimulated by beta-adrenergic agonists that do not affect secretion. The capacity of beta-adrenergic agonists to inhibit rat peritoneal mast cell secretion in vivo (Koopman et al., 1970) suggests that uncoupling occurs during the process of mast cell isolation.

Only recently has the effect of sympathetic nerve stimulation in vivo on mast cell secretion been studied. Lazarus et al. (1979) challenged *Ascaris*-sensitive dogs in vivo with antigen and monitored histamine release before sacrificing the animals and measuring lung cyclic nucleotide levels. Release of mast cell mediators stimulated a rise in cyclic AMP and cyclic GMP in vivo as had been seen in human lung tissue in vitro (Platshon and Kaliner, 1978). Infusion of isoproterenol into the dogs increased lung cyclic AMP and reduced *Ascaris*-induced histamine release. Thus exogenous beta-agonists in dogs appeared to have the same actions in vivo as they had in vitro. More recently Garrity et al. (1985) demonstrated that sympathetic nerve stimulation during *Ascaris* challenge completely inhibited both mast cell degranulation and smooth muscle constriction in the same dog model. Thus endogenous beta-adrenergic discharge through nerve stimulation is also capable of inhibiting mast cell reactivity. Finally these studies have recently been extended to human asthmatics. Howarth et al. (1985) demonstrated that cromolyn, an agent that stabilizes mast cells and prevents antigen-induced asthma, not only inhibited experimental asthma in allergic asthmatics but also prevented concomitant increases in plasma histamine. In the same experiment, the $beta_2$-adrenergic agonist albuterol also prevented both bronchial obstruction and histamine release. Thus, exogenous beta adrenergic agonists act not only as bronchodilators but also to inhibit mast cell reactions in humans in vivo, confirming the data from in vivo and in vitro model systems.

The alpha-adrenergic agonist norepinephrine was found to increase human lung cyclic AMP and inhibit antigen-induced mast cell degranulation (Orange et al., 1971b). The capacity of propranolol to prevent both of these effects suggested that norepinephrine was acting as a beta-adrenergic agonist. The combination of norepinephrine plus propranolol reduced total lung cyclic AMP in association with enhanced mast cell mediator release. Phenylephrine also augmented mediator release in association with reduced cyclic AMP levels; these effects were prevented by phentolamine. Thus it appeared that selected alpha-adrenergic stimulation might facilitate mast cell reactivity.

These data suggest the possibility that mast cells have alpha-adrenergic receptors on their surface. Very few studies have examined this issue: rat peritoneal mast cells appear to have alpha-adrenergic receptors (Taniguchi et al., 1980), as do Furth mastocytoma cells (Moroni et al., 1977), while dog mastocytoma cells do not (Phillips et al., 1985). The importance of alpha-adrenergic influences in human asthma is unclear. A number of studies demonstrate that alpha-adrenergic antagonists given systemically or by inhalation are capable of preventing experimentally induced asthma. Moreover, there are several anecdotal reports of inhaled phentolamine in the treatment of asthma (Gross et al., 1974; Patel and Kerr, 1975; Black et al., 1978). However, most clinical trials of phentolamine in asthma have been unimpressive and there is some doubt that alpha-adrenergic discharge contributes to asthma.

The parasympathetic neurohormone acetylcholine, as well as carbachol, were found to enhance the immunologic release of mediators from human lung tissue (Kaliner et al., 1972). These agents were active in a physiological dose range(10^{-9}-10^{-12} M) and their effect was prevented by atropine, indicating the likely presence of muscarinic receptors on human lung mast cells. These data were extended to demonstrate a close relationship between carbachol-induced increases in total lung cyclic GMP and enhancement of the immunologic release of mediators (Kaliner, 1977a). In these studies, exposure of human lung to cholinergic agonists failed to stimulate mediator release, but instead facilitated immunologically stimulated mast cell degranulation.

Again very few studies have been reported analyzing the presence of cholinergic receptors on mast cells. One group has claimed the presence of muscarinic receptors on rat mast cells (Masini et al., 1983), while Phillips et al. (1985) failed to find such receptors on canine mastocytoma cells.

Antigen challenge of *Ascaris*-sensitive dogs causes bronchial constriction, which may be significantly reduced by atropine or cooling the vagus nerve (Gold et al., 1972). Antigen challenge causes stimulation of C-fibers, which might initiate a reflex arc resulting in vagally mediated muscle constriction (Sampson and Vidruk, 1975). Thus it appeared that canine asthma might be largely parasympathetic. However, not all investigators have been able to reproduce these findings (Krell et al., 1976). In humans, the effect of atropine appears to be largely as a bronchodilator, without a major effect on allergen-induced asthma or histamine release (Rosenthal et al., 1977; Fish et al., 1977; Howarth et al., 1985). Unfortunately, no analysis of the effect of cholinomimetics or vagal stimulation upon antigen-induced mediator release could be found in the literature.

The possible mechanisms by which alterations in cyclic AMP or cyclic GMP levels may influence mast cell degranulation include modulation of membrane-associated phospholipid methylation (Hirata and Axelrod, 1980; Ishizaka, 1981), suppression of membrane phospholipid turnover (Kennerly et al., 1979), and alterations in microtubule function (Kaliner, 1977b). An additional mechanism includes phosphorylation of essential proteins through activation of cyclic-AMP-dependent protein kinases (Holgate et al., 1980). Thus beta-adrenergic agents may interact with their appropriate receptor, stimulate phospholipid methylation, and increase membrane fluidity, facilitating receptor coupling to adenylate cyclase activation. Once hormone, receptor, and enzyme are combined, however, full activation of cyclase is also dependent on the presence of guanyl nucleotides and divalent cations such as magnesium and calcium (Steer, 1977).

Kinetic analysis of mast cells undergoing immunologically induced degranulation indicates that there is an initial reduction in total cyclic AMP associated with a depletion in cellular ATP (Kaliner and Austen, 1974). Subsequent investigators have demonstrated an earlier rise in cAMP followed by reductions (Sullivan et al., 1975a,b; Sullivan and Parker, 1976) or a biphasic elevation not accompanied by a reduction (Lewis et al., 1979). Thus, it is not possible to state definitely the relationship between mast cell cyclic AMP levels and secretion.

II. Influence of Neuropeptides on Mast Cells

In addition to the classic neurotransmitters, many nerves also contain neuropeptides that may function as transmitter substances. Some of the known neuro-

Table 3 Neuropeptides and Mast Cell Histamine Release

Mast cell origin	NT	SP	SST	VIP	Gastrin	Opioids
Rat peritoneum	+/–	+	+	+/[a]	–	+
Rat intestine	–	+	–	–	–	–
Rat pleura	+	+	?	?	?	?
Rat lung	?	?	?	?[a]	?	?
Rat basophilic leukemia	–	–	I/[a]	?	?	?
Monkey lung	–	+	–	–	–	–
Monkey intestine	–	+	–	–	–	–
Mouse bone-marrow-derived	?	?	I	?	?	?
Human skin	+	+	–	–	+	+
Human basophils	–	–	I/[a]	–	–	–

[a]Contains peptide.
I, inhibition of histamine release. +, activation of histamine release. ?, unknown or uncertain action. –, no activity on histamine release.

peptides are produced in neuroepithelial cells, others in autonomic nerves, and a variety of neuropeptides are found in the lung where they may act similarly to hormones. In recent years it became obvious that these neuropeptides may influence immunologic systems and particularly mast cells, but this research is still in its infancy. The published data on the influence of neuropeptides on mast cells mostly involve rat mast cells, although some work on humans and primates has been reported. Because the results for many neuropeptides are not yet confirmed, any conclusions must be drawn very cautiously, especially since the evidence strongly suggests that mast cell subtypes respond differently to the same stimulus (Table 3).

A. Neurotensin

One of the best studied peptides capable of influencing mast cells is neurotensin (NT). NT has neurotropic effects and, when applied systemically, brings about a variety of pharmacologically changes in rats: hypotension, gut contraction, increased vascular permeability, hypoinsulinemia, hyperglycemia, accentuation of the action of barbiturates, mediation of the release of prolactin and growth hormone from the pituitary, and increase in the plasma levels of adrenocorticotropin, luteinizing hormone, and follicle-stimulating hormone. Some of these actions can be reversed by the H1-histamine antagonist, diphenhydramine, suggesting a histamine-releasing effect of neurotensin on mast cells. Lazarus et al. (1977a,b) showed in specific ligand-binding experiments that neurotensin binds with its C-terminal portion to mast cells. The reaction is pH-, temperature-, and calcium-dependent. Of 18 different peptides tested, only bradykinin and xenopsin, a naturally occurring C-terminal analogue of neurotensin, were able to compete with the binding site. While this group could not find any competition of substance P for the NT-receptor, Foreman et al. (1982) proposed that NT is a partial agonist and substance P (SP) a full agonist for a common receptor. Foreman found that NT was a relatively weak histamine releaser compared to substance P. In these studies, the NT-receptor dissociation constant (1.8 μM Foreman; 0.15 μM Lazarus) was found to be quite different, perhaps because Foreman used a pure peritoneal mast cell population while Lazarus used a mixture of pleural and peritoneal mast cells. Indeed Krueger et al. (1982) demonstrated that pleural mast cells release much more histamine after NT treatment in vitro than do peritoneal mast cells. Taken together, these data suggest that pleural mast cells are distinct from peritoneal mast cells.

It is interesting that NT added simultaneously to mast cells with SP appeared to inhibit SP-induced histamine release, but had no effect on antigen- or ionophore-induced histamine release (Foreman et al., 1982). These data may indicate that NT does interact with the same receptor as SP and thereby antagonizes some SP actions. Along the same line of reasoning, Foreman found that NT partially reduced the wheal and flare reaction in human skin to SP. Thus, both NT and SP may interact with the same receptor, and their actions may vary depending on the mast cell type.

In order to address the issue of various responses by distinct mast cell subtypes, Shanahan et al. (1985) isolated rat intestinal mucosal mast cells and compared them to peritoneal cells. In their model, somatostatin was capable of causing degranulation of peritoneal cells at 10^{-6}-10^{-7} M, while vasoactive intestinal peptide (10^{-5}-10^{-6} M), and substance P (10^{-4}-10^{-5} M) were less active. NT was relatively ineffective, up to 5×10^{-4} M. The isolated mucosal mast cells were relatively unresponsive to all the agonists, although substance P (10^{-4} M) was most active. Barrett et al. (1986) compared the responses of mast cells isolated from monkey intestine or lung to substance P, NT, somatostatin, VIP, and pentagastrin. Only SP was able to induce some histamine release, with the amount released varying between individual animals.

A few studies have analyzed the effects of NT in vivo. Intradermal injection of NT increased capillary permeability and caused increased histamine release in rat skin slices. These effects are prevented by depletion of mast cell histamine with pretreatment with compound 48/80 (Cochrane et al., 1982; Carraway et al., 1982). The same investigators also demonstrated increased histamine levels after intravenous infusion of NT. Kerouac et al. (1984) found that NT infused into the rat hindquarter caused histamine release and that the C-terminal portion was responsible. NT was found to have no histamine releasing or inhibiting effect on anti-IgE challenge of basophils (Payan et al., 1984).

B. Substance P

The other neuropeptide that has been examined carefully is SP. The capacity of systemic SP to cause hypotension has been recognized since 1936 (Euler, 1936; Pernow, 1953). That this action is not solely due to a direct effect on smooth muscle was shown by Johnson and Erdoes (1973). They demonstrated that SP caused a mixture of pleural and peritoneal mast cells to release histamine. This observation was confirmed by Kitada et al. (1980), and Erjavec et al. (1981). Mazurek et al. (1981) and Fewtrell et al. (1982) demonstrated that histamine release was due to the N-terminal portion of the peptide, but that the C-terminal portion was required for the full effect. It was noted, however, that the histamine-releasing effect required a 1000-fold greater concentration of SP than that required to stimulate smooth muscles from the GI tract or secretion from the parotid gland. SP release of histamine requires intact oxidative phosphorylation and energy utilization, and the release is temperature- and pH dependent. Shibata et al. (1985) suggested that SP probably binds to negatively charged sites of membrane lipids, and subsequent penetration of the C-terminal portion into the hydrophobic core of lipid bilayer may induce an increase of membrane permeability and lead to histamine release. No effect of SP on human basophils has been observed (Payan et al., 1984).

SP induces wheal, flare, and itching in vivo on human skin (Haegermark et al., 1978; Piotrowski et al., 1984; Foreman and Jordan, 1982). The flare induced by SP is more inhibitable by antihistamines than is the wheal. Erjavec and Iskra (1984) found that carbachol, which does not cause histamine release by itself, potentiated the histamine-releasing effect of SP, suggesting a possible role of the cholinergic system in the regulation of SP responses.

Since SP-containing nerves are found throughout the body, and SP has other immunologic functions (Payan et al., 1985), it seems likely that SP may have in vivo functions in allergic reactions. Noxious stimuli may cause excitation of nerves in skin leading to antidromic release of SP, which might lead to histamine release. It is possible that such a phenomenon may apply to the lung as well.

C. Somatostatin

Although the tetradecapeptide somatostatin (SST) is best known for its inhibitory effects in somatotrophs and many other cells, it is a powerful stimulus to secretion in the rat peritoneal mast cell (Baxter and Adamik, 1978; Theoharides and Douglas, 1978, 1981). SST concentrations above 1 μg/ml are active in histamine release. Pretreatment of mast cells with dibutyryl cyclic AMP or 8-bromo-cyclic AMP substantially reduced the secretory response to SST. The data suggest that SST acts on the surface of mast cells, suggesting a receptor-mediated action. Further experiments have suggested that the orientation of the cationic moieties in SST and the mast cell secretagogue compound 48/80 could be similarly arranged spatially, thereby possibly explaining the ability of these compounds to induce mast cell secretion (Theoharides and Douglas, 1981). Diel et al. (1980) described a dose-related histamine release for synthetic cyclic SST on rat pleural mast cells, and Carraway et al. (1984) found the same for rat peritoneal cells.

In contrast to the secretory effects of SST on connective tissue mast cells, SST may actually inhibit secretion by mucosal mast cells. Renold et al. (1985) showed that SST could inhibit antigen-triggered histamine release in mouse bone-marrow-derived mast cells and rat basophilic leukemia cells. The immunologic release of LTC_4 from rat basophilic leukemia cells was also inhibited. Goetzl and Payan (1984) described reduced histamine and LTD_4 release after anti-IgE challenge of human basophils or rat basophilic cells with SST. In this study, SST had no secretagogue actions on its own. By contrast, Diel et al. (1983) studied a higher concentration of cyclic SST-14 (5×10^{-6} M) and found histamine release from basophils of allergic patients. Barrett et al. (1986) saw no effect of SST on monkey lung or intestinal mast cells. Shanahan et al. (1985) found the same for rat intestinal mast cells, while peritoneal mast cells did release histamine. Recently, SST-like substances have been found to be produced by rat basophilic leukemia cells (Goetzl et al., 1985), with the same inhibitory effect on immunologic mediator release from basophils.

D. Vasoactive Intestinal Peptide

Cutz et al. (1978) showed that rat peritoneal mast cells, rat and mouse lung mast cells, and rat intestinal mast cells contain vasoactive intestinal peptide (VIP). Undem et al. (1983) showed that VIP in high concentrations was able to inhibit antigen induced histamine release from guinea pig lung. However, because of the high concentration used (2 μM), the physiological significance of this observation is unknown. Barrett et al. (1986) was not able to induce any histamine release on monkey intestinal and lung cells by VIP. Shanahan et al. (1985) found no effect on rat intestinal mast cells, while peritoneal mast cells released histamine in response to VIP stimulation.

E. Gastrin

One study (Tharp et al., 1984) showed that gastrin and pentagastrin induced histamine release from human cutaneous mast cells. In rat peritoneal mast cells and mucosal intestinal mast cells (Shanahan et al., 1985) as well as in monkey intestinal and lung mast cells (Barrett et al., 1986), pentagastrin had no effect.

F. Bombesin

Bombesin (30 μM) in one study caused histamine release from rat peritoneal mast cells (Carraway et al., 1984), while no effect on either rat peritoneal mast cells or rat mucosal mast cells was seen in other studies (Barrett et al., 1986; Shanahan et al., 1985).

G. Opioids

Casale et al. (1984) induced mast cell degranulation in human skin by opiates and endogenous opioid peptides. Dynorphin [D-Ala^2, D-Leu^5]-enkephalin, beta-endorphin, and morphiceptin induced wheal and flare reactions in human skin in vivo. Hydroxyzine, a histamine receptor antagonist, inhibited the reactivity, suggesting that the mast cell is involved. Naloxone, a morphine receptor antagonist, blocked the morphine reaction, but not the response to dynorphin, suggesting both opiate and nonopiate receptor participation. In rat peritoneal mast cells (Shanahan et al., 1984) dynorphin, alpha-neoendorphin, and beta-endorphin had a dose-dependent histamine-releasing effect that was temperature- and energy-dependent. However, intestinal mucosal mast cells were unresponsive to opioids. Cromolyn partially blocked the secretory action. In this study naloxone blocked the reaction to opioids only at high concentrations, which also inhibited antigen-induced mediator release, suggesting that the inhibitory effect was not specific.

III. Conclusions

Many neuropeptides are found in nerves; SP and SST are found in skin, while SP and VIP are detected in the lung. SP has a role in pain perception and may influence several immunologic effector systems. As was suggested by Lundberg and Saria (1983) and by Kizawa and Takayanagi (1984), cigarette smoke and mechanical and chemical irritants are able to induce mucosal edema formation by increasing vascular permeability, which is preventable by capsaicin pretreatment, suggesting that SP plays a role. If SP is released, probably by antidromic excitation, the likelihood is that mast cells are involved in causing the vascular permeability. Thus, the link between nonspecific irritants and the release of SP and nonimmunologic activation of mast cells would provide a powerful inflammatory mechanism in the lung.

In the skin a close relationship between SP fibers and mast cell is very likely. Skin test results after capsaicin treatment have no flare reaction (Lundblad et al., 1985), suggesting that mast cell degranulation leads to SP release and the vasodilation response (flare). Conversely, injection of SP causes mast cell degranulation and there may be a cycle between SP release and mast cell activation. The possible role of SP in trauma-, cold- and exercise-induced anaphylactic reactions opens a new and exciting research field not only for SP but conceptually for all the other neuropeptides described above.

Acknowledgment

K. Sertl is a Fellow of the Max Kade Foundation.

Discussion

Barnes. While SP degranulates human skin mast cells in vivo, is there any evidence that it can degranulate lung mast cells?

Kaliner. SP has no effect on lung and nasal tissue unless protease inhibitors are added simultaneously, so an absence of effect may reflect SP breakdown. There may be several classes of mast cells, one of which, the mucosal mast cell, is unresponsive to SP as well as 48/80 and opioids.

Burnstock. There is clear evidence for transmitter effects as much as 1-2 μm from effector cells, so presumably they are likely to act on mast cells. The most likely possibilities are ATP released as a cotransmitter with norepinephrine, and SP from sensory nerve collaterals.

Kaliner. It seems likely that peptidergic transmission will be the major nonimmunologic trigger of mast cell degranulation.

Said. Do you think neuropeptides may be involved in exercise-induced anaphylaxis?

Kaliner. We have carefully analyzed seven lungs for mast cell morphology and, although there were some nerves near to mast cells in the bronchi, no specific association was noted. We can think of no other likely explanation for mast cell degranulation related to increased core temperature other than release of neuropeptides or possibly a peptide colocalized in parasympathetic nerves.

Vanhoutte. As core temperature increases, sympathetic tone is reduced and this might remove an inhibitory factor on mast cell degranulation.

Nadel. Do mast cells metabolize neuropeptides?

Kaliner. Mast cell granules contain a number of potent enzymes, including proteases and peptidases. There may, in addition, be membrane-associated enzymes.

References

Assem, E. S. K., and Schild, H. O. (1969). Inhibition by sympathomimetic amines of histamine release induced by antigen in passively sensitized human lung. *Nature* **224**:1028-1029.

Barrett, K. E., and Metcalfe, D. D. (1987). Heterogeneity of mast cells in the tissues of the respiratory tract and other organ systems. *Am. Rev. Respir. Dis.* **135**:1190-1195.

Barrett, K. E., Szucs, E. F., and Metcalfe, D. D. (1986). Mast cell heterogeneity in non-human primates. *Fed. Proc.* **45**:1105.

Baxter, J. H., and Adamik, R. (1978). Differences in requirements and actions of various histamine-releasing agents. *Biochem. Pharmacol.* **27**:497-503.

Black, J. L., Temple, D. M., and Anderson, S. D. (1978). Long term trial of an alpha-adrenoceptor blocking drug (Indoramin) in asthma. A preliminary report. *Scand. J. Respir. Dis.* **59**:307-312.

Carraway, R., Cochrane, D. E., Lansman, J. B., Leeman, S. E., Paterson, B. M., and Welch, H. J. (1982). Neurotensin stimulates exocytotic histamine secretion from mast cells and elevates plasma histamine levels. *J. Physiol.* **323**:403-414.

Carraway, R. E., Cochrane, D. E., Granier, C., Kitabgi, P., Leeman, E., and Singer, E. A. (1984). Parallel secretion of endogenous 5-hydroxytryptamine and histamine from mast cells stimulated by vasoactive peptides and compound 48/80. *Br. J. Pharmacol.* **81**:227-229.

Casale, T. B., Bowman, S., and Kaliner, M. (1984). Induction of human cutaneous mast cell degranulation by opiates and endogenous opioid peptides: evidence for opiate and nonopiate receptor participation. *J. Allergy Clin. Immunol.* **13**:775-781.

Cochrane, D. E., Emigh, C., Levine, G., Carraway, R. E., and Leeman, S. E. (1982). Neurotensin alters cutaneous vascular permeability and stimulates histamine release from isolated skin. *Ann. N.Y. Acad. Sci.* **400**:396-397.

Cutz, E., Chan, W., Track, N. S., Goth, A., and Said, S. I. (1978). Release of vasoactive intestinal polypeptide in mast cells by histamine liberators. *Nature* **275**:661-662.

Diel, F., Vangala, B., Neidhart, B., and Antweiler, H. (1980). Histamine liberation from rat mast cells caused by hazardous substances and cyclic somatostatin in-vitro. *Toxicol. Letts.* **SI 1**:205.

Diel, F., Bethge, N., and Opree (1983). Histamine secretion in leucocyte incubates of patients with allergic hypersensitivity induced by somatostatin-14 and somatostatin-28. *Agents Actions* **13**:216-218.

Donlon, M., Hunt, W. A., Catravas, G. N., and Kaliner, M. (1982). A characterization of beta-adrenergic receptors on cellular and perigranular membranes of rat peritoneal mast cells. *Life Sci.* **31**:411-416.

Erjavec, F., and Iskra, M. (1984). The interaction of cholinomimetics, peptides and compounds 48/80 on histamine secretion from the mast cell. *Agents Actions* **14**:373-375.

Erjavec, F., Lembeck, F., Florjanc-Irman, T., Skofitsch, G., Donnerer, J., Saria, A., and Holzer, P. (1981). Release of histamine by substance P. *Naunyn Schmiedebergs Arch. Pharmacol.* **317**:67-70.

Euler, U. S. v. (1936). Untersuchungen ueber Substanz P, die atropinfeste, darmerregende und gefaeszerweiternde Substanz aus Darm und Gehirn. *Naunyn Schmiedebergs Arch. Exp. Pathol. Pharmacol.* **181**:181-197.

Fewtrell, C. M. S., Foreman, J. C., Jordan, C. C., Oehme, P., Renner, H., and Stewart, J. M. (1982). The effects of substance P on histamine and 5-hydroxytryptamine release in the rat. *J. Physiol.* **330**:393-411.

Fish, J. E., Rosenthal, R. R., and Summer, W. R. (1977). The effect of atropine on acute antigen-mediated airway constriction in subjects with allergic asthma. *Am. Rev. Respir. Dis.* **115**:371-379.

Foreman, J., and Jordan, C. (1983). Histamine release and vascular changes induced by neuropeptides. *Agents Actions* **13**:105-116.

Foreman, J. C., Jordan, C. C., and Piotrowski, W. (1982). Interaction of neurotensin with the substance P receptor mediating histamine release from rat mast cells and the flare in human skin. *Br. J. Pharmacol.* **77**:531-539.

Garrity, E. R., Stimler, N. P., Munoz, N. M., Tallet, J., David, A. C., and Leff, A. R. (1985). Sympathetic modulation of biochemical and physiological response to immune degranulation in canine bronchial airways in vivo. *J. Clin. Invest.* **75**:2038-2046.

Goetzl, E. J., and Payan, D. G. (1984). Inhibition by somatostatin of the release of mediators from human basophils and rat leukemic basophils. *J. Immunol.* **133**:3255-3259.

Goetzl, E. J., Chernov-Rogan, T., Cooke, M. P., Renold, F., and Payan, D. G. (1985). Endogenous somatostatin-like peptides of rat basophilic leukemia cells. *J. Immunol.* **135**:2707-2712.

Gold, W. M., Kessler, G. F., and Yu, D. Y. (1972). Role of the vagus nerve in experimental asthma in dogs. *J. Appl. Physiol.* **33**:719-725.

Gross, G. N., Souhrada, J. F., and Farr, R. S. (1974). The long-term treatment of an asthmatic patient using phentolamine. *Chest* **66**:397-401.

Haegermark, Oe., Hoekfelt, T., and Pernow, B. (1978). Flare and itch induced by substance P in human skin. *J. Invest. Dermatol.* **71**:233-235.

Hirata, F., and Axelrod, J. (1980). Phospholipid methylation and biological signal transmission. *Science* **209**:1082-1090.

Holgate, S. T., Lewis, R. A., and Austen, K. F. (1980). 3′,5′-Cyclic adenosine monophosphate dependent protein kinase of the rat serosal mast cell and its immunological activation. *J. Immunol.* **124**:2093-2099.

Howarth, P. H., Durham, S. R., Lee, T. H., Kay, A. B., Church, M. K., and

Holgate, S. T. (1985). Influence of albuterol, cromolyn sodium and ipratropium bromide on the airway and circulating mediator responses to allergen bronchial provocation in asthma. *Am. Rev. Respir. Dis.* **132**:986-992.

Hughes, J. M., Seale, J. P., and Temple, D. M. (1983). Effect of fenoterol on immunological release of leukotrienes and histamine from human lung in-vitro: selective antagonism by beta-adrenoceptor antagonists. *Eur. J. Pharmacol.* **95**:239-245.

Ishizaka, T. (1981). Analysis of triggering events in mast cells for immunoglobulin E-mediated histamine release. *J. Allergy Clin. Immunol.* **67**:90-96.

Johnson, A. R., and Erdoes, E. G. (1973). Release of histamine from mast cells by vasoactive peptides. *Proc. Soc. Exp. Biol. Med.* **142**:1252-1256.

Kaliner, M. (1977a). Human lung tissue and anaphylaxis. I. The role of cyclic GMP as a modulator of the immunologically induced secretory process. *J. Allergy Clin. Immunol.* **60**:204-211.

Kaliner, M. (1977b). Human lung tissue and anaphylaxis. Evidence that cyclic nucleotides modulate the immunologic release of mediators through effects on microtubular assembly. *J. Clin. Invest.* **60**:951-959.

Kaliner, M., and Austen, K. F. (1974). Cyclic AMP, ATP, and reversed anaphylactic histamine release from rat mast cells. *J. Immunol.* **112**:664-674.

Kaliner, M., Orange, R. P., and Austen, K. F. (1972). Immunological release of histamine and slow reacting substance of anaphylaxis from human lung. IV. Enhancement of cholinergic and alpha adrenergic stimulation. *J. Exp. Med.* **136**:556-567.

Kaliner, M., Wasserman, S. I., and Austen, K. F. (1973). Immunologic release of chemical mediators from human nasal polyps. *N. Engl. J. Med.* **289**: 277-281.

Kennerly, D. A., Sullivan, T. J., and Parker, C. W. (1979). Activation of phospholipid metabolism during mediator release from stimulated mast cells. *J. Immunol.* **122**:152-159.

Kerouac, R., St-Pierre, S., and Rioux, F. (1984). Histamine release by neurotensin in the rat hindquarter: structure-activity studies. *Peptides* **5**: 695-699.

Kitada, C., Ashida, Y., Maki, Y., Fujimo, M., Hirai, Y., Yashura, Y., Nakajama, T., Takeyama, M., Koyama, K., and Yajima, H. (1980). Synthesis of granuliberin-R and various fragment peptides and their histamine releasing activities. *Chem. Pharmacol. Bull.* **28**:887-892.

Kizawa, Y., and Takayanagi, I. (1985). Possible involvement of substance P immunoreactive nerves in the mediation of nicotine-induced contractile responses in isolated guinea-pig bronchus. *Eur. J. Pharmacol.* **113**:319-323.

Koopman, W. J., Orange, R. P., and Austen, K. F. (1970). Immunochemical and biologic properties of rat IgE. III. Modulation of the IgE-mediated release of slow-reacting substance of anaphylaxis by agents influencing the level of cyclic 3′,5′-adenosine monophosphate. *J. Immunol.* **105**:1096-1102.

Krell, R. D., Chakrin, L. W., and Wardell, J. R. Jr. (1976). The effect of cholinergic agents on a canine model of allergic asthma. *J. Allergy Clin. Immunol.* **58**:19-30.

Krueger, P. G., Aas, P., Onarheim, J., and Helle, K. B. (1982). Neurotensin-induced release of histamine from rat mast cells in-vitro. *Acta Physiol. Scand.* **114**:467-469.

Lazarus, H. L., Perrin, M. H., and Brown, M. R. (1977a). Mast cell binding of neurotensin. I. Iodination of neurotensin and characterization of the interaction of neurotensin with mast cell receptor sites. *J. Biol. Chem.* **252**: 7174-7179.

Lazarus, H. L., Perrin, M. H., Brown, M. R., and Rivier, J. E. (1977b). Mast cell binding of neurotensin. II. Molecular conformation of neurotensin involved in the stereospecific binding to mast cell receptor sites. *J. Biol. Chem.* **252**:7180-7183.

Lazarus, S. C., Chesrown, S. E., Frey, M. J., Reed, B. R., Mjoerndal, T. O., and Gold, W. M. (1979). Experimental canine anaphylaxis: cyclic nucleotides, histamine, and lung function. *J. Appl. Physiol.* **45**:919-926.

Lewis, R. A., Holgate, S. T., Roberts, L. J., Maguire, J. F., Oates, J. A., and Austen, K. F. (1979). Effects of indomethacin on cyclic nucleotide levels and histamine release from rat serosal mast cells. *J. Immunol.* **123**:1663-1668.

Lundberg, J. M., and Saria, A. (1983). Capsaicin-induced desensitization of airway mucosa to cigarette smoke, mechanical and chemical irritants. *Nature* **308**:351-353.

Lundblad, L., Lundberg, J. M., Aenggard, A., and Zetterstroem, O. (1985). Capsaicin pretreatment inhibits the flare component of the cutaneous allergic reaction in man. *Eur. J. Pharmacol.* **113**:461-462.

Mann, S. P. (1971). The innervation of mammalian bronchial smooth muscle: the localization of catecholamines and cholinesterases. *Histochem. J.* **3**:319-331.

Marquardt, D. L., and Wasserman, S. I. (1982). Characterization of the rat mast cell beta-adrenergic receptor in resing and stimulated cells by radioligand binding. *J. Immunol.* **129**:2122-2127.

Masini, E., Fantozzi, R., Blandina, P., Brunelleschi, S., and Mannaioni, P. F. (1983). Muscarinic cholinergic receptor binding in rat mast cells. *Agents Actions* **13**:327-332.

Mazurek, N., Pecht, I., Teichberg, V. I., and Blumberg, S. (1981). The role of the N-terminal tetrapeptide in the histamine releasing action of substance P. *Neuropharmacology* **20**:1025-1027.

McNeill, R. S. (1964). Effect of a beta-adrenergic blocking agent, propranolol, on asthmatics. *Lancet* **2**:1101-1102.

Moroni, F., Fantozzi, R., Masini, E., and Mannaioni, P. F. (1977). The modulation of histamine release by alpha-adrenoceptors: evidences in murine neoplastic mast cells. *Agents Actions* **7**:57-61.

Newson, B., Dahlstroem, A., Enerbaeck, L., and Ahlman, H. (1983). Suggestive evidence for a direct innervation of mucosal mast cells. *Neuroscience* **10**: 565-570.

Orange, R. P., Kaliner, M. A., Laraia, P. J., and Austen, K. F. (1971a). Immunological release of histamine and slow reacting substance of anaphylaxis from human lung. II. Influence of cellular levels of cyclic AMP. *Fed. Proc.* **30**: 1725-1729.

Orange, R. P., Austen, W. G., and Austen, K. F. (1971b). Immunological release of histamine and slow reacting substance of anaphylaxis from human lung. I. Modulation by agents influencing cellular levels cyclic 3′,5′-adenosine monophosphate. *J. Exp. Med.* **134**(Suppl):136s-148s.

Partanen, M., Laitinen, A., Hervonen, A., Toivanen, M., and Laitinen, L. A. (1982). Catecholamine- and acetylcholinesterase-containing nerves in human lower respiratory tract. *Histochemistry* **76**:175-188.

Patel, K. R., and Kerr, J. W. (1975). Alpha-receptor-blocking drugs in bronchial asthma. *Lancet* **1**:348-349.

Payan, D. G., Levine, J. D., and Goetzl, E. J. (1984). Modulation of immunity and hypersensitivity by sensory neuropeptides. *J. Immunol.* **132**:1601-1604.

Pernow, B. (1953). Studies on substance P. Purification, occurrence and biological actions. *Acta Physiol. Scand.* **29**(Suppl. 105):1-90.

Peters, S. P., Schulman, E. S., Schleimer, R. P., Macglashan, D. W., Newball, H. H., and Lichtenstein, L. M. (1982). Dispersed human lung mast cells. Pharmacologic aspects and comparison with human lung fragments. *Am. Rev. Respir. Dis.* **30**:1034-1039.

Phillips, M. J., Barnes, P. J., and Gold, W. M. (1985). Characterization of purified dog masocytoma cells. Autonomic membrane receptors and pharmacologic modulation of histamine release. *Am. Rev. Respir. Dis.* **132**:1019-1026.

Piotrowski, W., Devoy, M. A. B., Jordan, C. C., and Foreman, J. C. (1984). The substance P receptor on rat mast cells and in human skin. *Agents Actions* **14**:420-424.

Platshon, L., and Kaliner, M. (1978). The effect of the immunologic release of histamine upon human lung cyclic nucleotide levels and prostaglandin generation. *J. Clin. Invest.* **62**:1113-1121.

Renold, F., Chernov, T., Lee, J., Payan, G. G., Furuichi, K., and Goetzl, E. J. (1985). Somatostatin (SOM-14) modulation of mediator release by mouse bone marrow-derived mast cells (BMMC), rat serosal, mast cells (SMC), and rat basophilic leukemia cells (RBL-2H3), *Fed. Proc.* **44**:1917.

Rosenthal, R. R., Norman, P. S., Summer, W. R., Permutt, S. (1977). Role of the parasympathetic system in antigen-induced bronchospasm. *J. Appl. Physiol.* **42**:600-606.

Sampson, S. R., and Vidruk, E. H. (1975). Properties of "irritant" receptors in canine lung. *Respir. Physiol.* **25**:9-22.

Schild, H. O. (1936). Histamine release and anaphylactic shock in isolated lungs of guinea pigs. *Q. J. Exp. Physiol.* **26**:165-179.

Seyle, H. *The Mast Cell.* Washington, D.C., Butterworth, 1965.

Shanahan, F., Lee, T. D. G., Bienenstock, J., and Befus, A. D. (1984). The influence of endorphins on peritoneal and mucosal mast cell secretion. *J. Allergy Clin. Immunol.* **74**:499-504.

Shanahan, F., Denburg, J. A., Fox, J., Bienenstock, J., and Befus, D. (1985). Mast cell heterogeneity: effects of neuroenteric peptides on histamine release. *J. Immunol.* **135**:1331-1337.

Shibata, H., Mio, M., and Tasaka, K. (1985). Analysis of the mechanism of histamine release induced by substance P. *Biochim. Biophys. Acta* **846**: 1-7.

Skofitsch, G., Savitt, J. M., and Jacobowitz, D. M. (1985). Suggestive evidence for a functional unit between mast cells and substance P fibers in the rat diaphragm. *Histochemistry* **82**:5-8.

Steer, M. L. (1977). Adrenergic receptors. In *Clinics in Endocrinology and Metabolism.* Edited by L. Landsberg. Philadelphia, Saunders, pp. 577-598.

Sullivan, T. J., Parker, K. L., Stenson, W., and Parker, C. W. (1975a). Modulation of cyclic AMP in purified rat mast cells. I. Response to pharmacologic, metabolic, and physical stimuli. *J. Immunol.* **114**:1473-1485.

Sullivan, T. J., Parker, K. L., Eisen, S. A., and Parker, C. W. (1975b). II. Studies on the relationship between intracellular cyclic AMP concentrations and histamine release. *J. Immunol.* **114**:1480-1485.

Sullivan, T. J., and Parker, C. W. (1976). Pharmacologic modulation of inflammatory mediator release by rat mast cells. *Am. J. Pathol.* **85**:437-463.

Taniguchi, T., Wang, J. K., and Spector, S. (1980). Properties of [^{3}H] diazepam binding to rat peritoneal mast cells. *Life Sci.* **27**:171-178.

Tauber, A. I., Kaliner, M., Stechschulte, D. J., and Austen, K. F. (1973). The immunologic release of histamine and slow reacting substances of anaphylaxis from human lung. V. Effect of prostaglandin on histamine release. *J. Immunol.* **111**:27-32.

Tharp, M. D., Thirlby, R., and Sullivan, T. J. (1984). Gastrin induces histamine release from human cutaneous mast cells. *J. Allergy Clin. Immunol.* **74**: 159-165.

Theoharides, T. C., and Douglas, W. W. (1978). Somatostatin induces histamine secretion from rat peritoneal mast cells. *Endocrinology* **102**:1647-1640.

Theoharides, T. C., Douglas, W. W. (1981). Mast cell histamine secretion in response to somatostatin analogues: structural considerations. *Eur. J. Pharmacol.* **73**:131-136.

Theoharides, T. C., Betchaku, T., and Douglas, W. W. (1981). Somatostatin-induced histamine secretion in mast cells. Characterization of the effect. *Eur. J. Pharmacol.* **69**:127-137.

Tuft, L., and Brodsky, M. L. (1936). The influence of various drugs upon allergic reactions. *J. Allergy* **7**:238-248.

Undem, B. J., and Buckner, C. K. (1984). Evidence that only one type of beta adrenergic receptor mediates inhibition of antigen-induced histamine release from guinea-pig minced lung. *J. Pharmacol. Exp. Ther.* **229**:391-398.

Undem, B. J., Dick, E. C., Buckner, C. K. (1983). Inhibition by vasoactive intestinal peptide of antigen-induced histamine release from guinea-pig minced lung. *Eur. J. Pharmacol.* **88**:247-250.

18

Bronchial Hyperreactivity
Neural Contributions

THOMAS B. CASALE

University of Iowa
Iowa City, Iowa

Abnormally increased responsiveness of the trachea and bronchi to various physical, chemical, and pharmacologic stimuli is a characteristic feature of asthma. This exaggerated responsiveness, or bronchial hyperreactivity, was first described in 1921 when Alexander and Paddock (1921) observed that asthmatics wheezed when given pilocarpine. The exact mechanisms underlying bronchial hyperresponsiveness are, however, still not known. It is likely that a variety of factors are involved including baseline airway geometry, autonomic nervous control of the smooth muscle, the smooth muscle cell itself, bronchial mucosal permeability, and epithelial damage and inflammation. These potential causes have been the subject of many previous reviews (Boushey et al., 1980; Nadel, 1983; Nadel and Holtzman, 1984; Barnes, 1985; Boushey, 1985). In this chapter, only neurogenic mechanisms will be considered.

Autonomic nervous system regulation of airway tone is complex and involves cholinergic, adrenergic, and nonadrenergic, noncholinergic mechanisms (Richardson, 1979; Nadel and Barnes, 1984; Barnes, 1984). This chapter briefly reviews normal autonomic airway control and describes possible imbalances in the excitatory and inhibitory nervous systems that could lead to bronchial hyperreactivity.

I. Parasympathetic Nervous System

The parasympathetic nervous system plays an intricate part in maintaining resting bronchial smooth muscle tone and in mediating acute bronchospastic responses. Thus, it seems likely that the parasympathetic nervous system might play an important role in the bronchial hyperreactivity of asthma. Detailed below is a description of the parasympathetic nervous innervation of the respiratory tract and a discussion of possible ways in which this nervous system might be involved in the development of bronchial hyperresponsiveness.

The vagus nerves provide the parasympathetic motor supply to airway smooth muscle. Morphologic and histochemical studies have demonstrated parasympathetic postganglionic fibers carried in the vagus nerves extending from the upper tracheobronchial tree to the level of the small airways (Richardson, 1979). Thus, electrical stimulation of the peripheral ends of cut vagal nerves induces diffuse narrowing of the airways from the trachea to large bronchioles (Colebatch and Halmagyi, 1963; Olsen et al., 1965). This response is blocked by atropine and potentiated by acetylcholinesterase inhibitors (Colebatch and Halmagyi, 1963; Olsen et al., 1965), indicating that the effect is produced by acetylcholine acting on muscarinic receptors. Light microscopic autoradiography has shown that the distribution of muscarinic receptors is greatest in the large airways and least in the peripheral airways (Barnes et al., 1983), which is consistent with the pattern of vagal-mediated airway constriction.

Stimulation of receptors in the nose (Nadel and Widdicombe, 1962a), larynx (Nadel and Widdicombe, 1962a), lungs (Widdicombe and Nadel, 1963), and airways (Nadel and Widdicombe, 1963), as well as chemoreceptors and baroreceptors located elsewhere (Nadel and Widdicombe, 1962b) induces changes in airway tone. That a reflex mechanism involving vagal efferent pathways is responsible for these changes is shown by studies that have separated the stimulation of the sensory endings from the smooth muscle effector (Boushey, 1985). For example, mechanical irritation of the larynx (Nadel and Widdicombe, 1962a) and delivery of sulfur dioxide only to the upper airways (Nadel et al., 1965) caused constriction of the lower airways that was abolished by cutting the sensory or motor nervous pathways or by atropine.

The observation that many of the stimuli that produce bronchoconstrictor responses in patients with asthma (e.g., histamine and sulfur dioxide) also stimulate vagal sensory nerve endings led to the hypothesis that enhancement of parasympathetic reflex activity could be responsible in part for the exaggerated bronchospastic responses in asthmatics (Simonsson et al., 1967). However, the exact involvement of a parasympathetic reflex in human bronchomotor responses has been difficult to define since it is not feasible to study the vagi directly. Researchers have indirectly studied the involvement of parasympathetic reflex pathways by comparing responses before and after treatment with cholinergic antagonists. Cholinergic antagonists have in some studies been found to block or decrease the bronchoconstrictor response to various stimuli including histamine, carbon dust, cold air, and citric acid (Simonsson et al., 1967), prostaglandins (Alanko and Poppius, 1974), and aerosols of propellant and surfactant (Sterling and Batten, 1969). Other studies, however, have reported muscarinic antagonists to be ineffective in inhibiting the bronchomotor effects of these stimuli (Itkin and Anand, 1970; Casterline et al., 1976). These variable results are probably due to differences in dosages of the stimuli and antagonists, as well as the mode of antagonist delivery.

If bronchial hyperreactivity is due to an enhancement of the transmission through the parasympathetic nervous pathway, this might be due in part to an increase in the number or affinity of muscarinic receptors on airway smooth muscle. Therefore, in order to inhibit cholinergic-induced bronchospasm, the antagonist would have to be administered in higher doses. Furthermore, increasing concentrations of cholinergic antagonists should inhibit acetylcholine-induced bronchoconstriction in a dose-dependent manner. Sheppard et al. (1982) showed that increasing concentrations of atropine did indeed inhibit cold-air-induced bronchoconstriction in a dose-dependent fashion. In a later study, however, ipatropium bromide inhibited cold-air-induced bronchoconstriction in only a subgroup of asthmatics, and then not in a dose-dependent manner (Tam et al., 1983). These data suggest, therefore, that nonparasympathetic mechanisms might also be involved in the bronchial hyperreactivity observed in some asthmatics.

Bronchial hyperreactivity could be due to an enhancement of the transmission through the parasympathetic nervous pathway at other loci as well. Asthmatics have been shown to respond to psychological stimuli with bronchoconstriction that is inhibited by atropine (McFadden et al., 1969). Neural output from the central nervous system could, therefore, contribute to increased vagal efferent activity, which, in turn, could lead to bronchial hyperreactivity.

Effects on vagal motor ganglia or any portion of the postganglionic pathways could also lead to enhanced vagal motor responses (Douglas et al., 1973). Serotonin, for example, potentiates the release of acetylcholine from parasympathetic efferent nerves (Sheller et al., 1982). It is conceivable, therefore, that other neurochemical agents may modulate the output of acetylcholine through prejunctional or ganglionic effects as well (Nadel, 1983). Further, since mast cell degranulation and inflammatory cell infiltration are frequently associated with exacerbations of asthma, these cells might lead to increased vagal nerve activity by releasing mediators that also facilitate efferent transmission of nervous impulses.

Inflammation of the airway epithelium could lead to bronchial hyperreactivity by other mechanisms as well. The hypothesis that increased airway responsiveness can be caused by airway inflammation was first suggested by the observation that each stimulus that has been used to cause airway hyperresponsiveness experimentally in humans may also cause airway inflammation or the release of inflammatory mediators (Nadel and Holtzman, 1984). For example, viral respiratory infections (Empey et al., 1976) and ozone (Golden et al., 1978; Holtzman et al., 1979) cause airway inflammation and bronchial hyperresponsiveness that are prevented by atropine. Laitinen and co-workers (1985) measured bronchial reactivity to inhaled histamine and histologically examined the bronchial biopsy specimens from eight asthmatics. These investigators found that epithelial destruction in the respiratory tract of the asthma patients with mild to severe bronchial hyperresponsiveness was prominent enough to expose the epithelial nerves for specific or nonspecific stimuli. Thus, inflammatory changes resulting in exposure of parasympathetic afferent nerves to nonspecific stimuli and released mediators could also contribute to the bronchial hyperresponsiveness noted in asthmatics.

Another possibility for cholinergically mediated bronchial hyperreactivity is changes in the efferent pathways at sites distal to the ganglion. To determine more precisely which site might be responsible for the increased bronchial reactivity in atopics, Holtzman and co-workers (1980) studied the effects of premedication with aerosols of hexamethonium, a ganglionic blocking agent, and atropine, a postganglionic blocking agent, on the bronchomotor responses to methacholine aerosols in five atopic subjects. After the administration of aerosolized atropine, baseline specific airway resistance decreased, and the increases in specific airway resistance produced by methacholine were prevented in each subject. The response to methacholine was unchanged by hexamethonium, however, indicating that ganglionic neural transmission was, therefore, not necessary. These findings suggest that inhaled methacholine acts directly at the smooth muscle muscarinic receptor site to cause bronchoconstriction, and that increased bronchomotor responses may be due to a change in the sensitivity or the responsiveness of the smooth muscle to acetylcholine-mediated parasympathetic nervous activity.

As previously mentioned, an increase in the number or binding affinity of the muscarinic receptors on bronchial smooth muscle might also lead to parasympathetically mediated bronchial hyperreactivity. In this case, the bronchomotor response to methacholine and other muscarinic agonists would be increased because they act by stimulating the smooth muscle receptors directly, and atropine would block the effect by competing for the receptor sites. In order to investigate whether increased cholinergic responsiveness might be due

Table 1 Possible Sites in the Parasympathetic Nervous Pathway that May be Involved in Bronchial Hyperreactivity

Vagal sensory endings
Sensory ganglion
Central nervous system
Vagal motor ganglion
Acetylcholine release from motor end plate
Smooth muscle muscarinic receptors

to increased receptor number or affinity, Mita and co-workers (1983) studied the effects of prolonged aerosol sensitization with low dose-antigen in ovalbumin-sensitized guinea pigs. These investigators found an increased number of lung muscarinic receptors in those animals that produced IgE antibodies to ovalbumin compared to normal control animals. These data suggest that atopic asthmatics may in part have bronchial hyperresponsiveness due to an increased number of airway cholinergic receptors.

Thus, bronchial hyperreactivity in some patients might be due to enhanced parasympathetic nervous transmission. Several possible sites in the parasympathetic pathway may be involved (Table 1). However, it does not appear that an imbalance in the cholinergic nervous system is the only cause of bronchial hyperreactivity; nonparasympathetic mechanisms might also play a role.

II. Sympathetic Nervous System

The sympathetic nerve supply to the lungs originates from the second to fourth thoracic preganglionic fibers that end in the extrapulmonary stellate ganglia. Postganglionic fibers enter the lungs at the hila, accompanying the vagus nerves. Although, there is marked variability in sympathetic innervation of airway smooth muscle among different species, it is generally sparse (Mann, 1971). Histochemical studies have demonstrated catecholamine-containing nerve fibers in human bronchial blood vessels and submucosal glands, as well as a few nerve fibers in airway smooth muscle (Partanen et al., 1982). Other studies, however, have failed to show the presence of adrenergic nerve fibers in human airway smooth muscle (Doidge and Satchell, 1982). Thus, the presence of adrenergic fibers in human airway smooth muscle is controversial and, even if they are present, they represent only a minor component of the total nerve fibers (Partanen et al., 1982).

Physiological studies are consistent with the anatomical findings of little or no direct adrenergic airway innervation. The usual response of airway smooth muscle to electrical stimulation of the thoracic sympathetic nerves is bronchodilation (Dixon and Ransom, 1912), an effect that is abolished by beta-adrenergic antagonists (Castro de la Mata et al., 1962; Cabezas et al., 1971). However, the bronchodilatory effect of sympathetic nerve stimulation depends upon preexisting vagally induced smooth muscle tone (Cabezas et al., 1971). This suggests that the bronchodilatory effect of the sympathetic nervous system may in part be due to inhibition of parasympathetic efferent nerve activity.

Although direct sympathetic innervation of airway smooth muscle does not appear to be a dominant factor in regulating bronchomotor tone, stimulation of smooth muscle adrenergic receptors may be. Both alpha- and beta-adrenergic receptors have been demonstrated in human lung by radioligand binding studies (Barnes et al., 1980a). Furthermore, both receptors have been localized to human and mammalian airway smooth muscle using autoradiography (Barnes et al., 1983; Carstairs et al., 1985). The density of beta- and alpha-adrenergic receptors is least in the larger airways and increases as the airways become smaller (Barnes et al., 1983; Carstairs et al., 1985).

The exact role of alpha-adrenergic receptors in regulating airway tone is not clear. Kneussl and Richardson (1978) demonstrated alpha-receptor-mediated contraction of airway smooth muscle obtained at autopsy from patients with chronic obstructive airway disease or bronchopneumonia, but not from normal control subjects. Alpha-responsiveness could be induced in the normal airway tissue by pretreatment with KCl or histamine (Kneussl and Richardson, 1978). In an in vivo study, histamine has also been shown to induce alpha-adrenergic contractions of canine trachealis muscle (Brown et al., 1983). Thus, alpha-adrenergically mediated airway constriction may only occur in abnormal states and not be a significant factor in controlling airway tone in normal subjects.

Human in vivo studies of the effects of alpha-agonists on airway tone have yielded similar results to the in vitro studies. Inhalation of alpha-agonists has been shown to increase airflow resistance in asthmatics, but not in normal subjects (Patel and Kerr, 1973; Snashall et al., 1978). However, Thomson and coworkers (1982) studied a group of asthmatics who exhibited a wide range of nonspecific bronchial hyperresponsiveness, and found no relationship between alpha-receptor responsiveness and nonspecific bronchial responsiveness. These investigators concluded that increased bronchial smooth muscle alpha$_1$-receptor activity is not the primary abnormality producing the variability between asthmatics in nonspecific bronchial hyperresponsiveness.

Another approach to delineating the role of alpha-receptors in bronchial hyperreactivity has been to assess the ability of alpha-antagonists to dilate the airways of patients with asthma and to prevent the bronchoconstriction induced by nonspecific stimuli. Alpha-antagonists have been shown to inhibit partially the bronchoconstriction provoked by histamine (Gaddie et al., 1972) and exercise (Beil and DeKock, 1978) in patients with asthma. However, the pharmacologic criteria for blockade of airway alpha-receptors were not critically established in these studies (Boushey et al., 1980). Furthermore, Barnes and co-workers (1981) have shown that prazosin, a potent and selective $alpha_1$-antagonist, produced no change in airflow resistance of asthmatics who responded to salbutamol with bronchodilation.

Since there is little evidence that sympathetic nerves directly innervate human airway smooth muscle, and because the bronchoconstricting effects of alpha-agonists and the bronchodilatory effects of alpha-antagonists are weak, it is doubtful that airway smooth muscle alpha-receptors play a significant role in bronchial hyperreactivity. It is possible, however, that alpha-receptors may modulate nervous transmission in a way that might predispose subjects towards bronchospasm. In this regard, sympathetic $alpha_2$-receptors have been found to inhibit nonadrenergic neurotransmission (Starke, 1981). Moreover, other studies have demonstrated that cholinergic neurons in the trachea and main bronchi of the guinea pig are regulated by inhibitory, prejunctional $alpha_2$-adrenoceptors (Grundström et al., 1981; Wikberg et al., 1982). If these later mechanisms are present in human airways, the use of $alpha_2$-agonists may have relevance in the inhibition of cholinergically mediated airway bronchoconstriction.

Stimulation of beta-adrenergic receptors in the respiratory tract results in bronchodilation. If the bronchodilatory effect mediated by beta-adrenoceptors was, therefore, diminished, unopposed cholinergic and alpha-adrenergic stimulation could result in bronchial hyperreactivity. In this regard, there have been many in vivo studies showing that allergic asthmatics may have intrinsic abnormalities in neurohormonal responsiveness to adrenergic and cholinergic stimuli (Lockey et al., 1967; Kirkpatrick and Keller, 1967; Middleton and Finke, 1968; Grieco et al., 1968; Kaliner et al., 1982). In 1968, Szentivanyi proposed the beta-adrenergic theory of bronchial asthma (Szentivanyi, 1968) as a unifying concept to explain partially many of the abnormal neurohormonal responses noted in asthmatics. Based on data derived from two animal models of asthma, Szentivanyi postulated that beta-adrenergic blockade may be a predisposing factor in the development of asthma.

Since its inception, the beta-adrenergic theory of blockade has been the subject of intense study by many investigators. Recent in vivo studies by Kaliner and co-workers (1982) showed that atopic asthmatics had beta-adrenergic hyporesponsiveness and alpha and cholinergic hyperresponsiveness that would, therefore, predispose them to bronchospasm. Barnes and co-workers (1980b), using a guinea pig model of asthma, found that the lungs of sensitized animals had increased alpha- and decreased beta-adrenoceptors in comparison to control animals. These studies have been extended to the use of circulatory leukocytes. Many investigators have reported that asthmatic patients have a lower density of beta receptors on leukocytes (Kariman, 1980; Brooks et al., 1979), and leukocytes of asthmatics generate less cyclic AMP in response to beta-agonists (Parker and Smith, 1973). Other investigators, however, have found reduced leukocyte beta-adrenergic responsiveness and decreased beta-receptor number only after continuous treatment with beta-agonists (Conolly and Greenacre, 1976; Morris et al., 1977; Galant et al., 1978; Bruynzeel et al., 1979). Thus, although controversial, there are data suggesting that beta-adrenergic hyporesponsiveness might contribute to the development of bronchial hyperresponsiveness in some asthmatics.

The possibility of a defect in the beta-adrenergically mediated bronchodilatory system has also been investigated by studying the effects of beta-antagonists on airway tone. In normal subjects, propranolol has been found to have either minimal (Townley et al., 1976) or no effect (Zaid and Beall, 1966; Tattersfield et al., 1973) on airway caliber or on bronchial responsiveness. In contrast, propranolol may cause acute bronchoconstriction in asthmatics (MacDonald et al., 1967; Grieco and Pierson, 1971), which may be blocked by atropine. Thus, it appears that unopposed cholinergic or alpha-adrenergic activity may be the main cause of propranolol-induced bronchoconstriction in asthmatics.

Overall, these data indicate that although direct sympathetic innervation of the airways may not play a dominant role in controlling airway tone, alterations in lung adrenergic receptors may very well be important in the development of bronchial hyperreactivity. Possible mechanisms by which the sympathetic nervous system might predispose towards bronchial hyperreactivity are listed in Table 2.

Table 2 Mechanisms by Which the Sympathetic Nervous System Might Lead to Bronchial Hyperreactivity

Increased airway alpha-receptors
Decreased inhibitory prejunctional alpha-receptors
Decreased airway beta-receptor density or affinity
Abnormal balance of airway cholinergic and adrenergic receptors (increased cholinergic and alpha-adrenergic with decreased beta-adrenergic receptors)

III. Nonadrenergic Noncholinergic Nervous Systems

A third division of the autonomic nervous system, which is neither adrenergic nor cholinergic, has recently been recognized in the airways (Barnes, 1984). This third nervous system consists of nonadrenergic inhibitory nerves and noncholinergic excitatory nerves.

A. Nonadrenergic Inhibitory Nerves

One of the most interesting observations concerning the neurogenic control of airway caliber has been the recent delineation of nonadrenergic inhibitory nerves which innervate human airways. The existence of a nonadrenergic nervous system was first recognized in the gastrointestinal tract, where stimulation of these nerve fibers inhibits smooth muscle contraction (Burnstock and Costa, 1973). Since the airways develop embryologically from the foregut, it is not surprising to find that nonadrenergic inhibitory nerves are also present in the lung.

The demonstration of this system in the airways is most easily shown by electrical field experiments. When adrenergic and cholinergic receptors are blocked, electrical field stimulation of human airway smooth muscle results in relaxation (Richardson and Beland, 1976). Tetrodotoxin, a nerve toxin, abolishes this relaxation response, thus indicating that it is mediated by postganglionic nerves. Since there is little anatomical or functional evidence for direct sympathetic innervation of human airway smooth muscle, this nonadrenergic inhibitory nervous system is likely the only, or predominant, neural bronchodilator mechanism in human airways.

The nonadrenergic inhibitory nervous system has been difficult to study because the neurotransmitter is not known with certainty, and no specific blockers are available. Recent evidence suggests that vasoactive intestinal peptide (VIP) may be the neurotransmitter for this system. Electrical field stimulation of tracheobronchial preparations results in the release of VIP, and the release is blocked by tetrodotoxin (Matsuzaki et al., 1980; Cameron et al., 1983). Furthermore, VIP mimics the effect of electrical field stimulation when it is added to airway smooth muscle preparations (Matsuzaki et al., 1980; Cameron et al., 1983). VIP has also been localized to neurons and nerve terminals supplying airway smooth muscle (Dey et al., 1981). Inhaled VIP has been shown to have an inhibitory effect on histamine-induced bronchospasm (Said et al., 1982; Barnes and Dixon, 1984). Thus, it appears likely that VIP may be the neurotransmitter for the nonadrenergic inhibitory nervous system, but definitive proof awaits the development of a specific antagonist.

It is possible that deficiencies in the nonadrenergic inhibitory nervous system might underlie bronchial hyperreactivity. There could be either a congeni-

Table 3 Possible Nonadrenergic, Noncholinergic Nervous System Pathway Abnormalities Leading to Bronchial Hyperreactivity

Deficiency of nonadrenergic inhibitory neurones
Reversible blockade of nonadrenergic inhibitory nervous system ganglia or nerve endings
Deficiency of airway VIP receptors
Increased noncholinergic excitatory nervous system activity

tal or acquired lack of the inhibitory neurons in the airways, analogous to that seen in Hirschsprung's disease (Frigo et al., 1973). Asthmatics may also have a reversible blockade of the inhibitory system at the level of the ganglia or nerve endings (Richardson, 1985), or a deficiency of airway VIP receptors, similar to the defect postulated to occur in beta-adrenoceptor function by Szentivanyi (1968).

B. Noncholinergic Excitatory Nerves

Electrical stimulation of guinea pig bronchi in vitro produces a component of bronchoconstriction that is not inhibited by atropine but is blocked by a substance P antagonist (Lundberg et al., 1983a). Furthermore, substance P and capsaicin, a chemical that induces the release of substance P from unmyelinated sensory nerves, contract airway smooth muscle (Lundberg et al., 1983b). However, the presence of a noncholinergic excitatory nervous system does not appear to be a universal finding in human airways (Lundberg et al., 1983b). Nevertheless, the presence of such a nervous system could contribute to bronchial hyperreactivity by releasing substance P, which is capable of inducing vascular permeability (Lundberg et al., 1983a) airway contraction (Lundberg et al., 1983a,b), mucus secretion (Lundberg and Saria, 1983), and mast cell degranulation (Shibata et al., 1985).

A summary of the possible ways in which the nonadrenergic and noncholinergic nervous systems might cause bronchial hyperreactivity is given in Table 3.

IV. Summary

Autonomic nervous system abnormalities may indeed underlie bronchial hyperreactivity. Imbalances between excitatory (parasympathetic, alpha-adrenergic, and noncholinergic excitatory) and inhibitory (beta-adrenergic and nonadrenergic inhibitory) nervous systems at one or more loci could lead to airway hyperreactivity. The data to date, however, do not clearly identify any single abnormality in the autonomic nervous system that is ubiquitous in all asthmatic patients. It appears that bronchial hyperreactivity results from many factors, and that distinct autonomic nervous system abnormalities may occur in individual subjects.

Acknowledgment

The author gratefully acknowledges the expert secretarial assistance of Kay Hammons and Darla Bartels in the preparation of this manuscript.

Discussion

Vanhoutte. The fact that propranolol causes bronchospasm in asthmatic patients argues sharply against a decreased beta-adrenergic sensitivity. Rather, it suggests that the sympathetic system is doing all it can to reduce bronchoconstriction.

Casale. There may be several explanations for the effect of propranolol. If there are less beta-receptors in patients with asthma, propranolol may induce bronchoconstriction more readily in asthmatics because there are less "spare receptors." Propranolol-induced bronchoconstriction in asthmatics may be blocked by atropine, suggesting that increased cholinergic activity may be the main mechanism, perhaps by acting on presynaptic receptors of cholinergic nerves.

Diamond. Another possible explanation for the bronchoconstrictor effect of propranolol in asthmatics is that there could be a defect of nonadrenergic inhibitory innervation in asthmatic airways, so that circulating catecholamines would play a more important role in maintaining airway patency in those individuals. Thus, a beta-blocker would result in an autonomic imbalance that results in parasympathetic bronchoconstriction.

Daniel. In several studies, blockade of alpha-adrenoceptors did not have any major effects on hyperresponsiveness in asthmatics.

Casale. Alpha-agonists cause bronchoconstriction in asthmatic subjects when given as single doses, suggesting that there may be increased alpha-adrenergic responsiveness in asthma.

Said. Is it possible that asthmatics may have a molecular abnormality in adrenoceptors of the airways?

Lefkowitz. Results of direct measurements of beta-receptors have been contradictory and inconclusive. My own opinion is that there is unlikely to be a specific structural defect in beta-receptors, and any defects are in some way secondary to another, as yet undefined, more general abnormality.

Barnes. Because bronchial hyperresponsiveness is nonspecific it seems unlikely that a single receptor defect could explain this phenomenon. The increased airway cholinergic responsiveness is a manifestation of this, but is not an isolated abnormality.

Nadel. Rather than looking at specific abnormalities of beta-adrenergic, cholinergic and alpha-adrenergic receptors, it may be more useful to examine why asthmatics have long-term hyperresponsiveness and why many stimuli caused increased responses in airway smooth muscle in experimental and clinical states of hyperresponsiveness in vivo but not in vitro. This could imply a humoral or neural effect on the muscle contractile process.

References

Alanko, K., and Poppius, H. (1974). Anticholinergic blocking of prostaglandin-induced bronchoconstriction. *Br. Med. J.* **1**:294.

Alexander, H. L., and Paddock, R. (1921). Bronchial asthma: response to pilocarpine and epinephrine. *Arch. Intern. Med.* **27**:184-191.

Barnes, P. J. (1984). The third nervous system in the lung: physiology and clinical perspectives. *Thorax* **39**:561-567.

Barnes, P. J. (1985). Adrenergic and non-adrenergic mechanisms in asthma. *Prog. Respir. Res.* **19**:159-164.

Barnes, P. J., Karliner, J. S., and Dollery, C. T. (1980a). Human lung adrenoceptors studied by radioligand binding. *Clin. Sci.* **58**:457-461.

Barnes, P. J., Dollery, C. T., and MacDermot, J. (1980b). Increased pulmonary alpha-adrenergic and reduced beta-adrenergic receptors in experimental asthma. *Nature* **285**:569-571.

Barnes, P. J., Ind, P., and Dollery, C. T. (1981). Inhaled prazosin in asthma. *Thorax* **36**:378-381.

Barnes, P. J., Basbaum, C. B., and Nadel, J. A. (1983). Autoradiographic localization of autonomic receptors in airway smooth muscle: marked differences between large and small airways. *Am. Rev. Respir. Dis.* **127**:758-762.

Barnes, P. J., and Dixon, C. M. S. (1984). The effect of inhaled vasoactive intestinal peptide on bronchial reactivity to histamine in humans. *Am. Rev. Respir. Dis.* **130**:162-166.

Beil, M., and DeKock, A. (1978). Role of alpha-adrenergic receptors in exercise-induced bronchoconstriction. *Respiration* **35**:78-86.

Boushey, H. A. (1985). Asthma and bronchial hyperreactivity: possible role of disturbance in autonomic regulation. *Prog. Respir. Res.* **19**:124-136.

Boushey, H. A., Holtzman, M. J., Sheller, J. R., and Nadel, J. A. (1980). State of the art. Bronchial hyperreactivity. *Am. Rev. Respir. Dis.* **121**:389-413.

Brooks, S. M., McCowan, K., Bernstein, I. L., Altenau, P., and Peagler, J. (1979). Relationship between numbers of beta-adrenergic receptors in lymphocytes and disease severity in asthma. *J. Allergy Clin. Immunol.* **63**:401-406.

Brown, J. K., Shields, R., Jones, C., and Gold, W. M. (1983). Augmentation of alpha-adrenergic contractions in the trachealis muscle of living dogs. *J. Appl. Physiol.* **54**:1558-1566.

Bruynzeel, P. L. B., Van den Berg, W., Hamelink, M. L., Van den Bogaard, W., Houben, L. A. M. J., and Kreukniet, J. (1979). Desensitization of the beta-adrenergic receptor on leukocytes after long term oral use of a beta-sympathicomimetic: its effect on the beta-adrenergic blockade hypothesis of Szentivanyi. *Ann. Allergy* **43**:105-109.

Burnstock, G., and Costa, M. (1973). Inhibitory innervation of the gut. *Gastroenterology* **64**:141-144.

Cabezas, G. A., Graf, P. D., and Nadel, J. A. (1971). Sympathetic versus parasympathetic nervous regulation of airways in dogs. *J. Appl. Physiol.* **31**:651-655.

Cameron, A. C., Johnston, C. F., Kirkpatrick, C. T., and Kirkpatrick, M. C. A. (1983). The quest for the inhibitory neurotransmitter in bovine tracheal smooth muscle. *Q. J. Exp. Physiol.* **68**:413-426.

Carstairs, J. R., Nimmo, A. J., and Barnes, P. J. (1985). Autoradiographic visualization of beta-adrenoceptor sybtypes in human lung. *Am. Rev. Respir. Dis.* **132**:541-547.

Casterline, C. L., Evans, R. III, and Ward, G. W. Jr. (1976). The effect of atropine and albuterol aerosols on the human bronchial response to histamine. *J. Allergy Clin. Immunol.* **58**:607-613.

Castro de la Mata, R., Penna, M., and Aviado, D. M. (1962). Reversal of sympathomimetic bronchodilation by dichloroisoproterenol. *J. Pharmacol. Exp. Ther.* **135**:197-203.

Colebatch, H. J. H., and Halmagyi, D. F. J. (1963). Effect of vagotomy and vagal stimulation on lung mechanics and circulation. *J. Appl. Physiol.* **18**:881-887.

Conolly, M. E., and Greenacre, J. K. (1976). The lymphocyte beta-adrenoceptor in normal subjects and patients with bronchial asthma. The effect of different forms of treatment on receptor function. *J. Clin. Invest.* **58**:1307-1316.

Dey, R. D., Shannon, W. A., and Said, S. I. (1981). Localization of VIP-immunoreactive nerves in airways and pulmonary vessels of dogs, cats and human subjects. *Cell Tissue Res.* **220**:231-238.

Dixon, W. E., and Ransom, F. (1912). Bronchodilator nerves. *J. Physiol. (Lond.)*. **45**:413-428.

Doidge, J. M., and Satchell, D. G. (1982). Adrenergic and non-adrenergic inhibitory nerves in mammalian airways. *J. Autonom. Nerv. Sys.* **5**:83-99.

Douglas, J. S., Dennis, M. W., Ridgway, P., and Bouhuys, A. (1973). Airway constriction in guinea pigs: interaction of histamine and autonomic drugs. *J. Pharmacol. Exp. Ther.* **184**:169-179.

Empey, D. W., Laitinen, L. A., Jacobs, L., Gold, W. M., and Nadel, J. A. (1976). Mechanisms of bronchial hyperreactivity in normal subjects after upper respiratory tract infection. *Am. Rev. Respir. Dis.* **113**:131-139.

Frigo, G. M., del Tacca, M., Lecchini, S., and Crema, A. (1973). Some observations on the intrinsic nervous mechanism in Hirschsprung's disease. *Gut* **14**:35-40.

Gaddie, J., Legge, J. S., Petrie, G., and Palmer, K. N. V. (1972). The effect of an alpha-adrenergic receptor blocking drug on histamine sensitivity in bronchial asthma. *Br. J. Dis. Chest* **66**: 141-146.

Galant, S. P., Duriseti, L., Underwood, S., and Insel, P. A. (1978). Decreased beta-adrenergic receptors on polymorphonuclear leukocytes after adrenergic therapy. *N. Engl. J. Med.* **229**:933-936.

Golden, J. A., Nadel, J. A., and Boushey, H. A. (1978). Bronchial hyperirritability in healthy subjects after exposure to ozone. *Am. Rev. Respir. Dis.* **118**:287-294.

Grieco, M. H., and Pierson, R. N., Jr. (1971). Mechanism of bronchoconstriction due to beta-adrenergic blockade. *J. Allergy Clin. Immunol.* **48**:143-152.

Grieco, M. H., Pierson, R. N., Jr., and Pi-Sunyer, F. X. (1968). Comparison of the circulatory and metabolic effects of isoproterenol, epinephrine and methoxamine in normal and asthmatic subjects. *Am. J. Med.* **44**:863-872.

Grundström, N., Andersson, R. G. G., and Wikberg, J. E. S. (1981). Prejunctional α_2-adrenoceptors inhibit contraction of tracheal smooth muscle by inhibiting cholinergic neurotransmission. *Life Sci.* **28**:2981-2986.

Holtzman, M. J., Cunningham, J. H., Sheller, J. R., Irsigler, G. B., Nadel, J. A., and Boushey, H. A. (1979). Effect of ozone on bronchial reactivity in atopic and non-atopic subjects. *Am. Rev. Respir. Dis.* **120**:1059-1067.

Holtzman, M. J., Sheller, J. R., DiMeo, M., Nadel, J. A., and Boushey, H. A. (1980). Effect of ganglionic blockade on bronchial reactivity in atopic subjects. *Am. Rev. Respir. Dis.* **122**:17-25.

Itkin, I. H., and Anand, S. C. (1970). The role of atropine as a mediator blocker of induced bronchial obstruction. *J. Allergy* **45**:178-186.

Kaliner, M., Shelhamer, J. H., Davis, P. B., Smith, L. J., and Venter, J. C. (1982). Autonomic nervous system abnormalities and allergy. *Ann. Intern. Med.* **96**:349-357.

Kariman, K. (1980). Beta-adrenergic receptor binding in lymphocytes from patients with bronchial asthma. *Lung* **158**:41-51.

Kirkpatrick, C. H., and Keller, C. (1967). Impaired responsiveness to epinephrine in asthma. *Am. Rev. Respir. Dis.* **96**:692-699.

Kneussl, M. P., and Richardson, J. B. (1978). Alpha-adrenergic receptors in human and canine tracheal and bronchial smooth muscle. *J. Appl. Physiol.* **45**:307-311.

Laitinen, L. A., Heino, M., Laitinen, A., Kava, T., and Haahtela, T. (1985). Damage of the airway epithelium and bronchial reactivity in patients with asthma. *Am. Rev. Respir. Dis.* **131**:599-606.

Lockey, S. D., Jr., Glennon, J. A., and Reed, C. E. (1967). Comparison of some metabolic responses in normal and asthmatic subjects to epinephrine and glucagon. *J. Allergy* **40**:349-354.

Lundberg, J. M., and Saria, A. (1983). Capsaicin-induced sensitization of the airway mucosa to cigarette smoke, mechanical and chemical irritants. *Nature* **302**:251-253.

Lundberg, J. M., Saria, A., Brodin, E., Rossell, S., and Folkers, K. (1983a). A substance P antagonist inhibits vagally induced increase in vascular permeability and bronchial smooth muscle contraction in the guinea pig. *Proc. Natl. Acad. Sci. U.S.A.* **80**:1120-1124.

Lundberg, J. M., Martling, C. R., and Saria, A. (1983b). Substance P and capsaicin-induced contraction of human bronchi. *Acta Physiol. Scand.* **119**:49-53.

MacDonald, A. G., Ingram, C. G., and McNeill, R. S. (1967). The effect of propranolol on airway resistance. *Br. J. Anaesth.* **39**:919-929.

Mann, S. P. (1971). The innervation of mammalian bronchial smooth muscle: the localization of catecholamines and cholinesterases. *Histochem. J.* **3**:319-331.

Matsuzaki, Y., Hamasaki, Y., and Said, S. I. (1980). Vasoactive intestinal peptide: a possible transmitter of nonadrenergic relaxation of guinea pig airways. *Science* **210**:1252-1253.

McFadden, E. R., Jr., Luparello, T., Lyons, H. A., and Bleecker, E. (1969). The mechanism of action of suggestion in the induction of acute asthma attacks. *Psychosom. Med.* **31**:134-143.

Middleton, E., Jr., and Finke, S. R. (1968). Metabolic response to epinephrine in asthma. *J. Allergy* **42**:288-299.

Mita, H., Yui, Y., Yasueda, H., and Shida, T. (1983). Changes of $alpha_1$ and beta-adrenergic and cholinergic muscarinic receptors in guinea pig lung sensitized with ovalbumin. *Int. Arch. Allergy Appl. Immunol.* **70**:225-230.

Morris, H. G., Rusnak, S. A., and Barzens, K. (1977). Leukocyte cyclic adenosine monophosphate in asthmatic children. Effects of adrenergic therapy. *Clin. Pharmacol. Ther.* **22**:352-359.

Nadel, J. A. (1983). Bronchial reactivity. *Adv. Intern. Med.* **28**:207-223.

Nadel, J. A., and Barnes, P. J. (1984). Autonomic regulation of the airways. *Annu. Rev. Med.* **35**:45-67.

Nadel, J. A., and Holtzman, M. J. (1984). Regulation of airway responsiveness and secretion: role of inflammation. In *Asthma. Physiology, Immunopharmacology, and Treatment.* Edited by A. B. Kay, K. F. Austen, and L. M. Lichtenstein. London, Academic Press, pp. 129-155.

Nadel, J. A., and Widdicombe, J. G. (1962a). Reflex effects of upper airway irritation on total lung resistance and blood pressure. *J. Appl. Physiol.* **17**:861-865.

Nadel, J. A., and Widdicombe, J. G. (1962b). Effect of changes in blood gas tensions and carotid sinus pressure on tracheal volume and total lung resistance to airflow. *J. Physiol. (Lond.)* **163**:13-33.

Nadel, J. A., and Widdicombe, J. G. (1963). Reflex control of airway size. *Ann. N.Y. Acad. Sci.* **109**:712-722.

Nadel, J. A., Salem, H., Tamplin, G., and Yokiwa, Y. (1965). Mechanisms of bronchoconstriction during inhalation of sulfur dioxide. *J. Appl. Physiol.* **20**:164-167.

Olsen, C. R., Colebatch, H. J. H., Mebel, P. E., Nadel, J. A., and Staub, N. C. (1965). Motor control of pulmonary airways studied by nerve stimulation. *J. Appl. Physiol.* **20**:202-208.

Parker, C., and Smith, J. W. (1973). Alterations in cyclic adenosine monophosphate metabolism in human bronchial asthma. I. Leukocyte responsiveness to beta-adrenergic agents. *J. Clin. Invest.* **52**:48-59.

Partanen, M., Laitinen, A., Hervonen, A., Toivanen, M., and Laitinen, L. A. (1982). Catecholamine- and acetylcholinesterase-containing nerves in human lower respiratory tract. *Histochemistry* **76**:175-188.

Patel, K. R., and Kerr, J. W. (1973). The airways response to phenylephrine after blockade of alpha and beta receptors in extrinsic bronchial asthma. *Clin. Allergy* **3**:439-448.

Richardson, J., and Beland, J. (1976). Nonadrenergic inhibitory nervous system in human airways. *J. Appl. Physiol.* **41**:764-771.

Richardson, J. B. (1979). State of the art. Nerve supply to the lungs. *Am. Rev. Respir. Dis.* **119**:785-802.

Richardson, J. B. (1985). Nonadrenergic inhibitory nervous system in relation to asthma. In *Bronchial Asthma: Mechanisms and Therapeutics.* Edited by E. B. Weiss, M. S. Segal, and M. Stein. Boston, Little, Brown, pp. 123-125.

Said, S. I., Geumi, A., and Hara, N. (1982). Bronchodilator effect of VIP *in vivo*: protection against bronchoconstriction induced by histamine or prostaglandin $F_{2\alpha}$. In *Vasoactive Intestinal Peptide.* Edited by S. I. Said. New York, Raven Press, pp. 185-191.

Sheller, J. R., Holtzman, M. J., Skoogh, B. E., and Nadel, J. A. (1982). Interaction of serotonin with vagal- and Ach-induced bronchoconstriction in canine lungs. *J. Appl. Physiol.* **52**:964-966.

Sheppard, D., Epstein, J., Holtzman, M. J., Nadel, J. A., and Boushey, H. A. (1982). Dose-dependent inhibition of cold air-induced bronchoconstriction by atropine. *J. Appl. Physiol.* **53**:169-174.

Shibata, H., Mio, M., and Tasaka, K. (1985). Analysis of the mechanism of histamine release induced by substance P. *Biochem. Biophys. Acta* **846**: 1-7.

Simonsson, B. G., Jacobs, F. M., and Nadel, J. A. (1967). Role of the autonomic nervous system and the cough reflex in the increased responsiveness of airways in patients with obstructive airway disease. *J. Clin. Invest.* **46**:1812-1818.

Snashall, R., Boother, F. A., and Sterling, G. M. (1978). The effect of alpha adrenergic stimulation on the airways of normal and asthmatic man. *Clin. Sci. Mol. Med.* **54**:283-289.

Starke, K. (1981). Presynaptic receptors. *Annu. Rev. Pharmacol. Toxicol.* **21**: 7-30.

Sterling, G. M., and Batten, J. C. (1969). Effect of aerosol propellants and surfactants on airway resistance. *Thorax* **24**:228-231.

Szentivanyi, A. (1968). The beta adrenergic theory of the atopic abnormality in bronchial asthma. *J. Allergy* **42**:203-225.

Tam, E., Sheppard, D., Epstein, J., Ancic, P., and Boushey, H. (1983). Effect of increasing doses of ipatropium bromide on dose-response curve to isocapnic hyperventilation with cold air in asthmatic subjects. *Am. Rev. Respir. Dis.* **127**:250.

Tattersfield, A. E., Leaver, D. G., and Pride, N. B. (1973). Effects of beta-adrenergic blockade and stimulation on normal human airways. *J. Appl. Physiol.* **35**:613-619.

Thomson, N. C., Daniel, E. E., and Hargreave, F. E. (1982). Role of smooth muscle alpha$_1$-receptors in nonspecific bronchial responsiveness in asthma. *Am. Rev. Respir. Dis.* **126**:521-525.

Townley, R. G., McGeady, S., and Bewtra, A. (1976). The effect of beta-adrenergic blockade on bronchial sensitivity to acetyl-beta-methacholine in normal and allergic rhinitis subjects. *J. Allergy Clin. Immunol.* **57**:358-366.

Widdicombe, J. G., and Nadel, J. A. (1963). Reflex effects of lung inflation on tracheal volume. *J. Appl. Physiol.* **18**:681-686.

Wikberg, J. E. S., Grundström, Visnovsky, P., and Andersson, R. G. G. (1982). Pharmacology of B-HT 920 in some isolated smooth muscles of the guinea pig. *Acta Pharmacol. Toxicol.* **50**:266-271.

Zaid, G., and Beall, G. N. (1966). Bronchial response to beta-adrenergic blockade. *N. Engl. J. Med.* **275**:580-584.

19

Control of Airway Smooth Muscle

EDWIN E. DANIEL

McMaster University
Hamilton, Ontario, Canada

Airway smooth muscle can be controlled by intrinsic myogenic, intrinsic and extrinsic neural, or chemical factors. Chemical factors can be derived from the circulation or locally from cells mediating immune responses or from other sources. Since neural control is dealt with elsewhere in this volume, I will focus on myogenic control and make some comments on the interactions of myogenic and immune mediators. It is probable that all these controls interact in producing both normal and abnormal responses in physiological as well as in pathophysiological conditions. Although it is certainly wrong to consider that they operate in isolation, it is convenient to describe their operation in isolation and to begin with consideration of the structures that determine whether putative control systems may exist and operate or not. Although important, I will leave aside discussion of biochemistry of contractile proteins and contractile mechanics.

I. Myogenic Control

A. Structure

Airway smooth muscle possesses a diversity of structures relevant to myogenic activity (defined here as electrical activity initiated by smooth muscle and initiating or modulating contraction). Cell-to-cell junctions are required for intercellular communication and such communication is essential if myogenic activity is to have a control function. There are several main types of junctions: gap junctions (see below), intermediate contacts or desmosome-like contacts, and close appositions. Intermediate contacts, as seen in the electron microscope, are characterized by a parallel orientation of cell membranes about 60 nm (40-80 nm) apart with an electron-dense line in the basement membrane region between cells and often with electron-dense structures associated with the cytoplasmic surface of the plasma membrane. Close appositions (sometimes peg and socket arrangements) involve appositions of the cell membranes of two cells at a distance of about 20-30 nms. These have been described in smooth muscle in several publications (Henderson et al., 1971; Henderson, 1975; Gabella, 1976, 1981) and I will focus only on the gap junction because more is known of its role in cell-to-cell communication in smooth muscle (Daniel et al., 1976; Kannan and Daniel, 1978; Sims et al., 1982; Cole et al., 1985; Kannan et al., 1983).

The gap junctions are composed of arrays of membrane proteins, connexons, which, when aligned in apposed membranes of each of two cells and when open, provide channels between cells. These channels are low in electrical resistance and capable of passing molecules up to 800-1200 daltons (Flagg-Newton, 1980; Flagg-Newton and Loewenstein, 1979; Simpson et al., 1977). Obviously, they provide a basis for the communication of electrical signals as well as metabolic signals. Figure 1A shows, in thin sections, gap junctions between two human tracheal smooth muscle cells. The appearance of a gap junction in a freeze fractured smooth muscle cell membrane (p-face) is shown in Figure 1B-D; each of the hillocks is presumed to represent a single connexon (Revel et al., 1985), left behind when the external component of the cell membrane bilayer was fractured away.

Gap junctions can be regulated in two ways. First the conductance of gap junctions can be regulated (Table 1). Second, the synthesis or assembly of gap junction protein can be regulated (Table 2). Considerable attention has been paid in simpler systems than airway smooth muscle to regulation of conductance through gap junctions and the findings recently reviewed (Sheridan and Atkinson, 1985; Spray and Bennett, 1985). Simpler systems are usually cells from invertebrates, in which each of two large adjacent cells can be impaled with two microelectrodes and coupling measured by passing current into one cell while both cells are voltage clamped at a common holding potential using independent clamp currents. On application of a command pulse to one cell, current from the other cell is recorded along with the applied voltage from the first cell to yield transjunction resistance by Ohm's law (see Spray and Bennett, 1985). With the advent of whole cell voltage clamp through a patch, it has become possible to clamp and measure current or voltage and, hence,

Table 1 Control of Gap Junction Conductance

Physiological variables
pH: low pH, low conductance (pK <7; Hill coefficient ~ 1)
pCa: high Ca, low conductance (pK >40-$80\ \mu M$)
Voltage gradient: no effect in mammalian cells
Pharmacologic variables
c-AMP ↑, conductance ↑
Alcohols ↑, conductance ↓ (octanol)
Phorbol esters ↑, conductance ↓

Table 2 Control of Gap Junction Numbers (G.J. No.)

Physiological variables
Sex steroids in myometrium: estrogen ↑, G.J. No. ↑; progesterone ↑, G.J. No. ↓
Unknown factors in embryologic development
Pharmacologic variables
c-AMP in several cell types: c-AMP ↑, G.J. No. ↑
PGE_2, PEI_2; PG ↑, G.J. No. ↑
Glibenclamide on beta cells of pancreas: G.J. No.↑
Pathologic variables
Certain tumors: G.J. No. ↓
Inflammation ???

Source: Spray and Bennett, 1985; Sheridan and Atkinson, 1985.

coupling with a single electrode in each of two smaller cells (Spray and Bennett, 1985; White et al., 1985), but this has not been done in any smooth muscle cells.

The present consensus from studies in invertebrate and a few mammalian cell symptoms is that changes in intracellular pH, especially local changes near the gap junction, play the most important role. Low pH (Spray et al., 1981; Turin and Warner, 1980; Spray and Bennett, 1985) reduces or abolishes gap junction conductance and in mammalian heart pH above 7.0 retains or restores full conductance. The effect of low pH may involve changes in Ca^{2+} binding in

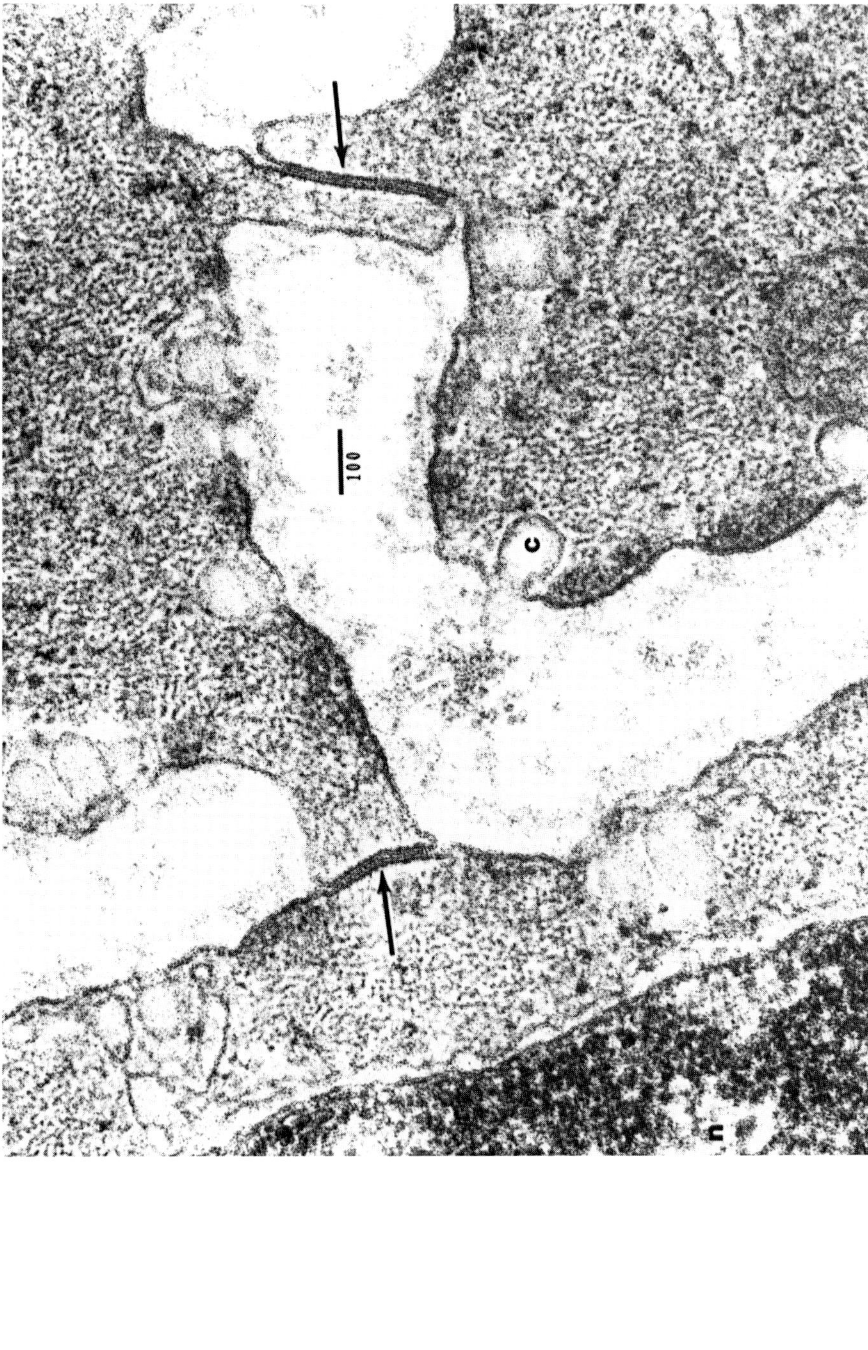

(A)

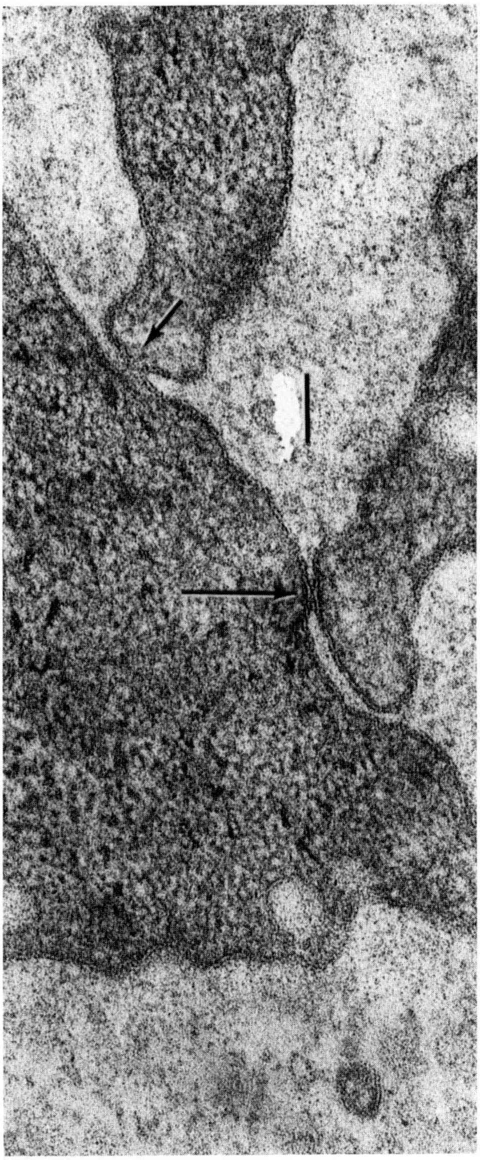

(B)

Figure 1 Two gap junctions (arrows) from human trachea. Note their typical seven-lined structure, including a 2 nm gap with an overall width of about 20 nm on cell appendages or on the main portion of the cell (near the nucleus, n). These cells have prominent caveolar (c). The bar is approximately 100 nm (from Daniel et al., 1986a). (B) Two nexuses (arrows between human bronchial smooth muscle cells. Note the absence of a detectable gap (compare to A). The nexus shown with the longer arrow is more clearly seen than the other (short arrow). Most of those observed resembled the latter. The bar is approximately 75 nm (from Daniel et al., 1986a).

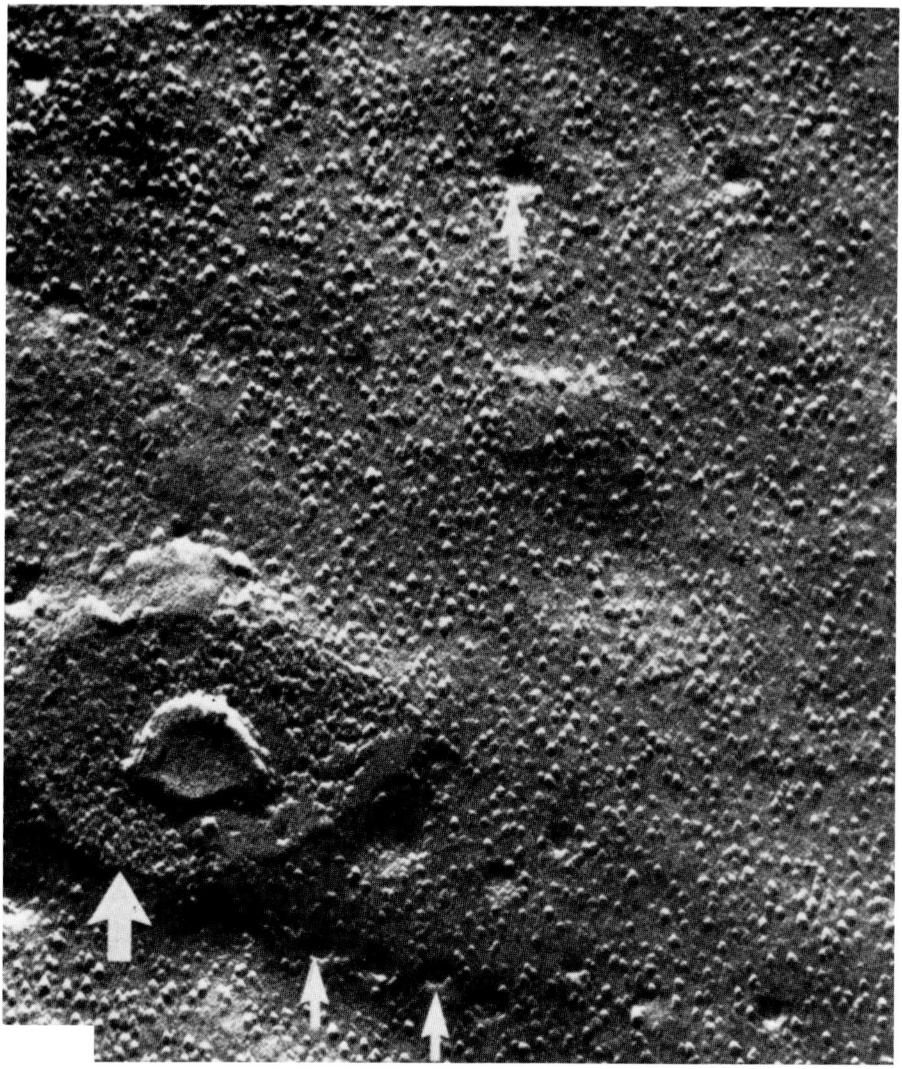

(C)

Figure 1 (continued) (C) Two large gap junctions (large arrows) in parturient rat myometrium seen in freeze-fracture replicas of the PFC fracture face (protoplasmic face) of the cell membrane. Note numerous necks of caveolae and membrane particles (small arrows). It is clear that not all membrane particles or small assemblies of particles can be identified as connexons (from Garfield et al., (1978).

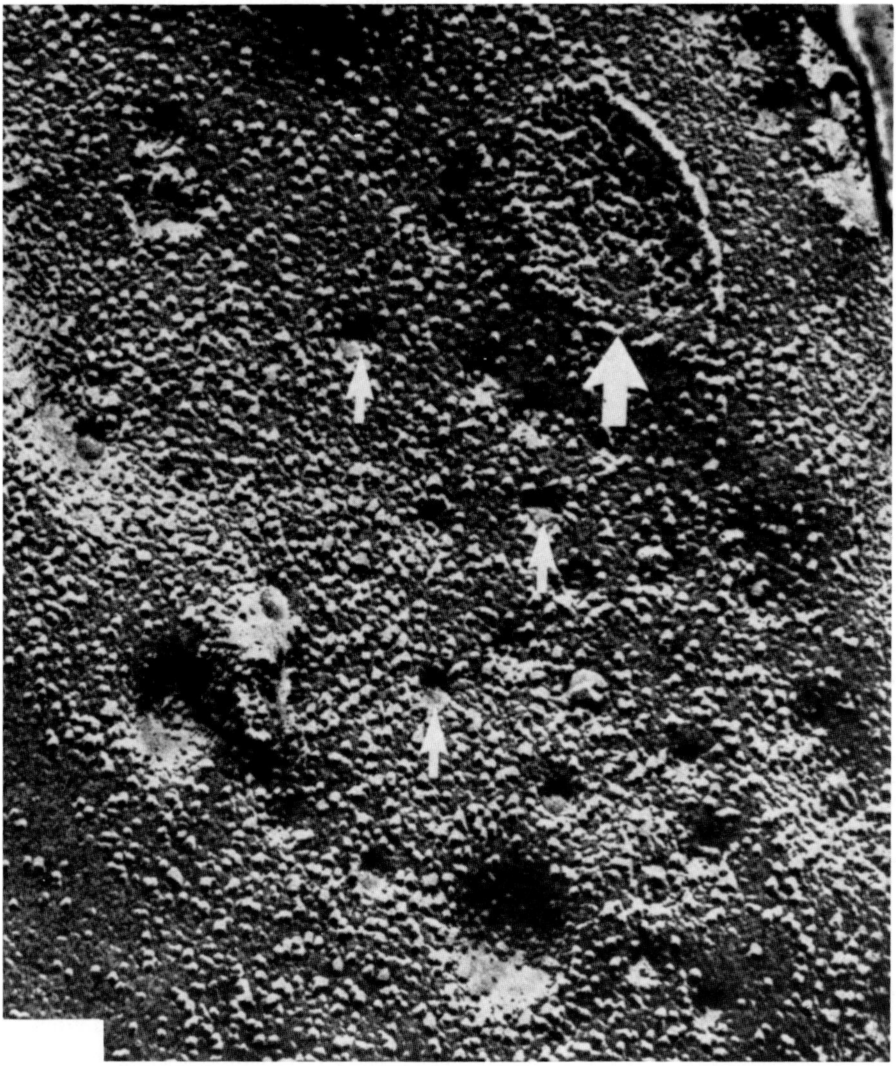

(D)

Figure 1 (continued)

or near the connexon. Certainly marked elevations (40-70 μM) of Ca_i^{2+} levels also inhibit gap junction conductance (Rose et al., 1977), but most evidence available to date suggests (see Spray and Bennett, 1985) that Ca_i^{2+} changes required to inhibit connexon coupling are unlikely to be achieved in normally functioning cells with Ca-handling machanisms intact. However, this conclusion may not be final because it ignores the fact that local Ca_i^{2+} concentrations near the connexon may be much higher than in the bulk cytosol (Rose and Loewenstein, 1975).

In several invertebrate systems, a voltage gradient across the gap junction may influence junctional conductance (Spray et al., 1979; Spray and Bennett, 1985). However, evidence to date suggests that the control system is absent in mammalian cells (White et al., 1985; Spray and Bennett, 1985). To what degree a voltage gradient affects coupling directly or through other mechanisms (e.g., pH) in the gap is unclear.

Recently, evidence has accumulated that elevation of c-AMP may enhance junctional permeability in several non-smooth-muscle systems (Flagg-Newton et al., 1981; Flagg-Newton and Loewenstein, 1981; Azarnia et al., 1981) as well as increase junctional particles. Also PGE_1 and catecholamines have these effects (Radu et al., 1982) and may operate through c-AMP. Studies in smooth muscle are lacking.

B. Distribution of Gap Junctions in Airway Smooth Muscle

Although the presence of gap junctions as structures observed after fixation does not prove the existence of low resistance contacts between living cells (Spray and Bennett, 1985), it certainly implies that they may be present. There has been considerable discussion and disagreement about whether the functional state of gap junctions can be determined by the disposition (irregularity) of the arrays of connexons seen after freeze fracture (see Peraccia, 1980) and it is certain that fixation by glutaraldehyde uncouples them (see Spray and Bennett, 1985). Certainly their appearance in thin sections after fixation cannot be used to distinguish their functional state. However, it seems reasonable to presume that structural gap junctions, when observed consistently between airway smooth muscle cells, represent at least in most instances the sites of functional gap junctions in life. That is because normal smooth muscle cells maintain a low intracellular Ca^{2+} ($< 10^{-7}$ M) and a pH probably slightly higher than 7 (Spray and Bennett, 1985); however, in acidosis or in the presence of sufficient Ca^{2+} entry to overwhelm Ca sequestration or pumping mechanisms (and perhaps during extreme contractions), connexons may be close. For the purposes of the following discussion, I will assume that those found in airway muscle are mostly open.

Humans

In humans (Richardson and Furguson, 1980; Daniel et al., 1980, 1986a), gap junctions in airway muscle are found in high density in trachea and first and second order bronchi (Fig. 1A). However, when smaller (approximately fourth to seventh order) bronchi are studied, typical gap junctions are absent (Daniel et al., 1986). Instead, very small areas of membrane apposition (nexuses) are present (Fig. 1B); no gap can be discerned but this may result from the technical problem of examining a small assembly of connexons (perhaps 10-20) with an overall diameter of 60 nm or less using ordinary electron microscopic examination of thin sections, which are themselves 50-70 nm thick (Fry et al., 1977; Gabella, 1981). Only when the gap junction is nearly perfectly aligned (its plane at right angles to the plane of section) throughout the thickness of the section can its characteristic 2 nm gap be seen clearly in thin sections. Obviously, this is unlikely when such small assemblies of connexons are present. Studies of freeze-fractured membranes might be helpful but none have been reported using these tissues. Also, the existence of a small assembly of membrane protein particles in a given cell membrane face after fracturing does not establish that these are connexons or that they were properly aligned with connexons in an adjacent cell. For the purpose of this discussion, I will consider these nexuses in small human bronchi to be true gap junctions. If they are, it is clear from present data (Daniel et al., 1986) showing that they are less frequent as well as smaller; thus they will provide far less coupling than normal-sized gap junctions (profiles averaging 100 nm diameter as seen in sections of human trachea; diameters possibly up to 300 nm of junctions in the cell).

Dogs

In dogs, we (Daniel, E. E., Berezin, I., Posey-Daniel, V., Hirshman, C. A., unpublished) have just completed a study of muscle from trachea and bronchi down through fourth order in normal and hyperresponsive dogs (Hirshman et al., 1984). In contrast to the human airway, the smooth muscle of both types had gap junctions of average size down through the fourth order bronchi. This is the case even though, as in the human, there is a dramatic increase in the density and closeness of the innervation in bronchi beginning in second order bronchi. Therefore, on structural grounds, canine airways appeared to be tightly coupled throughout the bronchial tree studied to date.

Cows

Bovine trachea resemble human and canine trachea in possessing numerous gap junctions (Cameron et al., 1982). Like the trachea from other species, it lacks a dense or close innervation. However, structures of bronchi from bovine airway have not been reported.

Guinea Pig

As far as I am aware, the ultrastructure of only the trachea of guinea pig has been examined, so comparisons between trachea and bronchi are not possible in this species. Guinea pig tracheas have gap junctions but the number is less than in dogs (Jones et al., 1980, Hoyes and Barber, 1980). There is, however, a very dense innervation, as in human and dog bronchi.

C. Functional Studies of Coupling

There are, to date, few direct functional studies of cell-to-cell coupling in bundles of airway smooth muscle. A major unsolved problem is: How should such studies be carried out? One widely used method has been the application of extracellular currents across plate electrodes forming a compartment in a partitioned bath (the Abe and Tomita [1986] method; see Sims et al., 1982; Kannan et al., 1983). Currents are applied across silver chloride electrodes set up as plates to form a compartment into which the tissue strip protrudes through a small hole. Outside the compartment microelectrodes are used to measure current spread (first recording during current passing in the extracellular fluid to eliminate certain artifacts and then recording inside cells at various distances from the plates). A result such as shown in Figure 2 is usually found for well-coupled tissues such as canine trachea. From these findings and from the rate of rise and fall of the potential changes within cells, space and time constants can be calculated (2 mm and 300 msec for canine trachea measured along the muscle bundles). Similar values were obtained in bovine trachea (Kirkpatrick, 1975, 1981). Figure 3 illustrates these data as affected by tetraethylammonium ion, 4-amino-pyridine, and acetylcholine. A space constant measures in a leaky biological cable the distance a voltage displacement spreads before its value decays to 1/e of its initial value and is directly related to the square root of the ratio of the membrane resistance divided by the longitudinal (myoplasmic plus junctional) resistance. A time constant reflects the passive electrical properties of the cable that determine the time course of the delay with which membrane potential differences follow applied potential differences. A long time constant implies a slow membrane response to an instantaneously applied voltage.

The use of this technique has been seriously questioned (Sperelakis, 1969; Sperelakis and MacDonald, 1974) on the grounds that the currents applied extracellularly are, in fact, transmitted at least in major part within the extracellular spaces of the muscle bundle, as well as within cells. It was assumed in applying the method that the current entered the cells and was transmitted nearly ex-

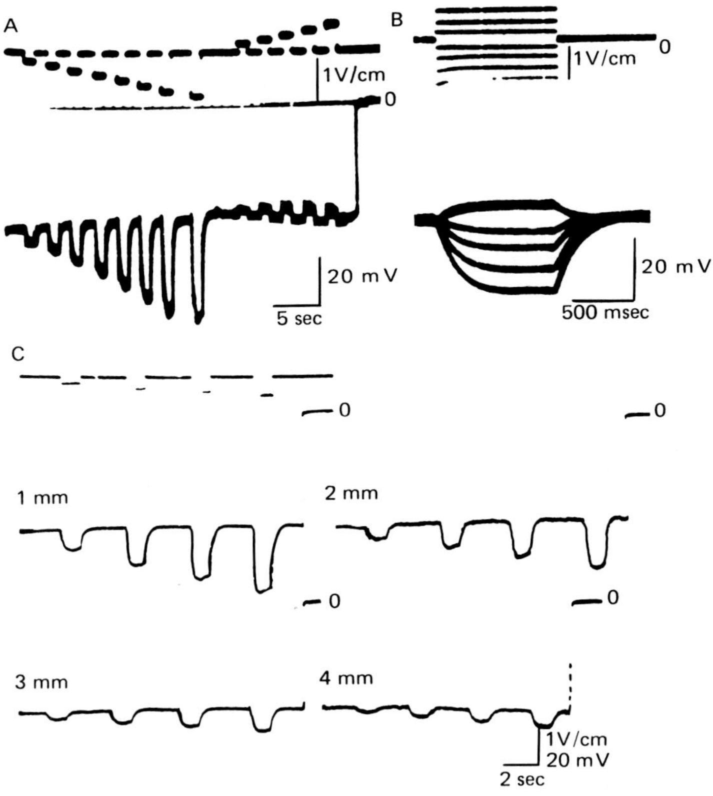

Figure 2 Membrane responses of canine tracheal smooth muscle to extracellular current injection in Abe-Tomita bath. Top traces are output of the current monitor (0 shows zero current output) and bottom traces are the membrane responses intracellularly. A and B show membrane responses to hyperpolarizing and depolarizing current pulses at slow and fast oscilloscope sweep speeds. The smaller and limited membrane responses to depolarizing (cathodal) currents illustrate the rectification observed. (C) Membrane responses to hyperpolarizing pulses recorded at increasing distance from the stimulatory electrodes (0 designates the zero membrane potential found on withdrawal of the microelectrode). Such data are plotted as log voltage change against distance from the stimulating electrodes to obtain the space constant. (From Kannan et al., 1983.)

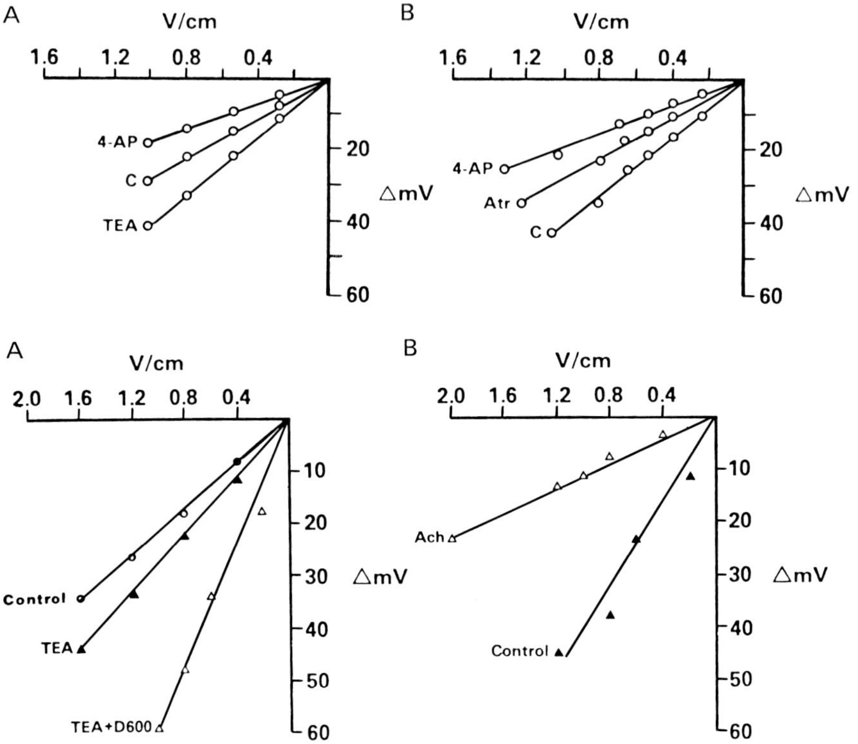

Figure 3 Data from study of canine trachea in the Abe-Tomita bath compared membrane responses by hyperpolarizing current pulses of different sizes (standardized as V/cm) under different conditions, recorded at the same distance from the stimulating electrode. Note that TEA (30 mM) increases the slope of the plot compared to control (c); that is, it increases apparent resistance since now a larger voltage change is produced by a given current. In contrast 4-AP (5 mM) and acetylcholine (10^{-7} M) decrease apparent resistance. Atropine pretreatment reverses the effect of 4-AP. The effect of TEA to increase resistance is enhanced if D600 is present to prevent Ca from entering via voltage operation channels opened when TEA depolarizes cells. This Ca probably opens K^+ channels and contributes to membrane inductance. (From Kannan et al., 1983.)

clusively within them. However, the longitudinal resistance to current flow in the extracellular space of a smooth muscle bundle is about 1/10 to 1/20 of the transverse resistance; thus its extracellular space also constitutes a cable (Sperelakis and MacDonald, 1974). Such a criticism, if correct, readily explains why space constants measured transverse to the long axis of the cells and bundles are very short ($<$ 1 mm) while those measured in the long axis are much longer 1.5 to 3.5 mm (e.g., see Cheung and Daniel, 1980). Gap junctions are usually found all along smooth muscle cells and not just at the ends, and different bundles usually have intersected branches, so the distribution of gap junctions and separation of bundles does not fully explain this finding. A spread of current in the extracellular space of muscle bundles may also explain why space constants in some smooth muscles lacking or having very few gap junctions still equal 1-3 mm in the long axis of the cell (Daniel et al., 1976; Gabella, 1981) and smooth muscle bundles appear to transmit currents across the sucrose compartment in a sucrose gap after the gap junctions have disappeared (Daniel et al., 1986b). In the latter case, spread of current is probably along the region of fixed charges and counterions at the cell surface.

Recently, a simplified (steady state) computer model using both the extracellular and the cellular cables has been tested (Sperelakis and Picone, 1986) and the results revealed that the basic premise of extracellular current flow seemed correct and also that varying the junctional resistance between cells in the cellular cable, from that found without any gap junctions to that found with many gap junctions or even to zero, had little effect of the estimated space constant. The authors concluded that results from methods using extracellular current applications should be reexamined and questioned.

Another concern about extracellular current injection techniques (partitioned bath or sucrose gap) is that they give values for space and time constants different from those obtained by intracellular current injections (Abe and Tomita, 1968; Holman, 1968; Tomita, 1966, 1969, 1970; Ohba et al., 1976; Sims et al., 1982); the latter method gives very short values.

A modification of the extracellular current injection technique involves use of alternating currents of various frequencies to assess impedance of a tissue in a narrow tube between two current-passing (say Pt-black) electrodes. To compel the current to pass through the tissue rather than around it, the physiological saline is replaced with sucrose solution and changes in impedance measured over time covering the frequency range of 0-1000 Hz. This method or related ones have been applied to some smooth muscles (Tomita, 1969; Ohba et al., 1976; Sims et al., 1982; Bortoff and Gilloteaux, 1980) but not to trachea. However, two of the smooth muscles studied have very few or no gap junctions (i.e., nonpregnant myometrium: Sims et al., 1982; Bortoff and Gilloteaux, 1980) and guinea pig taenia coli (Ohba et al., 1976, Sims et al., 1982) but longitudinal junctional resistances of quite low values (e.g., 300 ohm cm) were calculated. The assumption was that the impedance at very low frequencies represents the sum of longitudinal myoplasmic and junctional resistance, while that at very high frequencies represents that of the myoplasmic resistance, the junctional resistance have been bypassed at high frequencies because of a presumed capacity in the junction in parallel with the junctional resistance. If this proposed model is correct, the junctional impedance represents the difference between values found at low and high frequencies. Various ways of handling the data have been used (see previous references) but all depend on the above assumption about the equivalent circuit of the tissue in the sucrose gap (i.e., capacity in parallel to the resistance in junctions between cells). Also, all assume no significant current flow occurs in the extracellular space or along cell surfaces.

Recently, some concerns have emerged about how the current flow in a sucrose gap or in a tissue exposed to sucrose for impedance analysis (Pooler and Oxford, 1972; Pooler and Valenzeno, 1983). These include evidence that the cell membrane becomes leaky in sucrose. We recently found (Daniel et al., 1986b) that gap junctions are damaged and then disappear in sucrose, even though the performance of the tissue is normal (or improved in terms of size of membrane potentials and junction potentials to nerve stimulation) at the time the gap junctions are being lost (0.2-2 hr). These observations suggest that the fundamental assumptions described above to partition impedance also need reexamination and that current flows through the sucrose gap may be around rather than within the cells and may follow a current path in a thin layer of fixed charges and counterions at the cell surface. In a sense, these findings support the assumption that extracellular current flow may be important in longitudinal coupling and that the results obtained with the sucrose gap also require further evaluation to test this possibility.

The use of two microelectrodes, one for current passing and/or voltage clamping and the other for recording of membrane potential changes associated with spread if the current between the site of current injection and the recording site, has also been tried in some smooth muscles (see Kobayashi et al., 1967; Sperelakis and Tarr, 1965; Tarr and Sperelakis, 1964; Sperelakis, 1969, for comments). Ideally the system should have the capacity for voltage clamping of each cell as well as current passing and recording, but this requires two electrodes in the cells. Patch clamping with a single electrode for voltage clamping and current passing is now possible, but has not been applied to tracheal muscle. The currents passing electrode should be able to pass a wide range of currents, which is impossible when high resistance microelectrodes are used. The technique is difficult and contradictory results have so far been obtained (Kobayashi et al., 1967; Abe and Tomita, 1968; Tarr and Sperelakis, 1964; Sperelakis and Tarr, 1965; Sperelakis, 1969). Moreover, it has been suggested (Tomita, 1970) that the technique will not be applicable to a well-coupled tissue because the many low resistance junction coupling the injected cell to its neighbors will function as a large set of parallel pathways, each with low resistance to divide the current. Thus, any single cell coupled to the site of current injection will receive only a very small current and the resultant voltage drop across its cell membrane will be small, even negligible. In fact, when this technique was applied in guinea pig taenia coli (Abe and Tomita, 1968; Tomita, 1970) very little voltage charge was produced in the injected cell or in adjacent cells. Depolarizing currents did not usually produce action potentials in the injected cell and this was explained on similar grounds; that is, the sums of parallel resistances to current flow out of the injected cell are very low, so very little voltage drop occurs across the cell membrane. These interpretations are disputed by other workers (Sperelakis, 1969; see also Tarr and Sperelakis, 1964; Sperelakis and Tarr, 1965; Sperelakis and Picone, 1986). The irony is that very vew or no gap junctions can be found in taenia coli (Fry et al., 1977; Gabella, 1976, 1981) to account for the low resistance junctions. Recently, however, White et al. (1985) showed that low resistance junctions formed readily between adult mammalian myocytes studied in pairs, showing that such junctions can exist. This problem needs reexamination using single cell voltage clamping by way of a patch since this new technique provides better voltage control and allows passing of large currents, if isolated cells are used and allowed to form low resistance junctions.

If cells can generate active electrical currents (i.e., an action potential), the spread of these currents (velocity and distance) provides a crude index of coupling. The limitations of this technique are numerous, especially when applied to a multicellular system, and include the possibility that changes in the geometry of muscle bundle organization (degree of branching and interconnection) may have a significant effect on spread of action potentials without difference in coupling. Also, no airway muscle studied to date can produce action potentials under physiological conditions (see below).

My conclusion is that no straightforward electrical method exists to measure coupling of airway smooth muscle as it exists in bundles. If several measures (space constants and junctional impedances) agree in showing the same change in coupling, and if structural changes provide a basis for the observed changes, I am inclined to accept them qualitatively with serious reservations as to the absolute values obtained.

One less equivocal way to measure cell-to-cell coupling is by the analysis of the spread of intracellular labeled metabolites that cannot cross the cell membrane. One of these is 2-deoxyglucose, which is transported into smooth muscle and other cells by a Na-coupled transport system for glucose, is phosphorylated inside the cell, and then is unable to return either via the carrier or via diffusion. A recent study (Cole et al., 1985) in myometrium utilized a partitioned bath like that used by Abe and Tomita. The [^{3}H] deoxyglucose was applied in the compartment corresponding to theone by which current is applied and the spread of the labeled compound into the cells outside this compartment was followed over time and space. Control for leakage of label, into the other compartment by way of interstitial pathways, was provided by adding [^{3}H] sucrose or [^{3}H] mannitol, which do not readily enter cells, instead of [^{3}H] deoxyglucose. In the study mentioned, when gap junctions were numerous, [^{3}H] 2-deoxyglucose spread much further (diffusivity increased from 0.20-1.9 cm^2/sec) than when gap junctions were rare). However, sucrose or mannitol spread only approximately as predicted from a theoretical distribution in the extracellular space and this distribution did not change with the appearance of gap junctions. There seems to be a real difference in the spread of intracellular metabolite (Cole et al., 1985) and extracellularly applied current (Sims et al., 1982) when gap junctions were rare in these myometrial tissues. Electrical currents spread further in the absence of gap junctions than did an intracellular metabolite, and the change in appearance of gap junctions was less, possibly because the bundles also served as cables.

One method that may not measure coupling in airway muscle needs to be identified. The dose-response curve obtained in vitro when muscle strips are studied in a bath is such a method. It is possible that responsiveness might improve when cell-to-cell coupling is better, if activation of a given cell then leads to better transmission of active current (excitation) to other cells. One would then expect each concentration of a drug to cause a higher proportion of cells to be activated than in the absence of improved coupling and thus cause a larger contraction (Daniel et al., 1980). The maximum contraction would, of course, not change unless this was due to improved synchrony of responses.

However, this theoretical mechanism requires the operation of active currents initiated by a depolarizing agent (e.g., acetylcholine) at some cells; the spread of these currents would be enhanced. The normal canine, bovine, and guinea pig trachea (see below) cannot produce action potentials because of the strong rectification produced by activation of K^+-channels and efflux of K^+ induced by depolarizations (see below). In fact, in such circumstances, when only passive currents are transmitted electronically, improved coupling could interfere with spread of activation by tending to hold or clamp the membrane potential of cells coupled to those that are partly depolarized because they are near hot spots of mediator release (see below) close to the membrane potential of the rest of the bundle. This mechanism also might initially limit the excitation of muscle in the bath as effective drug concentrations are achieved first at the periphery of the tissue. It is worth remembering that c-AMP elevation in some cells increased the number and conductance of gap junctions (see above) and that many bronchodilators raise c-AMP levels in airway muscle. Interference with spread of depolarization from local hot spots might be involved in the action of these bronchodilators.

In any case, in the muscle bath eventually all cells would be exposed to the bath drug concentration so that the final effect achieved would depend upon coupling only if there were cells capable of activation by current spread but not by the drug. Recently, we (Mansour, S., and Daniel, E. E., unpublished) studied the effect of acute ovalbumin sensitization on gap junctions in guinea pig trachea and found, to our surprise, a marked reduction (2.5-0.6/100 cells in cross-section of membrane). However, there was no change in responses to cholinergic agonists, adrenergic agonists, histamine, autocoids (5-HT, prostaglandins, leukotrienes, etc.), or high K^+. We concluded that it was likely that none of these stimulus strength-response curves reflected the presumed alteration in cell-to-cell coupling.

II. Myogenic Electrical Activity: Canine and Bovine Trachea

The electrical activity of human airway smooth muscle studied by a reliable technique has not been reported. In unstimulated canine and bovine trachea, the cells are electrically silent (Suzuki et al., 1976; Kroeger and Stephens, 1975; Kirkpatrick and Tomita, 1978; Kannan et al., 1983; Kirkpatrick, 1975, 1981). However, Kirkpatrick (1981) reported that some preparations of bovine trachea were spontaneously active, producing slow waves. Usually, depolarization by applied currents does not lead to significant active currents and stretch does not cause activation of membrane currents or contraction (see Stephens et al., 1975). Applied depolarizing currents are strongly rectified (Suzuki et al., 1976; Kroeger and Stephens, 1975; Kirkpatrick and Tomita, 1978; Kannan et al., 1983; Kirkpatrick, 1975, 1981). However, these cells clearly have voltage-dependent Ca-channels and are capable of initiating action potentials. If K^+-channels are blocked by tetraethylammonium ion (TEA), depolarization ensures, rectification is diminished or abolished, and spontaneous action potentials (Ca^{2+}-ion-induced) are produced (Suzuki et al., 1976; Kroeger and Stephens, 1975; Kirkpatrick and Tomita, 1978; Kannan et al., 1983; Kirkpatrick, 1975, 1981). Figure 4 shows such potentials in canine trachea. The mechanisms whereby TEA causes those changes have been proposed to be blockade of potassium channels partly open at rest (to account for the depolarization) and those responsible for the rectification of depolarizing currents (although these may be the same channels). It appears probable that some Ca^{2+}-activated or other K^+ channels are not blocked by TEA, since repolarization of the action potentials produced by this agent is fairly rapid. However, this point has not been studied by voltage

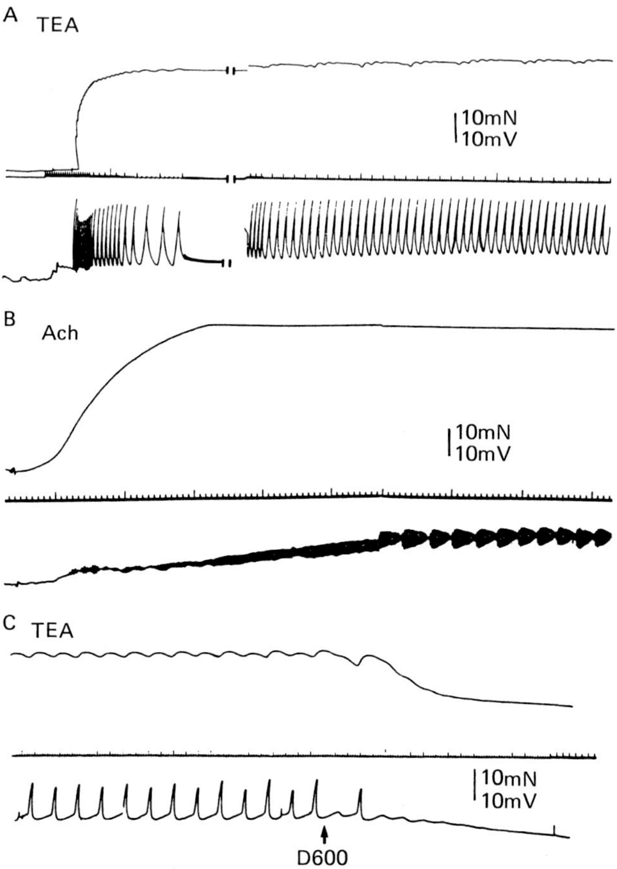

Figure 4 Responses to TEA (30 mM) and acetylcholine (Ach 10^{-7} M) in the single sucrose gap. Mechanical responses are shown in upper traces and electrical responses in lower traces. (A) Note the action potentials induced by TEA and associated with a large contraction (note changes in recording speed). (B) Note that Ach depolarizes and produces contraction; oscillations of membrane potential (individual oscillations cannot be distinguished) occur superimposed on the depolarization. (C) Note that D600 abolishes the action potentials induced by TEA and partially repolarizes the membrane while relaxing the contraction. Time marker: 1 min between larger lines and 10 sec between shorter lines as shown in the middle tracing. (From Kannan and Daniel, 1980 and Kannen et al., 1983.)

clamp or patch clamp techniques, and inactivation of Ca^{2+}-channels may also contribute to repolarization following each action potential.

Acetylcholine added to the bath or released from nerves also causes depolarization in bovine and canine trachea (Suzuki et al., 1976; Coburn, 1977, 1979; Farley and Miles, 1977, 1978; Kannan et al., 1983; Sharma et al., 1986; Kirkpatrick, 1975, 1981; Cameron and Kirkpatrick, 1977; Kirkpatrick and Tomita, 1978); on the plateau of depolarization membrane oscillations ensue (Fig. 4). The excitatory junction potential (EJP), when studied in the double sucrose gap, appears to be accompanied by increased membrane conductance, to have a reversal potential at 22 mv in our studies in canine trachea in the double sucrose gap, and to be dependent on Na^+ (Daniel et al., 1987). It appears possble that increase in conductance to anions is involved with Cl^- making a large contribution because of its outwardly directed electrochemical gradient. However, the conductance changes very early in the EJP cannot be measured in the double sucrose gap because of the long time constant of the membrane. Ca-entry leading to increased conductance through unblocked Ca-dependent K^+-channels may occur secondarily and contribute to the overall conductance increase.

It is of interest that contractions are often initiated along with EJP in the sucrose gap, even though no action potentials are produced. However, in our studies (Jager et al., 1986; Sharma et al., 1986) using the sucrose gap, we regularly find that contractions following EJPs in response to pulse trains are more closely associated with a second depolarization (Fig. 5) than with the EJP. A similar event can be detected in some records from bovine trachea (Fig. 18.3, Kirkpatrick, 1981). The nature of the increased conductance underlying these second potentials is unknown, but they show reversal potentials similar to EJPs and possibly reflect delayed or persistent Ach release (unpublished). It should be noted that EJPs can be produced by submaximal stimuli or by single pulses (Ito and Tajima, 1981; Inoue et al., 1984) that can summate, are sometimes associated with contraction (Daniel et al., 1987), but are not usually followed by secondary depolarizations.

When acetylcholine is applied endogenously or released by 4-aminopyridine in canine trachea (Daniel et al., 1987a,b; Fig. 6) there is a sustained depolarization and contraction in which membrane oscillations associated with phasic contractions occur. Similar observations were made recently in bovine trachea (Cameron and Kirkpatrick, 1977; Kirkpatrick, 1981). The conductance changes underlying these oscillations are unknown but they also may represent periodic openings of Ca^{2+} channels. Thus, active currents (after EJPs and during prolonged exposure to acetylcholine) can be produced even though action potentials are not, unless K^+-channels are blocked. Obviously, the nature of these active currents and the conditions that allow them to be initiated and

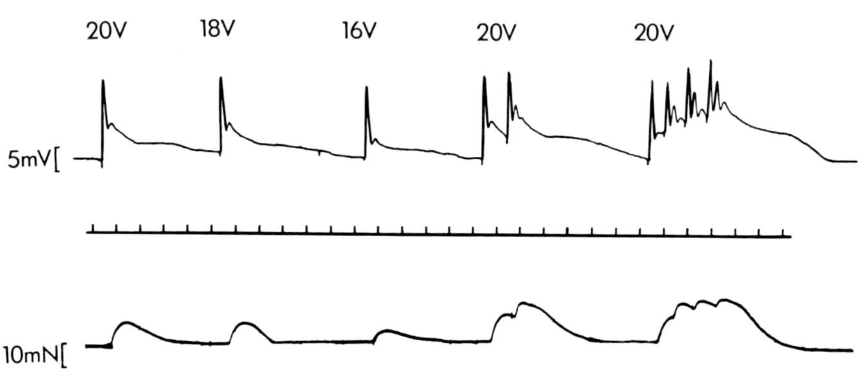

Figure 5 Membrane potential changes and contractions to pulse trains at various voltages that stimulate nerves of canine trachea, recorded in the single sucrose gap Note that contraction varies in amplitude as does the second slower potential following the EJP. (From Daniel et al., 1987.)

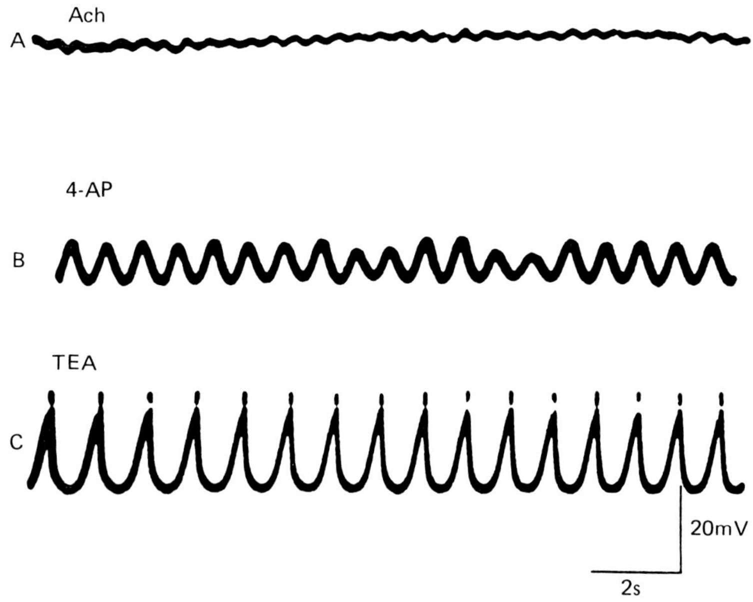

Figure 6 Membrane oscillations recorded intracellularly in canine trachea to Ach (10^{-7} M), 4-AP (5 mM), or TEA (30 mM) (as in Fig. 2). (From Kannan et al., 1983.)

propagated, as well as their relationship to slow waves of bovine trachea, need to be elucidated if we are to understand how contractions are initiated and coordinated in large airways with sparse innervation, such as canine trachea.

According to some reports (Coburn and Yamaguchi, 1977; Coburn, 1979; Farley and Miles, 1977, 1978), there is a component of pharmacomechanical coupling in the contractile response to acetylcholine or serotonin (5-HT). One group of investigators (Farley and Miles, 1977) found that low concentrations (10^{-7} M) of acetylcholine caused contraction without sufficient depolarization (judged by the relationship between K^+ depolarization and contraction) to initiate contraction. They concluded that at low concentrations acetylcholine had purely pharmacomechanical coupling of its action to contraction. Later, when they studied the effects of zero Ca^{2+} (Farley and Miles, 1978), they found that contractions of these low acetylcholine concentrations were more dependent on extracellular Ca^{2+} than were contractions to higher acetylcholine concentrations and suggested that they were dependent on Ca influx from a loosely bound Ca store, initiated by depolarization. Another investigator also found membrane-potential-independent contraction to acetylcholine, in the sense that depolarization for a given tension was smaller than with K^+ elevation (Coburn, 1979). However, acetylcholine in all effective concentrations caused depolarization. Furthermore, Coburn found that Ca channel antagonists (verapamil, D600, and La^{3+}) were more effective in inhibiting K^+- than acetylcholine-induced contractions caused contractions in Ca-free solutions and after depolarization, implying an independence of these effects from Ca entrance through voltage-dependent Ca channels (Kirkpatrick et al., 1975; Kirkpatrick, 1975). The roles of receptor-operated Ca channels vs. tightly bound extracellular Ca^{2+} in so-called pharmacomechanical coupling of excitation to contraction and other problems still need study.

If pharmacomechanical coupling is important when acetylcholine is released from nerves, it is difficult to know how acetylcholine released from a few scattered and distant (Kannan and Daniel, 1980b) nerve endings could lead to propagated coordinated contractions. However, like Coburn (1979), we (Daniel et al., 1987) find no evidence of pure pharmacomechanical coupling with acetylcholine (all concentrations caused some depolarization) in sucrose gap experiments.

In summary, it is clear that previous and our own studies do not clarify how depolarization induced by acetylcholine is coupled to contraction under physiological circumstances when the transmitter is released from sparse and distant nerves. First, the EJPs associated with acetylcholine can be up to 20 or 30 mV when elicited by maximal stimuli and are routinely 10-20 mV. These values are of course attenuated from those near transmitter release sites by electrotonic current spread and by the attenuation inherent in the sucrose gap method (see Bolton et al., 1981). Moreover, our studies suggest that channels other than Ca channels are involved in the EJP depolarization (based on a reversal potential at 20 mV of depolarization and Cl^--dependence of the EJP). Furthermore, the contractions may not be determined by the EJP directly but also by a second slow depolarization. The ionic mechanism causing and the mode of activation initiating this second potential are unknown but may be related to delayed release of acetylcholine. Therefore, comparisons of the voltage dependence of acetylcholine- and K^+-induced contractions may be irrelevant to propagation of responses to nerve stimulation. Finally, the possibility has not been fully explored whether receptor-operated Ca channels are opened by acetylcholine, allow Ca influx, and contribute to contraction when cells are exposed to normal external Ca^{2+}. Acetylcholine may release internal Ca^{2+}. However, it is unclear how opening of such channels or release of Ca^{2+} could lead to propagation of activation to cells not directly affected by the transmitter.

In contrast to bovine (in most preparations) and canine trachea, several studies have been shown the existence of myogenic activities of guinea pig trachea. Recordings either with microelectrodes or surface pore electrodes reveal spontaneous electrical oscillations (sometimes called slow waves) (Small, 1982; Dixon and Small, 1983; Foster et al., 1983a,b, 1984; McCaig and Souhrada, 1980). Sometimes with special recording techniques there are spontaneous contractions as well (Souhrada and Dickey, 1976). An important question is whether or not these slow waves per se can initiate opening of Ca channels, Ca influx, and contraction or whether (as is often the case in the gut: see Daniel and Sarna, 1978; Tomita, 1981) an interaction with other depolarizing events (e.g., release of acetylcholine from nerves) during the depolarized phase of the oscilliation if necessary to initiate contractions. So far, no evidence of such an interaction has been found and it is unclear whether and how slow waves might act as pacemakers for the phasic mechanical responses reported to occur in guinea pig trachea at similar frequencies (Souhrada and Dickey, 1976).

The most systematic studies of myogenic activity in guinea pig trachea have been made by Small and his colleagues (Small, 1982; Dixon and Small, 1983; Foster et al., 1983a,b, 1984). They record slow (about 1-1.5/sec) oscillations of membrane potential in guinea pig trachea using both extracellular pore electrodes and intracellular electrodes (Fig. 7). This tissue produces active tone, probably owing to PGE_2 production in vitro; abolition of slow waves by D600 reduces tone but does not abolish it (Foster et al., 1984). Since endogenous PGE_2 is a likely initiator of basal active tension in this tissue, but its contractile effects are not abolished by verapamil (Foster et al., 1984), it is likely that residual tone in the absence of slow waves is due to a pharmacomechanical effect of this prostaglandin.

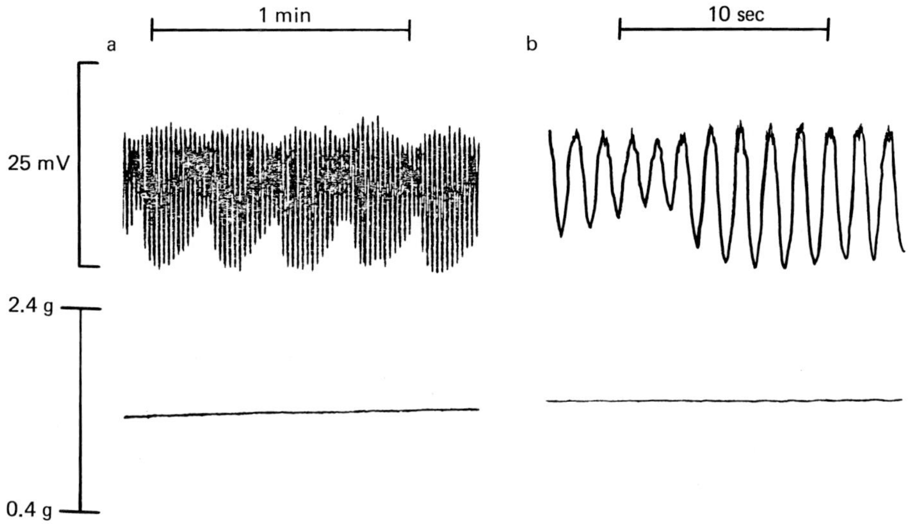

Figure 7 Intracellular membrane potential recordings (upper trace) and mechanical activity recording (lower tissue) in guinea pig trachea. The two traces were obtained from contiguous segments of guinea pig trachea. Recordings from the same cell at two different chart speeds are shown. Note small rapid oscillations on top of individual slow waves (right) and waxing and waving of slow wave amplitude (left). (From Small, 1982.)

However, there is no established temporal connection between electrical and tension change (Fig. 8) even when large phasic contractions are occurring after TEA. A major problem is that slow waves are recorded from one tracheal muscle bundle while tension is recorded from an adjacent one. Since there is poor coupling between adjacent tracheal muscle bundles (Dixon and Small, 1983), it seems possible that absence of a clear temporal connection between electrical and mechanical events recorded in this way should be anticipated. A further impediment is the effect of the tracheal cartilage, which is always present in these studies and may dampen phasic mechanical responses. Thus, it is unclear how these tracheal slow waves regulate contractile activity. In general, it seems that relaxants of tension (isopropylnorepinephrine, nitrite, adenosine, ATP and D600) abolish slow waves, but it is unclear whether this is always or sometimes accompanied by hyperpolarization. Excitants that depolarize (elevated K^+, acetylcholine, and histamine) enhance slow wave amplitude (and sometimes frequency) when depolarizations are modest (Small, 1982; Foster et al., 1983b, 1984) and abolish them when large depolarizations are produced (Ahmad et al., 1984). Recently,

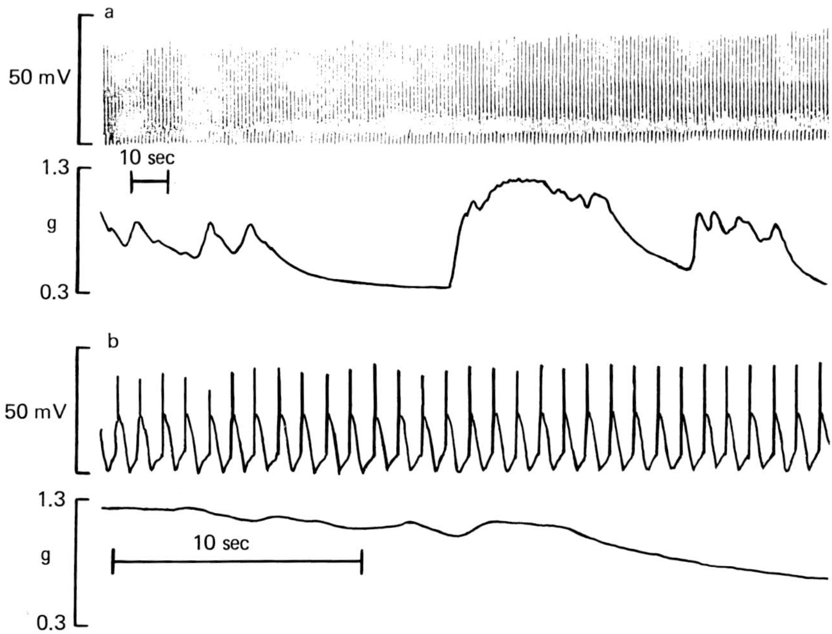

Figure 8 Intracellular recordings of membrane potentials (top traces) and tension (bottom traces) taken from contiguous segments of guinea pig trachea after action potentials were induced by TEA (15 mM). (From Dixon and Small, 1983.)

these investigators reported (Ahmad et al., 1984) that at high degrees of depolarization following acetylcholine the slow waves are replaced with a high-frequency, low-voltage, electrical noise apparently of myogenic origin. The significance of this noise also remains to be elucidated.

As in bovine and canine trachea, TEA blocks K^+ channels in guinea pig trachea, depolarizes them, and leads to myogenic initiation of action potentials that often have a plateau phase (Small, 1982; Dixon and Small, 1983; Foster et al., 1983a, 1984) (Figs. 8 and 9). These are associated with vigorous contractions (still there is no temporal connection between individual action potentials or bursts of them and tension development in adjacent tracheal bundles). Since the TEA-induced action potentials (Foster et al., 1983a, 1984; Ahmad et al., 1985) are sensitive to organic and inorganic Ca-channel antagonists, are accompanied by an increase in the La^{3+} resistant Ca fraction (presumed to be the intracellular Ca; see Daniel et al., 1979 for critique), and are abolished in Ca-free Ringer's solution

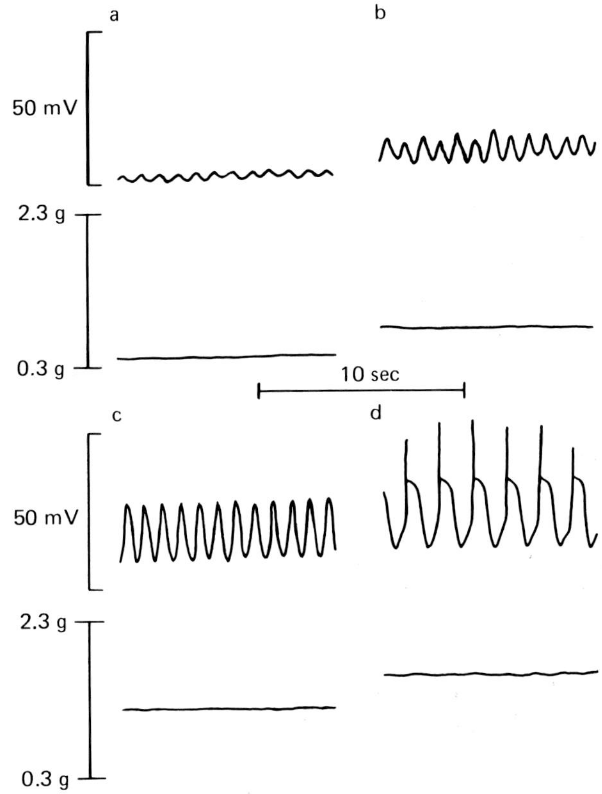

Figure 9 Intracellular recording of effects of increasing concentrations of TEA on membrane potential and tension in guinea pig trachea (see Fig. 7 for details). a: control; b: 2 mM TEA; c: 4 mM TEA; d: 8 mM TEA. (From Foster et al., 1983a.)

(no EGTA), it is assumed that TEA acts to depolarize the cells, blocking voltage-dependent K channels open at rest and causing rectification of depolarizing currents, this then leads to opening of Ca channels, repetitive action potentials, Ca entry, and contraction. Conductance changes and rectification have not been measured directly in this tissue. TEA contractions are postulated to be independent of release of intracellular Ca stores (Foster et al., 1983a; Ahmad et al., 1985). Elevated K^+ also caused contraction and an increase in the La^{3+}-resistant Ca fraction, which is likewise abolished in Ca-free medium or by Ca channel antagonists. Contractions from these two substances are not affected by TTX or by receptor antagonists and are therefore taken to be myogenic (Foster et al., 1983b).

In contrast, although acetylcholine and histamine cause depolarization (Small, 1982; Ahmad et al., 1984), they are resistant to removal of Ca, to Ca-chennel antagonists, and are not accompanied by an increase in the La^{3+}-resistant calcium fraction. There are postulated to act by release of internal Ca^{2+}.

Thus, as in bovine and canine trachea, guinea pig trachea normally do not produce action potentials, but are capable of doing so when TEA blocks K^+-channels. These action potentials involve voltage-dependent Ca channels. However, transmitters such as acetylcholine and histamine also depolarize and cause contraction, but Ca entry dependence of the contractile response cannot be demonstrated. To date, there is no information on how acetylcholine or histamine released endogenously affects membrane conductance, membrane potential or mediate contraction. Thus, it seems premature to speculate on how they initiate depolarization in guinea pig trachea, and how cell-to-cell coupling may participate in activation of the guinea pig trachea under physiological conditions. The dense innervation of this smooth muscle compared to canine, bovine, and human trachea may minimize the need for such coupling.

There are so far no convincing data that show whether spontaneous contractile activity occurs in airways in vivo, except in guinea pig and rabbit trachea (Dickey and Souhrada, 1976). The above-mentioned studies of slow waves in guinea pig trachea indicate the possibility that it may be occurring regularly but may not be recorded because of the lack of sensitivity and time resolution in the methods usually used.

The total lack of information on myogenic activities in vitro on smaller airways and the need for technical developments to allow it to be obtained emphasize our ignorance of these important questions.

III. Control Over Cell-to-Cell Coupling in Airways by Autocoids

Several years ago, we tested whether K^+-conductance blocking agents (TEA ion or 4-amino-pyridine [4-AP]) affected the number of gap junctions in canine trachea (Kannan and Daniel, 1980a). This was motivated by earlier observations that TEA increased the space constant of canine tracheal muscle measured by the Abe and Tomita bath technique in the longitudinal axis of the muscle bundles. This was originally explained by Kroeger and Stephens (1975) as owing to the resultant decrease (from K^+-conductance inhibition) in transmembrane conductance, confining currents flowing along cells more effectively within them and extending the distance such currents spread in the long axis of the cells. However, we found that gap junctions were approximately doubled in number, but unchanged in size within 20 min after exposure to TEA or 4-AP. The process did not require protein synthesis. Also, in the case of 4-AP, a presumed K^+-channel blocker, gap junction formation did not initiate any contractions, at least when 4-AP was given after atropine. TEA did cause contractions as well as increased gap junctions and these effects were unaffected by atropine. We concluded that these agents increased gap junctions by inhibiting the degradation or promoting the assembly of connexons but that this was not clearly related to initiation of myogenic activity.

Initially, we presumed that K^+-conductance channel closure somehow promoted gap junction formation. However, subsequent studies revealed that concentrations of 4-AP that cause a marked increase in gap junctions actually caused an increase in conductance, as did acetylcholine (Fig. 3), and this change was reduced or blocked by atropine (Kannan et al., 1983) without any effect on the increase in gap junctions (Kannan and Daniel, 1980). Since previous work in our laboratory had shown that rapid gap junction formation at term in mammalian myometrium depended upon endogenous prostanoids (Garfield et al., 1983), we proposed that TEA and 4-AP might affect gap junctions in trachea by releasing prostanoids. We tested this hypothesis using 4-AP.

The role of arachidonate metabolism was tested (Agarwal and Daniel, 1986) by giving selective or nonselective inhibitors of cyclooxygenase and lipoxygenase. Alone indomethacin has no effect, but it prevented the increase in gap junctions by 4-AP treatment; in fact, it reversed the action of this substance so that it caused a small but significant decrease in numbers of gap junctions. On the other hand, 5,8,11,14-eicosatetraynoic acid and nordihydroguariatric acid had no effect alone on gap junctions but prevented such an increase and any decrease produced by 4-AP. If arachidonic acid was added instead of 4-AP, trachea again showed a large increase in gap junctions that was blocked and reversed by indomethacin pretreatment. Further PGE_2 (10^{-6} M) and PGI_2 (10^{-6} M) each increased gap junctions, the former agent more than any other procedure. PGE_2 alone among the agents tested also increased gap junction size. It was concluded that agents that may release arachidonate, as well as arachidonate itself, rapidly increase tracheal gap junctions, probably by increasing production of PGE_2 or PGI_2. It was speculated that selective cyclooxygenase inhibition might cause arachidonate to be metabolized by 5′-lipoxygenase to leukotrienes or other products that inhibited gap junction formation. However, the leukotriene C_4 and D_4 antagonist FPL 55712 had no effect on the decrease in gap junctions produced by 4-AP in the presence of indomethacin. The results also implied, since selective and nonselective antagonists of cyclooxygenase and lipoxygenases had no effect on basal numbers of gap junctions, that endogenous PGs or leukotrienes were not affecting them. These results require confirmation but they raise the possibility that gap junctions are modulated locally and rapidly by products of inflammation or other procedures that release arachidonic acid.

This possibility was further emphasized when, in another study (Mansour, S., and Daniel, E. E., unpublished), we found that acute sensitization of guinea pigs to ovalbumin caused a marked reduction in numbers of gap junctions (from 2.5 to 0.6/100 smooth muscle cells) without causing any significant change in their size (average profile diameter, 0.2 μm). There was no change in these tissues in the concentration-response relationships between autonomic mediators, autocoids, or elevated K^+ in tissues from the same animals. Whether acute sensitization led to any inflammation or to local release of arachidonate or to other autocoids is unknown; however, our tissues were clearly sensitive to the antigen.

These new and preliminary findings raise many questions and answer none. But they do focus attention on the possible rapid modulation of gap junctions by procedures such as release of inflammatory mediators affecting airway responsiveness. They imply clearly the need to assess changes in gap junctions in conditions of inflammation or altered release of arachidonate or of its products. Also, since in other cell types elevation of c-AMP increased gap junction particle number and conductance (Spray and Bennett, 1985), it seems possible that beta-adrenoreceptor agonists and theophylline have similar actions in the airways.

There are no electrophysiological studies that would relate these findings to those about functional cell-to-cell coupling or to airway responsiveness. It is of interest that after acute sensitization of guinea pig with a combination of ovalbumin and *Bacillus pertussis* antigens, McCaig and Souhrada (1980) and Souhrada and Souhrada (1981) reported membrane hyperpolarization in tracheal muscle cells studied in vitro. This was in contrast to a marked depolarization of these cells seen after repeated exposure to antigens. Regular slow waves were much reduced in incidence, especially in the latter cells. This could reflect uncoupling owing to loss of gap junctions after repeated release of leukotrienes or it could result merely from the depolarization (see above). The hyperpolarization with acute sensitization might reflect better cell-to-cell coupling, but our own studies showed a reduction of gap junctions with acute sensitization to ovalbumin alone.

IV. General Conclusions

A. Structural Similarity and Diversity

It is evident that trachea of all species studied to date have gap junctions and cells are likely to be well coupled to one another. In human, canine, and bovine trachea, there is a paucity of innervation, which is located at the periphery of nerve bundles and not close ($>$ 1-5 μm) to smooth muscle. In contrast, guinea pig trachea has more numerous nerves, many within as well as at the periphery of nerves, and some very close ($<$30 nm) to muscle.

In contrast to trachea, human bronchi (fourth to seventh order) have only small nexuses, presumably gap junctions, between cells and probably cells are less well coupled to one another. Also in contrast to trachea, human bronchi have a dense innervation of muscle bundles, with nerves within as well as at the periphery of muscle bundles. Some of the nerve profiles are very close (<30 nm) to smooth muscle. Thus, in several respects, they resemble guinea pig trachea.

Canine bronchi (down to fourth order) have numerous gap junctions, in contrast to human bronchi, but are, like small human bronchi, densely innervated.

B. Functional Similarity and Diversity

Trachea of all species studied to date (dog, cow, guinea pig) are unable to initiate action potentials under physiological conditions because of the rectifying effect of potassium channels that open on depolarization. The guinea pig trachea alone among these muscles regularly generates slow waves when studied in vitro, which are often of considerable magnitude (up to 20 mV) and occur (1-2/sec) at a frequency too fast to explain spontaneous activity in vitro. These slow waves may be much smaller and some cells do not produce them or produce irregular fluctuations of membrane potential. The ionic mechanisms underlying these slow waves are uncertain and the accompanying conductance changes are unknown, but they depend upon external calcium and functioning Ca-channels and are influenced in size (and frequency to a lesser extent) by membrane potential.

All these tissues can produce action potentials if some K^+ channels are blocked by tetraethylammonium ion. These action potentials are Ca^{2+}-mediated and initiate contractions.

C. The Puzzle of Neural Activation of Tracheal Muscle

Acetylcholine from cholinergic nerves mediates contraction in canine and bovine trachea associated with excitatory junction potentials which do not initiate action potentials. The EJP appears to be associated with opening of ionic channels that are apparently selective for chloride ions. There may be a second slow depolarization in canine trachea that is more closely associated with the contraction than is the EJP and is also accompanied by conductance increase.

Since acetylcholine given into a bath medium may initiate contraction in part at least by pharmacomechanical coupling, it is so far unclear how the EJP associated with acetylcholine release initiates contraction. Since the EJP is normally unable to provoke action potentials, it is also unclear how the release of acetylcholine from a sparse, relatively remote, set of peripherally located nerves can lead to coordinated contractions.

D. The Problem of Functional Assessment of Cell-to-Cell Coupling

There is at present no straightforward and accepted method for assessing cell-to-cell coupling when smooth muscle cells are organized in bundles. Recent findings have stressed uncertainties about the interpretation of results using extracellular current injection. Intracellular current injections have also failed to provide this information in a smooth muscle bundle, but recent technical advances suggest re-examination of this technique. New approaches are also needed, such as study of spread of substances confined intracellularly, such as 2-deoxyglucose. Since airway responsiveness may be markedly influenced by the degree of cell-to-cell coupling in vivo, it is vital to develop these methods.

E. Cell-to-Cell Coupling May Be Modulated by Inflammatory Mediators

Recent finds suggest that PGE_2 and PGI_2 increase the number of gap junctional particles in canine trachea and that some nonprostanoid, possibly a leukotriene, may decrease the number. However, there is no evidence so far about the functional significance of these findings in relative to cell-to-cell coupling or airway responsiveness.

F. The Future

We need new techniques to study the cellular mechanisms underlying airway responsiveness: valid and reliable methods to study cell-to-cell coupling, to study ionic mechanisms in the cell membrane, and to study excitation-contraction coupling seem to me to be very urgently needed. To discover how these are changed in hyperresponsive airways is a challenge for those who study airway smooth muscle.

Discussion

Kaliner. How rapidly do gap junctions form and how long do they persist?

Daniel. After addition of arachidonate or PGE_2, gap junctions form within 5-10 min and we suspect that they may persist for hours.

Burnstock. We have previously reported that gap junctions may be more frequent in poorly innervated tissues. Does that seem to be the case in airway muscles?

Daniel. There is a generalized relationship that smooth muscle with many nerves has fewer or no gap junctions, while those with few nerves have many gap junctions. In Chagas disease we found a decrease in nerve fibers and an increase in gap junctions.

Diamond. Why is a decrease in number of gap junctions not associated with a change in concentration response curve to agonists?

Daniel. This could occur in vivo, since mediators are released at precise sites (nerve varicosities or cells) and activation must spread from these sites by diffusion or electrical propagation. In vitro this may not be seen since diffusion of agonist in the medium is complete and all cells exposed to it would respond.

Barnes. Is it possible to label gap junctions by specific immunocytochemical markers to make quantification easier?

Daniel. It is possible by using antibodies to gap junction proteins to label them and visualize them using a second antibody or protein A-gold. We have had no success with this in smooth muscle since there may be a loss of antigenicity of the junction proteins on fixation and processing.

Laitinen. What nerve profiles have you identified in human airway smooth muscle?

Daniel. In trachea most have small agranular vesicles with a few large granular vesicles. These cannot be assumed to be cholinergic since a variety of transmitters are contained in such nerves. In bronchi there is a higher proportion of nerve varicosities with small granular vesicles, which are possibly adrenergic.

Burnstock. I agree that we cannot confidently identify cholinergic nerve profiles since a number of such nerves are immunoreactive for peptides (Loesch and Burnstock, *J. Neurocytol.* **14**:327-335, 1985.

Daniel. The problem is complicated by the high probability that several mediators coexist in such nerves; thus VIP may be localized to the large granular vesicles.

References

Abe, Y., and Tomita, T. (1968). Cable properties of smooth muscle. *J. Physiol. (Lond.)* **196**:87-100.

Agrawal, R., and Daniel, E. E. (1986). Control of gap junction formation in canine trachea by arachidonic acid metabolites. *Am. J. Physiol. (Cell Physiol)* **250**, C495-C505.

Ahmad, F., Foster, R. W., Small, R. C., and Weston, A. H. (1984). Some features of the spasmogenic actions of acetylcholine and histamine in guinea pig isolated trachealis. *Br. J. Pharmacol.* **83**:227-233.

Ahmad, F., Foster, R. W., and Small, R. C. (1985). Some effects of nefedipine in guinea pig isolated trachealis. *Br. J. Pharmacol.* **84**:861-869.

Azarnia, R., Dahl, G., and Loewenstein, W. R. (1981). Cell junction and cyclic AMP. III. Promotion of junction membrane permeability and junctional membrane particles; in a junction-deficient cell type. *J. Membr. Biol.* **63**: 133-146.

Bolton, T. B., Tomita, T., and Vassort, G. (1981). Voltage clamp and the measurement of ionic conductances in smooth muscle. In *Smooth Muscle* II. *An Assessment of Current Knowledge.* Edited by E. Bulbring, A. F. Brading, A. W. Jones, and T. Tomita. London, Edward Arnold, pp. 47-64.

Bortoff, A., and Gilloteaux, J. (1980). Specific tissue impedance of estrogen and progesterone treated rabbit myometrium. *Am. J. Physiol.* **238**:C34-C42.

Cameron, A. R., and Kirkpatrick, C. T. (1977). A study of excitatory neuromuscular transmission in the bovine trachea. *J. Physiol.* (*Lond.*) **270**:733-745.

Cameron, A. R., Bullock, C. G., and Kirkpatrick, C. T. (1982). The ultrastructure of bovine tracheal muscle. *J. Ultrastruct. Res.* **81**:290-305.

Cheung, D. W., and Daniel, E. E. (1980). Comparative study of the smooth muscle layers of the rabbit duodenum. *J. Physiol.* (*Lond.*) **309**:13-27.

Coburn, R. F. (1977). The airway smooth muscle cell. *Fed. Proc.* **36**:2692-2697.

Coburn, R. F. (1979). Electromechanical coupling in canine trachealis muscle: acetylcholine contractions. *Am. J. Physiol.* **236**:C177-C184.

Coburn, R. F., and Yamaguchi, T. (1977). Membrane potential dependent and independent tension in canine tracheal muscle. *J. Pharmacol. Exp. Ther.* **201**:276-284.

Cole, W. R., Garfield, R. E., and Kirkaldy, J. S. (1985). Gap junctions and direct intercellular communication between rat uterine smooth muscle cells. *Am. J. Physiol.* (*Cell Physiol.*) **249**:C20-C31.

Daniel, E. E., Daniel, V. P., Duchon, G., Garfield, R. E., Nichols, M., Malhotra, S. K., and Oki, M. (1976). Is the nexus necessary for cell-to-cell coupling of smooth muscles? *J. Membr. Biol.* **28**:207-239.

Daniel, E. E., Kwan, C. Y., and Crankshaw, D. J. (1979). Intracellular sources of calcium for activation of smooth muscle. In *Trends in Autonomic Pharmacology,* Vol. 1. Edited by S. Kalsner. Germany, Urgan and Schwarzenberg, pp. 443-484.

Daniel, E. E., Davis, C., Jones, W. R., and Kannan, M. S. (1980). Control of airway smooth muscle. In *Airway Reactivity.* Edited by F. R. Hargreave. Mississauga, Ontario, Astra Pharmaceuticals, pp. 80-109.

Daniel, E. E., Jager, L. P., Inoue, F., Jury, J., and Serio, R. (1987). Electropharmacological characterization of contractile responses of canine trachealis muscle elicited by stimulation of intramural nerves. *J. Physiol.* (*Lond.*) (submitted)

Daniel, E. E., Kannan, M. S., Davis, C., and Posey-Daniel, V. (1986a). Ultrastructural studies on the neuromuscular control of human tracheal and bronchial muscle. *Respir. Physiol.* **63**:(in press).

Daniel, E. E., Posey-Daniel, V., Jager, L. P., Berezin, I., and Jury, J. (1986b). Structural effects of exposure of smooth muscle in the sucrose gap apparatus. Does the gap work as assumed. *Am. J. Physiol.* (*Cell Physiol.*) Accepted.

Daniel, E. E., Davis, C., and Sharma, V. (1987). Effects of endogenous and exogenous PGE_2 in neurotransmission in canine trachea. *Can. J. Physiol. Pharmacol.* (In press)

Dixon, J. S., and Small, R. C. (1983). Evidence of poor conduction of muscle excitation in the longitudinal axis of guinea-pig isolated trachea. *Br. J. Pharmacol.* **79**:75-83.

Farley, J. M., and Miles, P. R. (1977). Role of depolarization in acetylcholine-induced contractions of dog trachealis muscle. *J. Pharmacol. Exp. Ther.* **201**:199-205.

Farley, J. M., and Miles, P. R. (1978). The sources of calcium for acetylcholine-induced contractions of dog tracheal smooth muscle. *J. Pharmacol. Exp. Ther.* **207**:340-346.

Flagg-Newton, J. (1980). The permeability of the cell-to-cell membrane channel and its regulation in mammalian cell junction. *In Vitro* **16**:1043-1048

Flagg-Newton, J., and Loewenstein, W. R. (1979). Experimental depression of junctional permeability in mammalian cell culture. A study with tracer molecules in the 300 to 800 dalton range. *J. Membr. Biol.* **50**:65-100.

Flagg-Newton, J. L., and Loewenstein, W. R. (1981). Cell junction with cyclic AMP. II. Modulations of junctional membrane permeability, dependent on serum and cell density. *J. Membr. Biol.* **63**:123-131.

Flagg-Newton, J. L., Dahl, G., and Loewenstein, W. R. (1981). Cell junction and cyclic AMP. I. Upregulation of junctional membrane permeability and junctional membrane particles by administration of cyclic nucleotide or phosphodiesterase inhibitor. *J. Membr. Biol.* **63**:105-121.

Foster, R. W., Small, R. C., and Weston, A. H. (1983a). Evidence that the spasmogenic action of tetraethylammonium in guinea pig trachealis is both direct and dependent on the cellular influx of calcium ion. *Br. J. Pharmacol.* **79**:255-263.

Foster, R. W., Small, R. C., and Weston, A. H. (1983b). The spasmogenic action of potassium chloride in the guinea pig trachealis. *Br. J. Pharmacol.* **80**: 553-559.

Foster, R. W., Okpaluzo, B. I., and Small, R. C. (1984). Antagonism of Ca^{2+} and other actions of verapamil in guinea pig isolated trachealis. *Br. J. Pharmacol.* **81**:499-507.

Fry, G. N., Devine, C. E., and Burnstock, G. (1977). Freeze-fracture studies of nexuses between smooth muscle cells. Close relationships to sarcoplasmic reticulum. *J. Cell. Biol.* **72**:26-34.

Gabella, G. (1976). Quantative morphological study of smooth muscle cells of the guinea-pig taenia coli. *Cell Tissue Res.* **170**:161-186.

Gabella, G. (1981). Structure of smooth muscles. In *Smooth Muscle, An Assessment of Current Knowledge.* Edited by E. Bulbring, A. F. Brading, A. W. Jones, and T. Tomita. London, Edward Arnold, pp. 1-46.

Garfield, R. E., Sims, S. M., Kannan, M. S., and Daniel, E. E. (1978). Possible role of gap junctions in activation of myometrium during parturition. *Am. J. Physiol.* **235**:C168-C179.

Garfield, R. E., Kannan, M. S., and Daniel, E. E. (1980a). Gap junction formation in myometrium: control by estrogens, progesterone and prostaglandins. *Am. J. Physiol.* (*Cell Physiol.*) **238**:C81-C84.

Garfield, R. E., Merrett, D., and Grover, A. K. (1980b). Gap junction formation and regulation in myometrium. *Am. J. Physiol.* (*Cell Physiol.*) **239**:C217-C228.

Garfield, R. E., Daniel, E. E., Dukes, M., and Fitzgerald, J. D. (1983). Changes in gap junctions in myometrium of guinea pig at parturiation and abortion. *Can. J. Physiol. Pharmacol.* **60**:638-643.

Henderson, R. M. (1975). Cell-to-cell contacts. In *Methods in Pharmacology,* Vol. 3. Edited by E. E. Daniel and W. D. Paton, New York, Plenum.

Henderson, R. M., Duchon, G., and Daniel, E. E. (1971). Cell contacts in duodenal smooth muscle layers. *Am. J. Physiol.* **221**:564-572.

Hirshman, C. A., Downes, H., and Vieth, O. L. (1984). Airway responses if offspring of dogs with and without hyperreactivity. *J. Appl. Physiol.* **56**:1272-1277.

Holman, M. (1968). Introduction to the electrophysiology of visceral smooth muscle. In *Handbook of Physiology. Alimentary Canal,* 4. Edited by C. F. Code. Washington, D.C., American Physiological Society, pp. 1165-1708.

Hoyes, A. D., and Barber, P. (1980). Innervation of the trachealis muscle in the guinea pig: a quantitative ultrastructural study. *J. Anat.* **130**:789-900.

Inoue, T., Ito, Y., and Takeda, K. (1984). Prostaglandin-induced inhibition of acetylcholine release from neuronal elements of dog tracheal tissue. *J. Physiol.* (*Lond.*) **394**:533-570.

Ito, Y., and Tajima, K. (1981). Actions of indomethacin and prostaglandins on neuro-effector transmission in the dog trachea. *J. Physiol.* (*Lond.*) **319**: 379-382.

Jones, T. R., Kannan, M. S., and Daniel, E. E. (1980). Ultrastructural study of guinea pig tracheal smooth muscle and its innervation. *Can. J. Physiol. Pharmacol.* **58**:974-983.

Kannan, M. S., and Daniel, E. E. (1978). Formation of gap junctions by treatment *in vitro* with potassium conductance blockers. *J. Cell. Biol.* **78**: 338-348.

Kannan, M. S., and Daniel, E. E. (1980). Structural and functional study of control of canine tracheal muscle. *Am. J. Physiol.* **238**:C27-C33.

Kannan, M. S., Jager, L. P., Daniel, E. E., and Garfield, R. E. (1983). Effects of 4-aminopyridine and tetraethylammonium on the electrical activity and cable properties of canine tracheal smooth muscle. *J. Pharmacol. Exp. Ther.* **227**:706-715.

Kirkpatrick, C. T. (1975). Excitation and contraction in bovine tracheal smooth muscle. *J. Physiol. (Lond.)* **244**:263-281.

Kirkpatrick, C. T. (1981). Tracheobronchial smooth muscle. In *Smooth Muscle: An Assessment of Current Knowledge.* Edited by E. Bulbring, A. F. Brading, A. W. Jones, and T. Tomita. London, Edward Arnold, pp. 385-395.

Kirkpatrick, C. T., and Tomita, T. (1978). The spread of neural excitation compared with passive current spread in tracheal smooth muscle. *Ir. J. Med. Sci.* **147**:80-81.

Kirkpatrick, C. T., Jenkinson, H. A., and Cameron, A. R. (1975). Interactions between drugs and potassium-rich solutions in producing contractions in bovine tracheal smooth muscle: studies in normal and calcium-depleted tissues. *Clin. Exp. Pharmacol. Physiol.* **2**:559-570.

Kobayashi, M., Prosser, C. L., and Nagai, T. (1967). Electrical properties of intestinal muscle as measured intracellularly and extracellularly. *Am. M. Physiol.* **213**:275-286.

Kroeger, E. A., and Stephens, N. L. (1975). Effect of tetraethylammon ion on tonic airway smooth muscle: initiation of phasic electrical activity. *Am. J. Physiol.* **228**:633-636.

McCaig, D. J., and Souhrada, J. F. (1980). Alteration of electrophysiological properties of airway smooth muscle from sensitized guinea pigs. *Respir. Physiol.* **41**:49-60.

Peracchia, C. (1980). Structural correlates of gap junction permeation. *Int. Rev. Cytol.* **66**:81-146.

Pooler, J. P., and Oxford, G. S. (1972). Low membrane resistance in the sucrose gap—a parallel leakage path. *Biochim. Biophys. Acta* **255**:681-684.

Pooler, J. P., and Valenzeno, D. P. (1983). Reexamination of the double sucrose gap technique for the study of lobster giant axons. Theory and experiments. *Biophys. J.* **44**:261-269.

Ohba, M., Sakamoto, Y., Tokuno, H., and Tomita, T. (1976). Impedence components in longitudinal direction in the guinea-pig taenia coli. *J. Physiol. (Lond.)* **256**:527-540.

Radu, A., Dahl, G., and Loewenstein, W. R. (1982). Hormonal regulation of cell junction permeability: upregulation by catecholamine and prostaglandin E_1. *J. Membr. Biol.* **70**:239-251.

Revel, J.-P., Nicholson, B. J., and Yancy, S. B. (1985). Chemistry of gap junction. *Annu. Rev. Physiol.* **49**:263-279.

Richardson, J. B., and Furguson, C. C. (1980). Neuromuscular structure and function in the airways. *Fed. Proc.* **38**:202-208.

Rose, B., and Loewenstein, W. R. (1975). Calcium ion distribution in cytoplasm visualized by aequorin: diffusion in cytoplasm restricted by energized sequestering. *Science* **190**:1204.

Rose, B., Simpson, I., and Loewenstein, W. R. (1977). Calcium ion produces graded changes in permeability of membrane channels in cell junction. *Nature* **267**:625-627.

Sheridan, J. D., and Atkinson, M. K. (1985). Physiological roles of permeable junctions: some possibilities. *Annu. Rev. Physiol.* **47**:337-353.

Simpson, J., Rose, R., and Loewenstein, W. R. (1977). Size limit of molecules permeating the junctional membrane channels. *Science* **195**:294-296.

Sims, S. M., Daniel, E. E., and Garfield, R. E. (1982). Improved electrical coupling in uterine smooth muscle is associated with increased numbers of gap junctions at parturition. *J. Gen. Physiol.* **80**:353-376.

Small, R. C. (1982). Electrical slow waves and tone of guinea pig isolation trachealis muscle: effects of drugs are temperature change. *Br. J. Pharmacol.* **77**:45-54.

Souhrada, J. F., and Dickey, D. W. (1976). Mechanical activities of trachea as measured *in vitro* and *in vivo*. *Respir. Physiol.* **26**:27-40.

Souhrada, M., and Souhrada, J. F. (1981). Reassessment of electrophysiological and contractile characteristics of sensitized airway smooth muscle. *Respir. Physiol.* **46**:17-27.

Sperelakis, N. (1969). Lack of electrical coupling between contiguous myocardial cells of vertebrate hearts. In *Comparative Physiology of the Heart: Current Trends.* Edited by F. V. McCann. Basel, Birkhauser Verlag.

Sperelakis, N., and MacDonald, R. L. (1974). Ratio of transverse to longitudinal resistivities of isolated cardiac muscle fiber bundles. *J. Electrocardiol.* **7**: 301-314.

Sperelakis, N., and Picone, J. (1986). Cable analysis in cardiac and smooth muscle bundles. *IEEE Trans. Biomed. Eng.* (accepted).

Sperelakis, N., and Tarr, M. (1965). Weak electrotonic interaction between neighbouring contiguous visceral smooth muscle cells. *Am. J. Physiol.* **66**: 119-134.

Spray, D. C., and Bennett, M. V. L. (1985). Physiology and Pharmacology of gap junctions. *Annu. Rev. Physiol.* **47**:281-303.

Spray, D. C., Harris, A. L., and Bennett, M. V. L. (1979). Voltage dependence of junctional conductance of early amphibian embryos. *Science* **204**:432-434.

Spray, D. C., Harris, A. L., and Bennett, M. V. L. (1981). Gap junctional conductance is a simple and sensitive function of intracellular pH. *Science* **211**:712-715.

Stephens, N. L., Kroeger, E., and Kromer, U. (1975). Induction of a myogenic response in tonic airway smooth muscle by tetraethylammonium. *Am. J. Physiol.* **228**:628-632.

Suzuki, H., Morita, K., and Kuriyawa, H. (1976). Innervation and properties of the smooth muscle of the dog trachea. *Jpn. J. Physiol.* **26**:303-320.

Tarr, M., and Sperelakis, N. (1964). Weak electrotonic interaction between contiguous cardiac cells. *Am. J. Physiol.* **207**:691-700.

Tomita, T. (1966). Membrane capacity and resistance of mammalian smooth muscle. *J. Theor. Biol.* **12**:216-244.

Tomita, T. (1969). The longitudinal tissue impedance of the smooth muscle of guinea pig taenia coli (1976). *J. Physiol.* (*Lond.*) **201**:145-159.

Tomita, T. (1970). Electrical properties of mammalian smooth muscle. In *Smooth Muscle.* Edited by E. Bulbring, A. F. Brading, A. W. Jones, and T. Tomita. London, Edward Arnold, pp. 197-243.

Tomita, T. (1981). Electrical activities (spikes and slow waves) in gastrointestinal smooth muscles. In *Smooth Muscle II. An Assessment of Current Knowledge.* Edited by E. Bulbring, A. F. Brading, A. W. Jones, and T. Tomita. London, Edward Arnold, pp. 127-156.

Turin, L., and Warner, A. E. (1980). Intracellular pH in early X. enopus embryos: its effect on current flow between blastomeres. *J. Physiol.* (*Lond.*) **300**:489-504.

White, R. L., Spray, D. C., Campos de Carvalho, A. C., Whittenberg, R. A., and Bennett, M. V. L. (1985). Some electrical and pharmacological properties of gap junctions between adult ventricular myocytes. *Am. J. Physiol.* (*Cell Physiol.*) **249**:C447-C455.

20

Nonneural and Neural Regulation of Plasma Exudation in Airways

CARL G. A. PERSSON

University Hospital of Lund
and AB Draco
Lund, Sweden

INGRID A-L. ERJEFÄLT

AB Draco
Lund, Sweden

An important sign of inflammation is vascular leakage of plasma. The increase in permeability that allows bulk flow of large solutes out of microvessels is an active process under physiological and pharmacologic control (Cohnheim, 1882; Majno and Palade, 1961; Majno et al., 1961, 1969; Wilhelm, 1962, 1973; Spector and Willoughby, 1963; Zweifach, 1973; Grega et al., 1981; Hurley, 1983; Persson and Svensjö, 1985). The present overview discusses neural and nonneural mechanisms that may regulate tracheobronchial microvascular leakage of macromolecules (Fig. 1). Plasma exudation into the wall and the lumen of lower airways has recently been suggested as an important factor in the pathogenesis of asthma (Dunnill, 1978; Persson, 1986), emphasizing the role of tracheobronchial microvessels in disease.

I. Plasma Exudation in Asthma

A. Edema

Edema is generally considered a characteristic sign of asthmatic airways (Dunnill, 1978; Middleton et al., 1981; Hogg, 1984; Sybert and Weiss, 1985). However, few reports actually demonstrate edema (Dunnill, 1978; Hogg, 1984). Many

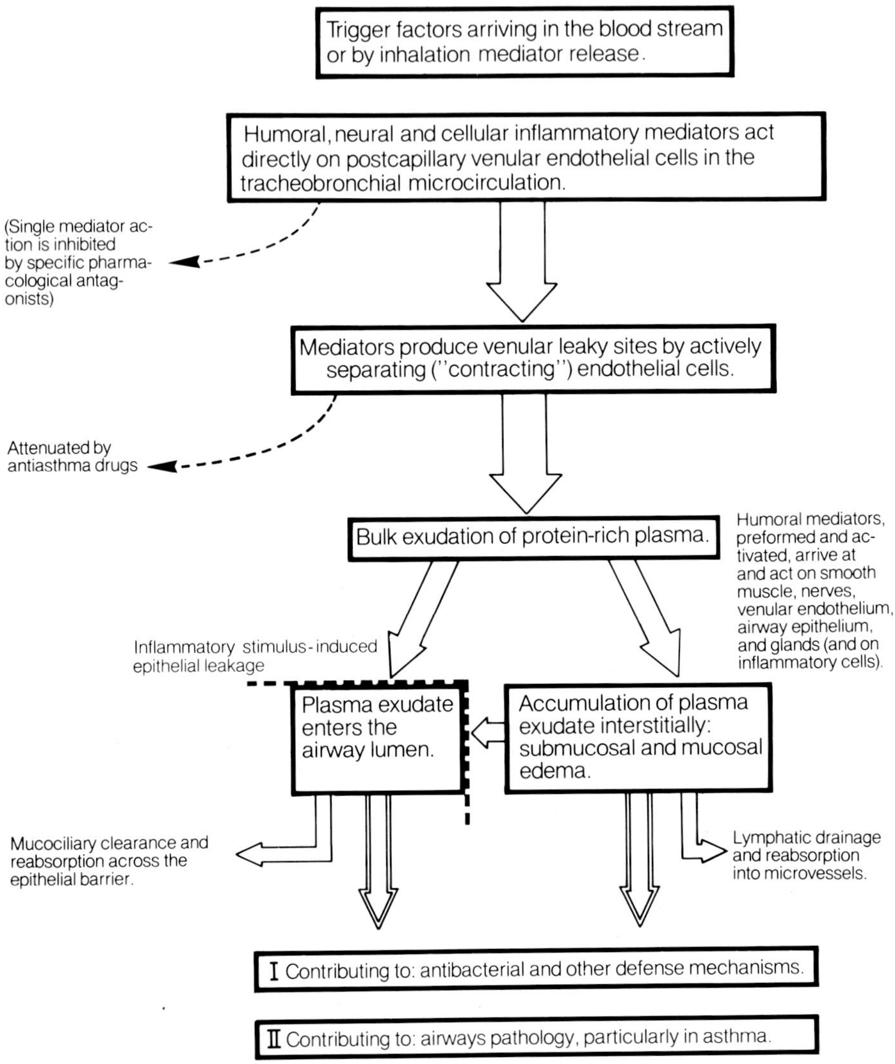

Figure 1 This scheme may illustrate a sequence of events initiated by the release or arrival of inflammatory mediators in the vicinity of tracheobronchial microvessels. Several proposed mediators of asthma are known to act directly on postcapillary venular endothelial cells to produce large intercellular gaps through which a bulk flow of protein-rich plasma into the interstitium occurs. The entry into the wall and the lumen of the airways by exudate with its preformed and readily activated protein mediators and other factors may be of importance in the pathogenesis of asthma (see text). Plasma exudation may also have a role in airway defense mechanisms (cf. Miles and Wilhelm, 1960; Spector and Willoughby, 1963; Hurley, 1983).

workers, who have done postmortem or biopsy examinations, have not identified edema in asthmatic airways (Huber and Koessler, 1922; Hilding, 1943; Houston et al., 1953; Cardell and Pearson, 1959; Williams and Leopold, 1959; Messer et al., 1960; Alexander, 1963; Salvato, 1968; Thurlbeck et al., 1970; Cutz et al., 1978). Lack of data on edema does not contradict the notion that plasma exudation is important in asthma. A slight mucosal swelling may produce airway hyperresponsiveness (Hutt and Wick, 1956) and a plasma exudate might enter the airway lumen and contribute to the pathology of asthmatic airways (Fig. 1).

Edema of tissues between the bronchial muscle and the epithelium would reduce the caliber of the airway lumen. Small changes in mucosal thickness may have a profound influence on the tendency for airways closure, as well as explaining the bronchoconstrictory hyperresponsiveness (Hutt and Wick, 1956). Airway edema including a peribronchial edema can be expected to reduce airway compliance. An increased tissue pressure caused by plasma exudation might also evoke vagal afferent activation (cf. Sellick and Widdicombe, 1969; Coleridge and Coleridge, 1977) but such a mechanism has not yet been demonstrated in tracheobronchial tissues. Airway edema and transepithelial passage of exuded plasma have been suggested by Dunnill (1960) as causing the shedding of epithelium seen in asthma (Moore, 1925; Hilding, 1943; Dunnill, 1960; Naylor, 1962; Sanerkin and Evans, 1965; Laitinen et al., 1985). Crenation of the mucosa during bronchoconstriction might also contribute (Houston et al., 1953; Naylor, 1962; Dunnill, 1978) and recent studies (Frigas et al., 1980) suggest a role for toxic proteins released from eosinophils in the shedding of epithelial cells.

B. Exudate in Airway Lumen

It seems well established that large amounts of plasma proteins can be found in sputa in airway diseases such as asthma (Huber and Koessler, 1922; Sanerkin and Evans, 1965; Ryley and Brogan, 1968; Brogan et al., 1975; Dunnill, 1978). Ryley and Brogan (1968) and Brogan et al. (1975) showed that the sol phase of asthmatic sputum contained larger amounts of plasma proteins (but not secretory proteins) than bronchitic sputum. They further distinguished a subgroup of cystic fibrosis patients with as high sputum concentrations of plasma proteins as were found in asthmatics (Brogan et al., 1975). Proteinaceous sputum and mucus plugs in asthma have repeatedly been demonstrated (Dunnill, 1960, 1978; Sanerkin and Evans, 1965) and a bronchial lavage that may selectively sample bronchial fluid has been found to contain 10-fold increased concentrations of albumin in asthmatic compared with control subjects (Lam et al., 1985). Proteins involved in the clotting mechanism may be present and fibrin formation would make the mucus viscous and obstructive (Huber and Koessler, 1922; Sanerkin and Evans, 1965; Don Barton and Lourenco, 1973; Middleton et al., 1981). Also, albumin and other solutes of the plasma exudate may interact with mucin to form viscous complexes (Forstner et al., 1977; List et al., 1975). Asthmatic sputum may produce smooth muscle contraction (Harkavy, 1930) and inhibition of ciliary motility (Dulfano and Luk, 1982). A plasma exudate in the airway lumen may move into peripheral airways and compromise surfactant activity, which may lead to narrowing of small airways (Macklem et al., 1970).

Movement of proteinaceous plasma from the vascular compartment into the airway lumen may occur soon after mediator challenge of the airway mucosa. We have used a nontraumatic technique for superfusing the guinea pig tracheal mucosa in vivo with defined concentrations of inflammatory agents and drugs (Erjefält et al., 1985). In this preparation such mediators as histamine, leukotrienes, tachykinins, and PAF-acether caused an acute exudation of plasma (Persson et al., 1985, 1986). It was further observed that charged (^{131}I-albumin) and uncharged (FITC-dextran, MW 70000-150000) vascular tracer molecules could be recovered in tracheal luminal fluid selectively collected within a few

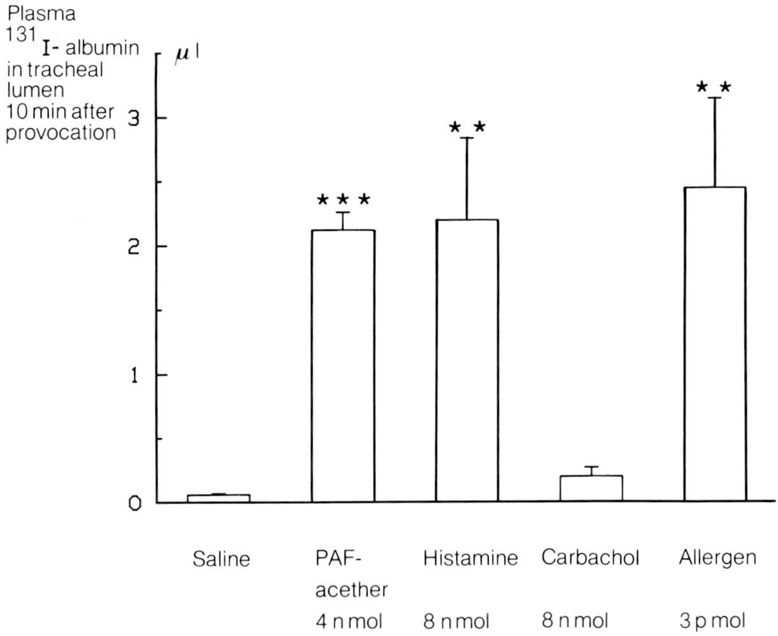

Figure 2 ^{131}I-Albumin (calculated as plasma clearance) recovered by lavage of the trachea 10 min after provocation (superperfusion of tracheal mucosal surface for 2 min) with saline, mediators, and allergen (ovalbumin in an IgE-driven reaction). **$p<0.01$; ***$p<0.001$ (comparisons with saline; n = 4–10).

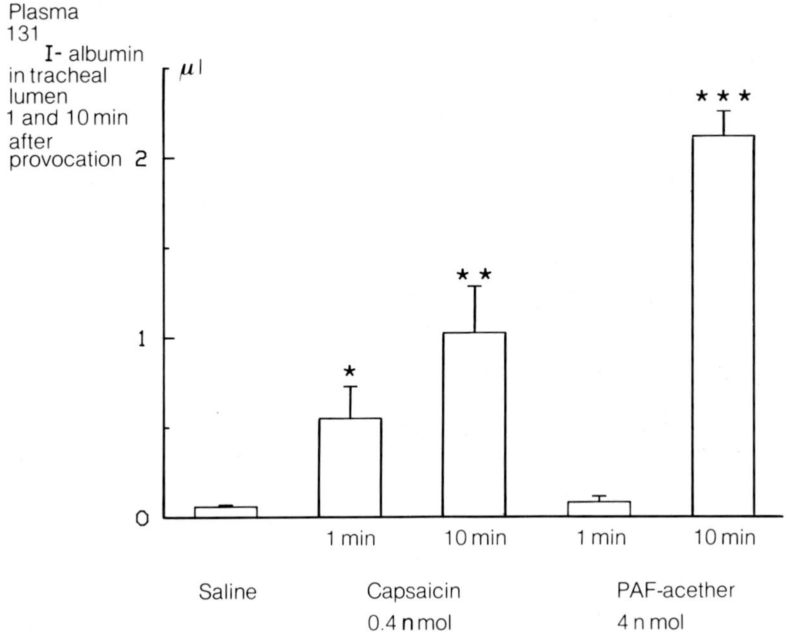

Figure 3 ^{131}I-Albumin (calculated as plasma clearance) recovered in tracheal lavage performed 1 and 10 min, respectively, after tracheal mucosal superperfusion (for 2 min) with saline, capsaicin, and PAF-acether. *$p<0.05$; **$p<0.01$; ***$p<0.001$ (comparisons with saline; n = 4–10).

minutes after mediator provocation (Persson and Erjefält, 1986; Figs. 2, 3). The volume of plasma exudate may increase the depth of the periciliary fluid layer and hence impair mucociliary transport (Wanner, 1985). Under physiological conditions there is a restricted intercellular transepithelial passage of plasma proteins such as albumin (Boucher et al., 1980). An intercellular route would also best explain the observations in guinea pigs of a rapid inflammatory leakage into the tracheal lumen of extravasated charged and uncharged macromolecules (Persson and Erjefält, 1986) (Fig. 3).

II. Tracheobronchial Circulation

Tracheal and bronchial arteries carrying systemic blood nourish the walls of the airways and their accompanying vessels. Species differences and variations within species exist for the origin and distribution of these arteries. Various types of anastomosis between the bronchial and pulmonary circulation have been demonstrated and there are different views as to how far the bronchial arteries travel in peripheral airways, but also the terminal bronchioles and alveoli may be supplied by these vessels (Florange, 1960; McLaughlin et al., 1961, 1966; Aviado, 1963; Pump, 1972). The bronchial circulation seems to receive about 1% of the cardiac output (Aviado, 1963; Baier et al., 1985). Studies in sheep suggest that a large fraction of bronchial blood flow goes to the airway submucosa (Parsons et al., 1985). The bronchial veins from the first two to three generations of bronchi drain into the azygous veins and then into the right heart. A large part of the bronchial blood drains into pulmonary capillaries and veins via anastomoses and enters the left heart (Bruner and Schmidt, 1947).

Different workers have demonstrated the presence of an extensive microvasculature in the trachea and bronchi (Miller, 1947; Sobin et al., 1963; Hughes, 1965, Nordin, 1977; Pietra and Magno, 1978; Parsons et al., 1985; Laitinen et al., Chap. 3). Pietra and Magno (1978), who studied dog airways, reported that on either side of the bronchial muscle layer there is an abundance of capillary-venular plexuses. In the larger bronchi the venular subepithelial plexuses are located mainly between the cartilage ring structures and in smaller bronchi the plexuses occupy the entire surface of the submucosal layer (Pietra and Magno, 1978). In close proximity to the bronchial microvascular plexus there is a system of lymphatic vessels (Pietra et al., 1979). McDonald (personal communication) has observed a similar distribution of venules in rat airways. Humans also seem to have a rich submucosal venular plexus in the tracheobronchial tree (Miller, 1947; Florange, 1960; Laitinen et al., Chap. 3). This superficial network of tracheobronchial microvessels suggests a role for the lower airways in inhaled air conditioning (Sobin et al., 1963; Hughes, 1965, Pietra et al., 1971; Baile et al., 1985). This function may be of particular relevance to asthmatic subjects who are sensitive to inhalation of cold and dry air (Anderson et al., 1982). Florey et al. (1932) induced airway inflammation and marked "transudation of vessel fluid" by blowing dry air through cat tracheas.

A number of vasodilator agents have been shown to produce an elevation of the mucosal surface in dog bronchi (Kyle et al., 1985; Laitinen et al., Chap. 3). A vasodilation-induced reduction of the lumen caliber and increased airway resistance can be expected to be readily reversed by topical application of sympathomimetic drugs, such as epinephrine, that reduce bronchial blood flow via α-receptor stimulation (Bruner and Schmidt, 1947) and have a blanching effect on the airways (Erjefält and Persson, 1982). Using bronchoscopy techniques, Herzog (personal communication) has observed that locally administered epinephrine can have a prompt effect in acutely swollen asthmatic airways. These drugs also may cause an exacerbation of the inflammatory response. In the rabbit skin, epinephrine (and norepinephrine) has been shown to convert mild bacterial endotoxin-induced inflammatory reactions into pronounced hemorrhagic lesions (Thomas, 1956; Gatling, 1958). The mechanism behind these injurious effects is unknown. Specific β_2-adrenoceptor agonists such as terbutaline lack α-receptor stimulant properties and are general vasodilators that by themselves might produce a slight swelling effect (Kyle et al., 1985). Since the clinical effectiveness of epinephrine does not seem to exceed that of β_2-receptor agonists, the contribution of swelling of submucosal vessels to airway resistance in asthma is in doubt.

Alterations in bronchial blood flow will affect the delivery of plasma and white cells, the perfused surface area, and the microvascular hydrostatic pressure. Accordingly, the degree of plasma exudation can be much affected by changes in the blood flow. The flow may be highly increased through tissue that is affected by inflammation (Aschheim and Zweifach, 1962), and with local hyperemia the hydrostatic pressure increases in the postcapillary venules (Zweifach, 1973) from which exudation takes place (see below).

Studies in animals have shown that the neural, hormonal, and pharmacologic regulation of bronchial flow has many of the general characteristics of a systemic circulation (Aviado, 1963; Zapata-Ortiz et al., 1967; Arowolo and Eyre, 1971; Bruner and Schmidt, 1947; Charan et al., 1985; Long et al., 1985; Baier et al., 1985; Parsons et al., 1985). Histamine increases bronchial blood flow (De Letona et al., 1961; Zapata-Ortiz et al., 1967; Charan et al., 1985; Long et al., 1985). Studies in dogs show that vagal stimulation produces cholinergic muscarinic receptor-mediated vasodilation and sympathetic nerve stimulation produces adrenergic α-adrenoceptor-mediated vasoconstriction (Bruner and Schmidt, 1947; Aviado, 1963). A noncholinergic, nonadrenergic vagal dilation of tracheobronchial vessels may also be important (Martling et al., 1985; see Laitinen et al., Chap. 3) (Fig. 4).

III. Inflammatory Extravasation of Macromolecules

Under physiological conditions fluid equilibrium is maintained by a balance between the hydrostatic pressure in the capillary bed, which tends to drive fluid out of the vascular compartment, and the counteracting force of an osmotic pressure of plasma proteins. During inflammation there are dramatic changes, in particular in the latter force. Julius Cohnheim (1882) concluded that the inflammatory extravasation of protein-rich fluid must be due to noxious stimuli acting directly on the microvascular wall to cause "eine moleculäre Aenderung der Gefässwandungen" (a molecular change in the vessel wall). Different workers have suggested that the intercellular material is loosened up by inflammation

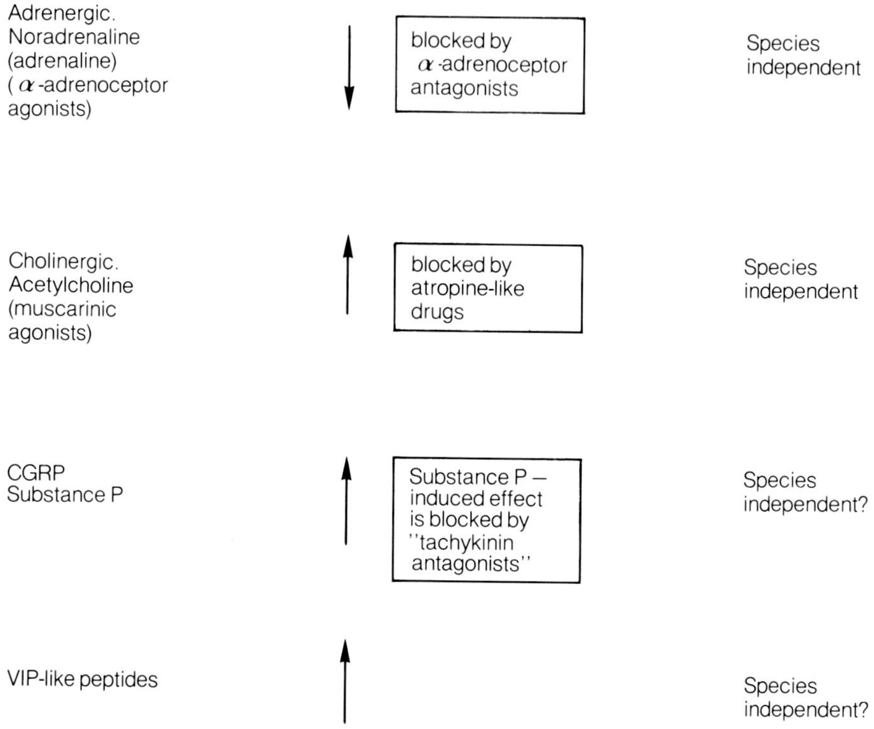

Figure 4 Neural effects on tracheobronchial blood flow (↑ increase; ↓ decrease). As well as its adrenergic vasoconstrictory and cholinergic vasodilatory effects, peptidergic neural actions may affect tracheobronchial blood flow. It remains to be established whether calcitonin gene-related peptide (CGRP), substance P, and vasoactive intestinal peptide (VIP) have a role in the regulation of airways blood flow. During inflammatory vascular leakiness, changes in blood flow may markedly affect the amount of plasma exudation.

producing an abnormal leakiness (Arnold, 1876; Cohnheim, 1882; Chambers and Zweifach, 1947). Ultrastructural, pathophysiological, and pharmacologic studies of systemic microvascular beds have now shown that inflammatory leakage of protein-rich plasma occurs in postcapillary venules (10-60 μm in diameter) through widened gaps between endothelial cells (Rous and Smith, 1931; Chambers and Zweifach, 1947; Miles and Wilhelm, 1960; Majno and Palade, 1961; Majno et al., 1961, 1969; Wilhelm, 1962, 1973; Spector and Willoughby, 1963; Zweifach, 1973; Grega et al., 1981; Hurley, 1983; Persson and Svensjö, 1985). Perhaps via contractile mechanisms mediators actively deform these cells, causing them to separate (Majno et al., 1969). At the sites of interendothelial gaps the

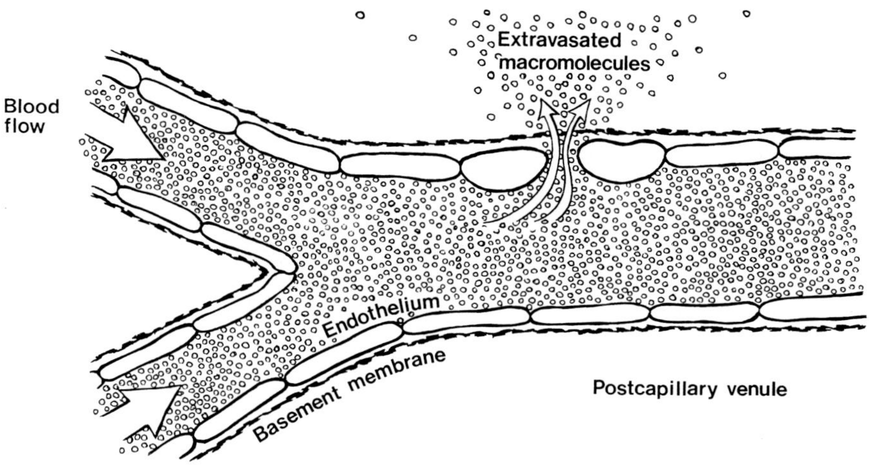

Figure 5 Schematic illustration of a leaky microvessel with free movement of large solutes from the vascular compartment into the interstitium. By active reversible deformation of endothelial cells in the postcapillary venules (10-60 μm in diameter), inflammatory mediators produce large interendothelial gaps. The mediators may actually produce a transient contraction of the endothelial cells. Since the basement membrane offers little resistance to molecules of the size of plasma proteins, a protein-rich plasma is exuded. In the inflamed airway macromolecular proteins may pass readily into the airway lumen.

transmural colloid osmotic pressure gradient is eliminated, plasma escapes, and filters through the endothelial basement membrane that offers little hindrance to plasma proteins (Fig. 5) (Zweifach, 1973). The concentration ratios of different proteins are similar in blood plasma and in inflammatory exudate (Ascheim and Zweifach, 1962; Baumgarten et al., 1985), supporting the view that there is a bulk flow of proteinaceous plasma out of leaky postcapillary venules.

IV. Inflammatory Mediators

A. Nonneural Mediators

Most of the traditional and newly identified proposed mediators of asthma have an ability to produce microvascular leaks in addition to their bronchoconstrictory capacity (Persson and Svensjö, 1983). However, bronchoconstriction and leakage may not always be linked. Figure 2 illustrates that PAF-acether, which is a poor constrictor of guinea pig trachea, is a powerful macromolecular leakage-inducing agent. Carbachol, on the other hand, is a potent tracheobronchial constrictor that does not increase leakiness (Fig. 2). The mediators may come from stationary and migrating inflammatory cells. In addition, airway epithelial cells (Nadel and Holtzman, 1984) and vascular endothelial cells (Prescott et al., 1984; Bult and Herman, 1985) may generate several of the inflammatory mediators. The preformed and dormant protein mediators that are circulating in the bloodstream must be considered important since they are supplied by the leaky venules themselves. The plasma proteins leaking through the venular gaps contain a number of powerful mediator systems, which may be activated during the transvascular passage and upon arrival in inflamed tissue by negative surface charges, proteases, and other factors (Spector, 1951; Miles and Wilhelm, 1955; Miles, 1964; Lewis, 1970; Gerdin and Saldeen, 1978; Movat, 1979; Ward et al., 1979; Wiggins et al., 1979).

B. Neural Mediators

Bruce (1910) examined inflammation in the skin and the eye and concluded that nerves and an axon reflex may have a major role in plasma exudation. Immunohistochemistry and other tools such as the tachykinin-depleting agent capsaicin have now identified tachykinins, including neurokinin A and substance P, as possible mediators of neurogenic microvascular leakage (Jancso et al., 1967, 1977; Nilsson et al., 1977; Lundberg et al., 1986). In guinea pig and rat airways capsaicin-sensitive innervation and tachykinins have been demonstrated by Lundberg and associates and others to produce significant plasma exudation and bronchoconstriction (Lundberg and Saria, 1982; Lundberg et al., 1983, 1985; Karlsson and Persson, 1983; Persson et al., 1986). Furthermore, McDonald (personal communication) has observed in rat trachea that vagal stimulation causes postcapillary venules to leak preferentially towards the epithelium and also that the epithelial cells were affected by the stimulation. These observations are consistent with the finding that capsaicin rapidly induced a movement of macromolecules from the blood into the tracheal lumen (Fig. 3) (Persson and Erjefält, 1986). The possibility of a neural reflex-mediated airway inflammatory response is intriguing and agrees with early thoughts of the nature of asthma (Salter, 1868). However, it is doubtful whether the findings made in guinea pig and rat are transferable to humans. Neural tachykinin-mediated inflammatory responses have, in fact, not been confirmed in the airways of nonrodent mammals (see Lundberg, Chap. 16) (Fig. 6). Human subjects, including asthmatics, responded to inhaled capsaicin with cough and negligible bronchoobstructive effects (Collier and Fuller, 1984; Fuller et al., 1985, and unpublished observations by Midgren, Simonsson, and Persson). Furthermore, substance P applied topically on human nasal mucosa does not increase nasal liquid production (through transudation or secretion), even when local doses were applied that produced flushing and significant increases in heart rate (Malm and Pettersson,

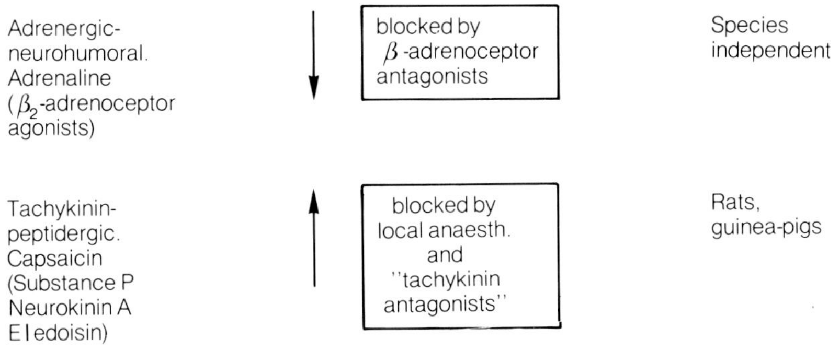

Figure 6 Neural effects on tracheobronchial venular permeability to macromolecules (↑ increased; ↓ decreased permeability). Sympathomimetic agents, through stimulation of β-receptors, may prevent the inflammatory stimulus-induced venular leakage of macromolecules. In select species capsaicin-sensitive innervation and putative tachykinin neurotransmitters have potent leakage-inducing effects.

1985). The role of the nervous system in the inflammatory process with an emphasis on "psychosomatic" aspects has been reviewed by Chapman and Goodell (1964). They discussed the possibility that "circumstances perceived as threatening in some individuals result in engorgement of the mucous membranes, increase in leukocytes and secretion of mucus, contraction of smooth muscle of the airways," and that such reactions may trigger various acute and chronic airway diseases, including asthma.

C. Interactions

Theoretically, the mediators of plasma exudation may interact at various levels. By additive or synergistic effects directly on the endothelial cells, the mediators may produce marked plasma exudation (Svensjö, 1978; Amelang et al., 1981). It has long been recognized that once permeability is increased, changes in blood flow will determine the degree of plasma exudation (Cohnheim, 1882; Wilhelm, 1962; Zweifach, 1962, 1973). The mediators may differ in effects on blood flow: histamine and substance P are vasodilators (Pernow, 1983; Long et al., 1985; Persson et al., 1986), whereas the leukotrienes may produce a transient vasoconstriction (Dahlén et al., 1981). Synergistic effects have been demonstrated in the skin between flow-increasing cyclooxygenase products or VIP and a permeability-increasing substance (see Williams, 1985). However, the degree of this kind of synergy may be unusually high in skin that has a low basal blood perfusion.

Other interactions concern recruiting and activation of inflammatory cells. Leukotriene B_4, the anaphylatoxins, and other factors are known to attract polymorphonuclear leukocytes (Ward et al., 1979; Dahlén et al., 1981; Bray et al., 1981; Kay and Lee, 1982). These cells have been suggested to be an important factor in increased microvascular permeability. The presence of polymorphonuclear leukocytes in experimentally inflamed airways has been documented (Holtzman et al., 1983; Nadel and Holtzman, 1984; Larsen, 1985; Behrens et al., 1985; Gordon et al., 1985; Hulbert et al., 1985) but their involvement in plasma exudation in this tissue remains to be elucidated. As with protein leakage, the leukocyte-endothelium interactions occur in postcapillary venules and the diapedesis is through endothelial intercellular junctions (Marchesi, 1961; Spector and Willoughby, 1963; Hurley, 1983). However, it is generally agreed that inflammatory extravasation of leukocytes and macromolecular solutes is induced via different mechanisms and can occur separately (Zweifach, 1973; Florey, 1970; Hurley, 1983).

D. Acute and Sustained Leakiness

The histologic and ultrastructural characteristics of the acute macromolecular leakage induced by various mediators appear identical (Majno and Palade, 1961; Majno et al., 1961, 1969; Svensjö, 1978; Hurley, 1983; Björk et al., 1985, 1985). Leakage of macromolecules is evident within 30-120 sec after application of a directly acting inflammatory agent on systemic microvascular beds including the tracheobronchial circulation (Miles and Wilhelm, 1960; Majno et al., 1961; Wilhelm, 1962, 1973; Spector and Willoughby, 1963; Pietra et al., 1971; Svensjö, 1978; Woodward et al., 1983; Persson and Svensjö, 1985; Persson et al., 1986; Persson and Erjefält, 1986) (Fig. 3). Normal low permeability is usually restored within 10-30 min and the affected tissue may partly be refractory to further permeability effects (Burke and Miles, 1958; Greaves and Shuster, 1967; Baumgarten et al., 1970; Svensjö and Joyner, 1984). In the skin of guinea pigs and humans responses to bradykinin were not reduced by prior application of bradykinin (Greaves and Shuster, 1967; Baumgarten et al., 1970) and it was concluded that prolonged formation of bradykinin may participate in delayed inflammatory reactions (Baumgarten et al., 1970). In the hamster cheek pouch model, Svensjö and associates (Svensjö and Joyner, 1984; and unpublished observations) have demonstrated that venular leakage disappears within 60 min despite the continued presence of an active concentration of histamine or bradykinin. They also showed that tachyphylaxis did not occur if these mediators were given as single applications at 30 min intervals, and that the venular gaps could be kept open for hours by giving different mediators in sequence or by gradually increasing the concentration of a single mediator.

Miles and co-workers (Elder and Miles, 1957; Burke and Miles, 1958; Craig and Miles, 1961) demonstrated biphasic as well as sustained permeability responses to bacterial toxins injected into guinea pig skin. Wilhelm (1973) described other types of injury that cause an immediate phase of leakiness that is followed after 1-2 hr by a late phase of sustained increased microvascular permeability. Tissue leukocytosis may be associated with the delayed response but a causal relationship between the two events has not been established (Willoughby and Spector, 1968; Willoughby and Giroud, 1969; Wilhelm, 1973). Some stimuli, for example, thermal injury, clearly produce leaks in both capillaries and venules (Miles, 1964). It seems that the capillary endothelium exhibits interendothelial gaps due to direct injury, whereas the venular leaks are produced by the action of inflammatory mediators (Hurley, 1983).

Sustained leakiness of tracheobronchial microvessels has not been investigated as yet. Tracheobronchial superfusion experiments in anesthetized guinea pigs have demonstrated that significant extravasation of uncharged dextran tracer molecules (MW 70,000-150,000) and ^{131}I-albumin is produced by leukotrienes C_4, D_4 at concentrations of 10^{-8} M. Histamine, substance P, neurokinin A, and capsaicin were active in concentrations around 10^{-6} M in the superfusate (Persson et al., 1985, 1986, Persson and Erjefält, 1986). However, these mediators apparently produced leakage of a brief duration. Preliminary data with locally applied PAF-acether and toluene diisocyanate suggest that these agents may induce prolonged vascular leakage (unpublished observations).

E. Antileakage Effects

Different antiasthma drugs may prevent the mediator-induced microvascular leakage, but this drug effect has so far only been studied in animal experiments with mediators inducing an acute leakage of brief duration. Glucocorticosteroids have been shown to inhibit or reduce mediator-induced vascular leakage. The latency time before the effect can be manifested is about 1 hr (Tsurufuji et al., 1980; Svensjö and Roempke, 1984) but the glucocorticoid drugs may need to be present in the target tissue only for a very brief period of time (5 min) in order to be effective (Svensjö and Roempke, 1984). Preliminary data obtained in guinea pigs suggest that budesonide could prevent mediator-induced exudative effects also in airways (Fig. 7). Ryley and Brogan (1968) found a relationship between a lowering of the albumin concentration in sputum, steroid therapy, and clinical improvement in an asthmatic subject. Also, based on serial measurements of neuraminic acid concentration (an indicator of bronchial secretion) in asthmatic sputum, Keal (1971) inferred that the effect of steroid therapy "lies in the reduction of transudate rather than in any change in the bronchial mucosal gland secretion."

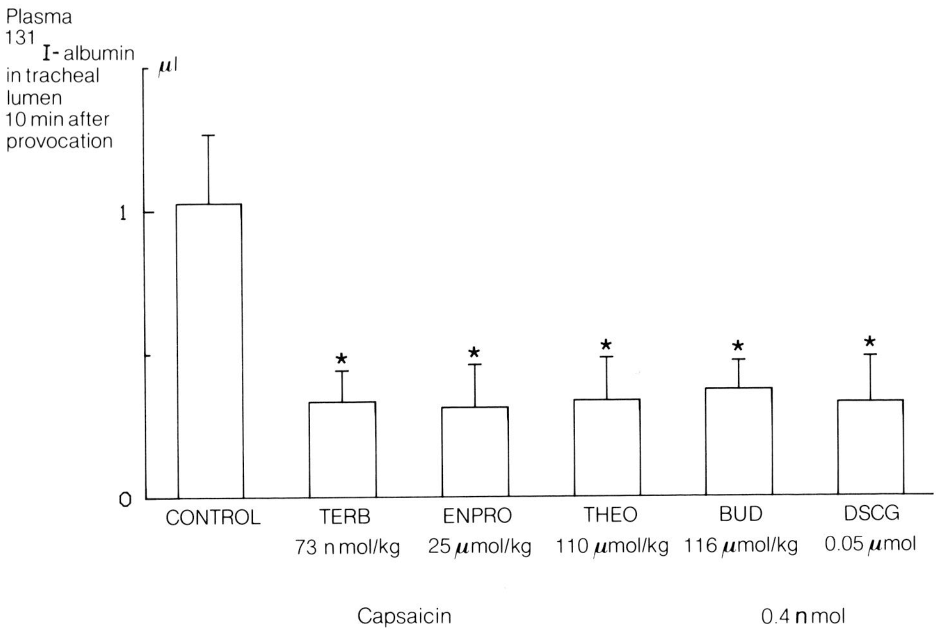

Figure 7 Different types of antiasthma drugs administered in regimens known to be effective in experimental guinea pig "asthma" are shown here to attenuate significantly capsaicin-induced leakage of macromolecules from the vascular compartment and into the tracheal lumen of anaesthetized guinea pigs. $*p<0.05$ (comparisons with capsaicin alone; n = 4–10); TERB, terbutaline; ENPRO, enprofylline; THEO, theophylline, all given intravenously 10 min before provocation; BUD, budesonide given intraperitoneally 24 hr before provocation; DSCG, cromoglycate given by a tracheal superfusion for 10 min just prior to provocation.

Antiasthma xanthines may be subdivided into adenosine-blockers such as theophylline and adenosine-nonblockers such as enprofylline (Persson, 1985; Persson and Karlsson, 1986). Included among the anti-inflammatory actions of these xanthines is a vascular antileakage effect that has variably been demonstrated in the hamster cheek pouch (Svensjö and Persson, 1984) and guinea pig trachea (Persson, 1985; Persson et al., 1986) (Fig. 7). Since enprofylline is as effective as theophylline, adenosine would not be involved in this response.

It cannot be excluded that an antiexudative effect has contributed to a portion of the protection provided by theophylline and enprofylline against late phase airway responses (after aeroallergen challenge in atopic asthmatics) (Pauwels et al., 1985). A third type of drug that is known to prevent late phase asthmatic responses is cromoglycate (Altounyan, 1980). Again, preliminary animal data suggest that it too may reduce plasma exudation and its entry into airways (Fig. 7).

It has been widely held that anti-inflammatory effects of sympathomimetic drugs reflect vasoconstriction and diminished blood flow to inflamed tissues. In addition, these drugs obviously exert a vascular antipermeability effect. The antileakage effect is β_2-adrenoceptor mediated and it more than outweighs the slightly proinflammatory blood flow increasing effect that also is produced by β_2-receptor agonists (Svensjö et al., 1977; see Persson and Svensjö, 1985). In experimental systems in which large doses of hypotensive inflammatory mediators are given, the vascular leakage effect may be significantly inhibited by endogenous epinephrine released from the adrenal medulla and acting on β-receptors (see Grega et al., 1981) (Fig. 6). β_2-Receptor agonists seemed particularly potent in preventing moderate effects of mediators on guinea pig tracheal microvasculature (Persson et al., 1986; Fig. 7). However, in guinea pig tracheas, where the microvascular baseline values had already been distorted by injury, a β_2-receptor agonist did not reduce a further inflammatory stimulus-induced leakage of macromolecules (Erjefält et al., 1985).

Different tachykinin antagonists were effective locally in the guinea pig trachea to antagonize a neurogenic inflammatory response (Persson et al., 1985), but the value of these antagonists as tools is in doubt since they exert nonspecific neurodepressant actions (Post et al., 1985). Low concentrations of the local anesthetic lidocaine also prevented the neurogenic exudative response in guinea pigs (Persson et al., 1985, 1986). However, local anesthetic drugs have not as yet been demonstrated to produce an acceptable clinical response in asthma (Griffin et al., 1982; Tullet et al., 1982; Sheppard et al., 1983).

Atropine and ipratropium bromide, which inhibit effects of cholinergic nerves on a variety of effector cells, have some antiasthma efficacy (Gross and Skorodin, 1984). However, antileakage effects are most likely not prominent in their action because acetylcholine and other muscarinic agonists, which are specifically antagonized by atropine-like drugs, do not seem to increase microvascular perviousness (Grega et al., 1980; Woodward et al., 1983; Fig. 2).

V. Conclusion

We conclude that inflammatory stimulus-induced plasma leakage from the tracheobronchial microvasculature may occur in asthma, and that the leakage-regulating postcapillary venular endothelium is an important effector cell in this disease. It is presently unclear if neural mechanisms, such as a capsaicin-sensitive innervation and neurally released tachykinins, can cause tracheobronchial microvascular leakage of macromolecules in mammalian species other than rats and guinea pigs. A neurohumoral β-receptor-mediated mechanism may be one of the factors involved in the reduction of macromolecular permeability of airway microvasculature.

Acknowledgment

We thank Professor Donald M. McDonald, Cardiovascular Research Institute, University of California, for helpful suggestions, and Mrs Ingegerd Källén for expert secretarial assistance.

Discussion

Daniel. You assume that microvascular leakage after capsaicin is caused by SP. Could it be acting as an irritant in some other way?

Persson. The potent inhibitory effect of lidocaine indicates that it is a neural response, and tachykinin antagonists markedly reduce the response to capsaicin and to vagal nerve stimulation. Lundberg and Saria (1982) have also shown that in animals depleted of SP-immunoreactivity there is no longer an inflammatory response to capsaicin.

Widdicombe. Does luminal capsaicin stimulate nerves in the epithelium with axon branches in the submucosa, with release of sensory neuropeptides at both sites? This might explain the changes in permeability at both venules and epithelium. It would be interesting to see the effect of luminal capsaicin in ferret, a species that lacks epithelial nerves.

Persson. McDonald (personal communication) has observed few nerves in rat epithelium, yet by nerve stimulation he observes venular leakiness as well as histologic changes in epithelium.

Barnes. With depletion of SP- and CGRP-immunoreactive nerves is there a reduction in the plasma exudation induced by inflammatory mediators, such as histamine and bradykinin, applied to the airway lumen?

Lundberg. The vascular permeability increase to both bradykinin and histamine are markedly reduced after capsaicin treatment. Together with recent data, suggesting that these two agents release tachykinins from the isolated perfused lung, this clearly indicates that the vascular permeability response to these agents is indirect due to the release of peptides from sensory nerves.

Said. What is the effect of VIP? As it stimulates cyclic AMP production it might be expected to reduce microvascular leakage.

Persson. VIP, in contrast to beta-2 agonists, may augment plasma exudation by increasing blood flow. Beta-2 agonists appear to have a specific microvascular antileak effect that may not be shared by VIP. The role of cyclic AMP in the regulation of venular leakage is unknown.

Nadel. Changes in permeability after vagal nerve stimulation are limited to trachea and mainstem bronchus.

Widdicombe. Are these changes seen in species other than rat and guinea pig?

Persson. Capsaicin-sensitive nerves are involved in the flare response in human skin. Apparently there is no evidence for neural effects on airway permeability in either dogs or cats.

References

Alexander, H. L. (1963). A historical account of death from asthma. *J. Allergy* **34**:305-313.

Altounyan, R. E. (1980). Review of clinical activity and mode of action of sodium cromoglycate. *Clin. Allergy* **10** (suppl):481-489.

Ameland, E., Prasad, C. M., Raymond, R. M., and Grega, G. J. (1981). Interactions among inflammatory mediators on edema formation in the canine forelimb. *Circ. Res.* **49**:298-306.

Anderson, S. D., Schoeffel, R. E., Follet, R., Perry, C. P., Daviskas, E., and Kendall, M. (1982). Sensitivity to heat and water loss at rest and during exercise in asthmatic patients. *Eur. J. Respir. Dis.* **63**:459-471.

Arnold, J. (1876). Uber die Kittsubstanz der Endothelien. *Virchows Arch. Pathol. Anat.* **66**:77-95.

Arowolo, R. A. O., and Eyre, P. (1971). Pharmacological comparison of isolated bronchial artery and pulmonary vein: possible functional relationships. *Res. Commun. Chem. Pathol. Pharmacol.* **26**:227-241.

Aschheim, E., and Zweifach, B. W. (1962). Quantitative studies of protein and water shifts during inflammation. *Am. J. Physiol.* **202**:554-558.

Aviado, D. M. (1963). Pharmacology of the bronchial circulation. In *First International Pharmacology Meeting.* Edited by B. Uvnäs. London, Pergamon Press, pp. 125-149.

Baier, H., Long, W. M., and Wanner, A. (1985). Bronchial circulation in asthma. *Respiration* **48**:199-205.

Baile, E. M., Dahlby, R. W., Wiggs, B. R., and Paré, P. D. (1985). Role of tracheal and bronchial circulation in respiratory heat exchange. *J. Appl. Physiol.* **58**:217-222.

Baumgarten, A., Melrose, G. J. H., and Vagg, W. J. (1970). Interactions between histamine and bradykinin assessed by continuous recording of increased vascular permeability. *J. Physiol.* **208**:669-675.

Baumgarten, C. R., Togias, A. G., Nacleiro, R. M., Lichtenstein, L. M., Norman, P. S., and Proud, D. (1985). Influx of kininogens into nasal secretions after antigen challenge of allergic individuals. *J. Clin. Invest.* **76**:191-197.

Behrens, B. L., Clark, R. A. F., Feldsien, D. C., Presley, D. M., Glezen, L. S., Graves, J. P., and Larsen, G. L. (1985). Comparison of the histopathology of the immediate and the late asthmatic and cutaneous responses in a rabbit model. *Chest* **87**:153S-155S.

Björk, J., Smedegård, G., Svensjö, E., and Arfors, K. E. (1984). The use of the hamster cheek pouch for intravital microscopy studies of microvascular events. In *Progress in Applied Microcirculation* 6. Edited by K. Messmer, F. Hammersen, and B. Zweifach. Basel, Karger, pp. 41-53.

Björk, J., Hugli, T. E., and Smedegård, G. (1985). Microvascular effects of anaphylatoxins C3a and C5a. *J. Immunol.* **134**:1115-1119.

Boucher, R. C., Bromberg, P. A., and Gatzy, J. T. (1980). Airway mucosal permeability. In *Airway Reactivity.* Edited by F. Hargreave. Mississauga, Ontario, Astra Canada, pp. 40-48.

Bray, M. A., Ford-Hutchison, A. W., and Smith, M. J. H. (1981). Leukotriene B_4: an inflammatory mediator in vivo. *Prostaglandins* **22**:213-222.

Brogan, T. D., Ryley, H. C., Neale, L., and Yassa, J. (1975). Soluble proteins of bronchopulmonary secretions from patients with cystic fibrosis asthma and bronchitis. *Thorax* **30**:72-79.

Bruce, A. N. (1910). Uber die Beziehung der sensiblen Nervenendigungen zum Entzündungsvorgang. *Arch. Exp. Pathol. Pharmakol.* **63**:424-433.

Bruner, H. D., and Schmidt, C. F. (1947). Blood flow in the bronchial artery of the anaesthetized dog. *Am. J. Physiol.* **148**:648-666.

Bult, H., and Herman, A. G. (1985). Vascular responses and their suppression: the role of endothelium. In *The Pharmacology of Inflammation. Handbook of Inflammation* 5. Edited by I. L. Bonta, M. A. Bray, and M. J. Parnham. Amsterdam, Elsevier-North Holland, pp. 83-105.

Burke, J. F., and Miles, A. A. (1958). The sequence of vascular events in early infective inflammation. *J. Pathol. Bacteriol.* **76**:1-19.

Cardell, B. S., and Pearson, R. S. B. (1959). Death in asthmatics. *Thorax* **14**:341-352.

Chambers, R., and Zweifach, B. W. (1947). Intercellular cement and capillary permeability. *Physiol. Rev.* **27**:436-463.

Chapman, L. F., and Goodell, H. (1964). The participation of the nervous system in the inflammatory reaction. *Ann. N.Y. Acad. Sci.* **116**:990-1017.

Charan, N. B., Turk, G. M., and Ripley, R. (1985). Measurement of bronchial arterial blood flow and bronchovascular resistance in sheep. *J. Appl. Physiol.* **59**:305-308.

Cohnheim, J. (1882). *Vorlesungen uber allgemeine Pathologie I.* Berlin, August Hirschwald, pp. 232-367.

Coleridge, H. M., and Coleridge, J. C. G. (1977). Afferent vagal C-fibres in the dog lung. Their discharge during spontaneous breathing and their stimulation by alloxan and pulmonary congestion. In *Krogh Centenary Symposium of Respiratory Adaptions, Capillary Exchange and Reflex Mechanisms.* Edited by A. S. Paintal and P. Gill-Kumar. Delhi, University of Delhi, pp. 396-406.

Collier, J. G., and Fuller, R. W. (1984). Capsaicin inhalation in man and the effect of sodium cromoglycate. *Br. J. Pharmacol.* **81**:113-117.

Craig, J. P., and Miles, A. A. (1961). Some properties of the iota-toxin of clostridium welchii including its action on capillary permeability. *J. Pathol. Bacteriol.* **81**:481-493.

Cutz, E., Levison, H., and Cooper, D. M. (1978). Ultrastructure of airways in children with asthma. *Histopathology* **2**:407-421.

Dahlén, S. E., Björk, J., Hedquist, P., Arfors, K. E., Hammarström, S., Lindgren, J. Å., and Samuelson, B. (1981). Leukotrienes promote plasma leakage and leukocyte adhesion in postcapillary venules: in vivo effects with relevance to the acute inflammatory response. *Proc. Natl. Acad. Sci. U.S.A.* **78**:3887-3891.

De Letona, J. M. L., De la Mata, R. C., and Aviado, D. M. (1961). Local and reflex effects of bronchial arterial injection of drugs. *J. Pharmacol. Exp. Ther.* **133**:295-303.

Don Barton, A., and Lourenco, R. C. (1973). Bronchial secretions and mucociliary clearance. *Arch. Intern. Med.* **131**:140-144.

Dulfano, M. J., and Luk, C. K. (1982). Sputum and ciliary inhibition in asthma. *Thorax* **37**:646-651.

Dunnill, M. S. (1960). The pathology of asthma with special reference to changes in the bronchial mucosa. *J. Clin. Pathol.* **13**:27-33.

Dunnill, M. S. (1978). The pathology of asthma. In *Allergy Principles and Practice II.* Edited by E. Middleton, C. E. Reed, and E. F. Ellis. St. Louis, C. V. Mosby, pp. 678-686.

Elder, J. M., and Miles, A. A. (1957). The action of the lethal toxins of gas-gangrene clostridia on capillary permeability. *J. Pathol. Bacteriol.* **74**: 133-145.

Erjefält I., and Persson, C. G. A. (1982). Effects of adrenaline and terbutaline on mediator-increased vascular permeability in the cat trachea. *Br. J. Pharmacol.* **77**:399P.

Erjefält, I. A. L., G-Wagner, Z., Strand, S. E., and Persson, C. G. A. (1985). A method for studies of tracheobronchial microvascular permeability to macromolecules. *J. Pharmacol. Methods* **14**:275-283.

Florange, W. (1960). Anatomie und Pathologie der Arteria bronchialis. In *Ergebnisse der allgemeinen Pathologie und pathologische Anatomi* 39.

Edited by P. Cohrs, W. Giese, and H. Meesen. Berlin, Springer Verlag, pp. 152-224.

Florey, H., Carleton, H. M., and Wells, A. Q. (1932). Mucus secretion in the trachea. *Br. J. Exp. Pathol.* **13**:269-284.

Florey, H. W. (1970). Inflammation. In *General Pathology* 4th Ed. Edited by H. W. Florey. London, Lloyd-Luke, pp. 22-123.

Forstner, J. F., Jabbal, I., Findlay, B. P., and Forstner, G. G. (1977). Interaction of mucins with calcium, H^+ ion and albumin. *Mod. Probl. Paediatr.* **19**: 54-65.

Frigas, E., Loegering, D. A., and Gleich, G. J. (1980). Cytotoxic effects of the guinea-pig eosinophil major basic protein on tracheal epithelium. *Lab. Invest.* **42**:35-40.

Fuller, R. W., Dixon, C. M. S., and Barnes, P. J. (1985). The bronchoconstrictor response to inhaled capsaicin in humans. *J. Appl. Physiol.* **85**:1080-1084.

Gatling, R. R. (1958). Altered reactivity to epinephrine in the hypersensitive rabbit. *J. Exp. Med.* **108**:441-451.

Gerdin, B., and Saldeen, T. (1978). Effect of fibrin degradation products on microvascular permeability. *Thromb. Res.* **13**:995-1006.

Gordon, T., Sheppard, D., McDonald, D., Distefano, S., and Scypinski, L. (1985). Airway hyperresponsiveness and inflammation induced by toluene diisocyanate in guinea-pigs. *Am. Rev. Respir. Dis.* **132**:1106-1112.

Greaves, M., and Shuster, S. (1967). Response of skin blood vessels to bradykinin, histamine and 5-hydroxytryptamine. *J. Physiol.* **193**:255-267.

Grega, G. J., Maciejco, J. J., Raymond, R. M., and Sak, D. P. (1980). The interrelationship among histamine, various vasoactive substances, and macromolecular permeability in the canine forelimb. *Circ. Res.* **46**:264-275.

Grega, G. J., Svensjö, E., and Haddy, F. J. (1981). Macromolecular permeability of the microvascular membrane: physiological and pharmacological regulation. *Microcirculation* **1**:325-341.

Griffin, M. P., McFadden, E. R., Ingram, R. H., and Pardee, S. (1982). Controlled-analysis of the effects of inhaled lignocaine in exercise-induced asthma. *Thorax* **37**:741-745.

Gross, N. J., and Skorodin, M. S. (1984). Anticholinergic, antimuscarinic bronchodilators. *Am. Rev. Respir. Dis.* **129**:856-870.

Harkavy, J. (1930). Spasm-producing substance in the sputum of patients with bronchial asthma. *Arch. Intern. Med.* **45**:641-646.

Hilding, A. C. (1943). The relation of ciliary insufficiency to death from asthma and other respiratory diseases. *Anal. Otol. Rhin. Laryng.* **52**:5-19.

Hogg, J. C. (1984). The pathology of asthma. *Clin. Chest Med.* **5**:567-571.

Holtzman, M. J., Fabbri, L. M., O'Byrne, P. M., Gold, B. D., Aizawa, H., Walters, E. H., Alpert, S. E., and Nadel, J. A. (1983). Importance of inflammation for hyperresponsiveness induced by ozone. *Am. Rev. Respir. Dis.* **127**:686-690.

Houston, J. C., De Navasquez, S., and Trounce, J. R. (1953). A clinical and pathological study of fatal cases of status asthmaticus. *Thorax* **8**:207-213.

Huber, H. L., and Koessler, K. K. (1922). The pathology of bronchial asthma. *Arch. Intern. Med.* **30**:689-760.

Hughes, T. (1965). Microcirculation of the tracheobronchial tree. *Nature* **4982**: 425-426.

Hulbert, W. H., McLean, T., and Hogg, J. C. (1985). The effect of acute airway inflammation on bronchial reactivity in guinea-pigs. *Am. Rev. Respir. Dis.* **132**:7-11.

Hurley, J. C. (1983). *Acute Inflammation,* 2nd ed. Edinburgh, Churchill Livingstone.

Hutt, G., and Wick, H. (1956). Bronchial-lumen und Atemwiderstand. *Z. Aerosol-Forsch. Ther.* **5**:131-140.

Intaglietta, M., Pawula, R. F., and Tompkins, W. R. (1970). Pressure measurements in the mammalian microvasculature. *Microvasc. Res.* **2**:212-220.

Jancso, N., Jancso-Gabor, A., and Szolcsanyi, J. (1967). Direct evidence for neurogenic inflammation and its prevention by denervation and by pretreatment with capsaicin. *Br. J. Pharmacol.* **31**:138-151.

Jancso, G., Kiraly, E., and Jancso-Gabor, A. (1977). Pharmacologically induced selective degeneration of chemosensitive primary sensory neurons. *Nature* **270**:741-743.

Karlsson, J. A., and Persson, C. G. A. (1983). Evidence against vasoactive intestinal polypeptide (VIP) as a dilator and in favour of substance P as a constrictor in airway neurogenic responses. *Br. J. Pharmacol.* **79**:634-636.

Kay, A. B., and Lee, T. H. (1982). Neutrophil chemotactic factor of anaphylaxis. *J. Allergy Clin. Immunol.* **70**:317-322.

Keal, E. E. (1971). Biochemistry and rheology of sputum in asthma. *Postgrad. Med. J.* **47**:171-177.

Kyle, H., Robinson, N. P., and Widdicombe, J. G. (1985). Changes in mucosal thickness in the dog trachea. *J. Physiol.* **362**:13.

Laitinen, L. A., Heino, M., Laitinen, A., Kava, T., and Haahtela, T. (1985). Damage of the airway epithelium and bronchial reactivity in patients with asthma. *Am. Rev. Respir. Dis.* **131**:599-606.

Lam, S., Leriche, J. C., Kijek, K., and Phillips, R. T. (1985). Effect of bronchial lavage volume on cellular and protein recovery. *Chest* **88**:856-859.

Larsen, G. (1985). Pulmonary inflammation–animal models. In *Inflammation.* Edited by P. Venge and A. Lindbom. Stockholm, Almquist Wicksell, pp. 425-444.

Lewis, G. P. (1970). Kinins in inflammation and tissue injury. In *Handbook of*

Experimental Pharmacology, vol. 25. Edited by E. G. Erdos. Berlin, Springer Verlag, pp. 516-530.

List, S. J., Findlay, B. P., Forstner, G. G., and Forstner, J. F. (1975). Enhancement of the viscosity of mucin by serum albumin. *Biochem. J.* **175**:565-571.

Long, W. M., Sprung, C. L., El Fawal, H., Yerger, L. D., Eyre, P., Abraham, W. M., and Wanner, A. (1985). Effects of histamine on bronchial artery blood flow and bronchomotor tone. *J. Appl. Physiol.* **59**:254-261.

Lundberg, J. M., and Saria, A. (1982). Capsaicin-sensitive vagal neurons involved in control of vascular permeability in rat trachea. *Acta Physiol. Scand.* **115**:521-523.

Lundberg, J. M., Brodin, E., and distribution of vagal capsaicin-sensitive substance P neurons with special reference to the trachea and lungs. *Acta Physiol. Scand.* **119**:243-252.

Lundberg, J. M., Saria, A., Theodorsson-Norheim, E., Brodin, E., Hua, X., Martling, C. R., Gamse, R., and Hökfelt, T. (1985). Multiple tachykinins in capsaicin-sensitive afferents: occurrence, release and biological effects with special reference to irritation of the airways. In *Tachykinin Antagonists.* Edited by R. Håkansson and F. Sundler. Amsterdam, Elsevier-North Holland, pp. 159-169.

Macklem, P. T., Proctor, D. F., and Hogg, J. C. (1970). The stability of peripheral airways. *Respir. Physiol.* **8**:191-203.

Majno, G., and Palade, G. E. (1961). Studies on inflammation I. *J. Biophys. Biochem. Cytol.* **11**:571-605.

Majno, G., Palade, G. E., and Schoefl, G. I. (1961). Studies on inflammation II. Site of action of histamine and serotonin along the vascular tree: a topographic study. *J. Biophys. Biochem. Cytol.* **11**:607-626.

Majno, G., Shea, S. M., and Levental, M. (1969). Endothelial contraction induced by histamine-type mediators. *J. Cell Biol.* **42**:647-672.

Malm, L., and Pettersson, G. (1985). Tachykinins and nasal secretion. In *Tachykinin Antagonists.* Edited by R. Håkansson and F. Sundler. Amsterdam, Elsevier-North Holland.

Marchesi, V. T. (1961). The site of leukocyte emigration during inflammation. *J. Exp. Physiol.* **46**:115-133.

Martling, C. R., Anggård, A., and Lundberg, J. M. (1985). Non-cholinergic vasodilation in the tracheobronchial tree of the cat induced by vagal nerve stimulation. *Acta Physiol. Scand.* **125**:343-346.

McLaughlin, R. F., Tyler, W. S., and Canada, R. O. (1961). Subgross pulmonary anatomy in various mammals and man. *JAMA* **175**:694-697.

McLaughlin, R. F., Tyler, W. S., and Canada, R. O. (1966). Subgross pulmonary anatomy of the rabbit, rat, and guinea-pig, with additional notes on the human lung. *Am. Rev. Respir. Dis.* **94**:380-387.

Messer, J. W., Peters, G. A., and Bennet, W. A. (1960). Causes of death and pathologic findings in 304 cases of bronchial asthma. *Dis. Chest* **38**:616-624.

Middleton, E. Jr., Atkins, F. M., Fanning, M., and Georgitis, J. W. (1981). Cellular mechanisms in the pathogenesis and pathophysiology of asthma. *Med. Clin. North Am.* **65**:1013-1031.

Miles, A. A. (1964). Large molecular substances as mediators of the inflammatory reaction. *Ann. N. Y. Acad. Sci.* **116**:855-890.

Miles, A. A., and Wilhelm, D. L. (1955). Enzyme-like globulins from serum reproducing the vascular phenomena of inflammation. *Br. J. Exp. Pathol.* **36**:71-81.

Miles, A. A., and Wilhelm, D. L. (1960). The activation of endogenous substances inducing pathological increases of capillary permeability. In *The Biochemical Response to Injury.* Edited by H. B. Stoner and C. J. Threlfall. Oxford, Blackwell, pp. 51-83.

Miller, W. S. (1947). The Lung. Springfield, Chas C Thomas, pp. 74-88.

Moore, W. F. (1925). Ciliary inhibition or destruction in tracheobronchial asthma. *Am. J. Med. Sci.* **169**:799-806.

Movat, H. Z. (1979). Kinins and the kinin system as inflammatory mediators. In *Chemical Messengers of the Inflammatory Process. Handbook of Inflammation* 1. Edited by J. C. Houck. Amsterdam, Elsevier-North Holland, pp. 47-112.

Nadel, J. A., and Holtzman, M. J. (1984). Regulation of airway responsiveness and secretion: role of inflammation. In *Asthma.* Edited by A. B. Kay, K. F. Austen, and L. M. Lichtenstein. London, Academic Press, pp. 129-153.

Naylor, B. (1962). The shedding of the mucosa of the bronchial tree in asthma. *Thorax* **17**:69-72.

Nilsson, G., Dahlberg, K., Brodin, E., Sundler, F., and Strandberg, K. (1977). Distribution and constrictor effect of substance P in guinea-pig tracheobronchial tissue. In *Substance P.* Edited by U. S. von Euler and P. Pernow. New York, Raven Press, pp. 57-81.

Nordin, U. (1977). The trachea and cuff-induced tracheal injury. *Acta Laryngol.* **83** (suppl 345):1-71.

Parsons, G. H., Kramer, G. C., Link, D. P., Lantz, B. M. T., Gunther, R. A., Green, J. F., and Cross, C. E. (1985). Studies of reactivity and distribution of bronchial blood flow in sheep. *Chest* **87**:180S-182S.

Pernow, B. (1983). Substance P. *Pharmacol. Rev.* **35**:84-141.

Persson, C. G. A. (1985). Experimental lung actions of xanthines. In *Anti-Asthma Xanthines and Adenosine.* Edited by K. E. Andersson and C. G. A. Persson. Amsterdam, Excerpta Medica, pp. 61-83.

Persson, C. G. A. (1986). Role of plasma exudation in asthmatic airways. *Am. Rev. Respir. Dis.* **2**:1126-1129.

Persson, C. G. A., and Erjefält, I. (1986). Inflammatory leakage of macromolecules from the vascular compartment into the tracheal lumen. *Acta Physiol. Scand.* **126**:615-616.

Persson, C. G. A., and Karlsson, J. A. (1986). In vitro responses to bronchodilator drugs. In *Asthma Therapy: Theory and Practice. Lung Biology in Health and Disease* (Lenfant, C., series ed.). Edited by J. W. Jenne and S. Murphy. New York, Marcel Dekker.

Persson, C. G. A., and Svensjö, E. (1983). Airway hyperreactivity and microvascular permeability to large molecules. *Eur. J. Respir. Dis.* (suppl 131) **64**: 183-214.

Persson, C. G. A., and Svensjö, E. (1985). Vascular responses and their suppression: drugs interfering with venular permeability. In *Handbook of Inflammation,* Vol. 5: *The Pharmacology of Inflammation.* Edited by I. L. Bonta, M. A. Bray, and M. J. Parnham. Amsterdam, Elsevier, North-Holland, pp. 61-81.

Persson, C. G. A., Erjefält, I., and Karlsson, J. A. (1985). Effects of tachykinins and tachykinin antagonists on the tracheobronchial microcirculation. In *Tachykinin Antagonists.* Edited by R. Håkanson and F. Sundler. Amsterdam, Elsevier, North-Holland, pp. 171-179.

Persson, C. G. A., Erjefält, I., and Andersson, P. (1986). Leakage of macromolecules from guinea-pig tracheobronchial microcirculation. Effects of allergen, leukotrienes, tachykinins, and antiasthma drugs. *Acta Physiol. Scand.* **127**:95-106.

Pietra, G. G., and Magno, M. (1978). Pharmacological factors influencing permeability of the bronchial circulation. *Fed. Proc.* **37**:2466-2470.

Pietra, G. G., Szidon, J. P., Leventhal, M. M., and Fishman, A. P. (1971). Histamine and interstitial pulmonary edema in the dog. *Circ. Res.* **29**:323-337.

Pietra, G. G., Magno, M., Johns, L., and Fishman, A. P. (1979). Bronchial veins and pulmonary edema. In *Pulmonary Edema.* Edited by A. P. Fishman and E. M. Renkin. Bethesda, American Physiological Society, pp. 196-206.

Post, C., Butterworth, J. F., Strichartz, G. R., Karlsson, J. A., and Persson, C. G. A. (1985). Tachykinin antagonists have potent local anaesthetic actions. *Eur. J. Pharmacol.* **117**:347-354.

Prescott, S. M., Zimmerman, G. A., and McIntyre, T. M. (1984). Human endothelial cells in culture produce platelet activating factor (1-alkyl-2-acetyl-sn-glycero-3-phosphocholine) when stimulated with thrombin. *Proc. Natl. Acad. Sci.* **81**:3534-3539.

Pump, K. K. (1972). Distribution of bronchial arteries in the human lung. *Chest* **62**:447-451.

Rous, P., and Smith, F. (1931). The gradient of vascular permeability. *J. Exp. Med.* **53**:219-241.

Ryley, H. C., and Brogan, T. D. (1968). Variation in the composition of sputum in chronic chest diseases. *Br. J. Exp. Pathol.* **49**:625-633.

Salter, H. H. (1868). *On Asthma: Its Pathology and Treatment,* 2nd ed. London, Churchill.

Salvato, G. (1968). Some histological changes in chronic bronchitis and asthma. *Thorax* **23**:168-172.

Sanerkin, N. G., and Evans, D. M. D. (1965). The sputum in bronchial asthma: pathognomonic patterns. *J. Pathol. Bacteriol.* **89**:535-541.

Sellick, H., and Widdicombe, J. G. (1969). The activity of lung irritant receptors during pneumothorax, hypertonea and pulmonary vascular congestion. *J. Physiol.* **203**:359-381.

Sheppard, D., Rizk, N. W., Boushey, H. A., and Bethel, R. A. (1983). Mechanism of cough and bronchoconstriction induced by distilled water aerosol. *Am. Rev. Respir. Dis.* **127**:691-694.

Sobin, S. S., Frasher, W. G., Tremer, H. M., and Hadley, G. G. (1963). The microcirculation of the tracheal mucosa. *Angiology* **14**:165-170.

Spector, W. G. (1951). The role of some higher peptides in inflammation. *J. Pathol. Bacteriol.* **63**:93-110.

Spector, W. G., and Willoughby, D. A. (1963). The inflammatory response. *Bacteriol. Rev.* **27**:117-154.

Svensjö, E. (1978). Bradykinin and prostaglandin E_1, E_2 and F_2-induced macromolecular leakage in the hamster cheek pouch. *Prostaglandins Med.* **1**:397-410.

Svensjö, E., and Joyner, W. L. (1984). The effects of intermittent and continuous stimulation of microvessels in the cheek pouch of hamsters with histamine and bradykinin on the development of venular leaky sites. *Microcirc. Endothel. Lymph.* **1**:381-396.

Svensjö, E., and Persson, C. G. A. (1984). Effects of two xanthines on histamine-induced microvascular permeability increase for large molecules. Role of adenosine antagonism. *Microcirc. Clin. Exp.* **3**:489.

Svensjö, E., and Roempke, K. (1984). Time-dependent inhibition of bradykinin and histamine-induced increase in microvascular permeability by local glucocorticosteroid treatment. In *Glucocorticosteroids: Inflammation and Bronchial Hyperreactivity.* Edited by J. C. Hogg, R. Ellul-Micallef, and R. Brattsand. Amsterdam, Excerpta Medica, pp. 136-144.

Svensjö, E., Persson, C. G. A., and Rutili, G. (1977). Inhibition of bradykinin-induced macromolecular leakage from postcapillary venules by a β_2-adrenoceptor stimulant, terbutaline. *Acta Physiol. Scand.* **101**:504-506.

Sybert, A., and Weiss, E. B. (1985). Status asthmaticus. In *Bronchial Asthma,*

2nd ed. Edited by E. B. Weiss, M. S. Segal, and M. Stein. Boston, Little, Brown, pp. 808-842.

Thomas, L. (1956). The role of epinephrine in the reactions produced by the endotoxins of gram-negative bacteria. *J. Exp. Med.* **104**:865-880.

Thurlbeck, W. M., Hendersson, J. A., Fraser, R. G., and Bates, D. V. (1970). Chronic obstructive lung disease. A comparison between clinical roentgenologic, functional and morphologic criteria in chronic bronchitis, emphysema, asthma and bronchiectasis. *Medicine* **49**:81-145.

Tsurufugi, S., Sugio, K., Takemasa, F., and Yoshisawa, S. (1980). Blockade by anti-glucocorticoids, actinomycin D and cycloheximide of anti-inflammatory action of dexamethasone against bradykinin. *J. Pharmacol. Exp. Ther.* **212**:225-231.

Tullett, W. M., Patel, K. R., Berkin, K. E., and Kerr, J. W. (1982). Effect of lignocaine, sodium cromoglycate, and ipratropium bromide in exercise-induced asthma. *Thorax* **37**:737-740.

Wanner, A. (1985). Mucociliary function in bronchial asthma. In *Bronchial Asthma,* 2nd ed. Edited by E. B. Weiss, M. S. Segal, and M. Stein. Boston, Little, Brown, pp. 270-279.

Ward, P. A., Hugli, T. E., and Chenoweth, D. E. (1979). Complement and chemotaxis. In *Chemical Messengers of the Inflammatory Process. Handbook of Inflammation* 1. Edited by J. C. Houck. Amsterdam, Elsevier, North-Holland, pp. 153-178.

Wiggins, R. C., and Cochrane, C. G. (1979). Hageman factor and the contact activation system. In *Chemical Messengers of the Inflammatory Process. Handbook of Inflammation* 1. Edited by J. C. Houck. Amsterdam, Elsevier, North-Holland, pp. 179-196.

Wilhelm, D. L. (1962). The mediation of increased vascular permeability in inflammation. *Pharmacol. Rev.* **14**:251-280.

Wilhelm, D. L. (1973). Chemical mediators. In *The Inflammatory Process,* 2nd ed. Edited by B. W. Zweifach, L. Grant, and R. T. McCluskey. New York, Academic Press, pp. 251-302.

Williams, T. J. (1985). Vascular responses and their suppression: vasodilation and edema. In *The Pharmacology of Inflammation. Handbook of Inflammation* 5. Edited by I. L. Bonta, M. A. Bray, and M. J. Parnham. Amsterdam, Elsevier, North-Holland, pp. 49-60.

Williams, D. A., and Leopold, J. G. (1959). Death from bronchial asthma. *Acta Allergy* **14**:83-86.

Willoughby, D. A., and Giroud, J. P. (1969). The role of polymorphonuclear leucocytes in acute inflammation in agranulocytic rats. *J. Pathol.* **98**:53-60.

Willoughby, D. A., and Spector, W. G. (1968). Inflammation in agranulocytotic rats. *Nature* **219**:1258.

Wilson, G. B., and Fudenberg, H. H. (1977). Ciliary dyskinesia factors in cystic fibrosis and asthma. *Nature* **266**:463-464.

Woodward, D. F., Weichman, B. M., Gill, C. A., and Wasserman, M. A. (1983). The effect of synthetic leukotrienes on tracheal microvascular permeability. *Prostaglandins* **25**:131-142.

Zapata-Ortiz, V., De la Mata, R. C., Fernandez, E., Gen, A., and Batalla, L. (1967). Bronchial circulation in high altitudes. *Am. J. Physiol.* **212**:1464-1468.

Zweifach, B. W. (1962). Pathophysiology of the blood vascular barrier. *Angiology* **13**:345-355.

Zweifach, B. W. (1973). Microvascular aspects of tissue injury. In *The Inflammatory Process,* 2nd ed. Edited by B. W. Zweifach, L. Grant, and R. T. McCluskey. New York, Academic Press, pp. 3-46.

21

Autonomic Control of Mucociliary Function

ADAM WANNER

University of Miami School of Medicine
Miami, Florida

The clearance of surface liquids from the normal tracheobronchial tree is governed by the interaction among the beating cilia, the rate at which secretions are elaborated by mucus cells, the net direction and rate of transepithelial water fluxes, and the rheologic features of the fluid layers covering the epithelial surface. A wealth of information has been generated on the structure and function of the airway epithelium and the factors that control mucociliary clearance in numerous species including humans; this has been reviewed in detail (Gray, 1928; Sleigh, 1962; Rivera, 1962; Kilburn and Salzano, 1966; Kinosita and Murakami, 1967; Hilding, 1967; Kilburn, 1968a,b; Okeson and Divertie, 1970; Asmundsson and Kilburn, 1973; Newhouse et al., 1976a,b; Wanner, 1977). One of the earliest questions regarding mucociliary transport has addressed the role of the autonomic nervous system in maintaining baseline function and in the response of the mucociliary apparatus to physiological and injurious stimuli. A mismatch between the net production and clearance of lower airway liquids must lead to their accumulation in the airway lumina and necessitate cough as a backup system to clear the tracheobronchial tree. These relationships are of importance in assessing the influence of the autonomic nervous system on mucociliary function. For example, cholinergic agonists have been shown to not only increase the volume of secretions, but also to increase ciliary beat frequency and mucus transport in the trachea (Wanner et al., 1975; King and Viires, 1979; Maurer et al., 1982). Thus, these individual effects of cholinergic agonists on the components of mucociliary interaction tend to defend the "normal" thickness of the airway liquid layers and prevent their buildup.

The influence of the adrenergic, cholinergic, and nonadrenergic, noncholinergic (peptidergic) nervous system on the mucociliary apparatus of the lower airways has been carefully examined. This review summarizes what is currently known on the autonomic control of mucociliary interaction.

I. Mucociliary Targets of Autonomic Nervous System

Several structures of the airway mucosa are believed to participate in mucociliary clearance. Since mucociliary clearance depends upon the interaction between cilia protruding from the epithelium and the liquids covering it, ciliated columnar cells, mucus cells, and possibly other epithelial cells involved in liquid transport must play important contributing roles. The anatomy of the airway mucociliary apparatus is distinctly different in large and peripheral airways, and this is reflected by differences in mucosal function between those sites. It is therefore useful to consider them separately.

A. Trachea

Lucas and Douglas (1934) proposed a two-layer principle for surface liquid transport in the airways. According to their concept, cilia are surrounded by a periciliary fluid layer (sol), and are covered by a mucus layer (gel) that interacts with the tips of the cilia. The presence of these two layers has been clearly demonstrated in several animal species (Nowell and Tyler, 1971). It is still being debated whether the mucus layer is a contiguous blanket covering the surface of the trachea or consists of discontinuous islands (Barclay and Franklin, 1937; Van As, 1977). Particle transport has been shown to fail in the absence of mucus, but transport can be restored by placing autologous or heterologous mucus on the ciliated epithelium (Sade et al., 1970). This requirement for mucus is consistent with either concept in that mucus could move as an entire blanket or as a small island. With respect to the latter mechanism, it has even been suggested that mucus is absent in the unstimulated airway and is only produced in response to irritation. For example, an inhaled particle would produce mucus secretion at the site of its deposition, be trapped in the mucus, and thus cleared from the airways (Van As, 1977).

In the trachea, most of the surface epithelium is ciliated, with focal areas as large as 1 mm in diameter devoid of cilia (Fig. 1) (Wanner, 1977). The ratio

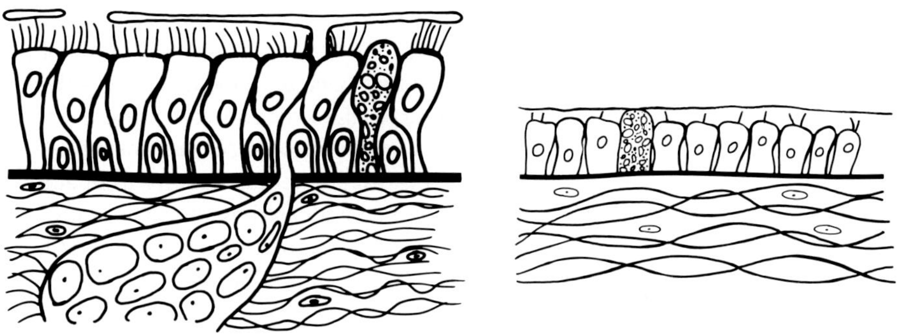

Figure 1 Schematic representation of the mucociliary apparatus in trachea (left) and bronchiole (right). Note the differences in the height of the epithelium and the extent of surface ciliation, the absence of submucosal gland and goblet cell, and of the surface mucus layer in bronchiole, and the presence of Clara cell (secretory cell) in bronchiole.

of ciliated columnar cells to nonciliated surface cells is between 5 and 10:1. Small areas of squamous metaplasia may be found. The surface of each ciliated columnar cell contains approximately 200 cilia with an average length of 6 μm and diameter of 0.2 μm. The cilia of human and other mammalian respiratory epithelia or cilia from lower animals are remarkably similar when compared by transmission and scanning electron microscopy (Roth and Shingenaka, 1964). Each cilium contains longitudinal microtubules that represent contractile elements. Two microtubules form a central core and nine doublets of microtubules are arranged in a circular fashion in the periphery of the cilium. The peripheral microtubules join to one structure towards the tip of the cilium. A basal body in the apex of the cell corresponds to each cilium. The pattern of ciliary motion is also uniform among different species. High-speed cinematography of isolated cilia or isolated ciliated cells has revealed that the beating of cilia occurs in one plane with a fast effective stroke (power stroke) and a slow recovery stroke (Sleigh, 1962; Wilson et al., 1985). The effective stroke is two to three times faster than the recovery stroke. The bending of cilia has been suggested to result from the sliding between the doublets of peripheral microtubules (Satir, 1974). Dynein arms bridging the space between the microtubules are thought to play an important role in this sliding motion. The force of the bending doublets is transferred to the ciliary membrane by connecting bridges. ATP has been identified as the energy source for ciliary motion, and ATP-ase has been found in the cytoplasm of the cilia (Usuki, 1959). Ciliary motion can be enhanced by adding ATP and other nucleoside triphosphates to the medium (Saavedra and Renaud, 1975).

It has been clearly established that the motion of adjacent cilia on an individual cell or the motion among cilia of adjacent cells is coordinated; however, the mechanisms responsible for this coordination have not been elucidated (Wanner, 1977). The ciliary coordination results in a metachronal wave propagation that appears to be a function of the recovery stroke velocity. The effective stroke of the ciliary motion is in the cephaled direction. The "normal" ciliary beat frequency ranges between 12 and 15 Hz in a wide variety of species including humans (Sleigh, 1962; Low et al., 1984).

Of the two liquid layers that line the tracheal epithelium, the mucus layer is between 5 and 10 μm deep while the periciliary fluid layer is more or less equal to the length of the ciliary shaft (approximately 6 μm) (Hulbert et al., 1982). It has been well established that the surface mucus is produced by goblet cells and submucosal glands. In contrast, the origin of the periciliary fluid has not been firmly established. The periciliary fluid could result from a liquifying effect of ciliary beating on mucus, represent alveolar or bronchiolar secretions, reflect the effects of varying pH values in the two layers on the gel point of glycoprotein containing respiratory secretions (Gatto, 1981), or result from active water and ion transport across the airway epithelium. This latter mechanism has been suggested by many investigators (Phipps, 1984).

In tracheostomized subjects, the daily volume of respiratory secretions eliminated through the trachea has been estimated to be between 10 and 100 ml (Wanner, 1977). It is not known what fraction of this total volume is produced in large airways and peripheral airways, and what fraction represents mucus gland products or epithelial water secretions. Of the various constituents of respiratory secretions, glycoproteins and water seem to be important in determining the rheologic properties of those secretions. In particular, disulfide cross-linking and hydrogen bonding between glycoprotein molecules and water have been found to influence the viscoelastic properties (Barton and Lourenco, 1973).

Theoretically, the thickness and rheologic properties of both the mucus layer and periciliary fluid layer govern the interaction between cilia and mucus and hence mucociliary transport. Studies of the ultrastructure of mucus in the upper and central airways of animals have revealed a heterogeneous basic fibrous network (Reissig et al., 1978). The luminal surface of the mucus layer appears smooth, whereas the underface in contact with cilia is irregular with the mucus penetrating a short distance between the ciliary shafts. This indentation, along with brushlike projections at the ciliary tips, may further facilitate the mechanical interaction between cilia and mucus. On the other hand, the importance of this contact between cilia and mucus has been called into question. For example, in vitro experiments utilizing the frog palate have suggested that a direct contact between the cilia and the mucus layer is not necessary to transmit the shear forces to the mucus (Winet et al., 1984). For a surface liquid 60 μm deep, the flow characteristics within the mucus layer were similar throughout the entire depth.

Theoretical considerations suggest that within a moderate range of deviation from "normal" and with ciliary beat frequency and wave velocity held constant, the mucus transport velocity is directly related to mucus elasticity and the depth of periciliary fluid and inversely related to mucus viscosity and the depth of the mucus layer (Ross and Corssin, 1974). Some of these factors have been tested experimentally. Thus, Stewart (1948) found that up to a weight of 20 mg/mm^2, the ciliated epithelium is capable of transporting test particles with out a decrease in their velocity. The relationship between the rheology and transportability of mucus has also been demonstrated by determining the viscosity and elastic modulus of artificial mucus or of sputum from patients, and measuring the transport rate of the same material on the frog palate. There appears to be an ideal viscosity/elasticity ratio for optimal mucociliary interaction, with an increase in viscosity and/or decrease in elasticity resulting in reduced transport rates. From a practical standpoint, both the depth and rheologic properties of mucus appear to have a major influence on mucociliary interaction; in contrast, changes in the rheologic properties of periciliary fluid, a sol, appear to be less important than changes in its depth.

Normal in vivo tracheal mucus transport rates have been reported to range between 2 and 20 mm/min (Wanner, 1977). This wide variability is probably due more to differences in technique than to interspecies differences. In any case, the clearance of particulate matter from the trachea is remarkably fast. In an adult human with a tracheal length of 12 cm and a mucus transport rate of 10 mm/min, it would take a particle deposited at the carina 12 minutes to reach the larynx.

B. Bronchioles

With an increase in airway generations, there is a decrease in the number of goblet cells and submucosal glands, and the number and length of cilia (Wanner, 1977). Submucosal glands are absent in noncartilaginous airways. In the most peripheral bronchioles, the surface epithelium is no longer psuedostratified, but characterized by flattened cells (Fig. 1). Distinct secretory cells (Clara cells) can be identified in most animal species (Breeze and Wheeldon, 1977). The mucus layer cannot be identified in normal peripheral airways, and little is known about the source and rheologic properties of the surface liquid.

Although ciliary beat frequency does not appear to be lower in smaller bronchi (at least as small as segmental bronchi) (Yager et al., 1980), mucus transport rates decline with increasing airway generation (Iravani and Van As, 1972; Serafini et al., 1976). It should be noted, however, that ciliary beat frequency is frequently measured by observing ciliated cells in vitro; this eliminates the natural milieu in which cilia beat, and the true in vivo ciliary beat frequency can therefore not be determined. For technical reasons, the beating pattern of cilia and the surface liquid transport characteristics in bronchioles have not been elucidated.

II. Autonomic Control of Mucociliary Apparatus

Autonomic neurotransmitters (agonists) can reach their receptors on target cells of the mucociliary system in two ways. First, the agonists can be released into the circulation at remote sites and gain access to the airway epithelium via the bronchial circulation. A classic example for this mode of action is epinephrine, which is secreted by neuroendocrine cells in the adrenal medulla. Second, autonomic agonists can be released from nerve endings in the vicinity of mucociliary targets within the airway wall. If the autonomic nervous system is to exert a local effect on mucociliary function, autonomic neurons should be demonstrable in the mucosa and submucosa of the tracheobronchial tree. While such a distribution of axons has, until recently, only been observed in lower air breathing animals, there is convincing new neuroanatomical evidence for an innervation of the mucociliary apparatus in mammals including humans. This new information can now be combined with physiological observations to allow us to understand better the autonomic control of mucociliary function.

A. Structure

In the large airways, sensory and motor nerve endings have been identified both within the mucosa and submucosa, presumably representing autonomic nerve fibers (Basbaum, 1984). Unmyelinated fibers have been shown to end at ciliated epithelial cells, but it has not been determined if these neurons are afferent fibers, efferent fibers, or both. In the submucosa, some nerve endings are in close relationship to the mucus glands. These observations have been made primarily in rodents and cats; the exact distribution of autonomic nerves in the human airway mucosa and submucosa remains to be described.

Immunohistochemical studies have revealed the presence of adrenergic, cholinergic, and peptidergic neurotransmitters in the nerve endings, and of alpha-adrenergic, beta-adrenergic, cholinergic, and peptidergic receptors in the epithelial and subepithelial tissues (Basbaum, 1984). Vasoactive intestinal peptide (VIP) and substance P are the best investigated peptidergic agonists in the airway wall, with VIP released from efferent and substance P possibly from afferent nerve fibers (Barnes, 1984). VIP immunoreactive nerves have been clearly identified in the airway walls of various species, mostly near airway smooth muscle and in vessel walls

(Dey et al., 1981). More importantly, submucosal glands are also surrounded by and the surface epithelium is in close relationship to VIP and substance P immunoreactive nerves (Uddman and Sundler, 1979; Pernow, 1983; Hakanson et al., 1983). The effects of neuropeptides on mucociliary targets seem to be species-dependent. Thus, VIP has been reported to increase immunoreactive cyclic adenosin monophosphate (c-AMP) in the submucosal mucus cells but not in ciliated cells of ferret trachea (Lazarus et al., 1983). In the dog trachea, on the other hand, VIP increased c-AMP in ciliated cells but not in goblet cells.

Nerve endings have also been described in peripheral airways. The nature of these neurons, their relation to ciliated and secretory (Clara) cells, and the types of agonists released at nerve endings are not known.

These and other investigations clearly establish the presence of autonomic nerve endings in the vicinity of ciliated epithelial cells, goblet cells, and submucosal gland cells; of neurotransmitters in those nerve fibers; and of receptors for those neurotransmitters on the ciliated epithelial, goblet, and submucosal mucus cells. The precise neural pathways to and from the mucociliary targets have not been completely described, particularly in humans. However, the immunohistochemical studies, which have also involved human tissues, form a solid morphologic basis for an autonomic control of airway mucociliary function.

B. Function

Several questions arise concerning the influence of the autonomic nervous system on mucociliary clearance. The first question is whether baseline mucociliary function is under autonomic control. The second question relates to the effect of autonomic nerve stimulation on the mucociliary apparatus. The third question addresses the actions of the various autonomic agonists on mucociliary clearance. Finally, one would like to know what effect these agonists have on the components of mucociliary interaction. These questions will be considered individually.

Baseline Function

There are essentially two ways to assess baseline autonomic mucociliary control physiologically: chemical or physical disruption of neural pathways and the administration of adrenergic, cholinergic, and peptidergic antagonists.

With the exception of the frog palate (Pohle, 1931), nervous control of baseline mucociliary transport has not been demonstrated when using autonomic nerve interruption techniques. While early workers strongly suggested a nervous control of ciliary beating in the mammalian trachea, based on circumstantial evidence (McDonald et al., 1928), more recent studies have failed to substantiate this (Gosselin, 1966; Iravani, 1969; Brody et al., 1971). Vagal section in dogs has been shown to have no effect on in vivo ciliary activity in the large airways (Lommel, 1908), and the sympathetic and parasympathetic nervous systems seem to lack an effect on baseline radiolabeled glycoprotein secretion in the cat (Gallagher et al., 1975).

Specific autonomic antagonists are capable of blocking the effects of electrical neural stimulation or exogenous autonomic agonists on ciliary activity, mucus and water secretion, and mucociliary clearance. However, in general these antagonists do not influence baseline mucociliary clearance and its component functions. The cholinergic antagonist atropine is a notable exception. Most investigators agree that atropine depresses mucociliary transport and inhibits ciliary activity in the airways. This has been demonstrated in vivo and in vitro, and in a wide variety of species including humans (Foster et al., 1976; Corssen and Allen, 1959). In contrast, atropine appears to have relatively little effect or no effect on baseline epithelial secretions. In the dog trachea, for example, atropine has no effect on baseline chloride and hence water secretion towards the luminal side (Marin et al., 1976). Likewise, atropine has been shown not to alter the volume or rheologic properties of submucosal gland secretions as assessed by single gland duct cannulation in the cat trachea (Leikauf et al., 1984). Similar results were obtained when total secretory material was examined in a canine tracheal pouch preparation; neither the secretory volume nor the viscoelastic properties of the secretions were changed by atropine in those experiments (Giordano et al., 1978). Somewhat different results have been reported by King et al. (1979; King and Angus, 1981), who found a decrease in the secretory volume in the canine trachea after atropine administration. This apparent change in secretory rate was not associated with significant changes in the viscosity/elasticity ratios of the secretions (unless the initial elasticity was low) or the transportability of those secretions on the frog palate. One might therefore conclude that atropine does not change the physical properties of airway secretions to an extent that they may interfere with mucociliary clearance. The impairment of mucociliary clearance by atropine in vivo is therefore likely to result from the above-mentioned cilioinhibition. This does not, however, explain the apparently incompatible results obtained with pharmacologic and mechanical vagal blockade, a decrease in mucociliary transport with the antimuscarinic agent atropine but not with section of the vagal nerve.

It is also unclear why there is a difference between atropine and its analogue, the quaternary ammonium compound ipratropium bromide with respect to mucociliary function. In contrast to atropine, ipratropium bromide up to a concentration of 10^{-3} g/ml has been shown to depress ciliary best frequency only minimally (less than 20%) in rat airways (Iravani, 1972). Likewise, ipratropium bromide given as an aerosol has been shown to have no effect on the volume or viscoelastic properties of tracheal mucus in dogs (King and Angus, 1981). Finally, tracheal mucus velocity has been found to be decreased by less than 20% after inhalation of 40 μg ipratropium bromide in contrast to a 60% decrease after inhalation of 750 μg atropine in anesthetized dogs (Sackner et al., 1977). Numerous studies have also demonstrated that inhaled ipratropium bromide up to a delivered dose of 200 μg fails to depress airway mucociliary clearance in normal subjects (Ruffin et al., 1978; Konietzko et al., 1974; Francis et al., 1977). No satisfactory explanation has thus far been offered for this intriguing difference between ipratropium bromide and atropine. Differences in the absorption of atropine and ipratropium bromide from mucosal surfaces is unlikely to account for this difference since inhaled ipratropium bromide has anticholinergic effects on airway smooth muscle. Possibly, the subtypes of muscarine receptors on the target cells of the mucociliary apparatus are selected for various antimuscarinic agents (Hammer and Giachetti, 1983).

All of these observations on baseline mucociliary function and its regulation by the autonomic nervous system were made in large airways or the entire tracheobronchial tree. No data exist on the autonomic control of steady state ciliary activity, secretory activity, and liquid transport in bronchioles.

Effects of Autonomic Nerve Stimulation

Although the autonomic nervous system seems to play a limited role in the control of baseline mucociliary clearance, an increase in efferent vagal or sympathetic nerve activity, for example, as a result of local afferent nerve stimulation, might alter airway mucosal function. It was originally suggested that sympathetic nerve stimulation augments ciliary activity of the frog palate while parasympathetic nerve stimulation depresses ciliary activity (McDonald et al., 1928). This concept of an opposing effect of the two classic autonomic nervous systems on mucociliary function was subsequently challenged and proven wrong. Thus, both vagal and sympathetic nerve stimulation produce an increased rate of mucus secretion and water transport toward the airway lumen in several species including humans (Phipps, 1984; Pack and Richardson, 1984; Barnes, 1984). Electrical sympathetic nerve stimulation in the cat has been shown to increase tracheal glycoprotein secretion, presumably mediated by beta-adrenergic receptor stimulation (Peatfield and Richardson, 1982). The neurotransmitters involved in vagally induced mucus hypersecretion seem to include acetylcholine as well as neuropeptides (Barnes, 1984; Peatfield and Richardson, 1983; Borson et al., 1982). For example, electrical stimulation of the vagus in the cat has been found to increase the secretion of radiolabeled mucus in the airways, and this was not inhibited by the alpha-adrenergic antagonist phentolamine and the beta-adrenergic antagonist propanolol (Hybbinette and Mercke, 1982). Atropine afforded only an attenuation but no complete blockade. By exclusion, nonadrenergic noncholinergic effects of electrical vagal stimulation (i.e., peptidergic neurotransmission) was therefore implicated as a contributing factor in vagally induced mucus secretions.

While sympathetic and parasympathetic nerve stimulation apparently has differential effects on the glycoprotein composition of submucosal gland secretions (Dische et al., 1970), it is not known whether these biochemical discrepancies translate into different rheologic properties. Such information would be of considerable interest in view of the influence of mucus rheology on mucociliary interaction.

Similarly, very little is known about the effects of autonomic nerve stimulation on ciliary activity or mucociliary clearance in the airways. Vagal stimulation in dogs does not appear to alter ciliary activity in the trachea (Lommel, 1908). However, similar information is lacking in other species. The influence of sympathetic nerve stimulation on ciliary beat frequency in mammals is also unknown. Finally, definitive studies on the actions of autonomic nerve stimulation on mucociliary transport have not been reported.

The significance of efferent autonomic nerve excitation on mucociliary activity would be in relation to reflex responses to local and possibly remote exogenous or endogenous stimuli. One might expect irritation of the airway mucosa to cause reflex stimulation of mucus secretion and clearance. This has not been examined in humans. However, in the maxillary sinus of the rabbit, ciliary wave motion has been reported to increase upon cigarette smoke exposure, with the effect being partially blocked by atropine and an antagonist of substance P and completely blocked by the pretreatment with both antagonists (Lindberg, 1985). The prior administration of capsaicin, which is capable of releasing substance P, also attenuated the effect of cigarette smoke in ciliary wave motion. The authors suggested on the basis of these observations that both acetylcholine and substance P mediated cigarette-smoke-induced autonomic reflex ciliary stimulation.

One might therefore conclude from the currently available data on the autonomic regulation of mucociliary activity in the airways that (1) baseline function is controlled by vagal nerves via ciliary activity rather than the rate of secretion and rheologic features of surface liquids, (2) vagal and sympathetic nerve stimulation causes hypersecretion of water and mucus of variable rheologic properties with unknown effects on mucociliary clearance, and (3) autonomic reflex mechanisms stimulate ciliary activity via cholinergic and peptidergic pathways.

The response of the bronchiolar mucosa to vagal and sympathetic nerve stimulation is, to our knowledge, unknown.

Effects of Autonomic Agonists

The target cells of the mucociliary apparatus clearly contain receptors for adrenergic, cholinergic, and peptidergic agonists, and most information on the autonomic control of mucociliary function has been derived from studies involving the use of exogenous autonomic agonists and their analogues. It must be pointed out that such experiments merely demonstrate the presence of receptors on the various cells of the mucociliary apparatus and the physiological consequences of stimulating those receptors. The concentration of endogenous neurotransmitters at these receptor sites is unknown, regardless of whether the neurotransmitters are released from nerve endings in the airway wall or from other sites and gain access to the receptors via the bronchial circulation. Therefore, a comparison between the tissue concentrations of exogenous and endogenous autonomic agonists is not possible. This may partially explain the apparent discrepancies between the effects of autonomic nerve stimulation and exogenous autonomic agonists. For example, inhaled acetylcholine has been shown to increase airway mucociliary clearance in dogs (Wanner et al., 1975) while vagal stimulation has no effect (Lommel, 1908).

Ciliary Activity

The response of ciliary activity to autonomic agonists has been extensively studied in isolated epithelial cells, tracheal or bronchial explants, and in intact animals and humans (Wanner, 1977). Nearly all materials thus examined have exhibited stimulatory effects, and there is an excellent agreement among the results reported by various investigators (Fig. 2). Cholinergic agonists (acetylcholine, methacholine) stimulate ciliary activity in a dose-dependent manner in vitro and in vivo, and this effect can be blocked by atropine pretreatment (Kordik et al., 1952; Bulbring et al., 1953; Corssen and Allen, 1959; Hybbinette and Mercke, 1982; Maurer et al., 1982). In vivo and in tracheal explants, the administration of the cholinesterase inhibitor eserin is also capable of augmenting ciliary activity, which suggests that denervated airway tissues synthesize acetylcholine in the absence of an identifiable stimulus and contain cholinesterase (Kordik et al., 1952; Corssen and Allen, 1959).

The adrenergic agonists have differential effects on ciliary activity; beta-adrenergic agonists increase ciliary beat frequency in vitro and in vivo while alpha-adrenergic agonists do not appear to influence it. The ciliostimulatory actions of beta-adrenergic agonists have originally been questioned, but recent studies have clearly demonstrated a dose-dependent increase in ciliary beat frequency by such agents, including those that stimulate preferentially beta-2 receptors (Kordik et al., 1952; Blair and Woods, 1969; Van As, 1974; Verdugo et al., 1980; Yanaura et al., 1981; Maurer et al., 1982). Ephedrine has been reported to have similar effects by some but not all investigators (Melville et al., 1976; Saketkhoo et al., 1978). In contrast, norepinephrine is incapable of changing ciliary beat frequency (Kordik et al., 1952).

Substance P seems to stimulate ciliary activity in intact respiratory epithelia, presumably through a direct effect on the ciliated epithelial cells (Lindberg, 1985). The clearly demonstrated ciliostimulatory effect of analogues of cyclic AMP is noteworthy with respect to the actions of beta-adrenergic and peptidergic agonists on ciliary function (Yanaura et al., 1981). Both classes of agonists are

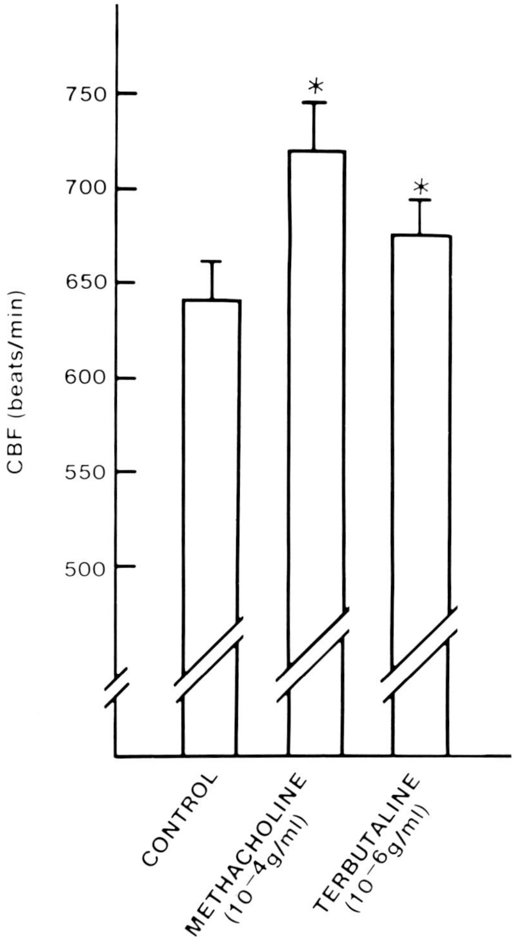

Figure 2 Effect of methacholine and terbutaline on ciliary beat frequency (CBF) in vitro. Values are means of 10 preparations with the brackets depicting S.E. *, Different from control ($p < 0.05$). (Constructed with data from Maurer et al., 1982.)

thought to exert their actions on target tissues via the generation of intracellular cyclic AMP.

The ciliary activity of bronchiolar epithelium and its modification by autonomic agonists have not been specifically examined. Considering the uniform ciliary responsiveness to such agents throughout the animal kingdom, peripheral airway cilia in humans are unlikely to differ from those of central airways in this regard.

Secretory Function

Again, nearly all experiments dealing with the effects of autonomic agonists on the production and rheology of airway liquid have involved the trachea. In most species, cholinergic, alpha-adrenergic, beta-adrenergic, and peptidergic agonists increase tracheal mucus and water secretion. Similar results have been obtained with a variety of experimental approaches in vivo and in vitro including (1) collection of total respiratory secretions (Reasor et al., 1978; Giordano et al., 1978; King et al., 1979; King and Viires, 1979; King and Angus, 1981), (2) volumetric measurements of single submucosal gland duct secretions using micropipettes (Leikauf et al., 1984), (3) secretory rate of radiolabeled macromolecules (glycoproteins) (Gallagher et al., 1975; Chakrin et al., 1973; Peatfield and Richardson, 1982; Phipps et al., 1982; Peatfield et al., 1983; Coles et al., 1984; Hartman et al., 1984), (4) determination in respiratory secretions of enzymes responsible for glycoprotein synthesis or of specific sugars (Baker et al., 1975, 1977; Limjuco and Hartmann, 1985), (5) morphologic evaluation of the extrusion of secretory granules using autoradiography or other staining methods (Sturgess and Reid, 1972; Coles et al., 1981; Basbaum et al., 1981), and (6) epithelial ion (and hence water) transport (Marin et al., 1976; Davis et al., 1979a,b; Al-Bazzaz and Cheng, 1979; Nathanson et al., 1983; Al-Bazzaz et al., 1985). Long-term stimulation of the mucociliary apparatus with cholinergic and beta-adrenergic agonists has even been shown to increase the number of goblet cells and/or cause submucosal gland hypertrophy in some experiments (Sturgess and Reid, 1973; Jones and Reid, 1979). Among the peptidergic agonists, VIP and substance P have similar effects and seem to influence mucus and ion secretory function directly, since they are not blocked by standard cholinergic and adrenergic agonists.

Several autonomic agonists are also capable of altering the rheologic properties and transportability of airway secretions. Total tracheal fluid in dogs has been shown to exhibit dose-dependent deviations in viscosity/elasticity ratios from baseline after methacholine administration, with a decrease in the transportability of the fluid (King et al., 1979; King and Viires, 1979). In contrast, the beta-adrenergic agents terbutaline and salbutamol have minimal or no effect on the rheologic properties of tracheal secretions (Giordano et al., 1978; King and Angus, 1981). With the micropipette technique, the examination of submucosal gland secretions in cat trachea has also revealed only minimal changes in mucus rheology after the administration of autonomic agents (Leikauf et al., 1984). Acetylcholine had no effect, while phenylephrine slightly decreased viscosity and isoproterenol slightly decreased elasticity with corresponding small deviations in the viscosity/elasticity ratios from baseline. It appears therefore that autonomic agonists have more profound effects on the volume than the rheology of airway secretions.

In the larger bronchi where, at least in the dog, the unstimulated epithelium absorbs water (rather than secreting water as in the trachea), acetylcholine reduces water absorption while adrenergic agents have no effect (Boucher and Gatzy, 1982). In the bronchioles of rats, both isoproterenol and pilocarpine have been shown to decrease the number of Clara cell granules in vivo, indicating secretion from these cells (Massaro et al., 1979, 1981). It is of interest that the secreta-

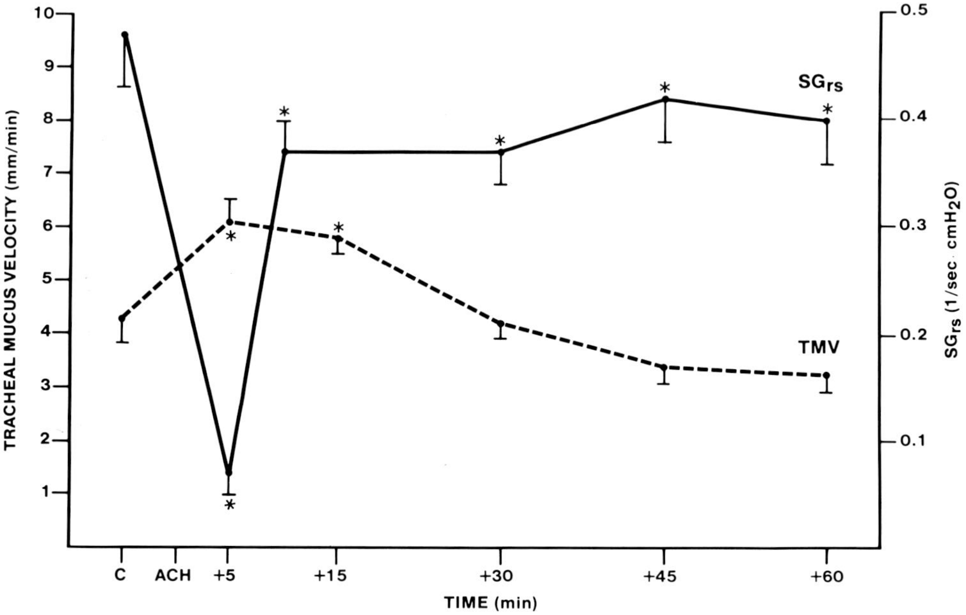

Figure 3 Effect of inhaled acetylcholine (ACH) (1% solution) on mean tracheal mucus velocity (TMV) and specific respiratory system conductance (SG_{rs}) in anesthetized dogs (n = 8). Brackets reflect S.E. *, Different from baseline control (C) at $p < 0.05$. (Constructed with data from Wanner et al., 1975).

gogue effect of pilocarpine was no longer seen in the excised lung; indeed, pilocarpine now had an inhibitory effect on isoproterenol-induced secretion. Thus, differences seem to exist between the trachea and bronchi in terms of baseline secretory functions and their responses to autonomic agonists.

Mucociliary Clearance

In various animal species and humans, the effects of exogenous autonomic agents on mucociliary clearance have been evaluated by surface markers and radioaerosol techniques, and with administration by inhalation, by mouth, or by injection (Figs. 3 and 4). Almost all studies have found an enhancement of mucociliary clearance by cholinergic and beta-adrenergic agonists (Camner et al., 1974, 1976; Konietzko et al., 1975; Wanner et al., 1975; Foster et al., 1976; Sackner et al., 1976, 1979; Lafortuna and Fazio, 1984). Alpha-adrenergic agents have not been evaluated with respect to their action on tracheobronchial mucociliary clearance. However, phenylephrine and tetrahydrozoline have been observed to increase nasal mucus transport by as much as 60% after local application (Saketkhoo et al.,

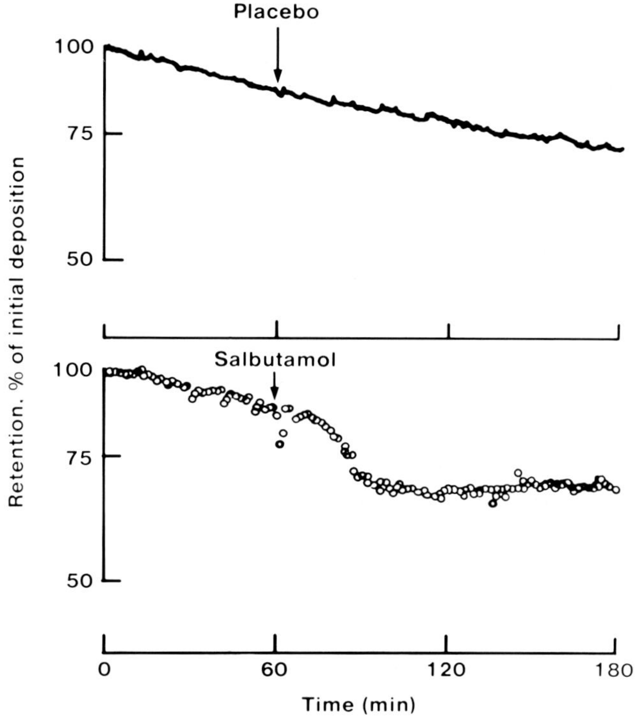

Figure 4 Stimulation of radioaerosol clearance from the tracheobronchial tree of a normal subject (expressed as retention of initially deposited aerosol) by inhaled albuterol (500 μg). (From Lafortuna and Fazio, 1984.)

1978). The effect of exogenous peptidergic neurotransmitters on airway mucociliary clearance remains to be determined.

III. Summary

Although the results of the numerous investigations concerned with the autonomic regulation of airway mucociliary clearance may show quantitative and occasionally qualitative differences related to methodologic and interspecies variabilities, several conclusions can be drawn. The mucosa and submucosa of large airways are innervated by the autonomic nervous system, and nerve endings seem to be located in the vicinity of ciliated epithelial cells and mucus cells all of which contribute to mucociliary interaction. Cholinergic, adrenergic, and peptidergic neurotransmitters are released at these sites and receptors exist for those neurotransmitters or their analogues on mucociliary target cells.

Baseline ciliary, but not secretory, function appears to be under cholinergic control, and atropine is capable of decreasing mucociliary transport rates. Autonomic nerve stimulation can increase the volume of airway secretions and the rate of mucociliary transport, with cholinergic, adrenergic, and peptidergic neurotransmitters all playing a role.

Exogenous cholinergic, alpha-adrenergic, beta-adrenergic, and peptidergic agonists enhance mucus and water secretions, with variable effects on their rheologic properties. Cholinergic and beta-adrenergic agonists have also been shown to increase ciliary activity and mucociliary clearance.

In peripheral airways, secretory functions seem to be regulated by autonomic agonists, but no information exists on ciliary or liquid transport functions in those airways.

These observations only pertain to the normal airway. In airway disease, the role of the autonomic nervous system in controlling baseline mucociliary function and in participating in the response to stimuli may markedly differ from that in normal airways. This may have major therapeutic implications, in terms of the beneficial and adverse effects of autonomic agents and their antagonists.

Discussion

Bousquet. Why does atropine have such a potent inhibitory effect on mucociliary clearance when ipratropium bromide does not?

Wanner. In vitro ipratropium bromide and atropine have been shown to be equipotent in blocking acetylcholine-induced smooth muscle contraction but ipratropium does not depress ciliary activity, whereas atropine does. Differences in absorption from mucosal surfaces or preferential binding to subtypes of muscarinic receptors are possible explanations.

Burnstock. Acetylcholine may be derived from cells other than nerves, since choline acetyltransferase immunofluorescence has been shown recently within vascular endothelial cells (Parnavelas et al., *Nature* **316**:724-725), and could perhaps also arise from airway epithelial cells.

Vanhoutte. What subtype of beta-adrenoceptor is involved in mucociliary clearance?

Wanner. Beta-2 agonists appear to be as potent as isoproterenol in increasing ciliary beat frequency and mucociliary clearance, suggesting that an important component is mediated by beta-2 receptors.

Burnstock. ATP stimulates cilia in other systems via a P2-purinoceptor. Has this been examined in airways?

Wanner. It is possible that ATP represents the energy sources for ciliary beating rather than binding to a specific receptor. The effect of ATP as an agonist on mucociliary clearance has not been studied.

References

Al-Bazzaz, F. J., and Cheng, E. (1979). Effect of catecholamines on ion transport in dog tracheal epithelium. *J. Appl. Physiol.* **47**:397-403.

Al-Bazzaz, F. J., Kelsey, J. G., and Kaage, W. D. (1985). Substance P stimulation of chloride secretion by canine tracheal mucosa. *Am. Rev. Respir. Dis.* **131**: 86-89.

Asmundsson, T., and Kilburn, K. H. (1973). Mechanisms of respiratory tract clearance. In *Sputum.* Edited by M. J. Dulfano. Springfield, IL, Chas. C Thomas, p. 107.

Baker, A. P., Chakrin, L. W., and Wardell, J. R. Jr. (1975). Chronic cholinergic stimulation of canine respiratory tissue: its effect on the activities of glycosyltransferases and release of macromolecules. *Am. Rev. Respir. Dis.* **111**:423-431.

Baker, A. P., Hillegass, L. M., Holden, D. A., and Smith, W. J. (1977). Effect of kallidin, substance P, and other basic polypeptides on the production of respiratory macromolecules. *Am. Rev. Respir. Dis.* **115**:811-817.

Barclay, A. E., and Franklin, K. J. (1937). The rate of excretion of India ink injected into the lungs. *J. Physiol.* **90**:482.

Barnes, P. J. (1984). The third nervous system in the lung: physiology and clinical perspectives. *Thorax* **39**:561-567.

Barton, A. D., and Lourenco, R. V. (1973). Bronchial secretions and mucociliary clearance. *Arch. Intern. Med.* **131**:140-144.

Basbaum, C. (1984). Innervation of the airway mucosa and submucosa. *Semin. Resp. Med.* **5**(4):308-313.

Basbaum, C. B., Ueki, I., Brezina, L., and Nadel, J. A. (1981). Tracheal submucosal gland serous cells stimulated *in ivtro* with adrenergic and cholinergic agonists. *Cell Tissue Res.* **220**:481-498.

Blair, A. M. J. N., and Woods, A. (1969). The effects of isoprenaline, atropine and disodium cromoglycate on ciliary motility and mucous flow measured *in vivo* in cats. *Br. J. Pharmacol.* **35**:379.

Borson, D. B., Charlin, M., Gold, B. D., and Nadel, J. A. (1982). Nonadrenergic noncholinergic nerves mediate secretion of macromolecules by tracheal glands of ferrets. *Fed. Proc.* **42**:1715.

Boucher, R. C., and Gatzy, J. T. (1982). Regional effects of autonomic agents on ion transport across excised canine airways. *J. Appl. Physiol.* **52**:893-901.

Breeze, R., and Wheeldon, E. B. (1977). The cells of the pulmonary airways. *Am. Rev. Respir. Dis.* **116**:705-777.

Brody, J. S., Waldhausen, J. A., and Kuhl, D. E. (1971). Mucociliary clearance in denervated bronchi. *Clin. Res.* **29**:507.

Bulbring, E., Burn, J. H., and Shelley, J. J. (1953). Acetylcholine and ciliary movement in the gill plates of *Mytilus edulis*. *Proc. R. Soc. Lond. (Biol.)* **141**:445-466.

Camner, P., Strandberg, K., and Philipson, K. (1974). Increased mucociliary transport by cholinergic stimulation. *Arch. Environ. Health* **29**:220.

Camner, P., Strandberg, K., and Philipson, K. (1976). Increased mucociliary transport by adrenergic stimulation. *Arch. Environ. Health* **31**:79-82.

Chakrin, L. W., Baker, A. P., Christian, P., and Wardell, J. R. Jr. (1973). Effect of cholinergic stimulation on the release of macromolecules by canine trachea *in vitro*. *Am. Rev. Respir. Dis.* **108**:69-76.

Chopra, S. K. (1978). Effect of atropine on mucociliary transport velocity in anesthetized dogs. *Am. Rev. Respir. Dis.* **118**:367-371.

Coles, S. J., Said, S. I., and Reid, L. M. (1981). Inhibition by vasoactive intestinal peptide of glycoconjugate and lysozyme secretion by human airways *in vitro*. *Am. Rev. Respir. Dis.* **124**:531-536.

Coles, S. J., Neill, K. H., and Reid, L. M. (1984). Potent stimulation of glycoprotein secretion in canine trachea by substance P. *J. Appl. Physiol.* **57**: 1323-1327.

Corssen, G., and Allen, C. R. (1959). Acetylcholine: its significance in controlling ciliary activity of human respiratory epithelium *in vitro*. *J. Appl. Physiol.* **14**:901-904.

Davis, B., Marin, M. G., Yee, J. W., and Nadel, J. A. (1979a). Effect of terbutaline on movement of Cl^-; and Na^+ across the trachea of the dog *in vitro*. *Am. Rev. Respir. Dis.* **120**:547-552.

Davis, B., Phipps, R. J., and Nadel, J. A. (1979b). A new method for studying tracheal secretion *in vitro*: effect of adrenergic agonists in cats. *Chest* **75**:224-225.

Dey, R. D., Shanon, W. A. Jr., and Said, S. I. (1981). Localization of VIP-immunoreactive nerves in airways and pulmonary vessels of dogs, cats, and human subjects. *Cell Tissue Res.* **220**:231-238.

Dische, Z., Kahn, N., Rothschild, C., Danilchenko, A., Licking, J., and Wang, S. C. (1970). Glycoproteins of submaxillary saliva of the cat: differences in composition produced by sympathetic and parasympathetic nerve stimulation. *J. Neurochem.* **17**:649-658.

Foster, W. M., Bergofsky, E. H., Bohning, D. E., Lippmann, M., and Albert, R. E. (1976). Effect of adrenergic agents and their mode of action on mucociliary clearance in man. *J. Appl. Physiol.* **41**:146-152.

Francis, R. A., Thomson, M. L., Pavia, D., and Douglas, R. B. (1977). Ipratropium bromide: mucociliary clearance rate and airway resistance in normal subjects. *Br. J. Dis. Chest* **71**:173-178.

Gallagher, J. T., Kent, P. W., Passatore, M., Phipps, R. J., and Richardson, P. S. (1975). The composition of tracheal mucus and the nervous control of its secretion in the cat. *Proc. R. Soc. Lond. B.* **192**:49-76.

Gatto, L. A. (1981). pH of mucus in rat trachea. *J. Appl. Physiol.* **50**:1226.

Giordano, A., Holsclaw, D., and Litt, M. (1978). Effects of various drugs on canine tracheal mucociliary transport. *Ann. Otol.* **87**:484-490.

Gosselin, R. E. (1966). Physiologic regulators of ciliary motion. *Am. Rev. Respir. Dis.* **93**:41.

Gray, C. (1928). *Ciliary Movement.* London, University Press.

Hakanson, R., Sundler, F., Moghimzadeh, E., and Leander, S. (1983). *Eur. J. Respir. Dis.* **64** (Suppl. 131):115-140.

Hammer, K., and Giachetti, A. (1983). Muscarinic receptor subtypes M_1 and M_2: biochemical and functional characterization. *Life Sci.* **31**:2991-2998.

Hartmann, J. F., Hutchison, C. F., and Jewell, M. E. (1984). Pig bronchial mucous membrane: a model system for assessing respiratory mucus release *in vitro. Exp. Lung Res.* **6**:59-70.

Hilding, A. C. (1967). The role of the respiratory mucosa. *Minn. Med.* **50**:915.

Hulbert, W. C., Forster, B. B., Laird, W., et al. (1982). An improved method for fixation of the respiratory epithelial surface with the mucous and surfactant layers. *Lab. Invest.* **47**:354-363.

Hybbinette, J-C., and Mercke, U. (1982). Effects of the parasympathomimetic drug methacholine and its antagonist atropine on mucociliary activity. *Acta Orolaryngol.* **93**:465-473.

Iravani, J. (1969). Koordination der Flimmerbewegung in Bronchialepithel der Ratte. *Pfluegers Arch.* **305**:199.

Iravani, J. (1972). Wirkung einiger bronchodilatierender Substanzen auf die Flimmeraktivitat unter besonderer Berucksichtigung von Berotec. *Int. J. Clin. Pharmacol.* Suppl. **4**:20-24.

Irvani, J., and Van As, A. (1972). Mucus transport in the tracheobronchial tree of normal and bronchitic rats. *J. Pathol.* **106**:81-93.

Jones, R., and Reid, L. (1979). B-agonists and rat airway secretory cell hyperplasia. *Fed. Proc.* **38**(3):1155.

Kilburn, K. H. (1968a). Theory and models for cellular injury and clearance failure in the lung. *Yale J. Biol. Med.* **40**:339.

Kilburn, K. H. (1968b). A hypothesis for pulmonary clearance and its implications. *Am. Rev. Respir. Dis.* **98**:449.

Kilburn, K. H., and Salzano, J. V. (1966). Symposium on structure, function and measurement of respiratory cilia. *Am. Rev. Respir. Dis.* **93**:184.

King, M., and Angus, G. E. (1981). Effect of aerosolized bronchodilators on viscoelastic properties of canine tracheal mucus. *Chest* **80**:852-854.

King, M., and Viires, N. (1979). Effect of methacholine chloride on rheology and transport of canine tracheal mucus. *J. Appl. Physiol.* **47**:26-31.

King, M., Cohen, C., and Viires, N. (1979). Influence of vagal tone on rheology and transportability of canine tracheal mucus. *Am. Rev. Respir. Dis.* **120**: 1215-1219.

Kinosita, H., and Murakami, A. (1967). Control of ciliary motion. *Physiol. Rev.* **47**:53.

Konietzko, N., Muller, N., and Adam, W. E. (1974). Studies of mucociliary clearance following the use of atrovent by healthy individuals and patients with chronic bronchitis. *Wien. Med. Wochenschr.* **124** (Suppl. 21):15-19.

Konietzko, N., Klopfer, M., Adam, W. E., und Matthys, H. (1975). Die mukociliare Klarfunktion der Lunge unter B-adrenerger Stimulation. *Pneumologie* **152**:203-208.

Kordik, P., Bulbring, E., and Burn, J. H. (1952). Ciliary movement and acetylcholine. *Br. J. Pharmacol.* **7**:67-79.

Lafortuna, C. L., and Fazio, F. (1984). Acute effect of inhaled salbutamol on mucociliary clearance in health and chronic bronchitis. *Respiration* **45**: 111-123.

Lazarus, S. C., Basbaum, C. B., Barnes, P. J., and Gold, W. M. (1983). Mapping of vasoactive intestinal peptide (VIP) receptors using cyclic AMP (cAMP) immunocytochemistry. *Am. Rev. Respir. Dis.* **127**(4):274.

Leikauf, G. D., Ueki, I. F., and Nadel, J. A. (1984). Autonomic regulation of viscoelasticity of cat tracheal gland secretions. *J. Appl. Physiol.* **56**:425-430.

Limjuco, G. A., and Hartmann, J. F. (1985). *In vivo* stimulation of glycoprotein secretion from the tracheobronchial tree of the laboratory rat. *IRCS Med. Sci.* **13**:718-719.

Lindberg, S. (1985). The regulation of mucociliary activity by substance P released from airway afferents. University Hospital, Lund, Sweden, Dept. of Oto-Rhino-Laryngology.

Lommel, F. (1908). Zur Physiologie und Pathologie des Flimmerepithels der Atmungsorgane. *Dtsch. Arch. Klin. Med.* **94**:365.

Low, P-M. P., Luk, C. K., Dulfano, M. J., et al. (1984). Ciliary beat frequency of human respiratory tract by different sampling techniques. *Am. Rev. Respir. Dis.* **130**:497-498.

Lucas, A. M., and Douglas, L. C. (1934). Principles underlying ciliary activity in the respiratory tract. *Arch. Otolaryngol.* **20**:518-541.

Marin, M. G., Davis, B., and Nadel, J. A. (1976). Effect of acetylcholine on Cl^- and Na^+ fluxes across dog tracheal epithelium *in vitro*. *Am. J. Physiol.* **231**:1546-1549.

Massaro, G. D., Paris, M., and Thet, L. A. (1979). *In vivo* regulation of secretion of bronchiolar Clara cells in rats. *J. Clin. Invest.* **63**:167-172.

Massaro, G. D., Fischman, C. M., Chiang, M-J., Amado, C., and Massaro, D. (1981). Regulation of secretion in Clara cells: studies using the isolated perfused rat lung. *J. Clin. Invest.* **67**:345-351.

Maurer, D. R., Sielczak, M., Oliver, W. Jr., et al. (1982). Role of ciliary motility in acute allergic mucociliary dysfunction. *J. Appl. Physiol.* **52**:1018-1023.

McDonald, J. F., Leisure, C. E., and Lenneman, E. E. (1928). Newly discovered controls of ciliary activity. *Am. J. Physiol.* **85**:395.

Melville, G. N., Horstman, G., and Iravani, J. (1976). Adrenergic compounds and the respiratory tract. A physiological and electron microscopial study. *Respiration* **33**:261.

Nathanson, I., Widdicombe, J. H., and Barnes, P. J. (1983). Effect of vasoactive intestinal peptide on ion transport across dog tracheal epithelium. *J. Appl. Physiol.* **55**:1844-1848.

Newhouse, M., Sanchiz, J., and Bienenstock, J. (1976a). Lung defense mechanisms (first of two parts). *N. Engl. J. Med.* **295**:990-998.

Newhouse, M., Sanchiz, J., and Bienenstock, J. (1976b). Lung defense mechanisms (second of two parts). *N. Engl. J. Med.* **295**:1045-1052.

Nowell, J. A., and Tyler, W. S. (1971). Scanning electron microscopy of the surface morphology of mammalian lungs. *Am. Rev. Respir. Dis.* **103**:313-328.

Okeson, G. C., and Divertie, M. B. (1970). Cilia and bronchial clearance: The effects of pharmacologic agents and disease. *Mayo Clin. Proc.* **45**:361.

Pack, R. L., and Richardson, P. S. (1984). The aminergic innervation of the human bronchus: a light and electron microscopic study. *J. Anat.* **138**:493-502.

Peatfield, A. C., and Richardson, P. S. (1982). The control of mucin secretion into the lumen of the cat trachea by α- and β-adrenoreceptors, and their relative involvement during sympathetic nerve stimulation. *Eur. J. Pharmacol.* **81**:617-626.

Peatfield, A. C., and Richardson, P. S. (1983). Evidence for non-cholinergic, non-adrenergic nervous control of mucus secretion into the cat trachea. *J. Physiol.* **342**:335-345.

Peatfield, A. C., Barnes, P. J., Bratcher, C., Nadel, J. A., and Davis, B. (1983). Vasoactive intestinal peptide stimulates tracheal submucosal and secretion in ferret. *Am. Rev. Respir. Dis.* **128**:89-93.

Pernow, B. (1983). Substance P. *Pharmacol. Rev.* **35**:85-141.

Phipps, R. J. (1984). Production of airway secretions. *Semin. Respir. Med.* **5**(4):314-318.

Phipps, R. J., Williams, I. P., Richardson, P. S., Pell, J., Pack, R. J., and Wright, N. (1982). Sympathomimetic drugs stimulate the output of secretory glycoproteins from human bronchi *in vitro*. *Clin. Sci.* **63**:23-28.

Pohle, K. (1931). Zur Frague der nervoesen Regulation des Flimmerepithels bei Wirbeltieren. *Arch. Exp. Pathol. Pharmakol.* **159**:452.

Reasor, M. J., Cohen, D., Proctor, D. F., and Rubin, R. J. (1978). Tracheobronchial secretions collected from intact dogs. II. Effects of cholinomimetic stimulation. *J. Appl. Physiol.* **45**:190-194.

Reissig, M., Bang, B. G., and Bang, F. B. (1978). Ultrastructure of the mucociliary interface in the nasal mucosa of the chicken. *Am. Rev. Respir. Dis.* **117**:327-341.

Rivera, J. A. (1962). *Cilia, Ciliated Epithelium and Ciliary Activity.* Oxford, Pergamon Press.

Ross, S. M., and Corrsin, S. (1974). Results of an analytical model of mucociliary pumping. *J. Appl. Physiol.* **37**:333-340.

Roth, L. E., and Shingenaka, Y. (1964). The structure and formation of cilia and filaments in rumen protozoa. *J. Cell Biol.* **20**:249-270.

Ruffin, R. E., Wolff, R. K., Dolovich, M. B., Eng. P., Rossman, C. M., Fitzgerald, J. D., and Newhouse, M. T. (1978). Aerosol therapy with Sch 100: short-term mucociliary clearance in normal and bronchitic subjects and toxicology in normal subjects. *Chest* **73**:501-506.

Saavedra, S., and Renaud, F. (1975). Studies on reactivated cilia. *Exp. Cell Res.* **90**:439-443.

Sackner, M. A., Epstein, S., and Wanner, A. (1976). Effect of beta-adrenergic agonists aerosolized by freon propellant on tracheal mucous velocity and cardiac output. *Chest* **69**:593-598.

Sackner, M. A., Chapman, G. A., and Dougherty, R. L. (1977). Effect of nebulized ipratropium bromide and atropine sulfate on tracheal mucous velocity and lung mechanics in anesthetized dogs. *Respiration* **34**:181-185.

Sackner, M. A., Yergin, B. M., Brito, M., and Januszkiewicz, A. (1979). Effect of adrenergic agonists on tracheal mucous velocity. *Bull. Europ. Physiopath. Respir.* **15**:505-511.

Sade, J., Eliezer, N., Silberberg, A., et al. (1970). The role of mucus in transport by cilia. *Am. Rev. Respir. Dis.* **102**:48-52.

Saketkhoo, K., Yergin, B. M., Januszkiewicz, A., Kovitz, K., and Sackner, M. A. (1978). The effect of nasal decongestants on nasal mucous velocity. *Am. Rev. Respir. Dis.* **118**:251-254.

Satir, P. (1974). The present status of the sliding microtube model of ciliary motion. In *Cilia and Flagella.* Edited by M. A. Sleigh. Oxford, Pergamon Press, p. 131.

Serafini, S. M., Wanner, A., and Michaelson, E. D. (1976). Mucociliary transport in central and intermediate size airways: effect of aminophylline. *Bull. Europ. Physiopath. Respir.* **12**:415.

Sleigh, M. A. (1962). *The Biology of Cilia and Flagella.* Oxford, Pergamon Press.

Stewart, W. C. (1948). Weight-carrying capacity and excitability of excised ciliated epithelium. *Am. J. Physiol.* **152**:1-5.

Sturgess, J., and Reid, L. (1972). An organ culture study of the effect of drugs on the secretory activity of the human bronchial submucosal gland. *Clin. Sci.* **43**:533-543.

Sturgess, J., and Reid, L. (1973). The effect of isoprenaline and pilocarpine on (a) bronchial mucus-secreting tissue and (b) pancreas, salivary glands, heart, thymus, liver, and spleen. *Br. J. Exp. Pathol.* **54**:388-403.

Uddman, R., and Sundler, F. (1979). Vasoactive intestinal peptide nerves in human upper respiratory tract. *Otorhinolaryngology* **41**:221-226.

Usuki, I. (1959). Effect of adenosine triphosphate on the ciliary activity and its histochemical demonstration in the oyster gill. *Sci. Rep. Res. Inst. Tohoku Univ.* (*Biol.*) **25**:65.

Van As, A. (1974). The role of selective B_2-adrenoceptor stimulants in the control of ciliary activity. *Respiration* **31**:146-151.

Van As, A. (1977). Pulmonary airway clearance mechanisms: a reappraisal. *Am. Rev. Respir. Dis.* **115**:721-726.

Verdugo, P., Johnson, N. T., and Tam, P. Y. (1980). B-adrenergic stimulation in respiratory ciliary activity. *J. Appl. Physiol.* **48**:868-871.

Wanner, A. (1977). Clinical aspects of mucociliary transport. *Am. Rev. Respir. Dis.* **116**:73-125.

Wanner, A., Zarzeki, S., Hirsch, J., and Epstein, S. (1975). Tracheal mucous transport in experimental canine asthma. *J. Appl. Physiol.* **39**:950-957.

Wilson, R., Pitt, T., Roberts, D., et al. (1985). A cilioinhibitory factor produced by *Pseudomonas aeruginosa. Am. Rev. Respir. Dis.* **131**(4):A226.

Winet, H., Yates, G. T., Wu, T. Y., et al. (1984). On the mechanics of mucociliary flows. III. Flow-velocity profiles in frog palate mucus. *J. Appl. Physiol.* **56**:785-794.

Yager, J. A., Ellman, H., and Dulfano, M. J. (1980). Human ciliary beat frequency at three levels of the tracheobronchial tree. *Am. Rev. Respir. Dis.* **121**:661-665.

Yanaura, S., Imamura, N., and Misawa, M. (1981). Effects of B-adrenoceptor stimulants on the canine tracheal ciliated cells. *Jpn. J. Pharmacol.* **31**: 951-956.

22

Respiratory Mucus

MICHAEL A. KALINER

National Institute for Allergic and Infectious Diseases
National Institutes of Health
Bethesda, Maryland

D. BENJAMIN BORSON and JAY A. NADEL

University of California
San Francisco, California

JAMES H. SHELHAMER

National Institutes of Health
Bethesda, Maryland

CARL A. PATOW

Uniformed Services University of the Health Sciences
Bethesda, Maryland

ZVI MAROM

Mt. Sinai Medical Center
New York, New York

Mucous membranes are so named because of their capacity to secrete mucus, the normal functions of which are noted in Table 1. In this discussion, we will focus on what is known about human respiratory tract mucus: its sources, biochemistry, recognized secretagogues.

The normal volume of tracheobronchial secretions is estimated to range from 10 to 100 ml/day. Alveolar type II cells, Clara cells, goblet cells, plasma cells, mucous and serous glandular cells, and probably other cell types, such as duct cells from submucous glands, produce components of this heterogeneous secretion. Microscopic examination shows that tracheobronchial secretions segregate into a sol phase, which is adjacent to the luminal surface of the epithelial lining cells, and a more superficial gel phase. This fluid blanket coats the airways from the alveoli to the trachea and is 2-5 μm thick.

The submucosal glands can be found throughout the respiratory tract, from the nose to airways containing cartilage (bronchi and trachea), whereas goblet cells exist throughout the respiratory tree to the level of the alveolar ducts, at which site Clara cells are found. The Clara cell has discrete granules that are electron dense and contain both protein and carbohydrate, and are secreted in response to secretory stimuli (Massaro et al., 1982).

Table 1 Functions of Respiratory Mucus

Functions
Protective functions
Lubrication
Humidification
Waterproofing
Insulation
Providing appropriate environment for ciliary action
Barrier functions
Selective macromolecular sieve
Entrapping of microorganisms
Extracellular surface for immunoglobulin action
Extracellular surface for enzyme actions
Neutralizing toxic gases
Transport function
Covering sheet for disposal of trapped materials (along with cilia)

(Reproduced with permission from Kaliner et al., 1984.)

Submucous glandular cells outnumber goblet cells by 40:1 in the normal bronchi and trachea. Submucosal glands are compound tubuloacinar glands consisting of a tubular duct from which multiple side tubes originate and terminate in acinar structures. The orifice of the duct is lined by epithelial cells that are ciliated, pseudostratified, and columnar; the collecting tube is lined by columnar epithelial cells; and the acinar structure is composed of discrete areas of mucous and serous cells. The columnar epithelial cells of the duct may contribute to the regulation of the water and electrolyte concentration of the secretions. Because both the staining characteristics and the histologic appearance of these cells are distinct from each other, it is very likely that the secretory products are also distinct. Monoclonal antibodies directed at mucous glycoproteins recognize mucous or serous gland cells or goblet cells selectively in several animal models (Basbaum et al., 1984), confirming the presence of antigenic differences in the secretory products of these cells. Goblet cells are the major nonciliated cell type found in the respiratory mucosa and are recognized by their goblet shape and the presence of multiple cytoplasmic vesicles that contain mucus. Specific biochemical characteristics of goblet cell secretions have not yet been described.

I. Biochemistry of Human Respiratory Mucous Glycoproteins

Tracheobronchial secretions line the luminal respiratory epithelium and are transported from the distal airways to the larynx by synchronized ciliary beating. The cilia beat in the aqueous layer of fluid, on top of which is a more gelatinous layer. By its very design, the system operates to clear trapped or discarded materials continuously from the airways and to maintain sterile conditions. It is not difficult to understand that this system might be overwhelmed by excessive secretion of respiratory mucus, an increase in transudated proteins or cells present in these secretions, an increase in the volume of secreted fluid, or by the presence of another fibrillar system added to the secretions, such as occurs when the DNA from dead neutrophils mixes with mucus in purulent secretions.

The composition of tracheobronchial secretions has been studied in laryngectomized patients and is about 95% water, 1% protein, 0.9% carbohydrate, and 0.8% lipid (Havez and Roussel, 1976). In the presence of inflammation or infection, these values may change with the finding that more protein, glycoprotein, or DNA is present in the secretions. Proteins found in tracheobronchial secretions may be present as a result of local production or reflect transudation of plasma proteins as a result of inflammation. Locally produced proteins include lysozyme and lactoferrin as well as immunoglobulins A and E. Transudated proteins identified in respiratory secretions include albumin, alpha-1 antitrypsin, alpha-2 macroglobulin, haptoglobin, and transferrin, as well as immunoglobulins M, G, and A.

The viscosity and elasticity characteristic of tracheobronchial secretions are due primarily to the presence of mucous glycoproteins (MGP). The rheologic characteristics of mucus are influenced by increases in DNA and other proteins in these secretions. Serum proteins such as albumin or lysozyme bind to MGP and also affect the physical characteristics of tracheobronchial secretions. This binding probably occurs via electrostatic bonding, although disulfide bonding may also occur.

Much of the information available about the biochemical characteristics of respiratory MGP is derived from analysis of expectorated sputum. These secretions are by definition a reflection of excessive mucus production as a result of inflammatory states (chronic bronchitis, asthma, and cystic fibrosis), and it is likely that these secretions are altered by the underlying disease process, by products released by inflammatory cells, or by substances in the saliva that always contaminate expectorated tracheobronchial secretions. In an attempt to obviate these problems, some recent studies have assessed the biochemical characteristics of MGP secreted in vitro from human airway organ cultures (Shelhamer et al., 1980). Secretory cells in human airways in organ culture will incorporate radiolabeled sugars, amino sugars, threonine, or sulfate into the secreted MGP, providing an intrinsically radiolabeled molecule for the study of MGP chemistry or physiology.

MGP is a macromolecule consisting of a protein core rich in serine, threonine, and proline (Fig. 1). Attached to the protein core are oligosaccharide side chains linked via an O-glycosidic bond between serine or threonine on the protein core and *n*-acetylgalactosamine on the oligosaccharide side chain. The length of the individual oligosaccharide chains varies and probably ranges from 1 to 20 monosaccharides. The monosaccharides that make up the carbohydrate portion of the molecule are typically composed of fucose, galactose, *n*-acetylneuraminic acid, *n*-acetylglucosamine, and *n*-acetylgalactosamine. Overall, the MGP molecule is 70 to 80% carbohydrate, about 20% protein, and 1 to 2% sulfate (Shelhamer et al., 1984). The sulfate is probably bound to the oligosaccharide side chains. The size of the MGP molecule, estimated by density gradient gradient techniques, ranges from 1.8 to 7 $\times$ 10^6 daltons. Column chromatography using Sephacryl S-1000 (Fig. 2) allows one to conclude that these molecules are not only very large but that a significant size heterogeneity exists as well; MGP filters with molecular sizes ranging from 0.2 to 20 $\times$ 10^6 daltons. While reduction and alkylation procedures, which break intermolecular and intramolecular disulfide bonds, have been effective in solubilizing gelatinous MGP, the effect of reduction and alkylation on solubilized fractions of MGP is variable. Treatment of MGP with the detergent sodium dodecylsulfate reduces the apparent size of MGP, but gel filtration still reveals a broad spread of molecular sizes. It has been suggested that the reduction and alkylation procedures break disulfide bonds primarily between MGP and other proteins while the effect of a detergent such as sodium dodecylsulfate may be to inhibit nonthiol interactions between MGP molecules. Despite the huge range in size of MGP, these molecules all express a similar acidic charge as manifested by adherence to diethylaminoethyl cellulose and elution by a linear salt gradient. Similarly, the acidic nature of these molecules is documented by isoelectric focusing procedures; MGP focuses on a single, sharp peak at pH 2.7 to 2.8.

II. Control of Airway Secretions in Experimental Animals

Many studies indicate that cholinergic nerves innervate and affect secretion from the airways (Fig. 3). Using a micropipette method for collecting secretions from individual glands, Ueki et al. found that stimulating the vagus nerves of cats caused the secretion of fluid, an effect mimicked by muscarinic agonists and

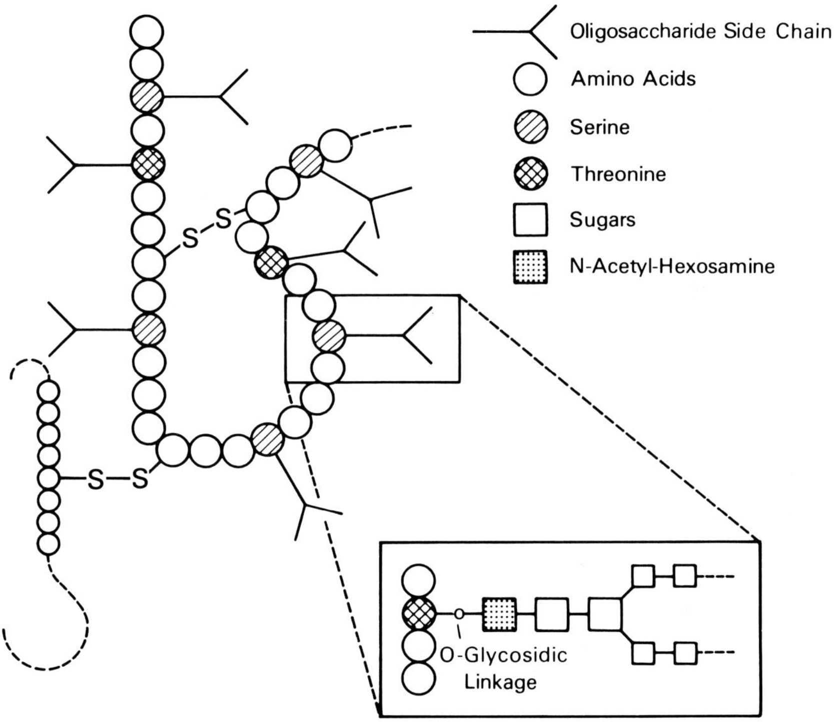

Figure 1 Schematic structure of human airway mucous glycoprotein. Circles indicate amino acids that are the protein core of the molecule. Threonine and serine are linkage points for O-glycosidic side chains, represented as branching lines. There may be intrachain and interchain disulfide linkages (–S–S) as well. (Reproduced with permission from Kaliner et al., 1984.)

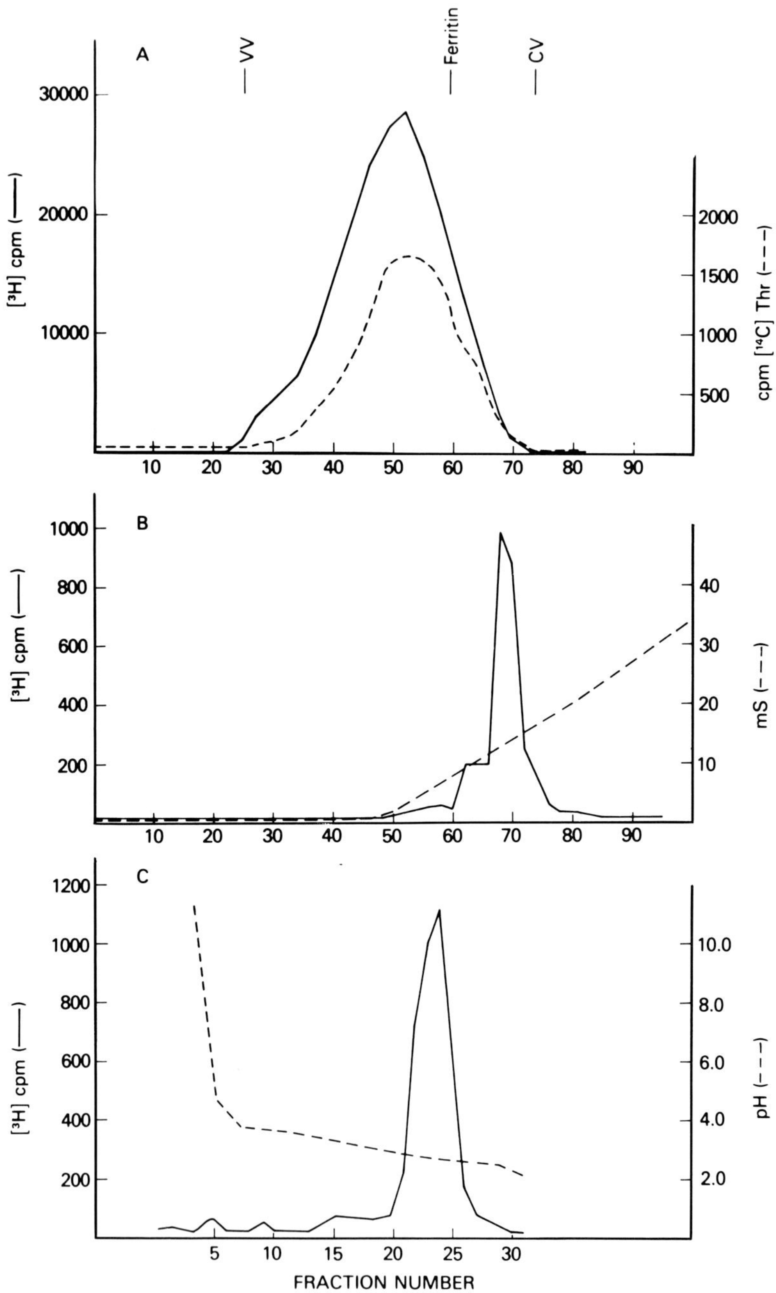
A
VV
Ferritin
CV
30000
20000
10000
[³H] cpm (——)
2000
1500
1000
500
cpm [¹⁴C] Thr (- - -)
10 20 30 40 50 60 70 80 90
B
1000
800
600
400
200
[³H] cpm (——)
40
30
20
10
mS (- - -)
10 20 30 40 50 60 70 80 90
C
1200
1000
800
600
400
200
[³H] cpm (——)
10.0
8.0
6.0
4.0
2.0
pH (- - -)
5 10 15 20 25 30
FRACTION NUMBER

prevented by the muscarinic antagonist atropine (Ueki et al., 1980). Stimulating the efferent cholinergic nerves also increased the secretion of $^{35}SO_4$-labeled macromolecules into the tracheas of cats and ferrets. Indicating that the secreted fluid contained mucins or proteoglycans. Various reflexes are mediated via vagal nervous pathways. Thus, laryngeal irritation, inhalation of SO_2, gastric distention, hypoxemia, and stimulation of bronchial c-fibers with capsaicin or bradykinin, reflexly stimulated secretion of fluid from glands via vagal pathways. Because secretion of both fluids and macromolecules was prevented by either injection of atropine or cutting the vagi, the effects observed were mediated by muscarinic-cholinergic nerves. However, baseline secretion is not completely under cholinergic control because atropine can reduce but not abolish resting secretion from submucosal glands.

Unlike cholinergic nerves, adrenergic nerves and their relationship with mucus-secreting glands have not been well studied. One study failed to show effects of adrenergic agonists on secretion of fluid from airways of rabbits, and this is probably due to the fact that this species does not have submucosal glands. However, close arterial injection in vivo of the alpha-adrenergic agonist phenylephrine stimulated fluid secretion from both cats (Ueki et al., 1980) and dogs, species that do have submucosal glands. Macromolecular secretion is also under adrenergic control. Stimulating the stellate ganglia of cats in vivo caused secretion of $^{35}SO_4$-labeled macromolecules (Gallagher et al., 1975). However, because it is difficult to stimulate sympathetic nerves without stimulating systemic reflexes and the release of circulating mediators, there are few studies of efferent adrenergic nerves. To overcome the problem of reflexes and the circulation, Borson et al. developed a method for stimulating nerves in vitro, and demonstrated that alpha-adrenergic neural mechanisms regulate fluid secretion (Borson et al., 1980), and that both alpha- and beta-adrenergic mechanisms regulate the secretion of $^{35}SO_4$-labeled

---

Figure 2 (A) Elution of radiolabeled MGP from 1 X 60 cm Sephacryl S-1000 column. The sample was obtained from human airways cultured in the presence of [^{3}H]glucosamine and [^{14}C]threonine. The culture medium was harvested, dialyzed against 6 M urea, and concentrated under pressure prior to chromatography. VV, void volume; CV, column volume. (B) Ion exchange chromatography on diethylaminoethyl cellulose of radiolabeled human MGP produced in vitro. The sample was applied to the diethylaminoethyl column in 6 M urea, 0.005 M phosphate buffer. The column was eluted with a linear salt gradient of 0–1.0 M sodium chloride. (C) Horizontal isoelectric focusing in Pevikon. Radiolabeled human MGP was purified over Sephacryl S-1000 and diethylaminoethyl cellulose before isoelectric focusing. (Reproduced with permission from Shelhamer et al., 1984.)

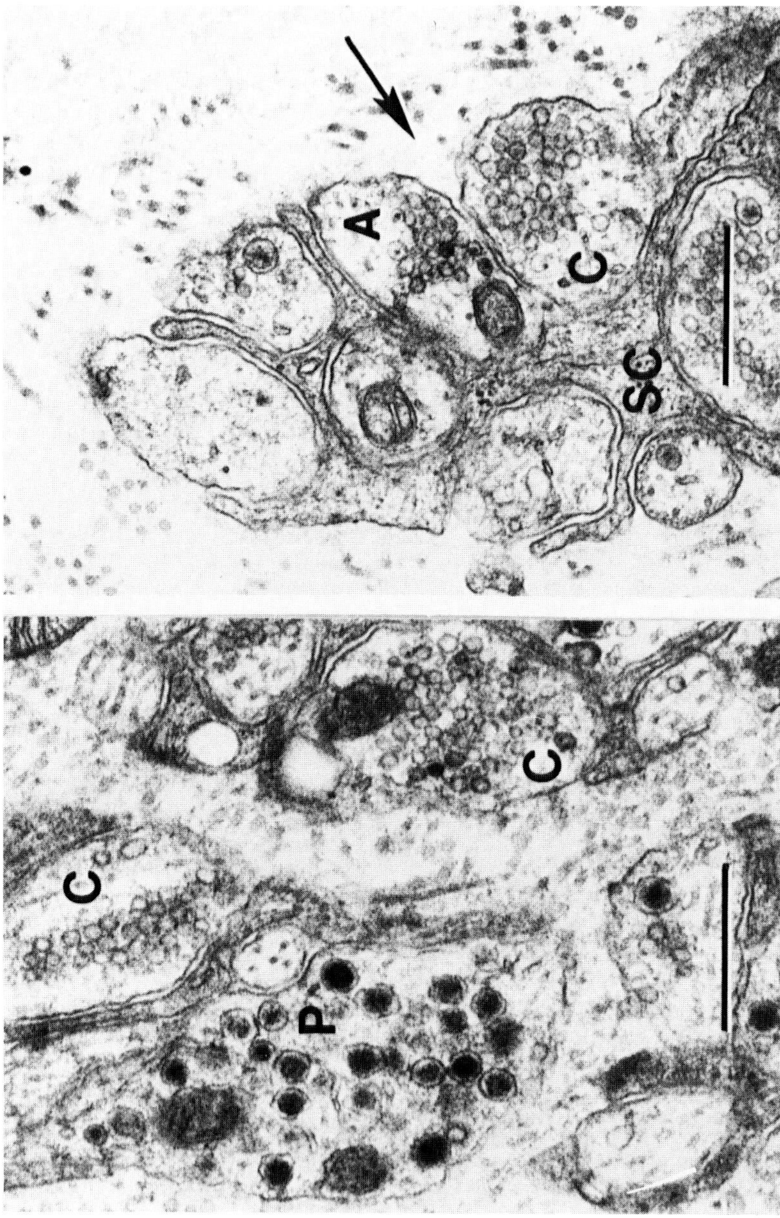
A
C
SC
C
C
P

Figure 3 Innervation of airway submucosal glands. Left. Electron micrograph of a nerve bundle near a submucosal gland of a ferret. Cholinergic nerve varicosities (C) contain small unfilled vesicles. Some nerves contain large, dense-cored vesibles characteristic of peptidergic nerves (P). (Photograph courtesy of C. Basbaum.) Right. Electron micrograph of another nerve bundle containing cholinergic nerves (C) and adrenergic nerves (A) with their characteristic small, dense-cored vesicles. At certain sites (arrow), cholinergic and adrenergic nerve terminals are found close together without process of a supporting cell (SC) between them. Neurotransmitters released by one nerve type (e.g., acetylcholine released from cholinergic nerves) may affect other nerve types (e.g., inhibit adrenergic neurotransmission). Bars, 0.5 μm. (Photograph from Basbaum et al., 1981, is reproduced with permission of the author and publisher.)

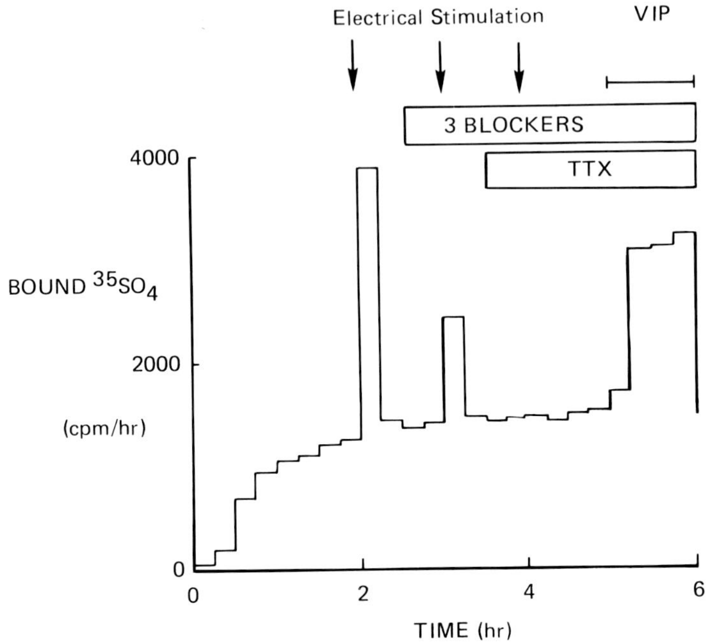

Figure 4 Effects of autonomic antagonists and nerve conduction blocker on secretion of $^{35}SO_4$-labeled macromolecules from tracheal blands of a ferret. Tissue was mounted in a chamber containing $^{35}SO_4$ for the duration of the experiment. Samples were collected from the luminal side. Tissue was stimulated electrically (↓) (intensity, 10 V; pulse duration, 0.5 ms; frequency, 5 cps for 5 min), first in the absence of drugs, again after inhibiting cholinergic and adrenergic neural effects with atropine, phentolamine, and propranolol together (3 BLOCKERS) each drug, 10^{-5} M). The neurally evoked secretion remaining, due to nonadrenergic noncholinergic nerves, was inhibited only after adding the nerve conduction blocker, tetrodotoxin (TTX) (10^{-7} M). To demonstrate that the glands were not inhibited, secretion was then stimulated by adding VIP (10^{-7} M).

macromolecules (Borson et al., 1984). Additionally, adrenergic drugs also cause the secretion of lysozyme from serous cells of submucosal glands, mostly via alpha-adrenergic mechanisms. Recent results obtained from cultured bovine serous gland cells indicate that beta-adrenergic agonists stimulate the release of chondroitin-sulfate proteoglycans (Basbaum et al., 1985), whose roles are unknown but may contribute to the viscoelastic properties of the secreted materials or provide a matrix within the secretory granules to bind cationic proteins such as lysozyme.

Nonadrenergic noncholinergic nerves can inhibit contraction of airway smooth muscle (Richardson and Beland, 1976), but the roles of these nerves in regulating secretion is poorly understood. The only study of nonadrenergic noncholinergic nerves on airway secretion in vitro relied on electrical field stimulation and $^{35}SO_4$ labeling of macromolecules. Using these methods, Borson et al. demonstrated the presence of nerve-mediated secretion that was not prevented by the combination of cholinergic and alpha- and beta-adrenergic antagonists (Fig. 4) (Borson et al., 1984). Although the transmitter that mediates this effect is not known, it is possible that neuropeptides are involved. Substance P (SP) is a possible candidate because it is present in nerves in the airways and caused secretion of macromolecules from dogs (Baker et al., 1977), ferrets, and humans. Vasoactive intestinal peptide (VIP) is another possible candidate because it is present in airways near glands, and exogenous VIP caused mucus secretion in certain species. For both SP and VIP, the peptide-induced secretion was associated with histologic evidence of degranulation of the serous cells in the glands (Gashi et al., 1986).

In addition to SP, the other tachykinins, neurokinins A and B, physalaemin, eledoisin, and kassinin, each stimulated secretion of radiolabeled macromolecules from the tracheas of ferrets (Borson et al., 1986). The response to tachykinins was markedly potentiated by thiorphan and phosphoramidon, inhibitors of enkephalinase (neutral endopeptidase; EC 3.4.24.11) (Borson et al., in press), but not inhibited by other peptidase or proteinase inhibitors. These results suggest that a major action of enkephalinase in the airway is to degrade SP and related peptides, and thus to play an important role in regulating peptide-induced reactions including modulation of mucus secretion.

Airway submucosal glands contain both serous and mucous cells. Muscarinic agonists stimulate the release of secretions from both cell types and thus show no cell selectivity (Basbaum et al., 1981). On the other hand, alpha- and beta-adrenergic agonists have more selective effects. A summary of their effects is shown in Table 2. Both agonists stimulated the release of radiolabeled macromolecules (Phipps et al., 1980). However, alpha-adrenergic agonists stimulated the production of fluid from glands, whereas beta-adrenergic agonists did not. Sampling from micropipettes also showed selectivity; alpha-adrenergic stimulation produced secretions with low protein and sulfur concentrations, whereas beta-adrenergic stimulation produced scanty fluid with higher concentrations of protein and sulfur. Lysozyme, a substance localized with serous but not mucous cells was released selectively by alpha adrenergic but not beta-adrenergic, stimulation, indicating that alpha-adrenergic agonists selectively caused secretion by stimulating serous cells. This was confirmed by Basbaum et al., who showed that alpha-adrenergic agonists preferentially depleted serous cells, leaving the mucous cells spared (Basbaum et al., 1981). With these differences, it is not surprising that the mucus produced varied in viscoelastic properties. Thus Leikauf et al. (1984) found that alpha-adrenergic agonists produced

Table 2 Effects of Adrenergic and Cholinergic Agonists on Properties of Tracheal Secretions in Animal Models

Effect	Alpha-adrenergic agonist	Beta-adrenergic agonist	Muscarinic agonist
Fluid secretion from glands	↑↑↑	↑	↑↑↑
Macromolecular secretion	↑↑↑	↑↑	↑↑↑
Protein concentration	↓	↑	→
Mucus viscosity	↓	↑	→
Mucus elasticity	→	↓	→

↑: increase; ↓: decrease; →: no change.

secretions of lower viscosity and elasticity than control. The evidence of selective adrenergic regulation of submucosal gland cells derives from studies employing several different species. However, because variations among species exist, extrapolation of these findings to human physiology needs to be done with caution.

The adrenergic responses can be elicited by release of adrenergic neurotransmitters locally or by the release of circulating catecholamines from chromaffin cells. Neural release of norepinephrine, a mediator with primarily alpha-adrenergic actions, would be expected to produce copious thin secretions. Such an action of sympathetic reflexes could assist in diluting inhaled irritating materials. On the other hand, circulating catecholamines include a higher concentration of epinephrine, which has more beta-adrenergic effects than norepinephrine, and presumably produces a more viscous gland secretion.

The close proximity of adrenergic and cholinergic varicosities without intervening supporting cells (Fig. 3) suggests that, in addition to secretory effects, the nerves might interact with each other. By measuring the release of $[^3H]$-norepinephrine in response to electrical field stimulation, Borson et al. found that physostigmine, a drug that potentiates the effects of stimulating cholinergic nerves by preventing the enzymatic degradation of acetylcholine, decreased the release of $[^3H]$norepinephrine evoked by electrical stimulation (Fig. 5) (Borson et al., 1981). Because this inhibition was reversed by the addition of atropine, the effect was mediated by muscarinic mechanisms. Conversely, there is evidence that adrenergic nerves can inhibit cholinergic neurotransmission to tracheal smooth muscle. Thus, autonomic nervous stimulation may affect glandular secretion directly or via effects on other nerves.

Until recently it has been difficult to study secretion from submucosal glands. By using cell-culture methods, Varsano and colleagues (1986) demonstrated that cultured airway epithelial cells take up and release $^{35}SO_4$-labeled macromolecules. The cells have a well formed glycocalyx, but contain no secre-

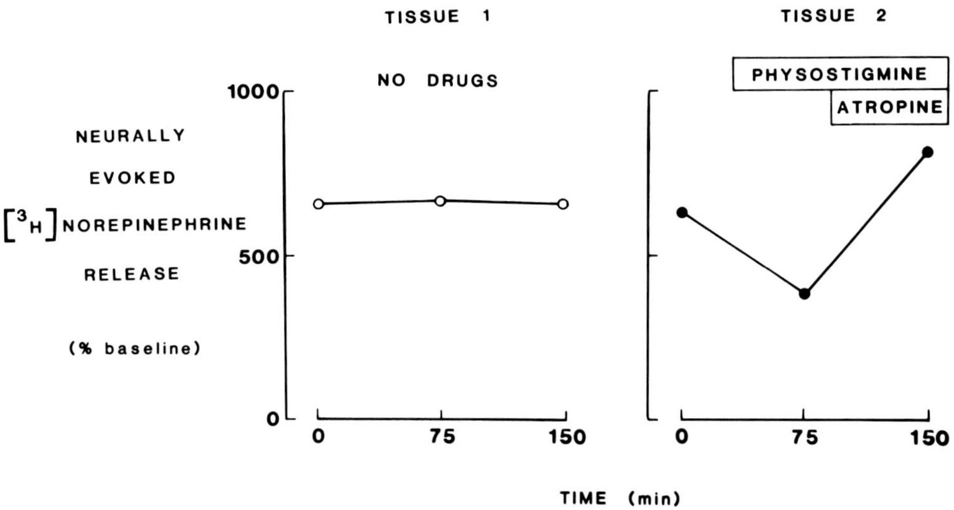

Figure 5 Effects of potentiating and inhibiting cholinergic nerves on electrically evoked release of [^{3}H]norepinephrine from adrenergic nerves to tracheal glands of a ferret. Two tissues were incubated with [^{3}H]norepinephrine for 90 min prior to washing out for 2 hr. Then each of the two tissues was stimulated electrically (intensity, 10 V; frequency, 10 Hz for 5 min) 3 times (at 75 min intervals). One tissue (left side) received no drugs; the other tissue (right side) was stimulated, first without drugs, then with physostigmine (10^{-6} M). Physostigmine decreased and atropine increased [^{3}H]norepinephrine release.

tory granules. A variety of endoproteinases can increase markedly the release of macromolecules. The materials released by proteinases were of high molecular weight ($> 10^6$ daltons), and were degraded by beta-galactosidase, keratanase, and beta-elimination, but were not degraded by chondroitinase ABC, heparinase, or heparan sulfate lyase. Furthermore, immunofluorescence studies using monoclonal antibodies directed to polylactosamine sequences demonstrated intense staining of the epithelial cell apical surface. These results suggest that most of the macromolecules released were proteoglycans whose glycosaminoglycan side chains contain polylactosamines characteristic of keratan sulfates. The precise roles of these proteoglycans in mucociliary clearance are not known, but they could possibly interact with each other or with mucins to contribute to the viscoelastic properties of the gel.

In asthma, the postmortem findings of mucous gland hypertrophy, increased numbers of goblet cells, and excessive airway secretions suggest that serious problems with mucociliary clearance exist in asthmatic subjects. In fact, delayed mucociliary clearance may be reported to occur in some people with asymptomatic asthma. Inhalation challenge with specific antigen decreased tracheal mucus velocity in sensitized dogs (Wanner et al., 1975) and in asthmatic subjects (Ahmed et al., 1981). The fact that the abnormal clearance was prevented by sodium cromolyn suggests that the release of mediators from mast cells is involved in the response, and the fact that the abnormal responses were also prevented by FPL-55712 suggests that lipoxygenase products of arachidonic acid were the active mediators.

There is a great deal of evidence that airway inflammation plays an important role in the increased bronchial responsiveness so characteristic of asthma (Nadel et al., 1984). Similarly, we suggest that inflammatory changes in asthma are responsible for many of the mucociliary changes in the disease (including status asthmaticus). Pathologic evidence indicates that inflammatory changes in asthma include the epithelium. Cough receptors are located superficially, just below the tight junctions of the epithelium. This probably explains why cough is often an early and persistent symptom of the disease. Because irritation of these receptors causes a reflex increase in submucosal gland secretions, perhaps chronic irritation in asthma is a cause of the abnormal mucociliary clearance and glandular hypertrophy that occur in this disease. Furthermore, if SP is present in afferent nerves in the airway, as it appears to be in the skin, stimulation of these nerves may result in the local release of SP or other neuropeptides that can cause mucus secretion and increases in vascular permeability. Inflammatory changes could also result in the production of bradykinin, which can stimulate mucus secretion directly, or indirectly by activating sensory bronchial c-fibers, thus producing reflex stimulation of submucosal gland secretion.

III. Studies on the Control of Mucus Secretion in Human Airways

Human airways may be cultured in the presence of radiolabeled sugars, amino acids, aminosugars, or sulfate, each of which is incorporated into newly synthesized and secreted MGP. Employing this technique for the measurement of the secretion of MGP from cultured human airways and nasal mucosa, we have studied the effects of various secretagogues (Table 3).

There is clear evidence of parasympathetic control of MGP secretion in animals and humans. The presence of parasympathetic nerve endings has been demonstrated around submucosal glands, and stimulation of the vagus nerve in experimental animals increases MGP secretion (Phipps, 1981). Inhalation of the cholinergic agonist acetylcholine in vivo induces sputum production (Lopez-Vidriero et al., 1977). Furthermore, the addition of the cholinergic agonist methacholine to human airways in organ culture results in increased MGP secretion (Shelhamer et

Table 3 Human Respiratory Mucus Secretory Responses

Agent	Airway mucus	Nasal turbinate mucus
Methacholine	↑	↑
Atropine	NE	NE
Methacholine + atropine	NE	NE
Alpha-adrenergic agonists	↑	↑
Beta-adrenergic agonists	NE	NE
Cyclic guanosine monophosphate	↑	NS
Cyclic adenosine monophosphate	NE	NS
Arachidonic acid	↑	NE
Prostaglandins E_1, $F_{2\alpha}$, D_2, I_2, A_2	↑	NE
Prostaglandin E_2	↓	NS
Aspirin	↑	NE
Indomethacin	↑	NE
Eicosatetraynoic acid	↓	NE
5-,8-,9-,11-, or 15-hydroxyeicosatetraenoic acid	↑	NE
5- and 9-hydroperoxyeicosatetraenoic acid	↑	NS
Leukotriene C_4 or D_4	↑	NE
Anaphylaxis	↑	↑
Histamine	↑	↑
Prostaglandin-generating factor	↑	NS
Macrophage or monocyte mucus secretagogue	↑	NS
C3a	↑	NS

NE = No net effect on mucus secretion.
NS = Not studied.

al., 1980; Patow et al., 1984). The cholinergic antagonist atropine blocks this secretory response. While atropine itself has no effect on MGP secretion in vitro, it has been reported to decrease sputum production in some patients with chronic sputum production (Lopez-Vidriero et al., 1975).

The role of adrenergic mediators in influencing MGP secretion is much less clear. In human tissue, alpha-adrenergic agonists appear to stimulate secretion. Beta-adrenergic stimulation has been variously reported to have no effect on human respiratory MGP secretion or to stimulate of MGP secretion. This variation may be due to differences in experimental design.

The airways are exposed to a variety of mediators released locally in immediate hypersensitivity or inflammatory reactions. Mast cell degranulation resulting from antigen interacting with cell-bound IgE results in the release of the mediators of anaphylaxis, including histamine, as well as the production and release of prostaglandins, leukotrienes, other lipoxygenase pathway products, and bradykinin.

Histamine given by inhaled aerosol induces sputum production in humans (Lopez-Vidriero et al., 1977). Histamine in micromolar concentrations stimulates MGP release from human airways or nasal mucosa in vitro (Shelhamer et al., 1980; Patow et al., 1984). However, other mediators may be as or even more important in the stimulation of MGP secretion. Among these are oxidative products derived from arachidonic acid and produced during immediate hypersensitivity reactions in lung tissue.

Arachidonic acid added to lung explants in vitro results in an increase in MGP secretion, an action presumably mediated by one of the metabolites of arachidonic acid (Marom et al., 1981). Products of the cyclooxygenase pathway of arachidonic acid metabolism include the prostaglandins, and prostaglandins A_2, D_2, E_1 and $F_{2\alpha}$, all stimulate MGP secretion in vitro when used in micromolar quantities. In addition, inhalation of prostaglandin $F_{2\alpha}$ has been shown to stimulate sputum production in humans. Inhibition of the production of cyclooxygenase pathway products in vitro by the addition of nonsteroidal anti-inflammatory agents, however, results in a substantial increase in MGP secretion, implying that lipoxygenase pathway products of arachidonic acid metabolism may be important in the regulation of MGP production. Lipoxygenase products include the monohydroxy- and the hydroperoxy-eicosatetraenoic acids as well as the leukotrienes. In fact, 5-, 8-, 11-, 12-, and 15-mono-hydroxyeicosatetraenoic acid all stimulate MGP secretion when present in nanomolar concentrations (Shelhamer et al., 1982; Marom et al., 1983). Two other lipoxygenase pathway products are even more potent. The slow-reacting substances of anaphylaxis, leukotriene C_4 and leukotriene D_4, when used in picomolar concentrations, are capable of stimulating MGP secretion from human airways in vitro (Marom et al., 1982). This effect is inhibited by the receptor antagonist of slow-reacting substances of anaphylaxis, FPL-55712. Arachidonic acid metabolite production may occur as a direct consequence of mast cell degranulation, or through the formation of a newly described mediator, prostaglandin-generating factor of anaphylaxis (Marom et al., 1984). It is certainly possible that other mediators produced in pulmonary hypersensitivity reactions may also be involved in MGP secretion.

References

Ahmed, T., Greenblatt, D. W., Birch, S., Marchette, B., and Wanner, A. (1981). Abnormal mucociliary transport in allergic patients with antigen-induced bronchospasm: role of slow reacting substance of anaphylaxis. *Am. Rev. Respir. Dis.* **124**:110-114.

Baker, A. P., Hillegass, L. M., Holden, D. A., and Smith, W. J. (1977). Effect of kallidin, substance P, and other basic polypeptides on the production of respiratory macromolecules. *Am. Rev. Respir. Dis.* **115**:811-817.

Basbaum, C. B., Mann, J., Chow, A., and Finkbeiner, W. E. (1984). Monoclonal antibodies as probes for unique antigens in secretory cells of mixed exocrine organs. *Proc. Natl. Acad. Sci. USA* **81**:4419-4423.

Basbaum, C. B., Paul, A., Finkbeiner, W. E., Mergey, M., Vessiere, D., and Picard, J. (1985). Biochemical characterization of glycoconjugates secreted by bovine tracheal gland cells in culture. *J. Cell Biol.* **101**:232a.

Basbaum, C. B., Ueki, I., Brezina, L., and Nadel, J. A. (1981). Tracheal submucosal gland serous cells stimulated in vitro with adrenergic and cholinergic agonists: a morphometric study. *Cell Tissue Res.* **220**:481-498.

Borson, D. B., Charlin, M., Gold, B. D., and Nadel, J. A. (1984). Neural regulation of $^{35}SO_4$-macromolecule secretion from tracheal glands of ferrets. *J. Appl. Physiol.* **57**:457-466.

Borson, D. B., Chinn, R. A., Davis, B., and Nadel, J. A. (1980). Adrenergic and cholinergic nerves mediate fluid secretion from tracheal glands of ferrets. *J. Appl. Physiol.* **49**:1027-1031.

Borson, D. B., Corrales, R., Varsano, S., Gold, M., Viro, N., Caughey, G., Ramachandran, J., and Nadel, J. A. (1987). Enkephalinase inhibitors potentiate substance P-induced secretion of $^{35}SO_4$-macromolecules from ferret trachea. *Exp. Lung Res.* (in press).

Borson, D. B., and Nadel, J. A. (1981). Cholinergic nerves inhibit adrenergic neurotransmission to tracheal submucosal glands of ferrets. *Fed. Proc.* **40**:254.

Gashi, A. A., Borson, D. B., Finkbeiner, W. E., Nadel, J. A., and Basbaum, C. B. (1986). Neuropeptides degranulate serous cells of ferret tracheal glands. *Am. J. Physiol.* **251** (*Cell Physiol.* **20**):C223-C229.

Havez, R., and Roussel, P. (1976). Bronchial mucus: physical and biochemical features. In *Bronchial Asthma: Mechanisms and Therapeutics.* Edited by Weiss, E. B., and Segal, M. S. Little, Brown and Company, Boston, pp. 409-422.

Kaliner, M., Marom, Z., Patow, C., and Shelhamer, J. (1984). Human respiratory mucus. *J. Allergy Clin. Immunol.* **73**:318-323.

Leikauf, G. D., Ueki, I. F., and Nadel, J. A. (1984). Autonomic regulation of viscoelasticity of cat tracheal gland secretions. *J. Appl. Physiol.* **56**:426-430.

Lopez-Vidriero, M. T., Costello, J., Clark, T. J., Das, I., Keal, E., and Reid, L. (1975). Effect of atropin on sputum production. *Thorax* **30**:543-547.

Lopez-Vidriero, M. T., Das, I., Smith, A. P., Picot, R., and Reid, L. (1977). Bronchial secretion from normal human airways after inhalation of prostaglandin F_{2alpha}, acetylcholine, histamine and citric acid. *Thorax* **32**:734-739.

Marom, Z., Shelhamer, J. H., and Kaliner, M. (1981). Effects of arachidonic acid, monohydroxyeicosatetraenoic acid and prostaglandins on the release of mucous glycoproteins from human airways *in vitro*. *J. Clin. Invest.* **67**:1695-1702.

Marom, Z., Shelhamer, J. H., Bach, M. K., Morton, D. R., and Kaliner, M. (1982). Slow-reacting substances, leukotrienes C_4 and D_4 increase the release of mucus from human airways *in vitro*. *Am. Rev. Respir. Dis.* **126**: 449-451.

Marom, Z., Sun, F., Shelhamer, J. F., and Kaliner, M. (1983). Human airway monohydroxyeicosatetraenoic acid generation and mucus release. *J. Clin. Invest.* **72**:122-127.

Marom, Z., Shelhamer, J. H., Steel, L., Goetzl, E. J., and Kaliner, M. (1984). Prostaglandin-generating factor of anaphylaxis increases mucous glycoprotein release and the formation of lipoxygenase products of arachidonate from human lung. *Prostaglandins* **28**:79-91.

Massaro, G. D., Fischman, C. M., Chiang, M. J., Amado, C., and Massaro, D. (1981). Regulation of secretion in Clara cells. *J. Clin. Invest.* **67**:345-351.

Patow, C. A., Shelhamer, J., Marom, Z., Logun, C., and Kaliner, M. (1984). Human nasal mucous glycoproteins: biochemical characterization and analysis of the effects of neurohormonal and immunologic stimulation. *Am. J. Otolaryngol.* **5**:334-343.

Phipps, R. J., Nadel, J. A., and Davis, B. (1980). Effect of alpha-adrenergic stimulation on mucus secretion and on ion transport in cat trachea in vitro. *Am. Rev. Respir. Dis.* **121**:359-365.

Phipps, R. J. (1981). The airway mucociliary system. In *International Review of Physiology. Respiratory Physiology III.* Edited by J. C. Widdicombe. Volume 23. Baltimore, University Park Press, pp. 213-260.

Richardson, J., and Beland, J. (1976). Nonadrenergic inhibitory nervous system in human airways. *J. Appl. Physiol.* **41**:764-771.

Shelhamer, J. H., Marom, Z., and Kaliner, M. (1980). Immunologic and neuropharmacologic stimulation of mucus glycoprotein release from human airways in vitro. *J. Clin. Invest.* **66**:1400-1408.

Shelhamer, J. H., Marom, Z., Sun, F., Bach, M., and Kaliner, M. (1982). The effects of arachanoids and leukotrienes on the release of mucus from human airways. *Chest* **81**:36S-37S.

Shelhamer, J. H., Marom, Z., Logun, C., and Kaliner, M. (1984). Human respiratory mucous glycoproteins. *Exp. Lung Res.* **7**:149-162.

Ueki, I., German, V. F., and Nadel, J. A. (1980). Micropipette measurement of airway subjucosal gland secretion. Autonomic effects. *Am. Rev. Respir. Dis.* **121**:351-357.

Varsano, S., Borson, D. B., Gold, M., Forsberg, L. S., Basbaum, C., and Nadel, J. A. (1986). Proteinases release $^{35}SO_4$-labeled macromolecules from cultured airway epithelial cells. *Fed. Proc.* **43**:786.

Wanner, A., Zarzecki, S., Hirsch, J., and Epstein, S. (1975). Tracheal mucus transport in experimental canine asthma. *J. Appl. Physiol.* **39**:950-7.

DEFINITIVE DISCUSSIONS

Innervation of the Tracheobronchial Circulation

John G. Widdicombe

St. George's Hospital Medical School, London, United Kingdom

The morphology of the tracheobronchial circulation consists of a double network of vessels. In the outer mucosa, under the epithelium, is a layer of capillaries, and somewhat deeper is an array of end-capillary venules. This seems to constitute the main vascular content of the mucosa and submucosa. Deeper, outside and around the cartilages, is a second network of arterioles and venules, supplied by larger arteries and drained by larger veins, which connects at intervals to the superficial network by arterioles and venules penetrating and passing around the airway smooth muscle. Physiologically the main drainage of the bronchial circulation is into the pulmonary vascular bed, via bronchopulmonary anastomoses; these have not been clearly defined structurally. About one-quarter to one-third of the bronchial venous drainage is into the azygus and hemiazygus veins. No systemic arteriovenous anastomoses have been identified definitely for the tracheal or bronchial circulations. The anatomy of the circulation and its control has been reviewed (Daly and Hebb, 1966; Baier et al., 1985; Fishman, 1985; Laitinen et al., 1987).

The main innervation of the tracheobronchial circulation is sympathetic and constrictor, as shown by nerve stimulation experiments. In addition, there is a parasympathetic dilator supply both to the bronchi and to the trachea (Widdicombe et al., 1986).

There have been few studies of the possibility of a nonadrenergic noncholinergic system to the airway vasculature, but its presence in the trachea has been demonstrated (Widdicombe et al., 1986); the mediator is unknown, but could be vasoactive intestinal peptide (VIP). The role of axonal reflexes in causing an airway vasodilatation is better established (Persson, Chap. 20) and, at least in the guinea pig, substance P seems to be the mediator. It can also be demonstrated for the dog trachea (Widdicombe et al., 1986). As implied above, there is some uncertainty as to the importance of neuropeptides in the control of the tracheobronchial vasculature but, at least for the dog, VIP and substance P are powerful dilators. Dilatation is also seen with PGE, bradykinin and histamine. $PGF_{2\alpha}$ has been described as causing either constriction or dilatation. The whole question of the innervation of the airway vasculature and its response to mediators is open, and research on this subject is only just beginning. Even less developed is our understanding of the reflex control of tracheobronchial blood flow. Recent studies (L. A. Laitinen, A. Laitinen and J. G. Widdicombe, unpublished; Laitinen et al., 1987) indicate that carotid sinus baroreceptor input causes a weak dilatation of tracheobronchial vessels, and that a similar dilatation is seen on activating afferent fibers from the larynx. Stimulation of lung C-fiber receptors causes a more powerful tracheal vasodilatation. It is likely that these reflexes are controlled mainly by modulation of sympathetic vasoconstrictor tone in the airways, and the role of the parasympathetic dilator innervation has not been studied.

A number of other stimuli have important actions on the tracheobronchial vasculature. Cooling the airways seems to increase blood flow, and this may be related to conditioning the air. Hypoxia usually increases airway blood flow. However, it is not clear to what extent these two responses depend on vascular innervation and reflexes. Irritation of the mucosal surface, for example, with cigarette smoke or capsaicin, sets up local axon reflexes producing vasodilatation, as well as systemic reflex responses associated with the afferent stimulation.

In summary, the lower airway vasculature is innervated, can be reflexly controlled, and its modification is of potential importance in both the physiology and the pathology of airway function.

References

Baier, H., Long, W. M., and Wanner, A. (1985). Bronchial circulation in asthma. *Respiration* **48**:199-205.

Daly, M. de B., and Hebb, C. (1966). *Pulmonary and Bronchial Vascular Systems.* London, Edward Arnold.

Fishman, A. P. (1985). Pulmonary circulation. In *Handbook of Physiology.* Section 3: The Respiratory System, vol. I. Edited by A. P. Fishman and A. B. Fisher. Washington, D. C., American Physiological Society, pp. 93-166.

Laitinen, L. A., Laitinen, A., and Widdicombe, J. G. (1987). Effects of inflammatory and other mediators on airway vascular beds. *Am. Rev. Respir. Dis.* (in press).

Widdicombe, J. G., Laitinen, A., and Laitinen, L. A. (1986). Parasympathetic nervous control of tracheal vascular resistance in the dog. *Fed. Proc.* **45**: 558.

Force of Capillarity Tending to Prevent Drying of Ciliary Mucosa

John G. Widdicombe

St. George's Hospital Medical School, London, United Kingdom

One force that would tend to prevent the drying of ciliary epithelium, which seems to have been neglected in previous discussions, is the force of capillarity that would tend to keep the ciliary layer waterlogged. It would behave like a sponge or a brush. In other words, as liquid tended to be absorbed from the periciliary layer, the liquid would exert a powerful surface tension due to capillary action.

Theoretical calculations indicate how powerful this force would be. Assuming a ciliary diameter of 0.25 μm, a density of 8 cilia/μm^2, a zero surface contact angle between liquid and ciliary wall, a surface tension of 0.04 N/m and the absence of any influence of ciliary curvature and movement, the total ciliary circumferential length would be 6.4×10^2 m/cm^2, and the surface force created along this length would be 2500 cm H_2O/cm^2 (2.5×10^5 N/m^2). Even allowing for inaccuracy in the selected values, and gross approximation of the assumptions, once liquid is withdrawn into the ciliary layer to set up a surface below the tips of the cilia, the force counteracting liquid withdrawal will be enormous. Provided there is liquid within the epithelial cells and the interstitium, it is difficult to see how the cilia could ever be dried out.

Molecular and Regulatory Properties of Adenylate Cyclase-Coupled Adrenergic Receptors

Robert J. Lefkowitz, Jeffrey L. Benovic, Ruth H. Strasser,* and Marc G. Caron

Duke University Medical Center, Durham, North Carolina

Membrane receptors for catecholamines, termed adrenergic receptors (AR), are of several pharmacologically distinct subtypes. The β_1 and β_2 receptors stimulate and α_2 receptors inhibit adenylate cyclase, while α_1 receptors are coupled to phosphatidylinositol turnover. G proteins are involved in coupling all of the AR to their effectors. We have purified each of these receptors to homogeneity using affinity chromatography and other techniques. The receptors are integral membrane glycoproteins. β_1, β_2 and α_2-AR are all of $M_r \cong 64{,}000$. The β_1 and β_2 receptors show strong immunologic cross-reactivity and very similar peptide maps, whereas α_2 receptors show weak immunologic reactivity with anti-β-receptor antibodies and quite different peptide maps. α_1-AR ($M_r \sim 80{,}000$) are quite distinct from the other types as assessed by antibodies or peptide mapping. The isolated receptors have been reconstituted in phospholipid vesicles with various G proteins and (for the β-AR) the adenylate cyclase and their function studied. The α_1 and β-AR action is regulated by phosphorylation, which results in desensitization. In addition to the cAMP-dependent protein kinase and protein kinase C, a newly discovered cAMP-independent kinase, the β-adrenergic receptor kinase (β-ARK), participates. The β-ARK phosphorylates only the agonist occupied form of the β-receptor and thus may be involved in agonist-specific desensitization. The β-ARK is a cytosolic enzyme, distinct from the cAMP, cGMP, Ca^{2+}-phospholipid, and Ca^{2+}-calmodulin-dependent protein kinases. When cells are desensitized by exposure to a β-agonist, β-ARK is rapidly translocated to the cell membrane. Prostaglandin-induced desensitization also leads to translocation of β-ARK to the plasma membrane. Thus β-ARK may phosphorylate a variety of adenylate-cyclase-coupled receptors. Phosphorylation of β-AR by β-ARK decreases its ability to interact with G_s in reconstituted systems. While β-ARK does not phosphorylate standard kinase substrates such as casein and histones, it does phosphorylate the "light receptor" rhodopsin, in a light-dependent fashion. Thus β-ARK may serve a function in hormone receptor systems in a manner analogous to rhodopsin kinase in the rod outer segments.

Discussion

Vanhoutte. Can beta-adrenoceptor-related kinase (BARK) phosphorylate other receptors, such as alpha-receptors or serotonin receptors?

Lefkowitz. The specificity of BARK is not yet certain.

**Present affiliation*: University of Heidelberg, Heidelberg, West Germany

Nadel. Rates of desensitization of beta-receptors in different tissues may vary; is there evidence that cystolic BARK concentrations vary correspondingly?

Lefkowitz. Tissue levels of BARK vary widely, but it is not certain whether this related to rates of desensitization.

Barnes. Do glucocorticoids or phospholipase $alpha_2$ inhibitors reduce BARK activity?

Lefkowitz. Glucocorticoids can attenuate or reverse beta-receptor desensitization, but whether BARK is involved remains to be determined.

Hahn. Can desensitization of beta-receptors occur at physiologically relevant concentrations of catecholamines?

Lefkowitz. In isolated cell systems the concentrations of beta-agonist necessary to desensitize are the same or lower than those required to activate the system.

Hahn. Is there a difference in the mechanisms of homologous and heterologus desensitization?

Lefkowitz. Heterologous desensitization probably involves multiple mechanisms, including receptor alterations and changes in other components of the system, such as guanine nucleotide regulatory proteins and adenylate cyclase. Phosphorylation of the receptor in heterologous desensitization may be due to the actions of cyclic-AMP-dependent kinase. In contrast, homologous desensitization appears to be associated with the actions of BARK. Since the effects of this kinase require agonist occupancy, homologous rather than heterologus desensitization results.

AUTHOR INDEX

Italic numbers give the page on which the complete reference is listed.

A

B

C

E

F

G

H

I

K

L

M

N

O

P

U

V

SUBJECT INDEX

N

X